Diagnosis and Treatment of Gastrointestinal Cancers

Editor: Donald Maxmilian

AMERICAN
MEDICAL PUBLISHERS
www.americanmedicalpublishers.com

AMERICAN
MEDICAL PUBLISHERS
www.americanmedicalpublishers.com

Cataloging-in-Publication Data

Diagnosis and treatment of gastrointestinal cancers / edited by Donald Maxmilian.
p. cm.
Includes bibliographical references and index.
ISBN 979-8-88740-058-7
1. Gastrointestinal system--Cancer. 2. Gastrointestinal system--Cancer--Diagnosis.
3. Gastrointestinal system--Cancer--Treatment. 4. Digestive organs--Cancer. I. Maxmilian, Donald.
RC280.D5 D53 2023
616.994 33--dc23

American Medical Publishers,
41 Flatbush Avenue,
1st Floor, New York,
NY 11217, USA

ISBN 979-8-88740-058-7 (Hardback)

Contents

Preface

It is often said that books are a boon to mankind. They document every progress and pass on the knowledge from one generation to the other. They play a crucial role in our lives. Thus I was both excited and nervous while editing this book. I was pleased by the thought of being able to make a mark but I was also nervous to do it right because the future of students depends upon it. Hence, I took a few months to research further into the discipline, revise my knowledge and also explore some more aspects. Post this process, I begun with the editing of this book.

Gastrointestinal cancer is a type of cancer that is characterized by malignant growth of cells in the gastrointestinal tract. This cancer targets the accessory organs of digestion such as esophagus, stomach, biliary system, pancreas, small intestine, large intestine, rectum and anus. There are several factors such as obesity, tobacco and alcohol use that lead to gastrointestinal cancer. Vomiting, poor digestion and visible swelling in the abdomen are some important symptoms of this type of cancer. Its diagnosis involves the examination of the lining of the stomach with a flexible lens containing tube called an endoscope. Other diagnostic methods include imaging techniques such as X-rays, computed tomography (CT) scans, and magnetic resonance imaging (MRI). The most effective way to treat gastrointestinal cancer is surgery along with radiation therapy and chemotherapy to relieve the symptoms. The objective of this book is to present advancements in the researches on gastrointestinal cancers. Different diagnostic approaches and treatment strategies for these type of cancers have been included herein. The book will serve as a valuable resource for medical professionals and students alike.

I thank my publisher with all my heart for considering me worthy of this unparalleled opportunity and for showing unwavering faith in my skills. I would also like to thank the editorial team who worked closely with me at every step and contributed immensely towards the successful completion of this book. Last but not the least, I wish to thank my friends and colleagues for their support.

Editor

1

NR2F1-AS1/miR-190a/PHLDB2 Induces the Epithelial–Mesenchymal Transformation Process in Gastric Cancer by Promoting Phosphorylation of AKT3

*Jinqi Lv[1,2,3,4], Simeng Zhang[1,2,3,4], Yang Liu[1,2,3,4], Ce Li[1,2,3,4], Tianshu Guo[1,2,3,4], Shuairan Zhang[1,2,3,4], Zenan Li[1,2,3,4], Zihan Jiao[1,2,3,4], Haina Sun[1,2,3,4], Ye Zhang[5] and Ling Xu[1,2,3,4]**

[1] Department of Medical Oncology, The First Hospital of China Medical University, Shenyang, China, [2] Key Laboratory of Anticancer Drugs and Biotherapy of Liaoning Province, The First Hospital of China Medical University, Shenyang, China, [3] Liaoning Province Clinical Research Center for Cancer, Shenyang, China, [4] Key Laboratory of Precision Diagnosis and Treatment of Gastrointestinal Tumors, Ministry of Education, Shenyang, China, [5] The First Laboratory of Cancer Institute, The First Hospital of China Medical University, Shenyang, China

***Correspondence:**
Ling Xu
cmuxuling@163.com

The median survival time of patients with advanced gastric cancer (GC) who received radiotherapy and chemotherapy was <1 year. Epithelial–mesenchymal transformation (EMT) gives GC cells the ability to invade, which is an essential biological mechanism in the progression of GC. The long non-coding RNA (lncRNA)-based competitive endogenous RNA (ceRNA) system has been shown to play a key role in the GC-related EMT process. Although the AKT pathway is essential for EMT in GC, the relationship between AKT3 subtypes and EMT in GC is unclear. Here, we evaluated the underlying mechanism of ceRNA involving NR2F1-AS1/miR-190a/PHLDB2 in inducing EMT by promoting the expression and phosphorylation of AKT3. The results of bioinformatics analysis showed that the expression of NR2F1-AS1/miR-190a/PHLDB2 in GC was positively associated with the pathological features, staging, poor prognosis, and EMT process. We performed cell transfection, qRT-PCR, western blot, cell viability assay, TUNEL assay, Transwell assay, cell morphology observation, and double luciferase assay to confirm the regulation of NR2F1-AS1/miR-190a/PHLDB2 and its effect on EMT transformation. Finally, GSEA and GO/KEGG enrichment analysis identified that PI3K/AKT pathway was positively correlated to NR2F1-AS1/miR-190a/PHLDB2 expression. AKT3 knockout cells were co-transfected with PHLDB2-OE, and the findings revealed that AKT3 expression and phosphorylation were essential for the PHLDB2-mediated EMT process. Thus, our results showed that NR2F1-AS1/miR-190a/PHLDB2 promoted the phosphorylation of AKT3 to induce EMT in GC cells. This study provides a comprehensive understanding of the underlying mechanism involved in the EMT process as well as the identification of new EMT markers.

Keywords: NR2F1-AS1, miR-190a, PHLDB2, EMT, AKT3

INTRODUCTION

Gastric cancer (GC) is the fifth most common cancer and the third leading cause of cancer-related death globally. Early GC has a good prognosis and can be treated with endoscopy and surgery. However, patients with advanced GC treated with radiotherapy and chemotherapy have a median survival time of <1 year and a 5-year overall survival rate of <5% (Smyth et al., 2020). The ability of GC cells to invade and metastasize is considered vital for GC progression. The epithelial–mesenchymal transformation (EMT) involves the conversion of epithelial cells into mesenchymal cell phenotype. The GC mesenchymal cells can undergo extensive migration and invasion, are anti-apoptotic, and can degrade the ECM. Thus, EMT is vital for acquiring the invasive ability (Yang et al., 2020).

The downregulated expression of E-cadherin (E-cad), upregulated expression of N-cadherin (N-cad), enhanced mesenchymal phenotype, decreased epithelial phenotype, and upregulated expression of VIM are all essential markers of EMT. The transcription factors ZEB, SNAI, and TWIST, are stimulated during EMT and play an important role in the process. The TGF/Smad pathway, Wnt/β-catenin pathway, PI3K/AKT pathway, Src pathway, IL-6/STAT3 pathway, Integrin pathway, Notch pathway, Hedgehog pathway, and NF-κB pathway are all known to be involved in the EMT process (Yang et al., 2020). Among them, the PI3K/AKT pathway is known to be vital for tumor cell EMT promotion and maintenance (Hoxhaj and Manning, 2020). The AKT family includes AKT1, AKT2, and AKT3; however, most studies study AKT as a single term (Fresno Vara et al., 2004); thus, the role of each subtype of the AKT family in EMT is unclear (Janku et al., 2018).

MicroRNA (miRNA) is a type of non-coding single-stranded RNA molecule approximately 22 nucleotides long, which can silence genes by binding to the mRNA. Studies have shown that miRNA plays a central role in the regulation of the EMT process in cancer progression and metastasis (Hur et al., 2013). Long non-coding RNA (lncRNA) (>200 bp) is an endogenous RNA molecule that does not encode a protein. Recent studies have found that lncRNA can function as a competitive endogenous RNA (ceRNA) by adsorbing miRNA to regulate target gene expression and regulate tumor occurrence and growth (Thomson and Dinger, 2016). LncRNAs are known to be closely related to the tumor's EMT, which affects the tumor's invasion and metastatic potential (Yuan et al., 2020). NR2F1-AS1, a type of lncRNA, has been shown to facilitate malignant tumor development (Zhang C. et al., 2020; Zhang Q. et al., 2020). MiR-190a has been shown to suppress the EMT pathway in cancers (Jin et al., 2020; Wang et al., 2020). PHLDB2 is a protein with a PH domain. PHLDB2 and CLASPS are known to form complexes at the cell edge to regulate cell migration and polarization, indicating that PHLDB2 plays an important role in tumor cell invasion and metastasis (Lim et al., 2016). However, the role of NR2F1-AS1/miR-190a/PHLDB2 in GC has not yet been reported. We used bioinformatics tools to identify a group of ceRNAs that were significantly related to the EMT process of GC cells. We aimed to investigate the regulatory impact of ceRNA composed of NR2F1-AS1/miR-190a/PHLDB2 on the EMT of GC as well as the relationship and mechanism between ceRNA, the AKT pathway, and GC cell EMT. It is of great significance for the acquisition of invasive phenotype of GC, the understanding of the EMT process, and the development of new EMT markers.

MATERIALS AND METHODS

Bioinformatics

The online website was used to call the GC data and clinical information in the TCGA database for bioinformatics analysis. We used Xiantao[1] to analyze the expression and correlation of mRNA in patients with GC, analyzed the prognosis of patients with GC, analyzed single-gene differential analysis, conducted visual GSEA analysis, analyzed the correlation with clinical information through binary logistics, drew Venn diagram, histogram, and heat map; GEPIA[2] (Tang et al., 2019) to analyze the expression of mRNA; Kaplan–Meier plotter[3] to analyze the prognosis of patients with GC (Nagy et al., 2018); Starbase[4] to predict target binding and correlation of 3′UTR between the miRNA and mRNA (Li et al., 2014); DAVID[5] for enrichment analysis of the gene sets (Huang da et al., 2009).

Cell Lines

BGC823, SGC7901, and HGC27 cells were purchased from the Shanghai Chinese Academy of Sciences. BGC823 and SGC7901 are poorly differentiated GC cells. HGC27 is undifferentiated GC. The cells were cultured under the standard cell culture conditions, including RPMI1640+ 10% fetal bovine serum (FBS) and 1% penicillin/streptomycin (Gibco). The cell lines were tested for mycoplasma every month using STR-DNA. The cells were passaged till the 12th generation.

Transfection

The target nucleic acid sequence was transfected into the GC cells using liposome 3000. The nucleic acid sequence included NR2F1-AS1 sequence of the plasmid vector, siRNA of NR2F1-AS1, PHLDB2-cDNA of the plasmid vector, siRNA for PHLDB2, miR-190a mimic, and inhibitor. **Supplementary Table 1** lists the transfection sequence. The transfection efficiency was detected by qPCR or western blot.

Lentivirus Infection

Lentivirus was used to construct AKT3-knockout GC cell lines. The siRNA targeting AKT3, which has been verified for knockout efficiency, was cloned into the lentiviral vector by GeneChem (Shanghai, China). Si-AKT3 lentivirus and Enhance infection enhancement solution were mixed and added to the culture medium for 10–12 h. Next, 72 h post-transfection, 5–10 μg/mL

[1] https://www.xiantao.love/products
[2] http://gepia2.cancer-pku.cn
[3] http://kmplot.com/
[4] http://starbase.sysu.edu.cn/
[5] https://david.ncifcrf.gov/

puromycin was added to screen the positively infected cells for 2 weeks. The silencing effect of AKT3 after lentivirus infection was detected by qPCR and western blot.

Western Blot Analysis

Western blot was performed using a previously described method (Xu et al., 2017a). The following antibodies were used to detect protein expression: PHLDB2 (1:1000, Abcam, ab234885, United States), GAPDH (1:1000, Proteintech,10494-1-AP, China), E-Cadherin (1:1000, Cst, 3195, United States), N-Cadherin (1:1000, Cst, 13116, United States), Vimentin (1: 1000, Cst, 5741, United States), ZEB1 (1:1000, Cst, 40098, United States), TWIST2 (1:1000, Proteintech, 11752-1-AP, United States), Akt3 (1:1000, Cst, 14982, United States), Akt (phosphor S472 + S473 + S474) (1:1000, Abcam, ab192623, United States), and PI3K (1:1000, Proteintech, 67071-1-Ig).

Immunofluorescence Analysis

Immunofluorescence was performed as previously described (Xu et al., 2017b). The cells were probed with anti-CDH2 and anti-VIM antibodies to assess their total expression and cellular localization.

qPCR

Total RNA of the cells was extracted *via* column RNA extraction, which was reverse transcribed to obtain single-stranded cDNA. The stem-loop method was used for reverse transcription and quantitative analysis of the miRNA. QuantStudio 3 was used to perform qRT-PCR. β-actin was used as the internal reference. The relative expression was calculated by the $2^{-\Delta\Delta CT}$ method. **Supplementary Table 1** lists all primers used in this study.

Cell Viability

The transfected cells were seeded in a 96-well plate (1 × 103 cells/well), and the blank medium was used as a control. Three secondary holes were performed in each experiment. We used the cell activity kit (China Wanshi, WLA074) to evaluate cell viability. The cell proliferation curve was drawn daily and was used to analyze the changes in cell proliferation ability.

TUNEL Assay

The TUNEL assay was used to detect apoptosis. The transfected cells were inoculated on cover slides, fixed using paraformaldehyde, permeated by Triton X-100, sealed in the dark using 3% H_2O_2, and stained for 90 min by TUNEL staining. The nucleus was stained with DAPI. The cells were observed and photographed using the BX51 fluorescence microscope.

Transwell Assay

The Transwell assay was performed using a previously described method (Xu et al., 2017a). Briefly, the transfected cells were placed in the upper chamber of the Transwell and invaded into the lower compartment through the filter membrane coated with Matrigel for 20 h. The invaded cells were photographed using a microscope (Olympus, Tokyo, Japan) and counted using the ImageJ software.

Cell Morphology

1×10^3 transfected cells were seeded in a six-well plate, and the morphology of a single cell was observed after 24 h of culture. The morphology of colony cells was photographed by BX51 microscope (Olympus, Tokyo, Japan).

Luciferase Assays

NR2F1-AS1 and PHLDB2-mRNA-3′-UTR with WT (Mut) type miR-190a binding site was cloned into the luciferase plasmid. The plasmid vector fragment was synthesized by Shanghai Obio. Next, the mimic-190a, Renilla plasmids, and constructed luciferase vector were transfected into cells for 48 h, and the luciferase activity was detected using a double luciferase reporter kit.

Statistical Analysis

The data are expressed as mean ± SD. All experiments were performed thrice independently. WB bands were quantified using the ImageJ software. We used the SPSS v17.0.1 software to perform the inter-group comparison using the students' double-tailed t-test. $P < 0.05$ implied a statistically significant difference between groups. The data sources and statistical methods of bioinformatics analysis are all on the website (see section "Bioinformatics").

RESULTS

Screening of the Long Non-coding RNA Related to the Epithelial–Mesenchymal Transformation Process of Gastric Cancer

The top 200 genes that were negatively correlated to CDH1 and positively correlated to CDH2, ZEB1, and TWIST2 were selected (**Supplementary Table 2**). We found that 22 genes were negatively correlated with CDH1 and positively correlated with CDH2, ZEB1, and TWIST2 (**Figure 1A**). Three of them were lncRNAs, which were MIR100HG, NR2F1-AS1, and MAGI2-AS3. Among them, MIR100HG (Li P. et al., 2020) and MAGI2-AS3 (Li D. et al., 2020) have been proved to promote the progression of GC; thus, here, we focused on NR2F1-AS1. However, NR2F1-AS1 expression was observed between GC and adjacent non-cancerous tissues, with the latter having slightly higher expression (**Supplementary Figure 1A**). Further analysis in the pathological features of GC showed that the expression of NR2F1-AS1 was significantly higher in ≤65 years old group, Asian group, *Helicobacter pylori* infection group, death group, poorly differentiated group, and G3 pathological staging group (**Figure 1B**). Also, we discovered that the expression of NR2F1-AS1 was linked to a poor prognosis in patients with GC (**Figure 1C**). NR2F1-AS1 and clinical data of GC patients in the TCGA database were determined

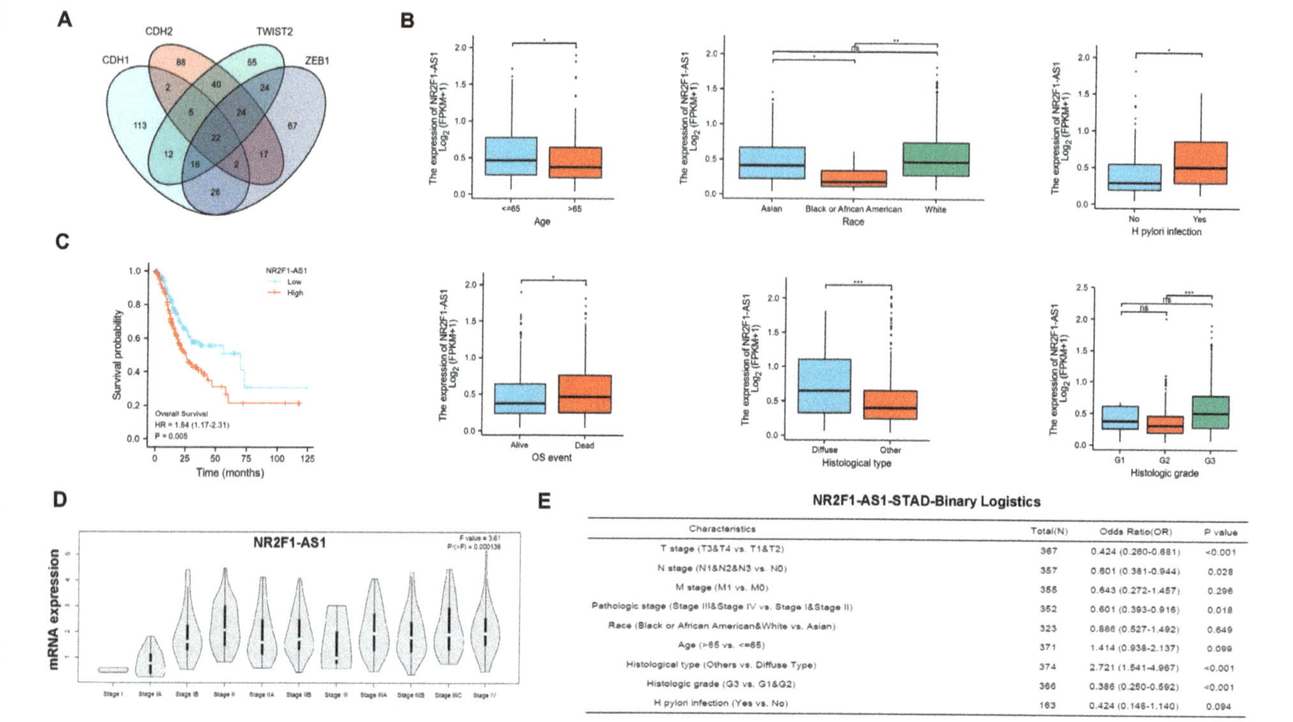

FIGURE 1 | Screening of EMT-related lncRNA in GC. **(A)** Xiantao was used to screen the correlation between CDH1, CDH2, ZEB1, TWIST2 and the whole genome in GC. The top 200 genes that were negatively related to CDH1 and positively related to CDH2/ZEB1/TWIST2 were selected and intersected. **(B)** The GC data of TCGA were classified according to clinical characteristics, and the expression of NR2F1-AS1 in each group was analyzed by Xiantao. **(C)** The effect of NR2F1-AS1 expression on the OS prognosis of patients with GC was analyzed by Xiantao. **(D)** GEPIA2 was used to analyze the expression of NR2F1-AS1 in different stages of GC. **(E)** Xiantao was used to analyze the correlation between NR2F1-AS1 and the clinical features by Binary Logistics. $^{*}p < 0.05$; $^{**}p < 0.01$; $^{***}p < 0.001$.

using GEPIA. We found that NR2F1-AS1 expression varied based on the stages of GC. The expression of NR2F1-AS1 was lowest during the early stages of GC and increased substantially with disease progression (**Figure 1D**). Finally, we used logistics to analyze the correlation between NR2F1-AS1 and pathological features of GC. We found that NR2F1-AS1 was significantly correlated with T/M stage, pathologic stage, diffuse histological type, and G3 histological grade of GC (**Figure 1E**). Even though the expression of NR2F1-AS1 was low in GC, NR2F1-AS1 played an important role in the invasion and progression of GC, which was probably related to the EMT process.

NR2F1-AS1 Promotes Malignant Phenotype, Poor Prognosis, and Epithelial–Mesenchymal Transformation Process of Gastric Cancer

We found that there was a high correlation between the elevated expression of NR2F1-AS1 and the EMT process through GSEA analysis (**Figure 2A**). We also discovered a close association between NR2F1-AS1 and markers of the EMT process in GC and drew a heat map. N-cadherin, VIM, ZEB1, and TWIST2 were positively correlated with the mesenchymal transformation markers, while E-cadherin and CLDN7 were negatively correlated with the epithelial phenotypic markers (**Figure 2B** and **Supplementary Figure 1B**). These results indicated that NR2F1-AS1 probably gained the ability to invade and metastasize by promoting the EMT process of GC cells.

When NR2F1-AS1-siRNA-1 and siRNA-2 were transfected, RNA expression was reduced by approximately 70 and 80%, respectively, compared with the transfected siRNA-control (**Figure 2C**). The NR2F1-AS1 mimic (NR2F1-AS1-OE) was transfected into the GC cell lines (SGC7901 and BGC823), and NR2F1-AS1 expression increased approximately 60 times compared to the blank plasmid vector (EV) (**Figure 2D**). The proliferation (**Figure 2E**) and anti-apoptotic (**Figure 2F**) potential decreased significantly after NR2F1-AS1 expression was reduced in SGC7901 and BGC823, based on the results of cell viability and TUNEL assays. After the overexpression of NR2F1-AS1, the ability of proliferation changed accordingly (**Supplementary Figure 1C**), the ability of apoptosis did not change significantly, and the cells were all in good condition (**Supplementary Figure 1D**). The results of the cell morphology assays (**Figure 2G**) and Transwell (**Figure 2H**) indicated an increase in NR2F1-AS1 expression in SGC7901 and BGC823 cells, the cell morphology shifted from epithelial to mesenchymal, and invasive capacity increased substantially. WB analysis revealed that with an increase in the expression of NR2F1-AS1 in SGC7901 and BGC823 cells, there occurred a significant change in the associated EMT markers. N-cadherin, VIM,

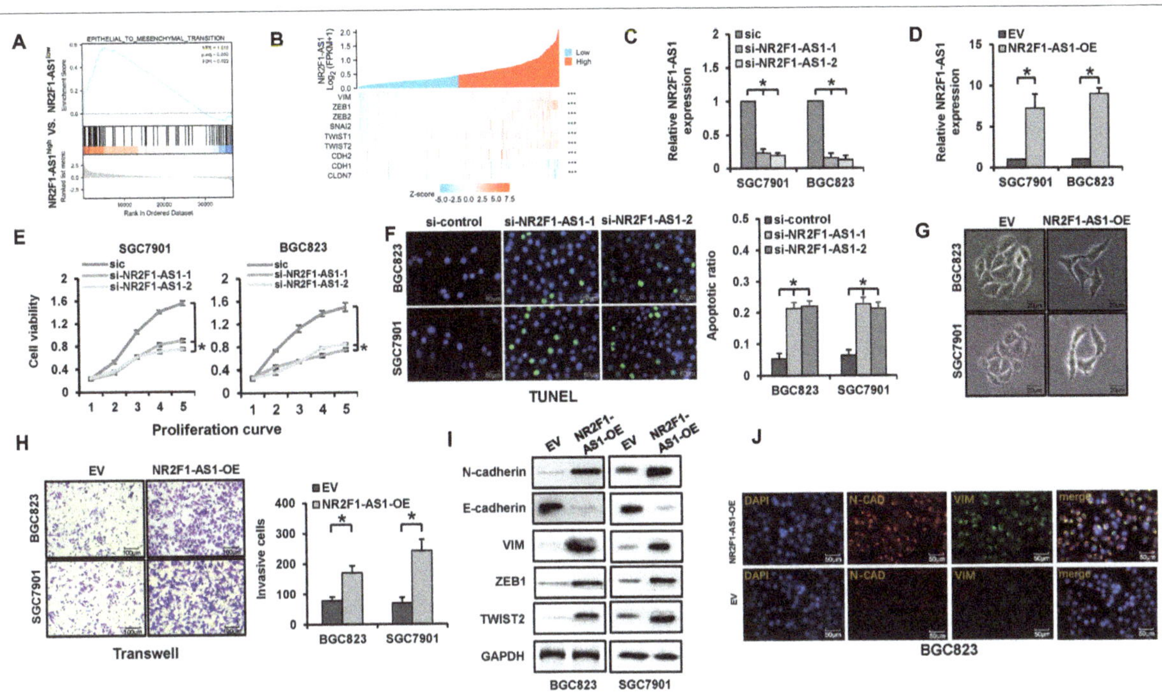

FIGURE 2 | NR2F1-AS1 promotes the poor prognosis and malignant phenotype of GC cells by activating EMT. **(A)** The data of TCGA GC were divided into two groups: low-expression group and high-expression group of NR2F1-A1. The whole genome expression of these two groups was enriched by GSEA and the enrichment in the EMT pathway was detected by Xiantao. **(B)** Xiantao was used to analyze the correlation between the expression of NR2F1-AS1 and EMT markers, and a heat map was drawn. **(C)** Si-control, si-NR2F1-AS1-1, and si-NR2F1-AS1-2 were transfected into BGC823 and SGC7901 cell lines to detect the expression of NR2F1-AS1 by qRT-PCR. **(E)** The cell proliferative ability by cell viability assay. **(F)** The proportion of apoptosis by TUNEL assay. **(D)** The expression of NR2F1-AS1 was detected by qRT-PCR after NR2F1-AS1-OE and EV were transfected in BGC823 and SGC7901 cell lines. **(G)** Transfect NR2F1-AS1-OE and EV into BGC823 and SGC7901 to detect the invasiveness of the cells by Transwell assay. **(H)** The morphology of cell colonies was observed after transfection of NR2F1-AS1-OE and EV in BGC823 and SGC7901. **(I)** After transfection of NR2F1-AS1-OE and EV in BGC823 and SGC7901, the expression of EMT markers was detected by WB. **(J)** After transfection of NR2F1-AS1-OE and EV in BGC823 and SGC7901, the expression of CDH2 and VIM was detected by immunofluorescence. $^{*}p < 0.05$; $^{**}p < 0.01$; $^{***}p < 0.001$.

ZEB1, and TWIST2, markers of mesenchymal transformation, increased substantially, while E-cadherin, a marker of epithelial phenotypic shift, decreased significantly (**Figure 2I**). The results of immunofluorescence showed that the overexpression of NR2F1-AS1 promoted the expression of EMT markers (**Figure 2J**). The experimental results of cell morphology assays (**Supplementary Figure 1E**), Transwell (**Supplementary Figure 1F**), and WB (**Supplementary Figure 1G**) in HGC27 showed that the silencing of NR2F1-AS1 inhibited the EMT process. These results suggested that NR2F1-AS1 expression probably resulted in malignant phenotypic transformation, staging progress, and poor prognosis of GC by promoting the EMT process.

Filtering of the Competitive Endogenous RNA Structure Composed of NR2F1-AS1

We used Starbase to analyze the RNA expression and clinical data of GC patients from the TCGA database. The miR-190a was screened out which was significantly negatively correlated with NR2F1-AS1 expression (**Figure 3B**), correlated with EMT (**Figure 4A**) and had a conservative target binding to NR2F1-AS1 (**Supplementary Table 3**). The PHLDB2 was screened out which was positively correlated with NR2F1-AS1 expression (**Figure 3B**), correlated with EMT (**Figure 5C**) and had conservative target binding to miR-190a (**Supplementary Table 3**). Both NR2F1-AS1 and PHLDB2 had regulatory targets for miR-190 (**Figure 3A**). According to the regulatory mechanism of ceRNA, miR-190 acted as the vector miRNA for NR2F1-AS1 to regulate the expression of PHLDB2. We analyzed the regulatory relationship between the NR2F1-AS1/miR-190a/PHLDB2 axes. After co-transfection of the wild-type (mutant) NR2F1-AS1, PHLDB2-3′-UTR double luciferase, and mimic-190a in BGC823, the results of double luciferase reporter assay showed that miR-190a expression significantly downregulated the luciferase activity of wt-NR2F1-AS1/wt-PHLDB2; however, there was no corresponding change in the mutant expression (**Figures 3C,D**). After transfection of NR2F1-AS1-OE into BGC823, the results of qPCR and WB showed that the expression of miR-190a was significantly decreased, and the expression of PHLDB2 was significantly increased compared with that of EV (**Figures 3F,G**). After the transfection of mimic-190a into BGC823, qPCR and WB analysis showed that the expression of NR2F1-AS1 and PHLDB2 decreased significantly compared with that of mimic-control transfection (**Figures 3E,H**). These results showed that NR2F1-AS1/miR-190a/PHLDB2 constituted the ceRNA regulatory population.

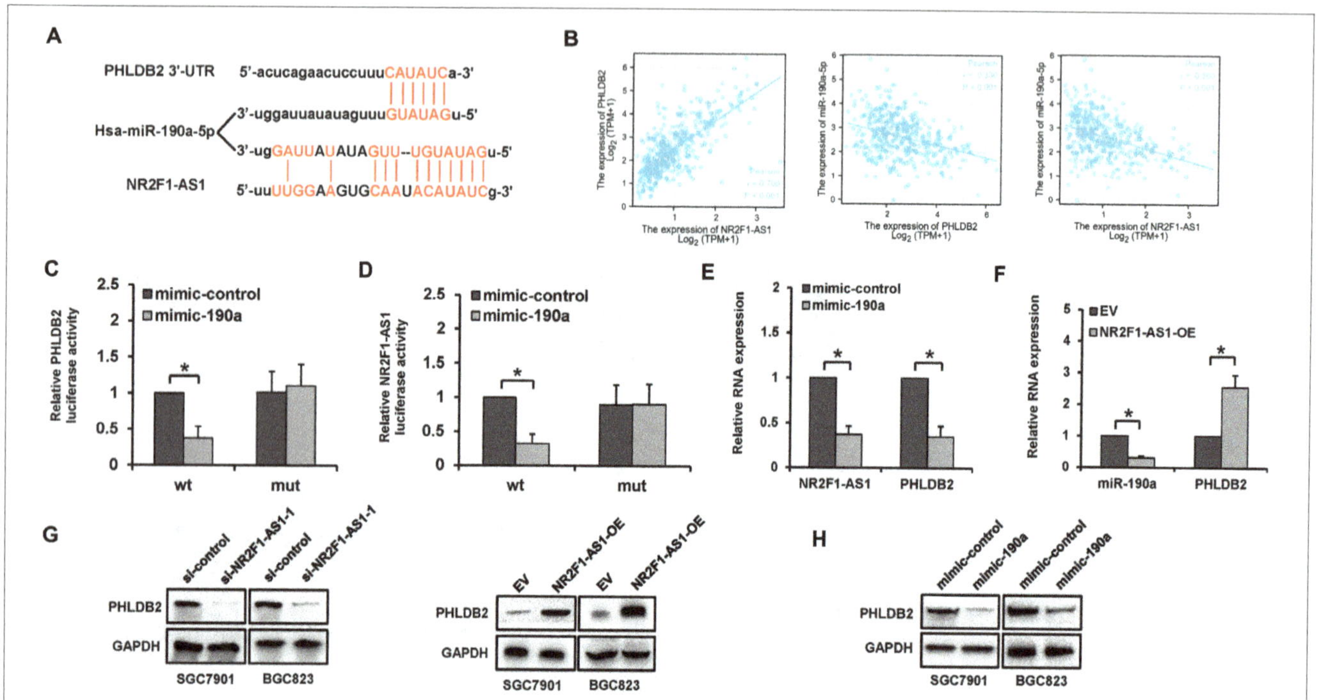

FIGURE 3 | NR2F1-AS1, miR-190a, and PHLDB2 may have formed ceRNA. **(A)** Starbase was used to analyze the interaction targets of miR-190a with NR2F1-AS1 and PHLDB2. **(B)** Xiantao was used to analyze the correlation between miR-190a and NR2F1-AS1 and PHLDB2 expression in GC. **(C)** BGC823 were transfected with mimic-190a, and PHLDB2 luciferase reporter plasmids (WT and MUT types) and dual-luciferase reporter assays were performed. **(D)** Luciferase reporter plasmids (WT and MUT types) of mimic-190a and NR2F1-AS1 were transfected into BGC823 cells. Luciferase activity was assessed *via* dual-luciferase reporter assays. **(E)** Mimic-190a and mimic-control were transfected into BGC823 and SGC7901 cell lines to detect the expression of NR2F1-AS1 and PHLDB2 by qRT-PCR. **(F)** NR2F1-AS1-OE and EV were transfected into BGC823 and SGC7901 cell lines to detect the expression of miR-190a and PHLDB2 by qRT-PCR. **(G)** After NR2F1-AS1-OE, EV, sic, and si-NR2F1-AS1 were transfected into BGC823, and SGC7901 cell lines, the expression of PHLDB2 was detected by WB. **(H)** The expression of PHLDB2 was detected by WB after transfection of mimic-190a and mimic-control into BGC823 and SGC7901 cell lines. $^{*}p < 0.05$.

MiR-190a Promotes Malignant Phenotype, Poor Prognosis, and Epithelial–Mesenchymal Transformation Process of Gastric Cancer

We analyzed the correlation between miR-190a and EMT markers and found that miR-190a was positively correlated to E-cadherin, an epithelial phenotypic marker, and negatively correlated to N-cadherin VIM, ZEB1, and TWIST2, the mesenchymal phenotypic markers (**Figure 4A**). Furthermore, we analyzed the relationship between miR-190a and the prognosis of patients with GC and found that the downregulated expression of miR-190a was significantly related to the poor prognosis of GC (**Figure 4B**). The mimic-190a was transfected into GC cell lines, SGC7901, and BGC823; we found that the expression of miR-190a increased by approximately 100 times compared with that of mimic-control (**Figure 4C**). The results of cell viability and TUNEL assay showed that the proliferation (**Figure 4D**) and anti-apoptotic ability (**Figure 4E**) of SGC7901 and BGC823 cells decreased significantly following an increase in miR-190a expression. The transfection of inhibitor-190a, an inhibitor of miR-190a, decreased the expression of miR-190a by approximately 70% compared with that of the control (**Figure 4F**). The results of cell morphology (**Figure 4G**) and Transwell assay (**Figure 4H**) showed that after the miR-190a expression of SGC7901 and BGC823 decreased, the cell morphology changed from epithelial type to mesenchymal type, and the invasive ability increased significantly. The results of WB showed that the EMT-related markers of SGC7901 changed significantly following a decrease in the expression of miR-190a. The mesenchymal transformation markers N-cadherin, VIM, ZEB1, and TWIST2, increased significantly, while the epithelial phenotypic marker E-cadherin decreased significantly (**Figure 4I**). Finally, we performed a rescue assay on the regulation of EMT by NRF1-AS1/miR-190a. We transfected mimic-190a into BGC823 cells overexpressing NR2F1-AS1 and found that the EMT process promoted by NR2F1-AS1 was significantly inhibited (**Supplementary Figures 3A–C**). These results suggested that NR2F1-AS1/miR-190a promoted the malignant phenotype and EMT process in the GC cells.

PHLDB2 Promotes Malignant Phenotype, Poor Prognosis, and Epithelial–Mesenchymal Transformation Process of Gastric Cancer

Elevated expression of PHLDB2 was significantly correlated to the poor prognosis of GC (**Figure 5A**). We found that there was a high correlation between the elevated expression of PHLDB2 and the EMT process through GSEA

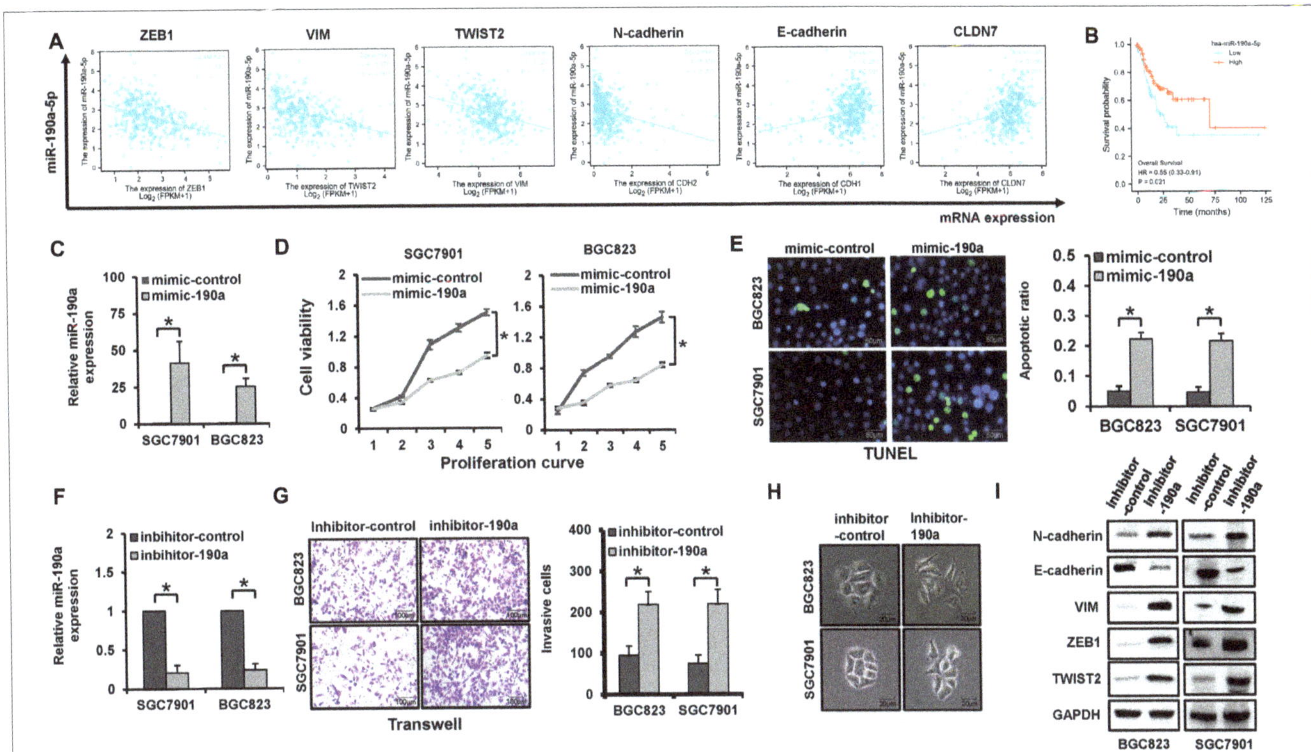

FIGURE 4 | MiR-190a promotes the poor prognosis and malignant phenotype of GC cells by activating EMT. **(A)** Xiantao was used to analyze the correlation between the expression of miR-190a and EMT markers in GC. **(B)** Xiantao was used to analyze the effect of miR-190a expression on the prognosis of patients with GC. **(C)** BGC823 and SGC7901 cell lines were transfected with mimic-190a and mimic-control to detect the expression of miR-190a by qRT-PCR. **(D)** BGC823 and SGC7901 cell lines transfected with mimic-190a and mimic-control were used to detect the cell viability by cell viability assay. **(E)** BGC823 and SGC7901 transfected with mimic-190a and mimic-control were used to detect the proportion of apoptosis by TUNEL assay. **(F)** BGC823 and SGC7901 cell lines were transfected with inhibitor-190a and inhibitor-control to detect the expression of miR-190a by qRT-PCR. **(G)** The invasiveness of cells was detected by Transwell after transfection of inhibitor-190a and inhibitor-control in BGC823 and SGC7901 cell lines. **(H)** BGC823 and SGC7901 cell lines were transfected with inhibitor-190a and inhibitor-control, and the morphology of the cell colonies was observed under the microscope. **(I)** BGC823 and SGC7901 cell lines were transfected with inhibitor-190a and inhibitor-control, the expression of EMT markers was detected by WB. $^{*}p < 0.05$.

analysis (**Figure 5B**). We also discovered a close association between PHLDB2 and markers of the EMT process in GC. N-cadherin, VIM, ZEB1, and TWIST2 were positively correlated with the mesenchymal transformation markers, while E-cadherin and CLDN7 were negatively correlated with the epithelial phenotypic markers (**Figure 5C** and **Supplementary Figure 2B**). We used GEPIA to analyze the mRNA expression and clinical data of GC patients from the TCGA database. The expression of PHLDB2 was the lowest during stage I of GC, and elevated expression was directly proportional to the enhanced metastatic progression of GC (**Figure 5D**). We used logistics to analyze the correlation between PHLDB2 and pathological features of GC. We found that PHLDB2 was significantly correlated with T/M stage, pathologic stage, diffuse histological type, and G3 histological grade of GC (**Figure 5E**). The expression of PHLDB2 in GC was slightly lower than that in adjacent non-cancerous tissues (**Supplementary Figure 2A**). Thus, there was a significant correlation between PHLDB2 expression and various markers of the EMT process in GC.

After transfection of PHLDB2-siRNA-1 and siRNA-2, the expression of PHLDB2 decreased by approximately 70 and 75% compared with that of transfected si-control (**Figure 5F**). The cDNA (PHLDB2-OE) of PHLDB2 was transfected into GC cell lines (SGC7901 and BGC823), and we found that the protein expression of PHLDB2 was significantly higher than that of the blank plasmid vector (EV) (**Figure 5G**). The results of cell viability assay (**Figure 5H**) and TUNEL assay (**Figure 5I**) showed that the proliferative and anti-apoptotic ability of SGC7901 and BGC823 cells decreased significantly in response to decreased PHLDB2 expression. After the overexpression of PGLDB2, the ability of proliferation changed accordingly (**Supplementary Figure 2C**), the ability of apoptosis did not change significantly, and the cells were in good condition (**Supplementary Figure 2D**). The results of cell morphology (**Figure 5J**) and Transwell assay (**Figure 6A**) showed that an increase in the expression of PHLDB2 in SGC7901 and BGC823 resulted in the change in cell morphology from epithelial type to mesenchymal type along with a significant increase in the invasive ability. The results of WB and immunofluorescence showed that the PHLDB2 expression of SGC7901 and BGC823 changed significantly after the expression of EMT-related markers. The mesenchymal transformation markers N-cadherin, VIM, ZEB1, and TWIST2, increased

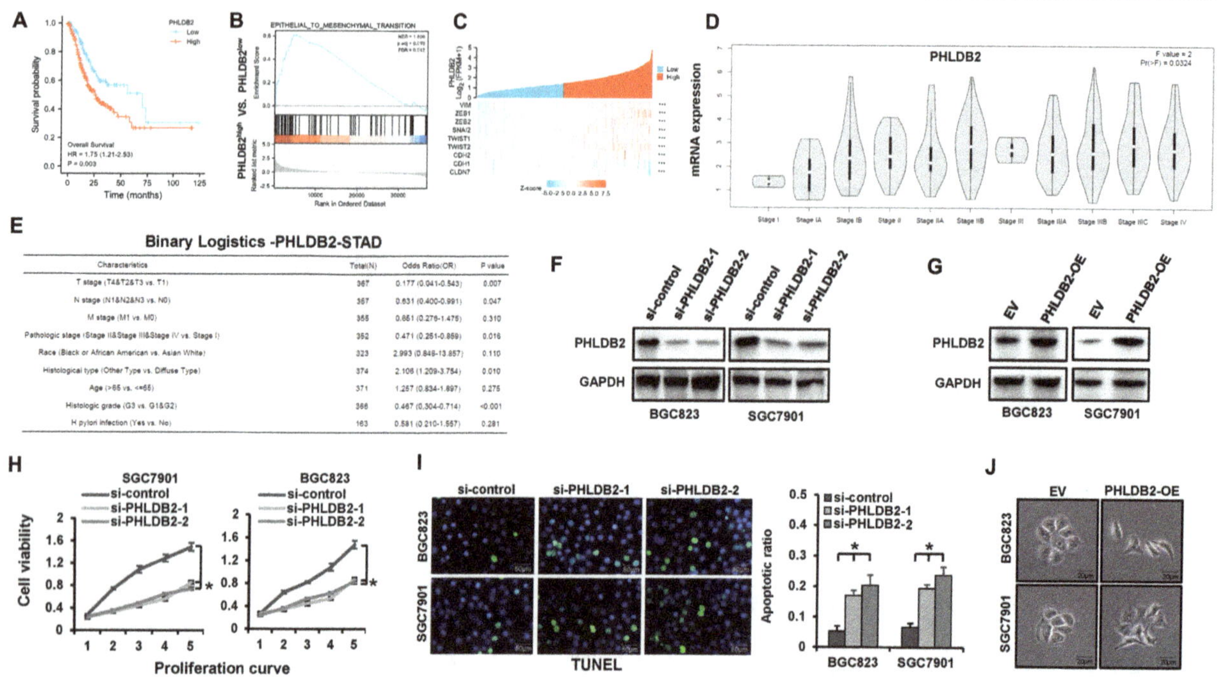

FIGURE 5 | PHLDB2 promotes the poor prognosis and malignant phenotype of GC cells by activating EMT. **(A)** Xiantao was used to analyze the effect of PHLDB2 expression on the prognosis of patients with GC. **(B)** The data of TCGA GC were divided into two groups: low-expression group and high-expression group of PHLDB2. The whole genome expression of these two groups was enriched by GSEA and the enrichment in the EMT pathway was detected by Xiantao. **(C)** Xiantao was used to analyze the correlation between the expression of NR2F1-AS1 and EMT markers, and a heat map was drawn. **(D)** GEPIA2 was used to analyze the expression of PHLDB2 in different stages of GC. **(E)** Xiantao was used to analyze the correlation between NR2F1-AS1 and clinical features by Binary Logistics. Si-control, si-PHLDB2-1, and si-PHLDB2-2 were transfected into BGC823 and SGC7901 to detect **(F)** the expression of PHLDB2 by WB. **(H)** The cell viability by cell viability assay. **(I)** The proportion of apoptosis by TUNEL assay. **(G)** BGC823 and SGC7901 cell lines were transfected with PHLDB2-OE and EV to detect the expression of PHLDB2 by WB. **(J)** The morphology of cell colonies was observed after transfection of PHLDB2-OE and EV in BGC823 and SGC7901 cell lines. *$p < 0.05$; **$p < 0.01$; ***$p < 0.001$.

significantly, while the epithelial phenotypic marker E-cadherin decreased significantly (**Figures 6B,C**). The experimental results of cell morphology assays (**Supplementary Figure 2E**), Transwell (**Supplementary Figure 2F**), and WB (**Supplementary Figure 2G**) in HGC27 show that the silencing of NR2F1-AS1 inhibited the EMT process. We performed a rescue assay on the regulation of EMT by miR-190a/PHLDB2. We transfected PHLDB2-OE into BGC823 cells overexpressing mimic-190a and found that the EMT process inhibited by mimic-190a was significantly restored (**Supplementary Figures 3D–F**). These results showed that ceRNA composed of NR2F1-AS1/miR-190a/PHLDB2 promoted the malignant phenotypic transformation, staging progress, and poor prognosis of GC caused by the EMT process.

NR2F1-AS1/miR-190a/PHLDB2 Promotes Epithelial–Mesenchymal Transformation by Promoting the Phosphorylation of AKT3

Next, we analyzed the regulatory relationship between NR2F1-AS1/miR-190a/PHLDB2 and the mechanism involved in the EMT process. The genes whose Spearmen correlation coefficients (**Supplementary Table 4**) were >0.7 between the whole genome expression and the expression of NR2F1-AS1 and PHLDB2 in the GC dataset were analyzed by GO/KEGG enrichment analysis. The results showed that the enrichment patterns of the genes related to NR2F1-AS1 and PHLDB2 were similar, and both were significantly enriched in the cancer pathway and PI3K/AKT pathway (**Figure 6D**). We found that there was a high correlation between the elevated expression of NR2F1-AS1/PHLDB2 and PI3K/AKT pathway through GSEA analysis (**Figure 6E**). We analyzed the expression of AKT1, AKT2, and AKT3 in GC using bioinformatics tools. AKT1 and AKT2 were significantly overexpressed in GC (**Supplementary Figures 4A, 5A**), and their high expression was significantly correlated with poor prognosis of GC (**Supplementary Figures 4B, 5B**), but not with staging, PHLDB2, and EMT-related markers (**Supplementary Figures 4C–E, 5C–E**). This suggested that the activation of the PI3K/AKT pathway by NR2F1-AS1/miR-190a/PHLDB2 axis might have a lower correlation with AKT1 and AKT2. However, the expression pattern of AKT3 was similar to that of PHLDB2, and there was no significant difference in the expression of AKT3 (**Supplementary Figure 6A**) between GC and the paracancerous tissues. The elevated expression of AKT3 was significantly related to the progression of GC stage (**Supplementary Figure 6B**), poor prognosis of GC (**Figure 7A**), the expression of EMT-related

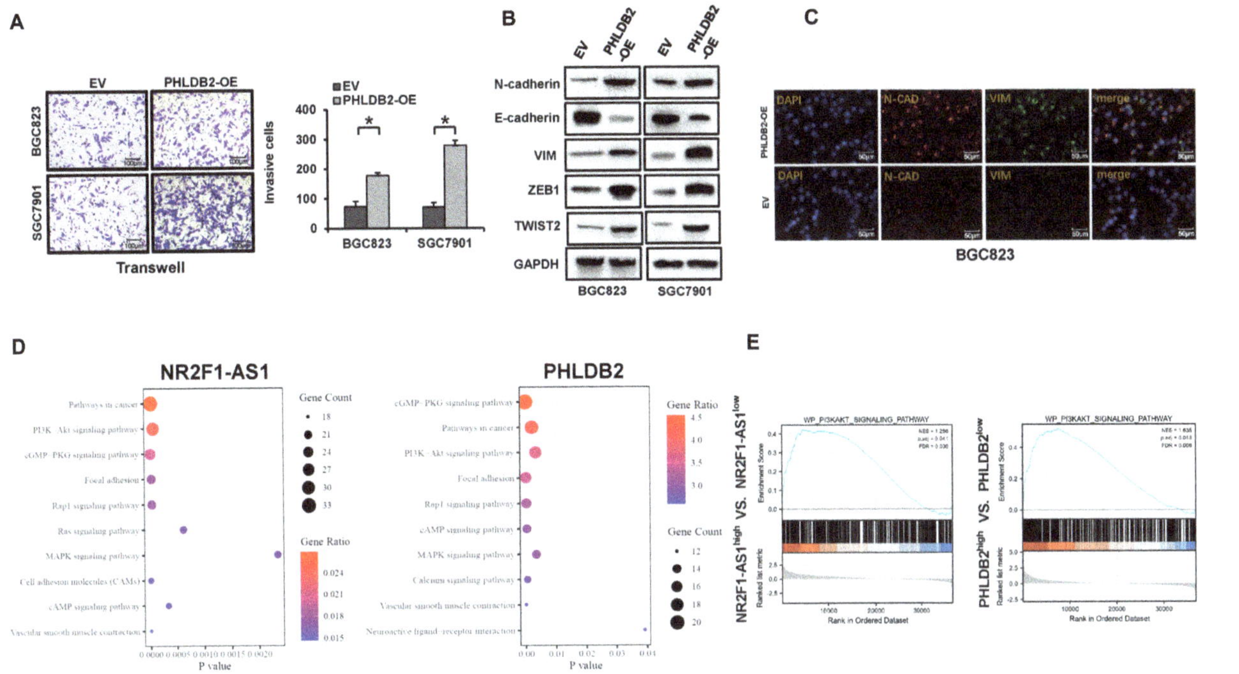

FIGURE 6 | NR2F1-AS1/PHLDB2 significantly enriched with PI3K/AKT pathway in GC. **(A)** BGC823 and SGC7901 cell lines were transfected with PHLDB2-OE and EV to detect the invasiveness of the cells by Transwell assay. **(B)** After PHLDB2-OE and EV were transfected into BGC823 and SGC7901 cell lines, the expression of EMT markers was detected by WB. **(C)** After transfection of PHLDB2-OE and EV in BGC823 and SGC7901, the expression of CDH2 and VIM was detected by immunofluorescence. **(D)** The correlation between the whole genome of GC and the expression of NR2F1-AS1 and PHLDB2 was analyzed by Xiantao, and the genes with Spearmen correlation coefficient >0.7 were analyzed by KEGG enrichment analysis using the DAVID website. **(E)** The enrichment of NR2F1-AS1/PHLDB2 expression in the PI3K/AKT pathway was analyzed by GSEA. $^{*}p < 0.05$.

markers (**Figure 7B** and **Supplementary Figure 6C**), NR2F1-AS1/miR-190a/PHLDB2 axis (**Figure 7D**) and EMT process (**Figure 7C**). Therefore, we speculated that the NR2F1-AS1/miR-190a/PHLDB2 axis promoted the EMT process of GC by regulating the expression of AKT3.

Finally, we investigated whether PHLDB2 promoted the EMT process through AKT3. We found that the overexpression of NR2F1-AS1 and PHLDB2 promoted expression of AKT3 and the phosphorylation of AKT but had no effect on the expression of PI3K (**Figures 7E,F**). We constructed an AKT3 stable knockout cell line using si-AKT3 lentivirus (**Supplementary Figure 6D**). The expression of EMT markers was detected *via* WB after transfecting PHLDB2-OE into the AKT3 stable knockout BGC823 cell line. The silencing of AKT3 prevented the phosphorylation of AKT and EMT transformation induced by PHLDB2 overexpression (**Figure 7G**). The results showed that the presence and phosphorylation of AKT3 was essential for promoting the transformation of EMT by PHLDB2.

CONCLUSION

Competitive endogenous RNA, NR2F1-AS1/miR-190a/PHLDB2 promoted the EMT process of GC cells, and PHLDB2 promoted the EMT process of GC cells by promoting the expression and phosphorylation of AKT3.

DISCUSSION

The purpose of this study was to explore the role and mechanism of ceRNA in the EMT process in GC cells. First, bioinformatics analysis revealed that the expression of the NR2F1-AS1/miR-190a/PHLDB2 axis varied considerably between carcinoma *in situ* and advanced GC, with a significant correlation between the expression of EMT-related markers. Furthermore, the NR2F1-AS1/miR-190a/PHLDB2 axis promoted EMT, which improved the ability of GC cells to proliferate, invade, and resist apoptosis. Next, KEGG enrichment analysis showed a close association between the NR2F1-AS1/miR-190a/PHLDB2 axis and the PI3K/AKT pathway. The highest correlation was found between the AKT family subtype AKT3 and the NR2F1-AS1/miR-190a/PHLDB2 axis. Further results showed that the expression and phosphorylation of AKT3 were required for the NR2F1-AS1/miR-190a/PHLDB2 axis to play a role in promoting EMT. Thus, the NR2F1-AS1/miR-190a/PHLDB2 axis facilitated GC cell proliferation, invasion, and anti-apoptosis by stimulating the AKT3 pathway to induce EMT.

NR2F1-AS1 is a type of lncRNA. NR2F1-AS1 has been shown to facilitate malignant tumor development in non-small cell lung cancer (Zhang C. et al., 2020), breast cancer (Zhang Q. et al., 2020), bone cancer (Li et al., 2019), thyroid cancer (Guo et al., 2019), and endometrial cancer (Wang et al., 2019), as well as tumor cell EMT in liver cancer (Ji et al., 2021)

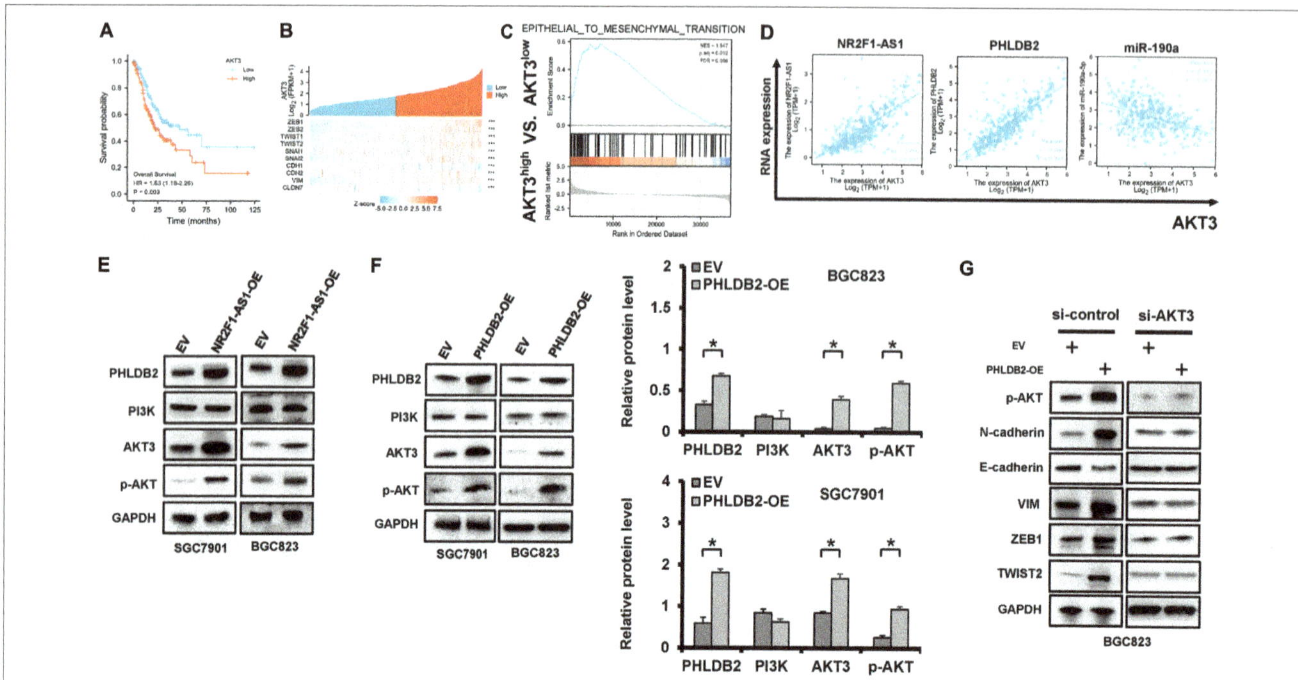

FIGURE 7 | PHLDB2 induces EMT by promoting phosphorylation of AKT3. **(A)** Xiantao website was used to analyze the effect of AKT3 expression on the prognosis of patients with GC. **(B)** Xiantao was used to analyze the correlation between the expression of AKT3 and EMT markers in GC. **(C)** The data of TCGA GC were divided into two groups: low-expression group and high-expression group of AKT3. The whole genome expression of these two groups was enriched by GSEA and the enrichment in the EMT pathway was detected by Xiantao. **(D)** Xiantao was used to analyze the correlation between AKT3 and NR2F1-AS1/miR-190a/PHLDB2 expression in GC. **(E,F)** The expression of PHLDB2, PI3K, AKT3, and p-AKT was detected by WB after transfection of PHLDB2-OE(EV) and NR2F1-AS1-OE(EV) into BGC823 and SGC7901 cell lines. **(G)** PHLDB2-OE and EV were transfected into BGC823 and SGC7901 with stable knockout-AKT3 or knockout-control to detect the expression of p-AKT and EMT markers by WB. $^{*}p < 0.05$; $^{**}p < 0.01$; $^{***}p < 0.001$.

and esophageal squamous cell cancer (Wang et al., 2019). However, the function and mechanism of NR2F1-AS1 in GC are unclear. This study found that NR2F1-AS1 promoted the malignant phenotypes of EMT and GC in GC cell lines. NR2F1-AS1 expression in GC *in situ* was considerably downregulated, and it increased dramatically following the increase in the invasive potential of GC cells. These findings indicated that NR2F1-AS1 played a small role in GC carcinogenesis but an important role in GC cell invasion, which probably explained the absence of substantial difference in NR2F1-AS1 expression between tumor cells and paracancerous tissues. Thus, the elevated expression of NR2F1-AS1 probably constituted the early biological mechanism by which the invasive potential of GC *in situ* was obtained *via* the EMT process. However, there are currently few studies on NR2F1-AS1, and the mechanism of its expression activation remains unknown. MiR-190a has been shown to suppress the EMT pathway in esophageal squamous cell carcinoma (Liang et al., 2020) and to have anti-tumor activity in triple-negative breast cancer (Wang et al., 2020), esophageal squamous cell carcinoma (Liang et al., 2020), glioma (Jin et al., 2020). In this research, we found that miR-190a inhibited EMT in GC cell lines. Also, miR-190a had regulatory targets for both NR2F1-AS1 and PHLDB2 and was also linked to EMT markers, indicating that miR-190a might be the medium by which NR2F1-AS1 regulated PHLDB2. PHLDB2 is a protein with a PH domain. Since PHLDB2 and CLASPS are known to form complexes at the cell edge to regulate cell migration and polarization, PHLDB2 could play an important role in tumor cell invasion and metastasis (Lim et al., 2016). PHLDB2 has been shown to promote carcinogenesis in renal cancer (Wang et al., 2021), colorectal cancer (Chen et al., 2019), and esophageal squamous cell cancer (Hoshino et al., 2016), as well as the process of EMT in colon cancer (Chen et al., 2019). PHLDB2 is known to play a tumor-promoting role as a downstream target of the Notch pathway and to stimulate the AKT pathway in GC (Kang et al., 2021). However, there are no active studies evaluating the relationship and mechanism between PHLDB2 and the EMT process in GC. Here, we showed that PHLDB2 could enhance EMT in GC cells. After confirming the relationship between NR2F1-AS1/miR-190a/PHLDB2 expression and regulation, we verified that ceRNA composed of NR2F1-AS1/miR-190a/PHLDB2 promoted the EMT process in GC. Also, bioinformatics findings suggested that the EMT process induced by the NR2F1-AS1/miR-190a/PHLDB2 axis was probably the first biological step in GC cells gaining invasive ability.

The mechanism of NR2F1-AS1/miR-190a/PHLDB2 supporting EMT is currently being investigated. KEGG enrichment analysis of genes related to NR2F1-AS1 and PHLDB2 expression showed that enrichment was significantly related to PI3K/AKT pathway. NR2F1-AS1 is known to be related to the activation of the PI3K/AKT pathway in endometrial cancer (Wang et al., 2019), and miR-190a has been shown to promote the activation of the PI3K/AKT pathway in gliomas (Jin et al., 2020). PHLDB2 was also found to be associated with AKT activation in GC cells (Kang et al., 2021). Therefore, the NR2F1-AS1/miR-190a/PHLDB2 axis might play a vital role in promoting EMT by activating the AKT pathway. AKT signaling pathway is known to promote tumorigenesis through a variety of downstream regulators (Janku et al., 2018). There are three molecules in the AKT family, AKT1, AKT2, and AKT3, whose amino acid structures are 80% similar. Thus, most studies analyze AKT1, AKT2, and AKT3 together (Kumar and Madison, 2005). Activated total AKT protein has been shown to activate EMT-related transcription factors to induce EMT transformation and promote tumor invasion and metastasis (Fresno Vara et al., 2004). The abnormal activation of AKT is also often found in epithelial cells with low metastatic ability. Thus each subtype of AKT has a different biological function (Xue and Hemmings, 2013; Hoxhaj and Manning, 2020). AKT3 has been found to be significantly associated with the EMT process of the thyroid (You et al., 2020), bladder (McNiel and Tsichlis, 2017), colorectal (Buikhuisen et al., 2021), and prostate cancer (Galbraith et al., 2021). This suggested that the EMT conversion induced by AKT might be largely dependent on specific AKT molecular subtypes. However, the relationship between AKT molecular subtypes and the EMT process in GC is unclear. In this study, we found that PHLDB2 had a low correlation with AKT1 and AKT2 but was highly correlated with the expression pattern of AKT3. The results of co-transfection showed that the expression and phosphorylation of AKT3 were critical for PHLDB2 to promote EMT. Therefore, we concluded that NR2F1-AS1/miR-190a/PHLDB2 activated the invasive ability of GC cells by promoting the phosphorylation of AKT3 to induce the EMT process.

In this study, we report that the upregulated expression of ceRNA composed of NR2F1-AS1/miR-190a/PHLDB2 axis promoted the EMT process, which might be the early biological process for GC cells to gain invasive ability. The newly discovered activation of AKT also promoted the upstream signal of EMT and finally clarified the important role of the AKT subtype, AKT3, in the process of EMT. This study enables a more comprehensive understanding of the EMT mechanism and the discovery of new EMT markers.

AUTHOR CONTRIBUTIONS

LX and YZ designed the research. JL and TG performed the data acquisition. HS and CL supervised the data and algorithms. ZJ and YL performed the data analysis and interpretation. ShZ and JL carried out the statistical analysis. ZL and JL performed the manuscript preparation. LX and SiZ participated in manuscript editing and review. All authors read and approved the final manuscript.

SUPPLEMENTARY MATERIAL

Supplementary Figure 1 | NR2F1-AS1 and EMT process in GC. **(A)** Xiantao was used to analyze the expression of NR2F1-AS1 in GC and paracancerous tissues. **(B)** Xiantao was used to analyze the correlation between the expression of NR2F1-AS1 and EMT markers in GC. NR2F1-AS1-OE and EV were transfected into BGC823 and SGC7901 cell lines to detect **(C)** the cell proliferative ability by cell viability assay. **(D)** The proportion of apoptosis by TUNEL assay. **(E)** The morphology of cell colonies was observed after transfection of si-control and si-NR2F1-AS1-1 in HGC27. **(F)** Si-control and si-NR2F1-AS1-1were transfected into HSC27 to detect the invasiveness of the cells by Transwell assay. **(G)** After transfection of si-control and si-NR2F1-AS1-1 in HGC27, the expression of EMT markers was detected by WB. $^*p < 0.05$.

Supplementary Figure 2 | PHLDB2 and EMT process in GC. **(A)** Xiantao was used to analyze the expression of PHLDB2 in GC and paracancerous tissues.**(B)** Xiantao was used to analyze the correlation between the expression of PHLDB2 and EMT markers in GC. PHLDB2-OE and EV were transfected into BGC823 and SGC7901 cell lines to detect **(C)** the cell proliferative ability by cell viability assay. **(D)** The proportion of apoptosis by TUNEL assay. **(E)** The morphology of cell colonies was observed after transfection of si-control and si-PHLDB2-1 in HGC27. **(F)** Si-control and si-PHLDB2-1 were transfected into HGC27 to detect the invasiveness of the cells by Transwell assay. **(G)** After transfection of si-control and si-PHLDB2-1 in HGC27, the expression of EMT markers was detected by WB. $^*p < 0.05$.

Supplementary Figure 3 | NR2F1-AS1 regulates the expression of PHLDB2 by adsorbing miR-190a, promoting the EMT process. Mimic-190a and mimic-control were transfected into BGC823 and HGC7901 overexpressing NR2F1-AS1 to detect **(A)** the invasiveness of the cells by Transwell assay. **(B)** The morphology of cell colonies. **(C)** The expression of EMT markers was detected by WB. PHLDB2-OE and EV were transfected into HGC27 overexpressing miR-190a to detect **(D)** the invasiveness of the cells by Transwell assay. **(E)** The morphology of cell colonies. **(F)** The expression of EMT markers was detected by WB. $^*p < 0.05$.

Supplementary Figure 4 | The expression of AKT1 in GC and its correlation with poor prognosis and EMT markers. **(A)** Xiantao was used to analyze the expression of AKT1 in GC and paracancerous tissues. **(B)** The effect of AKT1 expression on the prognosis of patients with GC was analyzed by the Kaplan–Meier plot website. **(C)** GEPIA2 was used to analyze the expression of AKT1 during different stages of GC. **(D)** Xiantao website was used to analyze the correlation between AKT1 and PHLDB2 expression in GC. **(E)** Xiantao website was used to analyze the correlation between the expression of AKT1 and EMT markers in GC. $^*p < 0.05$; $^{**}p < 0.01$; $^{***}p < 0.001$.

Supplementary Figure 5 | The expression of AKT2 in GC and its correlation with poor prognosis and EMT markers. **(A)** Xiantao website was used to analyze the expression of AKT2 in GC and paracancerous tissues. **(B)** The effect of AKT2 expression on the prognosis of patients with GC was analyzed by the Kaplan–Meier plot website. **(C)** GEPIA2 was used to analyze the expression of AKT2 during different stages of GC. **(D)** Xiantao website was used to analyze the correlation between AKT2 and PHLDB2 expression in GC. **(E)** Xiantao website was used to analyze the correlation between the expression of AKT2 and EMT markers in GC. $^*p < 0.05$; $^{**}p < 0.01$; $^{***}p < 0.001$.

Supplementary Figure 6 | The expression of AKT3 in GC and its correlation with poor prognosis and EMT markers. **(A)** Xiantao was used to analyze the expression of AKT3 in GC, and paracancerous tissues. **(B)** GEPIA2 was used to analyze the expression of AKT3 during different stages of GC. **(C)** Xiantao was used to analyze the correlation between the expression of AKT3 and EMT markers in GC.**(D)** WB were used to detect the expression of AKT3 in BGC823 and SGC7901 cell lines infected with si-AKT3 and si-control lentiviral vector.

REFERENCES

Buikhuisen, J. Y., Gomez Barila, P. M., Torang, A., Dekker, D., de Jong, J. H., Cameron, K., et al. (2021). AKT3 expression in mesenchymal colorectal cancer cells drives growth and is associated with epithelial-mesenchymal transition. *Cancers* 13:801. doi: 10.3390/cancers13040801

Chen, G., Zhou, T., Ma, T., Cao, T., and Yu, Z. (2019). Oncogenic effect of PHLDB2 is associated with epithelial-mesenchymal transition and E-cadherin regulation in colorectal cancer. *Cancer Cell Int.* 19:184. doi: 10.1186/s12935-019-0903-1

Fresno Vara, J. A., Casado, E., de Castro, J., Cejas, P., Belda-Iniesta, C., and González-Barón, M. (2004). PI3K/Akt signalling pathway and cancer. *Cancer Treat. Rev.* 30, 193–204. doi: 10.1016/j.ctrv.2003.07.007

Galbraith, L., Mui, E., Nixon, C., Hedley, A., Strachan, D., MacKay, G., et al. (2021). PPAR-gamma induced AKT3 expression increases levels of mitochondrial biogenesis driving prostate cancer. *Oncogene* 40, 2355–2366. doi: 10.1038/s41388-021-01707-7

Guo, F., Fu, Q., Wang, Y., and Sui, G. (2019). Long non-coding RNA NR2F1-AS1 promoted proliferation and migration yet suppressed apoptosis of thyroid cancer cells through regulating miRNA-338-3p/CCND1 axis. *J. Cell. Mol. Med.* 23, 5907–5919. doi: 10.1111/jcmm.14386

Hoshino, I., Akutsu, Y., Murakami, K., Akanuma, N., Isozaki, Y., Maruyama, T., et al. (2016). Histone demethylase LSD1 inhibitors prevent cell growth by regulating gene expression in esophageal squamous cell carcinoma cells. *Ann. Surg. Oncol.* 23, 312–320. doi: 10.1245/s10434-015-4488-1

Hoxhaj, G., and Manning, B. D. (2020). The PI3K-AKT network at the interface of oncogenic signalling and cancer metabolism. *Nat. Rev. Cancer* 20, 74–88. doi: 10.1038/s41568-019-0216-7

Huang da, W., Sherman, B. T., and Lempicki, R. A. (2009). Systematic and integrative analysis of large gene lists using DAVID bioinformatics resources. *Nat. Protoc.* 4, 44–57. doi: 10.1038/nprot.2008.211

Hur, K., Toiyama, Y., Takahashi, M., Balaguer, F., Nagasaka, T., Koike, J., et al. (2013). MicroRNA-200c modulates epithelial-to-mesenchymal transition (EMT) in human colorectal cancer metastasis. *Gut* 62, 1315–1326. doi: 10.1136/gutjnl-2011-301846

Janku, F., Yap, T. A., and Meric-Bernstam, F. (2018). Targeting the PI3K pathway in cancer: are we making headway. *Nat Rev. Clin. Oncol.* 15, 273–291. doi: 10.1038/nrclinonc.2018.28

Ji, W. C., Bao, G. J., Yang, F. W., Sun, L., and Han, R. (2021). Role of lncRNA NR2F1-AS1 and lncRNA H19 genes in hepatocellular carcinoma and their effects on biological function of Huh-7. *Cancer Manag. Res.* 13, 941–951. doi: 10.2147/CMAR.S284650

Jin, Z., Piao, L., Sun, G., Lv, C., Jing, Y., and Jin, R. (2020). Long non-coding RNA PART1 exerts tumor suppressive functions in glioma via sponging miR-190a-3p and inactivation of PTEN/AKT pathway. *Onco. Targets Ther.* 13, 1073–1086. doi: 10.2147/OTT.S232848

Kang, W., Zhang, J., Huang, T., Zhou, Y., Wong, C. C., Chan, R., et al. (2021). NOTCH3, a crucial target of miR-491-5p/miR-875-5p, promotes gastric carcinogenesis by upregulating PHLDB2 expression and activating Akt pathway. *Oncogene* 40, 1578–1594. doi: 10.1038/s41388-020-01579-3

Kumar, C. C., and Madison, V. (2005). AKT crystal structure and AKT-specific inhibitors. *Oncogene* 24, 7493–7501. doi: 10.1038/sj.onc.1209087

Li, D., Wang, J., Zhang, M., Hu, X., She, J., Qiu, X., et al. (2020). LncRNA MAGI2-AS3 is regulated by BRD4 and promotes gastric cancer progression via maintaining ZEB1 overexpression by sponging miR-141/200a. *Mol. Ther. Nucleic Acids* 19, 109–123. doi: 10.1016/j.omtn.2019.11.003

Li, J. H., Liu, S., Zhou, H., Qu, L. H., and Yang, J. H. (2014). starBase v2.0: decoding miRNA-ceRNA, miRNA-ncRNA and protein-RNA interaction networks from large-scale CLIP-Seq data. *Nucleic Acids Res.* 42, D92–D97. doi: 10.1093/nar/gkt1248

Li, P., Ge, D., Li, P., Hu, F., Chu, J., Chen, X., et al. (2020). CXXC finger protein 4 inhibits the CDK18-ERK1/2 axis to suppress the immune escape of gastric cancer cells with involvement of ELK1/MIR100HG pathway. *J. Cell. Mol. Med.* 24, 10151–10165. doi: 10.1111/jcmm.15625

Li, S., Zheng, K., Pei, Y., Wang, W., and Zhang, X. (2019). Long noncoding RNA NR2F1-AS1 enhances the malignant properties of osteosarcoma by increasing forkhead box A1 expression via sponging of microRNA-483-3p. *Aging* 11, 11609–11623. doi: 10.18632/aging.102563

Liang, X., Wu, Z., Shen, S., Niu, Y., Guo, Y., Liang, J., et al. (2020). LINC01980 facilitates esophageal squamous cell carcinoma progression via regulation of miR-190a-5p/MYO5A pathway. *Arch. Biochem. Biophys.* 686:108371. doi: 10.1016/j.abb.2020.108371

Lim, B. C., Matsumoto, S., Yamamoto, H., Mizuno, H., Kikuta, J., Ishii, M., et al. (2016). Prickle1 promotes focal adhesion disassembly in cooperation with the CLASP-LL5β complex in migrating cells. *J. Cell. Sci.* 129, 3115–3129. doi: 10.1242/jcs.185439

McNiel, E. A., and Tsichlis, P. N. (2017). Analyses of publicly available genomics resources define FGF-2-expressing bladder carcinomas as EMT-prone, proliferative tumors with low mutation rates and high expression of CTLA-4, PD-1 and PD-L1. *Signal Transduct. Target. Ther.* 2:16045. doi: 10.1038/sigtrans.2016.45

Nagy, Á, Lánczky, A., Menyhárt, O., and Győrffy, B. (2018). Validation of miRNA prognostic power in hepatocellular carcinoma using expression data of independent datasets. *Sci. Rep.* 8:9227. doi: 10.1038/s41598-018-27521-y

Smyth, E. C., Nilsson, M., Grabsch, H. I., van Grieken, N. C., and Lordick, F. (2020). Gastric cancer. *Lancet* 396, 635–648. doi: 10.1016/S0140-6736(20)31288-5

Tang, Z., Kang, B., Li, C., Chen, T., and Zhang, Z. (2019). GEPIA2: an enhanced web server for large-scale expression profiling and interactive analysis. *Nucleic Acids Res.* 47, 556–560. doi: 10.1093/nar/gkz430

Thomson, D. W., and Dinger, M. E. (2016). Endogenous microRNA sponges: evidence and controversy. *Nat. Rev. Genet.* 17, 272–283. doi: 10.1038/nrg.2016.20

Wang, H., Wang, L., Zheng, Q., Lu, Z., Chen, Y., Shen, D., et al. (2021). Oncometabolite L-2-hydroxyglurate directly induces vasculogenic mimicry through PHLDB2 in renal cell carcinoma. *Int. J. Cancer* 148, 1743–1755. doi: 10.1002/ijc.33435

Wang, L., Zhao, S., and Mingxin, Y. U. (2019). LncRNA NR2F1-AS1 is involved in the progression of endometrial cancer by sponging miR-363 to target SOX4. *Pharmazie* 74, 295–300. doi: 10.1691/ph.2019.8905

Wang, S., Liu, F., Ma, H., Cui, X., Yang, S., and Qin, R. (2020). circCDYL acts as a tumor suppressor in triple negative breast cancer by sponging miR-190a-3p and upregulating TP53INP1. *Clin. Breast Cancer* 20, 422–430. doi: 10.1016/j.clbc.2020.04.006

Xu, L., Zhang, Y., Qu, X., Che, X., Guo, T., Cai, Y., et al. (2017a). E3 ubiquitin ligase Cbl-b prevents tumor metastasis by maintaining the epithelial phenotype in multiple drug-resistant gastric and breast cancer cells. *Neoplasia* 19, 374–382. doi: 10.1016/j.neo.2017.01.011

Xu, L., Zhang, Y., Qu, X., Che, X., Guo, T., Li, C., et al. (2017b). DR5-Cbl-b/c-Cbl-TRAF2 complex inhibits TRAIL-induced apoptosis by promoting TRAF2-mediated polyubiquitination of caspase-8 in gastric cancer cells. *Mol. Oncol.* 11, 1733–1751. doi: 10.1002/1878-0261.12140

Xue, G., and Hemmings, B. A. (2013). PKB/Akt-dependent regulation of cell motility. *J. Natl. Cancer Inst.* 105, 393–404. doi: 10.1093/jnci/djs648

Yang, J., Antin, P., Berx, G., Blanpain, C., Brabletz, T., Bronner, M., et al. (2020). Guidelines and definitions for research on epithelial-mesenchymal transition. *Nat. Rev. Mol. Cell Biol.* 21, 341–352. doi: 10.1038/s41580-020-0237-9

You, A., Fu, L., Li, Y., Li, X., and You, B. (2020). MicroRNA-203 restrains epithelial-mesenchymal transition, invasion and migration of papillary thyroid cancer by downregulating AKT3. *Cell Cycle* 19, 1105–1121. doi: 10.1080/15384101.2020.1746490

Yuan, L., Xu, Z. Y., Ruan, S. M., Mo, S., Qin, J. J., and Cheng, X. D. (2020). Long non-coding RNAs towards precision medicine in gastric cancer: early diagnosis, treatment, and drug resistance. *Mol. Cancer* 19:96. doi: 10.1186/s12943-020-01219-0

Zhang, C., Wu, S., Song, R., and Liu, C. (2020). Long noncoding RNA NR2F1-AS1 promotes the malignancy of non-small cell lung cancer via sponging microRNA-493-5p and thereby increasing ITGB1 expression. *Aging* 13, 7660–7675. doi: 10.18632/aging.103564

2

Hypoxia-Induced ZWINT Mediates Pancreatic Cancer Proliferation by Interacting With p53/p21

Peng Chen[1,2†], *Zhiwei He*[1,2†], *Jie Wang*[1†], *Jian Xu*[1†], *Xueyi Jiang*[2], *Yankun Chen*[2], *Xinyuan Liu*[2] *and Jianxin Jiang*[1]*

[1]*Department of Hepatobiliary Surgery, Renmin Hospital of Wuhan University, Wuhan, China,* [2]*Department of Hepatic-Biliary-Pancreatic Surgery, The Affiliated Hospital of Guizhou Medical University, Guiyang, China*

Correspondence:
Jianxin Jiang
rm002979@whu.edu.cn

†*These authors have contributed equally to this work*

p53/p21 signaling plays a vital role in pancreatic cancer (PC) progression. ZWINT was shown to function as an oncoprotein in the progression of multiple cancers. However, the involvement of ZWINT and p53 activation in the progression of PC remains poorly understood. Bioinformatics and tissue array chip analyses were performed to evaluate ZWINT expression in pancreatic cancer. ZWINT mRNA and protein expression were evaluated in normoxia and hypoxia. CHIP was used to evaluate HIF1α interaction with the ZWINT promoter. CCK8, colony formation, EDU, and cell cycle analysis were used to examine PC cell proliferation. Immunoprecipitation and immunofluorescence were used to examine the interaction of ZWINT, MDM2, and p53. p53 activity was evaluated by q-PCR and luciferase assay. Protein degradation and ubiquitination assays were used to analyze the role of ZWINT in p53 ubiquitination. ZWINT was overexpressed in pancreatic cancer and induced in hypoxia. ZWINT promoted pancreatic cancer growth and cell cycle progression. Bioinformatic analysis revealed that ZWINT may regulate the p53 signal pathway. ZWINT interacts with p53 and promotes its ubiquitination and degradation. ZWINT promoted proliferation via p53/p21. Immunohistochemistry of clinical specimens revealed that that ZWINT expression was significantly negatively correlated with p53/p21. Our data showed that hypoxia regulates the expression of ZWINT, which activated p53/p21 signaling pathway to promote PC growth.

Keywords: ZWINT, pancreatic cancer, HIF1α, p53/p21, proliferation

INTRODUCTION

Pancreatic cancer (PC), one of the most serious gastrointestinal malignancies, is the fourth most frequent cause of cancer-associated death (Siegel et al., 2020). Because of the lack of precise diagnostic approaches, PC is usually diagnosed at advanced stage (The Lancet Gastroenterology and Hepatology, 2021). Patients with advanced PC can only receive chemotherapy instead of surgical resection (Perri and Katz, 2021). In the occurrence and development of pancreatic cancer, there are no more accurate early diagnosis and treatment methods. (Lee et al., 2020). Hence, studies of diagnostic markers and targeted therapies that inhibit the progression of PC have been key strategies to improve the treatment of PC.

Abbreviations: CCK-8, Cell Counting Kit-8; ChIP, Chromatin immunoprecipitation; PC, pancreatic carcinoma; mZWINT-1, ZW10-interacting kinetochore protein 1.

ZW10-interacting kinetochore protein 1 (ZWINT-1) is a centromere complex component necessary for the mitotic spindle checkpoint and participates in centromere function and cell development (Peng et al., 2019). ZWINT interacts with Zeste White 10 (ZW10), another centromere protein, to possibly regulate the relationship between ZW10 and centromeres (Woo et al., 2015). ZWINT-1 is a kinetochore component with a significant role in spindle assembly and kinetochore-microtubule attachment during meiosis and mitosis (Kasuboski et al., 2011). In addition, ZWINT-1 directly interacts with components of the KMN complex, specifically Ndc80 and Mis12, and functions as a bridge between the RZZ and KMN complexes necessary for kinetochore formation and spindle checkpoint activity (Zhang et al., 2015). As a mitotic checkpoint component, ZWINT-1 is required for the stable relationship between CENP-F and dynamitin and the kinetochore to guarantee precise chromosome segregation (Zhang et al., 2015).

Recent studies have indicated that ZWINT-1 may function as a biomarker for cancer due to its high expression in some human malignancies such as glioblastoma (Yang et al., 2020), breast cancer (Zhou G. et al., 2020), ovarian cancer (Zhao and Yu, 2020), bladder cancer, lung cancer (Yi et al., 2020), and hepatocellular carcinoma (Xie et al., 2020). In addition, knockdown of ZWINT-1 restrained the proliferation, migration, invasion, and colony formation abilities of pancreatic cancer cells and increased cell apoptosis (Kim et al., 2020). Another study showed that ZWINT interacts with Rab3C as a part of the MIS12 complex (Obuse et al., 2004). Endo et al. showed that cell proliferation in 293T cells and breast cancer MCF7 cells (Endo et al., 2012) were negatively regulated by ZWINT depletion by Terf/Trim (Endo et al., 2012). Together these findings suggest that ZWINT, which plays a role in the spindle filament and cell division, may function as an oncoprotein. However, the role of ZWINT in pancreatic cancer has remained unknown.

It was found that the aberrantly of ZWINT protein expression promoted PC pathogenesis as was a distasteful element. In addition, ZWINT promoted p53 ubiquitin degradation of p53 via interacting with MDM2, inactivating p53/p21 signaling, promoting the transition of cell cycle and cell development in PC. Our findings indicate that ZWINT functions as an oncoprotein and modulates p53/p21 to promote pancreatic cancer pathogenesis.

MATERIALS AND METHODS

Specimen Source and Clinical Materials

This study included 92 pancreatic cancer samples, including tumors and adjacent non-tumor tissues. The pancreatic cancer tissues were obtained from surgical specimens from inpatients in our hospital from 2016 to 2020.

5-Ethynyl-2′-Deoxyuridine Assay

Cells in a 24-well plate were incubated with 200 μl of EDU medium (5 μM) for 2 h and then fixed with 50 μl phosphate buffer saline (PBS) containing 4% paraformaldehyde for 30 min at room temperature. Cells were then incubated with 50 μl of glycine (2 mg/ml) for 5 min, followed by a 10-min treatment of 200 μl of osmotic agent (PBS containing 0.5% Triton X-100), a 30-min treatment of 200 μl of IX Apollo staining solution at room temperature in the dark, and two to three rinses with 200 μl of osmotic agent (PBS containing 0.5% Triton X-100; 10 min each time). Cells were counterstained with 4′, 6 diamidino-2-phenylindole (DAPI) for 5 min for nuclear staining and then examined using a fluorescence microscope.

TABLE 1 | The RNA primers used in the PCR.

Gene name	Sequences
ZWINT (NM_001005413)	F:AGGACACTGCTAAGGGTCTCG R:GCCTCTACGTGCTCCCTGTA
P53 (NM_001126118)	F:ACAGCTTTGAGGTGCGTGTTT R:CCCTTTCTTGCGGAGATTCTCT
P21 (NM_078467)	F:TGTCCGTCAGAACCCATGC R:AAAGTCGAAGTTCCATCGCTC
CDK4 (NM_000075)	F:ATGGCTACCTCTCGATATGAGC R:CATTGGGGACTCTCACACTCT
CDK6 (NM_001145306)	F:GCTGACCAGCAGTACGAATG R:GCACACATCAAACAACCTGACC
CyclinD1 (NM_053056)	F:GCTGCGAAGTGGAAACCATC R:CCTCCTTCTGCACACATTTGAA
CyclinE1 (NM_004864)	F:ACCTGCACCTGCGTATCTCT R:CGGACGAAGATTCTGCCAG
GAPDH (NM_001256799)	F:ACAACTTTGGTATCGTGGAAGG R:GCCATCACGCCACAGTTTC

Luciferase Reporter Assays

It is predicted that the human DNA sequences of the p21 promoter are bound with transcription element p53 cloned into a pGL3 vector. Cells were transfected with luciferase plasmids along with ZWINT or control lentivirus for x h. Cell lysates were obtained and luciferase activity was detected using the dual-luciferase reporter system according to the manufacturer's instructions (Promega, Madison, WI, United States).

RT-PCR

RNA was extracted from cells using Trizol based on the manufacturer's instructions, and a UV spectrophotometer was used to determine the purity and concentration of the RNA. RNA was reverse transcribed into cDNA using the RT-PCR kit TAKARA047A (Takara Bio, Inc., Shiga, Japan) of the Super Script III First-Strand Synthesis System. The BioRad Real-Time PCR system was used for real-time PCR amplification. The primers for ZWINT, p53, p21, CDK4, CDK6, Cyclin D1, Cyclin E1, and GAPDH mRNAs are shown in **Table 1**.

Immunohistochemistry

Immunohistochemistry was performed on 5-μm-thick paraffin sections. Monoclonal antibody against ZWINT was used at a 1:50 dilution (HAP022264, Sigma). After dewaxing, immunostaining permeation solution was applied to the samples. The presence of brown particles in the nucleus and cytoplasm indicated positive staining.

Chromatin Immunoprecipitation

The EZ-ChIPTM Chromatin Immunoprecipitation Kit (Millipore, Billerica, MA, United States) was used to perform

TABLE 2 | The siRNA sequence used in the transfection assay.

Gene	sequence (5′→3)
si-ZWINT#1	GCACGTAGAGGCCATCAAA
si-ZWINT#2	GAACCAGTGGCAGCTACAA
si-P53	GTACCACCATCCACTACAA
si-P21	GATGGAACTTCGACTTTGT

ChIP assays following the manufacturer's instructions. Rabbit anti-FLAG (Cell Signaling Technology, United States), anti-RNA polymerase II antibodies (Abcam, United Kingdom) and related rabbit-IgG (Cell Signaling Technology, United States) was applied as controls.

Cell Culture

The pancreatic cancer cell lines (AsPC-1, BxPC-3, MIA PaCa-2, SW 1990, PANC-1 and PANC03.27) and the HPDE normal pancreatic cell line were purchased from the ATCC. MIA PaCa-2, SW 1990, and PANC-1 cells were cultured in conventional DMEM medium (GIBCO, United States) containing 10% fetal bovine serum (BI, United States). AsPC-1, PANC03.27 and HPDE cells were cultured in RPMI 1640 medium (GIBCO) containing 10% fetal bovine serum. Cells were cultured at 37°C, 5% CO_2 with saturated humidity.

Cell Transfection and Lentivirus Infection

The liposome method (Lipo 3000 transfection kit, Invitrogen) was used to transfect small interfering RNA (siRNA) into PANC-1 and MIA PaCa-2 cell lines (siRNA sequences were shown in **Table 2**). Cells were harvested at 48 h and analyzed by RT-PCR and western blotting to determine the effect of siRNA transfection. **Table 2** shows the siRNA sequences of ZWINT, p53, p21, and that of the negative control (Ruibio, Guangzhou, China). The virus-mediated transfection and oncogene overexpression were applied to infect PANC-1 and MIA PaCa-2 cell lines. Cells were cultured in flasks at a density of 2×10^4 cells/culture flask the day before infection. After overnight culture, the medium was replaced with DMEM (without serum) containing lentivirus (MOI = 25) at 37°C. After 8–12 h, the medium was replaced with complete medium.

Western Blot

Cells were lysed using RIPA buffer for 30 min at 4°C, followed by centrifugation at 12,000×g at 4°C for 30 min. The BCA method was used to determine the protein concentration of supernatants. Denatured protein samples were separated by 10% sodium dodecyl sulfate-polyacrylamide gel electrophoresis (SDS-PAGE) and transferred to polyvinylidene difluoride (PVDF) membranes (Millipore, United States). The membrane was blocked with 5% milk or bovine serum albumin (BSA) for 2 h and then incubated with primary antibodies at 4°C overnight. After washes with Tris-buffered saline (TBST), membranes were incubated with secondary antibody (1:2000, abclone, Wuhan, China) for 2 h, followed by washes with TBST. The ECL reagent (Thermo Scientific ECL) was used to visualize bands. The experiment was performed three times.

Cell Counting Kit-8

Cell proliferation ability was assessed by CCK-8 (Dojindo Molecular Technologies, Inc., Kyushu, Japan) based on the manufacturer's instructions. Cells were seeded into 96-well culture plates at 2×10^3 cells per well the day before transfection or infection. The viability of pancreatic cancer cells was evaluated from five replicates in three independent experiments after indicated treatments for 6, 24, 48, and 72 h.

Cell Cycle Analysis

Cells were fixed with 70% ethanol overnight at 4°C. A staining working solution of 500 μl PI/RNase (PI:RNaseA prepared at 9:1) (KeyGen Biotech, Nanjing, China) was added when centrifugation was used to remove the ethanol in the following day. Cells were stained for 3 min at 4°C in the dark. Stained cells were then examined using a flow cytometer (US BD company).

Immunoprecipitation and Co-Immunoprecipitation

Anti-ZWINT antibody (1 μg) (Sigma: HAP022264) or anti-rabbit IgG antibody (Abcam: ab190492) was added to protein lysates (500 μg) and the samples were incubated at 4°C overnight. Next, 40 μl protein A/G PLUS-Agarose beads (Santa Cruz: sc-2003) was added and samples were incubated at 4°C for 6 h. After adding 2 × loading buffer, the immunoprecipitated protein complex was boiled and denatured. Samples were then analyzed by western blot. 1 μg of the anti-ZWINT primary antibody was employed to perform the same approach, so as to precipitate p53 and MDM2, and western blotting with the anti-p53 and anti-MDM2 primary antibody was conducted to detect the precipitated protein.

Immunofluorescence

Cells on glass coverslips were fixed with 4% paraformaldehyde for 20 min at room temperature. After 15 min incubation with immunostaining permeation solution (Triton X-100, P0096, Beyotime), PBS containing 5% BSA was used to block cells for 30 min. Cells were then incubated with primary antibody against ZWINT (1:50, diluted in blocking buffer) at 4°C overnight and then with Alexa Fluor 488-goat anti-mouse IgG (1:100) secondary antibody for 2 h. Cells were then rinsed with PBS for 15 min, and DAPI was applied for 5 min for nuclei staining. In some experiments, cells were incubated with anti-p53 and anti-p21 primary antibody and the anti-ZWINT primary antibody (1:50, Sigma) simultaneously. Alexa Fluor 488-goat anti-mouse and Alexa Fluor 594-goat anti-mouse were used as secondary antibodies.

Nude Mouse Xenograft Model

Twelve 4-week-old female BALB/cA-nu nude mice were obtained from Beijing Huafukang Biosciences (Beijing, China) and kept in pathogen-free conditions. PANC-1 cells (5×10^6) expressing either ZWINT or control vector in 150 μl of PBS were subcutaneously injected into the left flank of mice ($n = 5$ per group). The rate of tumor formation, number of tumors, tumor diameter, tumor mass and mouse body weight were measured every 7 days. Tumor volume was calculated as $V = 1/2 \times L \times W^2$. Mice were killed after 37 days. Tumors were fixed in 4% paraformaldehyde and embedded in paraffin.

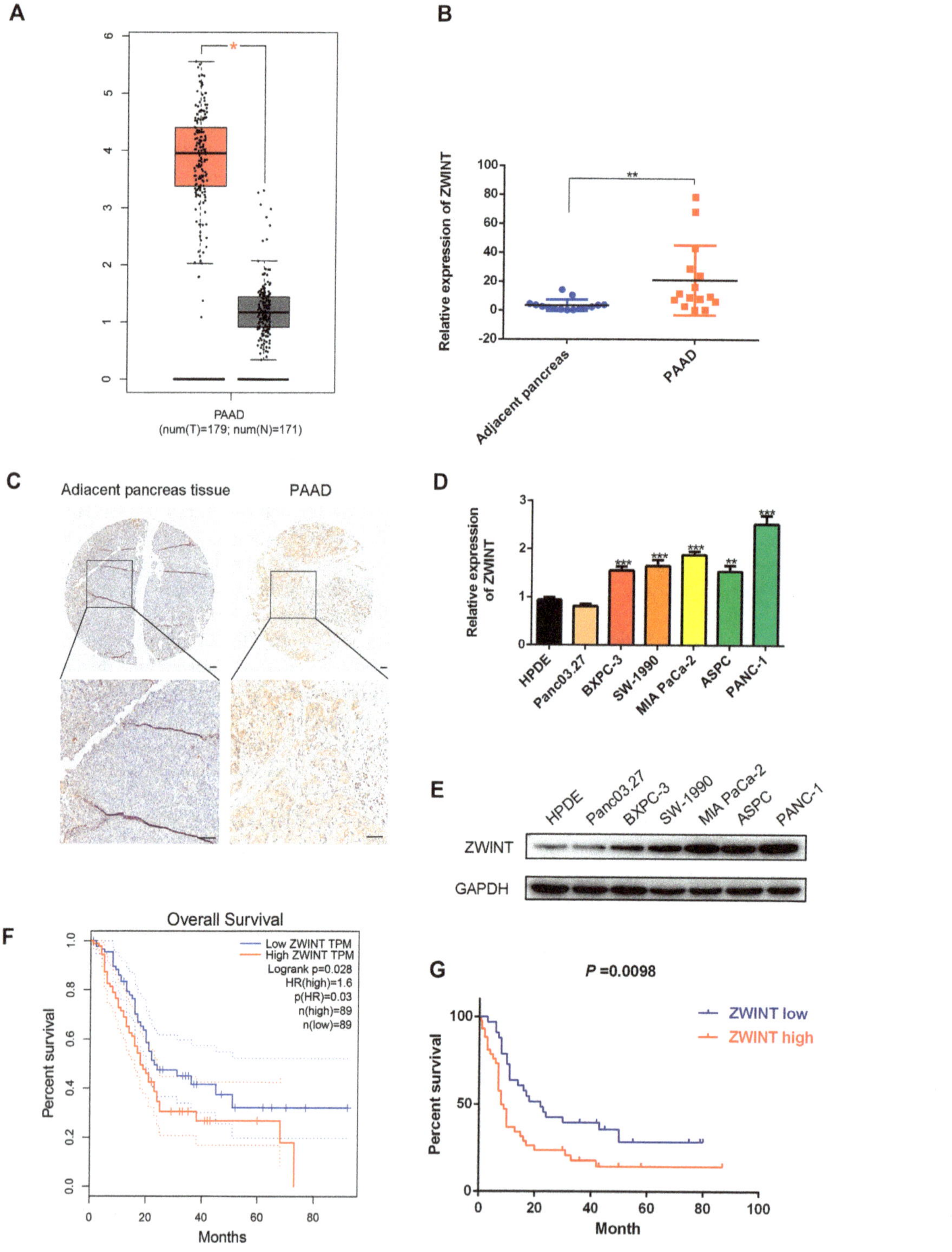

FIGURE 1 | ZWINT was upregulated in pancreatic cancer. **(A)**. ZWINT expression in TCGA-LIHC database. **(B)** ZWINT expression in 16 PC tissue samples and paired normal tissue samples by q-RT-PCR. **(C)** ZWINT expression in tissue microarrays, including 92 pairs of PC samples and adjacent normal tissues. **(D, E)** q-RT-PCR and western-blot quantitatively analysis of ZWINT expression in normal and PC cell lines. **(F)** Data in the TCGA database showed the overall survival of the two groups of patients with high ($n = 60$, red line) or low ($n = 32$, blue line) PC expression in colon cancer tissues. **(G)** Kaplan–Meier representation of the overall survival of the two groups of patients with high ($n = 60$, red line) or low ($n = 32$, blue line) ZWINT expression in our cohort. **(H)** ROC analysis of the correlation of ZWINT expression and survival time. All data are the mean ± SD of three independent experiments. $^{*}p < 0.05$.

Statistical Analysis

The x^2 test and Fisher's exact probability tests were used to analyze data, and the single-element analysis of variance was employed to measure the data. The t test was used to determine statistical variations between two groups, and more than two groups were compared using the one-way analysis of variance analysis. A two-tailed p value of <0.05 was regarded statistically significant.

RESULTS

ZWINT is Upregulated in Pancreatic Cancer

To determine the role of ZWINT in pancreatic cancer tumorigenesis, a bioinformation analysis was performed using TCGA database. The results indicated that ZWINT was significantly upregulated in pancreatic cancer tissue (**Figure 1A**). We next performed qRT-PCR assay using 16 pairs of PC and adjacent non-tumor tissues and found that ZWINT mRNA was highly expressed in PC tissues (**Figure 1B**). ZWINT was further examined in a tissue microarray that included 92 paired PC samples. The average expression of ZWINT was increased in PC tissues compared with levels in nearby non-tumor tissues (**Figure 1C**). The positive ZWINT expression rate was 65.2% (60/92) in PC tissue samples. Further analyses of PC cell lines by qPCR and western blot assay demonstrated that ZWINT mRNA and protein level was upregulated in PC cell lines (**Figures 1D,E**). Based on the GEPIA (http://gepia.cancer-pku.cn/) and survival data from the cohort, Kaplan-Meier analysis, ROC analysis results indicated that ZWINT expression was negatively correlated with PC patient overall survival (**Figures 1F,G**). We further analyzed the relationship between ZWINT expression and clinicopathological features in PC tissue samples (**Table 3**). ZWINT expression was positively related to tumor size, differentiation and Vessel invasion in PC tissues. Together these results indicate that low ZWINT expression is related to progression and poor prognosis in human PC.

ZWINT Enhances PC Cell Proliferation and Induces G1/S Phase Transition *in Vitro*

To clarify the role of ZWINT in regulating PC cell phenotype, we performed loss-of-function and gain-of-function assays in PC cells (**Figures 2A,B**). CCK-8 and colony formation assays showed that PC cell proliferation was reduced by ZWINT knockdown, while increased proliferation was observed in cells with overexpression of ZWINT (**Figures 2C,D**). EDU assay also showed that ZWINT overexpression significantly promoted PC cell proliferation (**Figure 2E**). We next evaluated the role of ZWINT in cell cycle regulation of PC cells using flow cytometry assays. We detected a significant increase in the G1/S phase population of ZWINT-depleted PC cells compared with the control group (**Figure 2F**). qPCR and western blot further demonstrated that ZWINT promoted cell cycle–associated gene and protein expression (**Figures 2G,H**). These findings indicate PC cell proliferation induces G1/S phase arrest was enhanced by ZWINT, making contribution to PC progression.

Hypoxia Micro-Environment Induce ZWINT Upregulation

We next explored the elements that induced high ZWINT expression in PC. Promoter sequence analysis tools (UCSC

TABLE 3 | The General clinical pathological characteristics of pancreatic cancer patients.

Clinical epidemiology and clinicopathologic feature	N	ZWINT Low expression	ZWINT High expression	*p value*
All cases	92	32	60	
Age				0.0871
≤60	25	5	20	
>60	67	27	40	
Gender				0.2586
Male	58	23	35	
Female	34	9	25	
Diameter of tumor				0.0330
≤3	29	15	14	
>3	63	17	46	
Tumor differentiation				0.0387
Well/moderate	30	15	15	
Poor	62	17	45	
Pathological T				0.6620
T1/T2	51	19	32	
T3/T4	41	13	28	
Lymph node metastasis				0.5045
N0 (negative)	55	21	34	
N1 (positive)	37	11	26	
Vessel invasion				0.0121
Negative	69	29	40	
Positive	23	3	20	

Note: Low/high by the sample median, used fisher's exact test.
**p < 05 was considered to be statistically significant.*

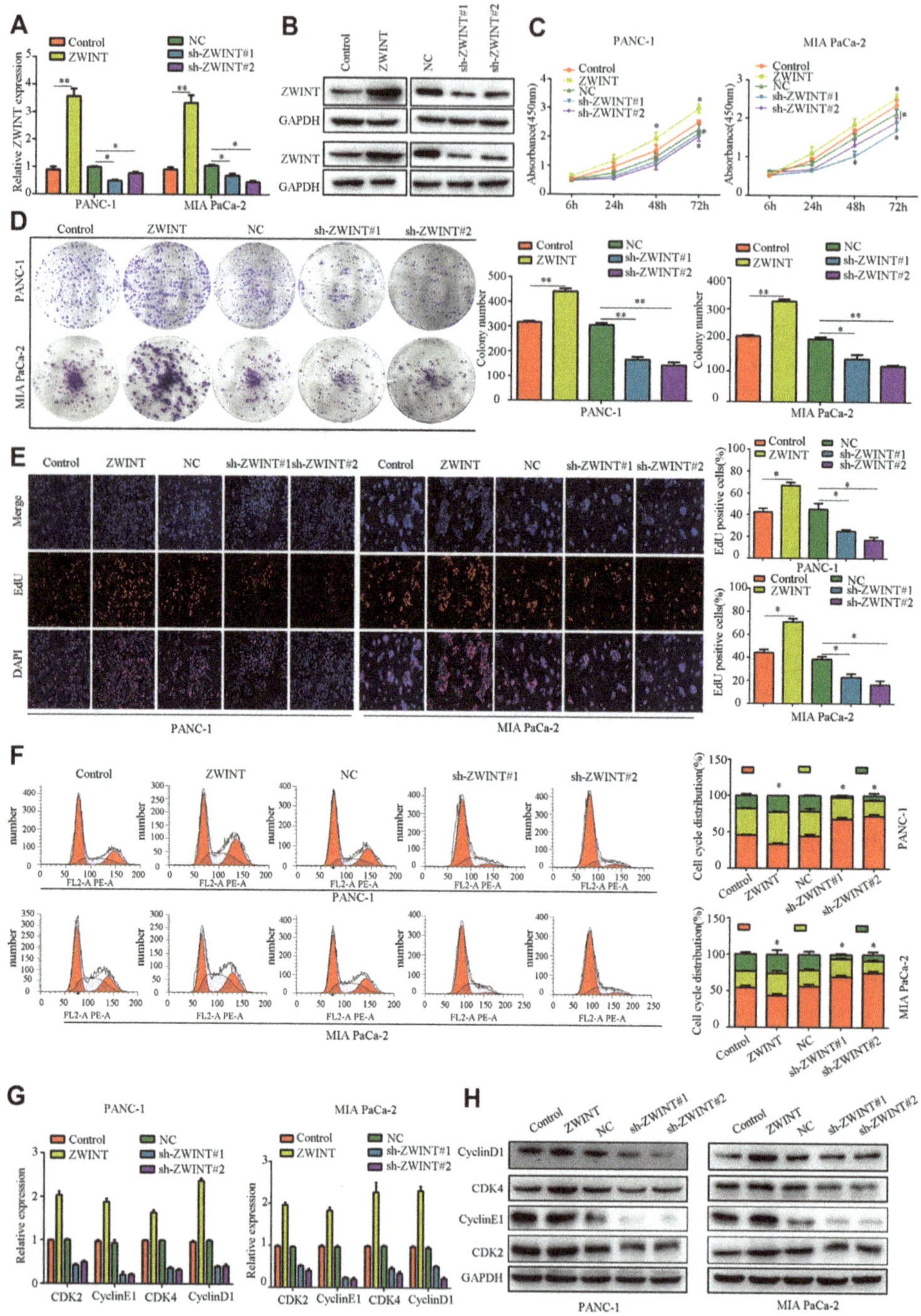

FIGURE 2 | ZWINT enhances PC cell proliferation induces G1/S phase transition in vitro. **(A,B)** q-RT-PCR and western-blots confirmed the knockdown and overexpressed of ZWINT. **(C,D)** CCK-8 and plated formation analysis of the growth ability of PC cell. **(E)** EDU assay was performed to analysis the proliferation of PC cell. **(F)** Cell cycle analysis showed the effects of ZWINT on PC cell cycle regulation. **(G-H)**. q-RT-PCR and western-blots analysis of the cell cycle associated genes expression.

and JASPAR) (**Figure 3A**) were used to inspect the genomic region (~2 kb upstream) upstream of the ZWINT gene. The results showed two putative HIF1α binding sites within the ZWINT promoter area (**Figure 3B**). We next performed ChIP-qPCR assay and confirmed that HIF1α directly bound to the chromatin fragments of the two predicted ZWINT promoter areas (**Figure 3C**). Luciferase assays also demonstrated that wild-type (WT) ZWINT promoter activity was significantly upregulated by HIF1α, while the mutant construct with mutations in the putative HIF1α-binding sequences showed no changes in response to HIF1α expression (**Figure 3D**). We performed q-RT-PCR analysis for ZWINT and HIF1α mRNA in PC tissues and the pearson analysis results revealed a positive correlation (**Figure 3E**). After 24 h treatment of hypoxia or the chemical inducer $CoCl_2$, the

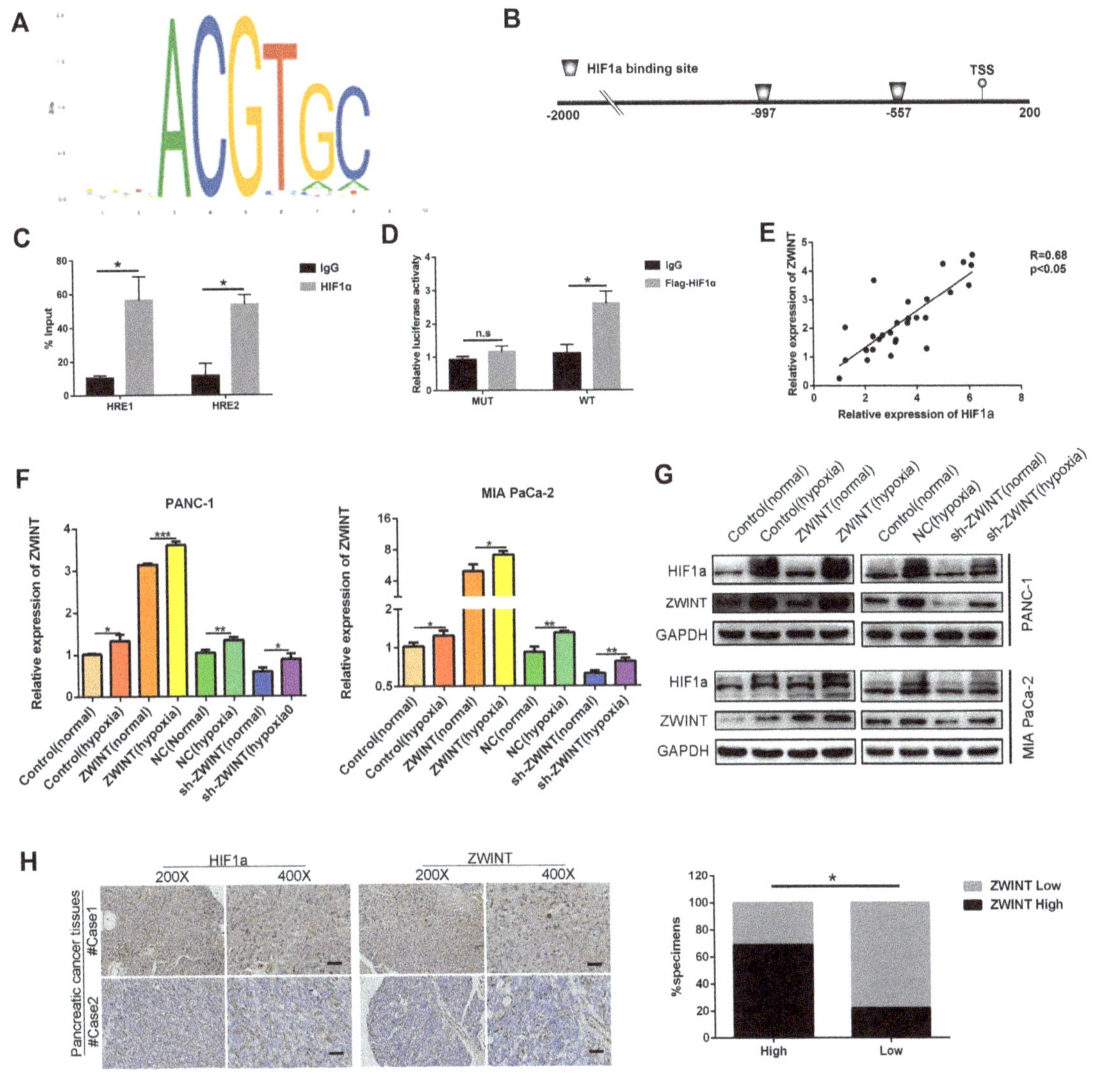

FIGURE 3 | ZWINT was a direct transcriptional target of HIF-1α. **(A)** Bioinformation analysis the promoter sequence region. **(B)** Schematic diagram indicated the potential promoter binding region. **(C)** HEK293 cells were transfected with pGL3 reporter vector containing ZWINT wide-type promoter (HRE-WT), or mutant-type promoter (HRE-MUT), respectively. Those transfected cells were further treated under normoxia or hypoxia. After 48 h, firefly luciferase activity was detected and normalized by renilla activity. **(D)** ChIP assay with anti-HIF-1α antibody was performed to verify the binding between HIF-1α and two HREs in ZWINT promoter in PANC-1 cells. **(E)** Pearson correlation analysis was performed to test the correlation between ZWINT and HIF1α. **(F, G)** The mRNA and protein expression levels of ZWINT and HIF-1α in PC cells were measured after culturing under normoxia, hypoxia ($CoCl_2$, 100 μM)) for 24 h by qRT-PCR and Western blot. **(H)** q-RT-PCR and IHC analysis the correlation of HIF-1α and ZWINT in the pancreatic cancer tissues. Data shown are mean ± SD (n = 3). ($^{*}p < 0.05$, $^{**}p < 0.01$, $^{***}p < 0.001$).

expression of ZWINT in PANC-1 and MIA PaCa-2 cells was increased on basis of upregulated HIF1α expression in the mRNA and protein level (**Figures 3F,G**). Immunohistochemistry of HIF1α and ZWINT in PC tissues showed that HIF1α and ZWINT expressions were positively correlated (**Figure 3H**). Together these data indicate that ZWINT is transcriptionally upregulated by HIF1α in the hypoxic tumor micro-environment. Subsequently, functional experiments were performed to measure the proliferation of PC cells in the condition of hypoxia compared with normoxia. The results suggested that hypoxia-mediated ZWINT overexpression significantly promoted cell proliferation compared with normoxia (**Supplementary Figure S1**).

ZWINT Negatively Regulates the p53/p21 Signal Pathway

To elucidate the downstream signal pathway of ZWINT, we analyzed the potential targeted pathways using the TCGA database. The results indicated that ZWINT likely regulates the cell cycle, DNA replication, and the p53 signaling pathway (**Figure 4A**). As ZWINT showed cell cycle regulation activity and p53 is a key regulator of the cell cycle, we next examined whether ZWINT affected p53 expression and activity. We first performed qRT-PCR to analyze p53 and p21 mRNA expression. ZWINT had no effect on p53 mRNA expression level and p21 expression was significantly upregulated in the ZWINT knockdown group (**Figures 4B,C**). Western blot assay revealed that

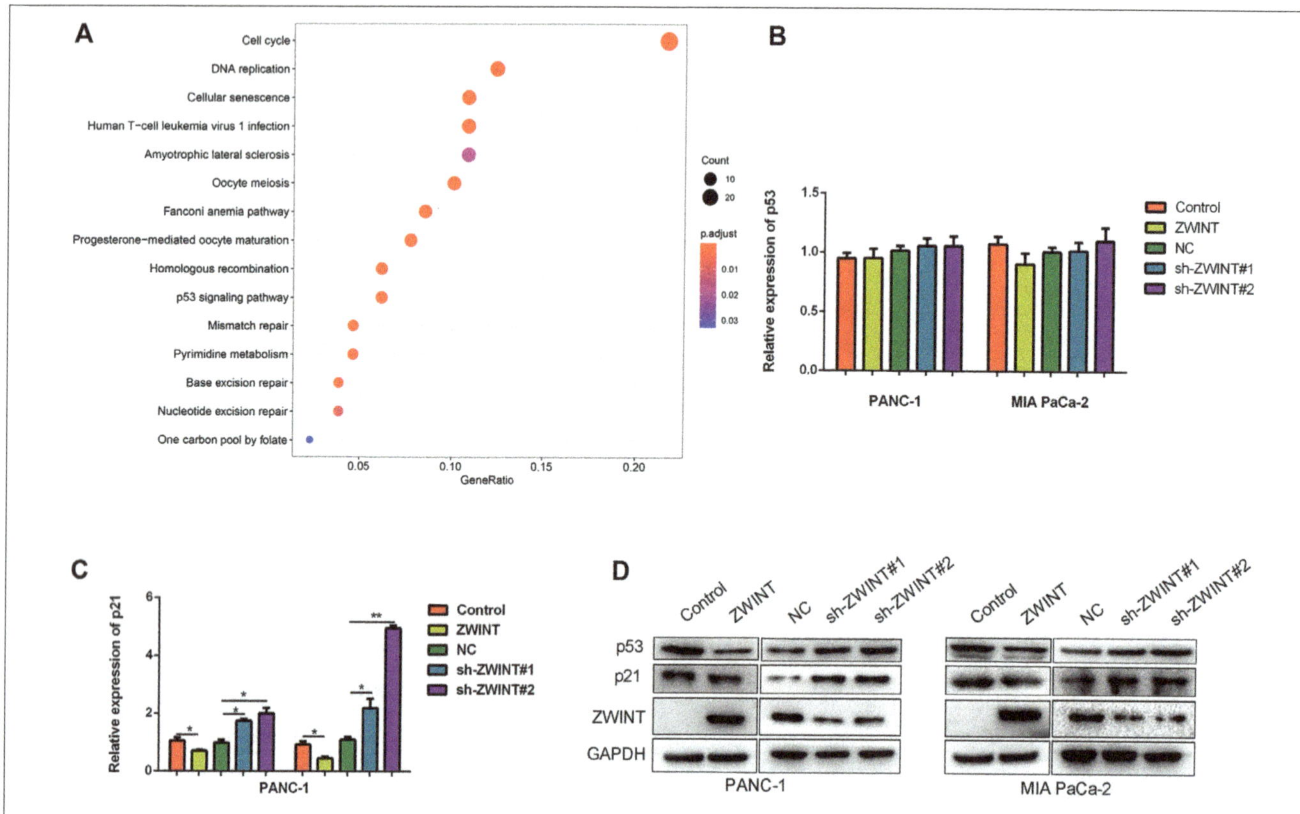

FIGURE 4 | ZWINT interacted and regulated p53/p21 signal pathway. **(A)** Bioinformatic analysis the downstream pathway of ZWINT based on the TCGA databse. **(B, C)** q-RT-PCR and western blot analysis the expression of p53 and p21 in mRNA level. **(D)** Western blot analysis the expression of p53 and p21 in protein level.

p53 and p21 were significantly downregulated in ZWINT-overexpressing pancreatic cancer cells (**Figure 4D**).

ZWINT Decreases p53 Expression by Promoting its Ubiquitination *via* Enhancing MDM2 Levels

Our results showed that ZWINT regulated p53 protein level. As p53 protein levels are regulated by MDM2-mediated ubiquitination, we further examined whether ZWINT interacted with MDM2 and p53 to affect p53 ubiquitination. We first analyzed the interactions between ZWINT, p53, and MDM2. Immunoprecipitation and immunofluorescence analysis indicated that ZWINT binds with and co-localizes with p53 and MDM2 (**Figures 5A,B**). Subsequently, western blot analysis showed that MDM2 expression was increased by the overexpression of ZWINT, while MDM2 levels were decreased by ZWINT knockdown (**Figure 5C**). We next examined whether ZWINT affect p53 ubiquitination and stability. Protein stability assay indicated that ZWINT significantly inhibited p53 stability and ubiquitination assay demonstrated that p53 ubiquitination was significantly increased in the ZWINT-upregulated group (**Figures 5D–F**). These results suggest that ZWINT promoting the effect of MDM2 and influences the ubiquitination, stability and expression level of p53 by decreasing the expression level of MDM2.

ZWINT Exerts Proliferation Effects by Directly Promoting the Transcription of p21

To investigate whether p53/p21 is necessary for ZWINT regulation of PC cell proliferation and cell cycle, we transfected p53 and p21 siRNA into ZWINT knockdown PC cells. CCK-8, colony formation assay and EDU proliferation assays showed that proliferation in ZWINT knockdown cells was enhanced upon p53 or p21 silencing (**Figures 6A–C**). qRT-PCR and western blot assays showed that p53 or p21 inhibition in PC cells abolished the inhibition of the expression of p53 and p21 reduced by ZWINT knockdown (**Figures 6D–G**).

ZWINT Promotes Pancreatic Cancer Growth *in Vivo*

To determine whether tumor growth is affected by ZWINT *in vivo*, we established a xenograft mouse model by subcutaneously injecting pancreatic cancer cells overexpressing ZWINT or controls into mice ($n = 5$, each group). After 6 weeks, mice were killed and tumor samples were harvested (**Figure 7A**). Tumor weight (**Figure 7B**) and volume (**Figure 7C**) from cells with knockdown of ZWINT were reduced compared with controls. Immunohistochemistry showed that Ki-67 and PCNA were highly expressed in tumors from the ZWINT upregulated group and downregulated in the knockdown group (**Figure 7D**). Together

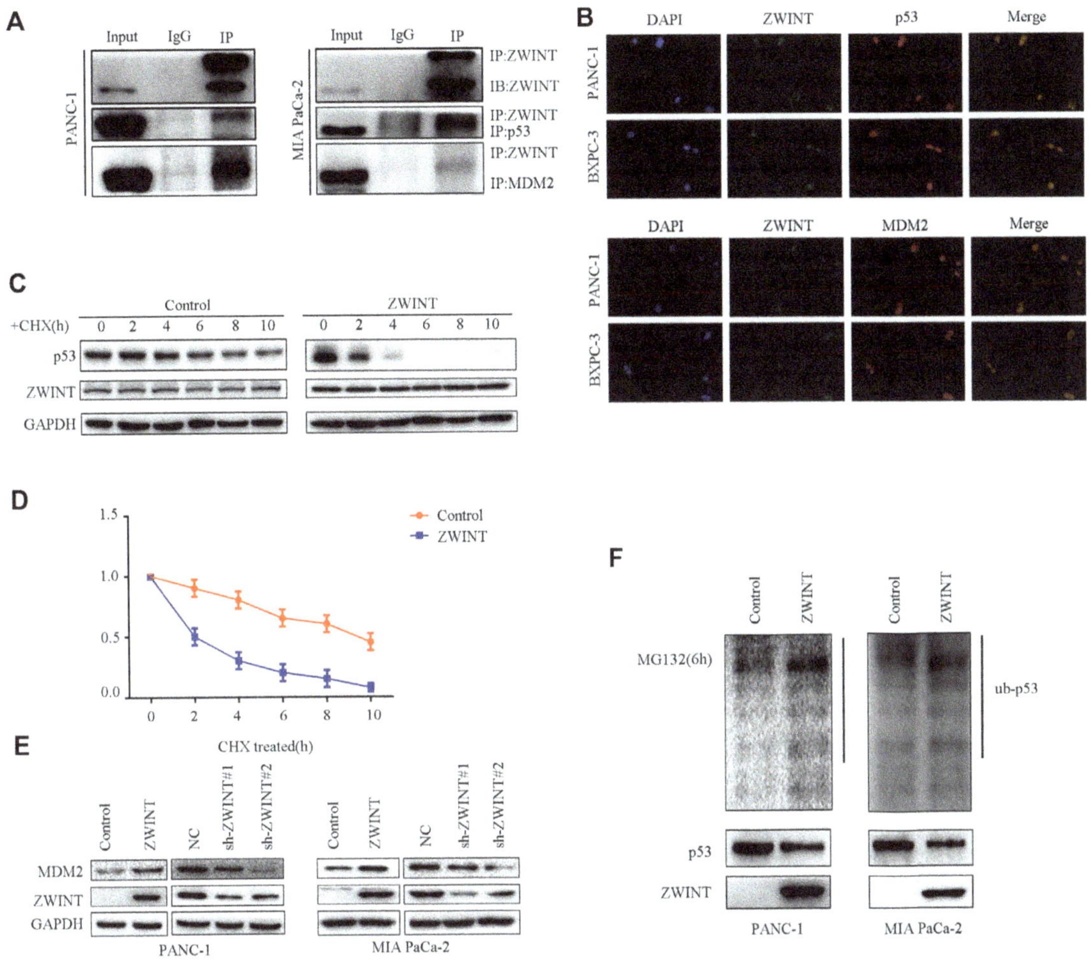

FIGURE 5 | ZWINT decreases p53 expression by promoting its ubiquitination via enhancing MDM2 function. **(A)** Immunoprecipitation analysis the interaction of ZWINT with p53 and MDM2. **(B)** Immunofluorescence analysis the interaction of ZWINT with p53 and MDM2. **(C)** Western blot analysis MDM2 expression in the ZWINT upregulated and knockdown group. **(D–E)** The protein stability analysis the p53 stability in the ZWINT upregulated group. **(F)** The ubiquitination assay analysis the p53 ubiquitination level in the ZWINT upregulated group.

these data indicate that ZWINT promoted pancreatic cancer growth *in vivo*.

DISCUSSION

In this study, we demonstrated that ZWINT, a centromere complex component, was significantly upregulated in PC tumor tissues and high expression of ZWINT was related to poor outcome in PC. ZWINT was recently reported to be an oncoprotein in multiple cancer types, including glioblastoma, breast cancer, lung adenocarcinoma. Kim JH found that ZWINT was upregulated in pancreatic cancer and promoted pancreatic cancer progression. however, the precise mechanism of its regulation was unknown (Kim et al., 2020). In this study, we focused on the mechanism of ZWINT, the interacting proteins and the downstream pathways involved in tumor regulation. Functional studies revealed that ZWINT promoted pancreatic cancer cell proliferation and cell cycle progression *in vitro* and enhanced tumor development *in vivo*. These findings suggest that ZWINT may promote PC progress.

To clarify the mechanisms by which ZWINT promotes pancreatic cancer progression, we analyzed the pathways associated with ZWINT using the TCGA database. The cell cycle and p53 signal pathway were the core targets regulator in ZWINT function. Consistent with the previous results, ZWINT could positively drive the pancreatic cancer cell cycle turning over. Abnormal cell cycle frequently occurs in cancer cells, resulting in accelerated cell division and growth in an uncontrollable rate and leading to tumor compression surrounding blood vessels and hypoxic microenvironment (Geismann and Arlt, 2020; Tao et al., 2021).

We further demonstrated that p53 expression and activity were significantly upregulated in ZWINT-knockdown pancreatic cancer cells. p53 is an upstream regulator of p21, and aberrant p53 expression and/or activity is a significant molecular hallmark

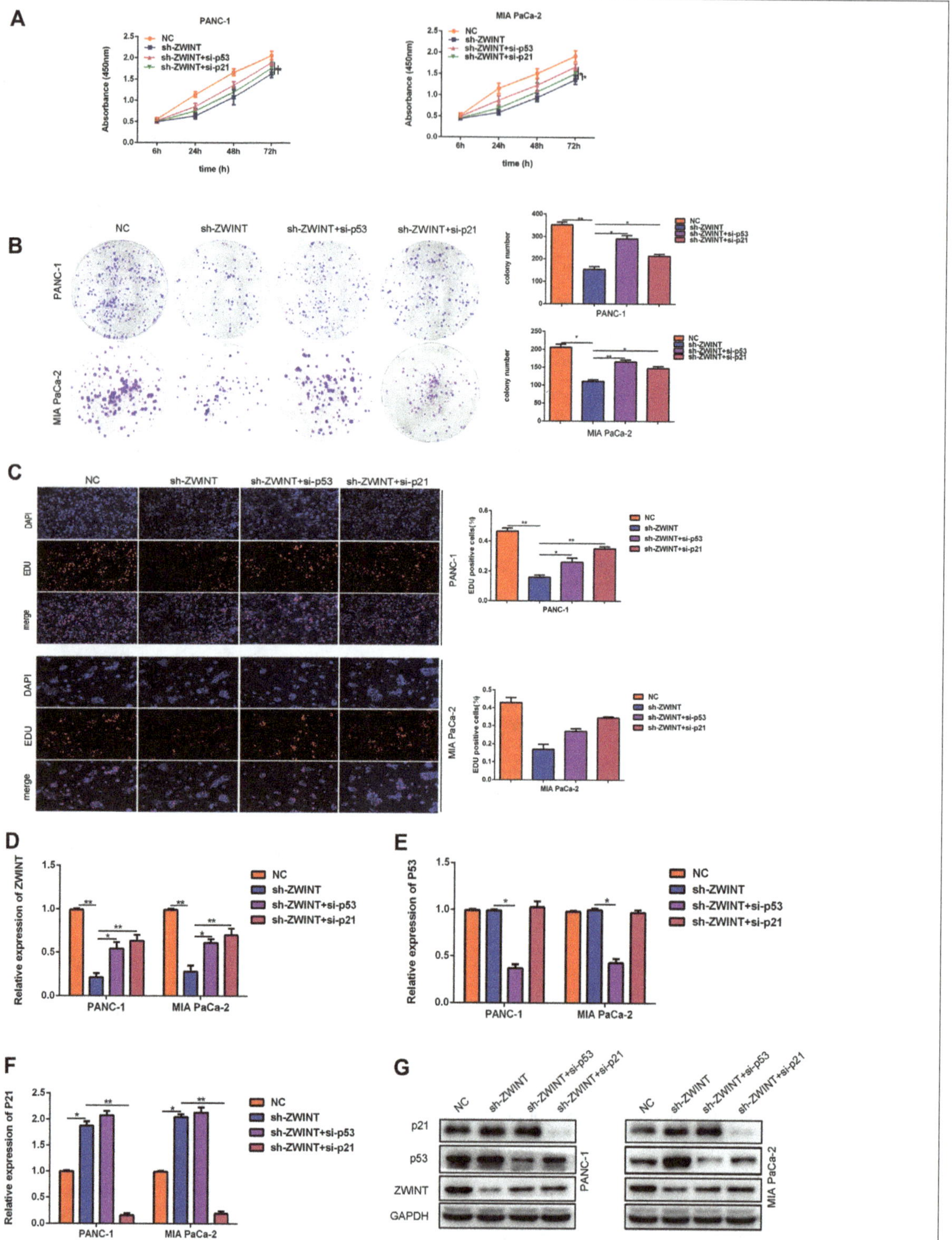

FIGURE 6 | ZWINT exerted proliferation effects by directly promoting the transcription of p21. CCK-8**(A)**, plate formation**(B)** and EDU**(C)** and assay analysis the proliferation of the cells in the ZWINT knockdown transfected with p53 or p21 siRNA. **(D–G)** qRT-PCR and western blot assays analysis the ZWINT, p53 and p21 expression of the cells in the ZWINT knockdown transfected with p53 or p21 siRNA.

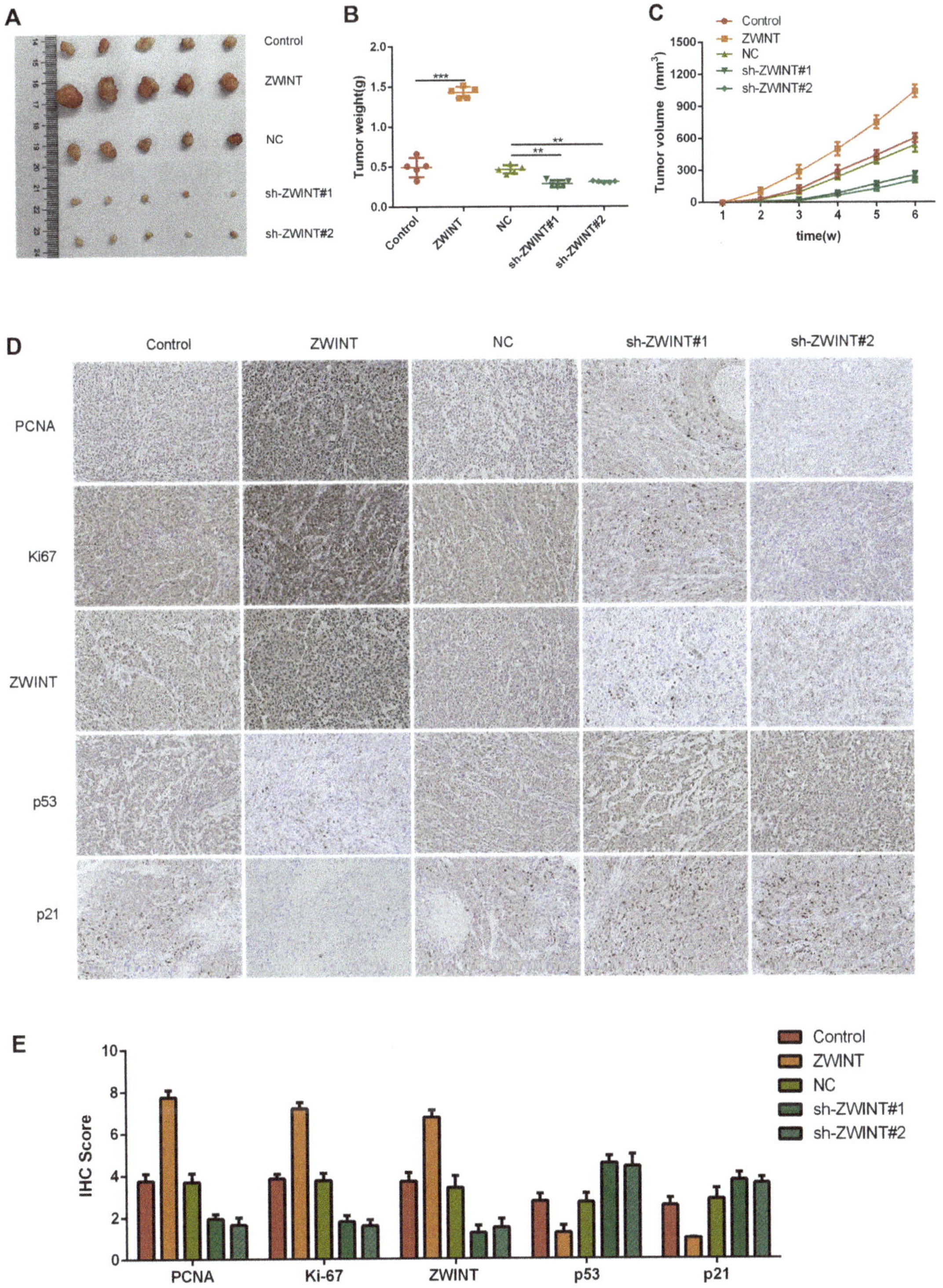

FIGURE 7 | ZWINT promoted pancreatic cancer growth *in vivo*. a Represent pictures of tumor formation of xenograft of PANC-1 **(A)** cells in nude mice ($n = 5$). **(B, C)** Weight and volume of tumors in the different group mice. **(D–E)** Representative images of KI-67 and PCNA staining of the xenograft. $^*p < 0.05$; $^{**}p < 0.01$.

of cancer (Amirinejad et al., 2020; Mansilla et al., 2020). p53 expression is typically downregulated in patients with wild-type p53, emphasizing the significance of its inhibited activity in cancer progression (Xu et al., 2021). Multiple studies have revealed various post-transcriptional modifications and regulation of p53 including phosphorylation, ubiquitination, and acetylation (Gencel-Augusto and Lozano, 2020). Ubiquitination-mediated proteasomal degradation is significant to stabilize p53 protein in post-translation (Zhou G. et al., 2020), while ubiquitination also plays role in p53 protein activation and nuclear location. Acetylation and phosphorylation play critical functions in enhancing p53 binding to its target genes (Yogosawa and Yoshida, 2018), and the cross-talk among these modifications may influence regulation of downstream target genes. Hence, according to our outcomes, the important role of p53 transcriptional regulation in the maintenance of the homeostasis of p53 expression is showed. Our results suggest that the ZWINT/p53 axis plays a key role in cell cycle regulation, cell proliferation, and tumorigenesis in PC. We also found that MDM2, the E3 ubiquitin ligase for p53 (Karakostis et al., 2020), interacts with ZWINT and we speculate that ZWINT interacts with MDM2 to influence the ubiquitination and degradation of p53. Further investigation shall be made to explore the precise mechanism by which p53 expression is regulated by ZWINT.

The stability of p53 is carefully regulated by the ubiquitin-proteasome system and p53 levels are finely tuned to respond to stressful conditions (Leu et al., 2020). Ubiquitination plays a role in the regulation of p53 expression for the regulation of cell cycle progression (Si et al., 2021). We examined the mechanism by which ZWINT regulated p53 expression and found that ZWINT inhibited p53 only at the protein level. Therefore, we speculate that ZWINT regulates p53 expression at the post-translation level. However, post-translation modifications of p53 including phosphorylation, ubiquitylation, acetylation can affect p53 expression, nuclear location, and transcriptionally activity (Sun et al., 2021).

To be different, according to our current research, our results suggest that ZWINT interacted with and restrained MDM2, to inhibit p53 protein stability by enhancing its degradation.

p21, a target gene of p53, inhibits cyclin D1 and CDK, resulting in G1/S arrest (Zhou et al., 2020b; Qi et al., 2021). Our results showed that p21 expression and transcriptional activity were inhibited in ZWINT knockdown pancreatic cancer cells. To our knowledge, this is the first data showing that ZWINT contributes to PC cell progression by regulating p53/p21 signaling.

Our data showed that hypoxia promoted the expression of ZWINT in pancreatic cancer, and ZWINT promoted pancreatic cancer proliferation *in vitro* and *in vivo*. In addition, ZWINT could inhibited p21 transcriptional activity by interacting with p53 mediated pancreatic progress.

ETHICS STATEMENT

The studies involving human participants were reviewed and approved by the Ethics Committees at Renmin Hospital of Wuhan University. The patients/participants provided their written informed consent to participate in this study. The animal study was reviewed and approved by the Animal Research Ethics Committees at Renmin Hospital of Wuhan University. Written informed consent was obtained from the individual(s) for the publication of any potentially identifiable images or data included in this article.

AUTHOR CONTRIBUTIONS

PC and JJ designed the study. ZH, JW, and JX completed the experiments and analyzed the data. PC, ZH, and JW wrote the manuscript and were responsible for language revisions. XJ, YC, and XL supervised the project. All authors reviewed the manuscript.

ACKNOWLEDGMENTS

We thank Gabrielle White Wolf, PhD, from Liwen Bianji, Edanz Editing China (www.liwenbianji.cn/ac), for editing the English text of a draft of this manuscript.

REFERENCES

Amirinejad, R., Rezaei, M., and Shirvani-Farsani, Z. (2020). An Update on Long Intergenic Noncoding RNA P21: a Regulatory Molecule with Various Significant Functions in Cancer. *Cell Biosci* 10, 82. doi:10.1186/s13578-020-00445-9

Endo, H., Ikeda, K., Urano, T., Horie-Inoue, K., and Inoue, S. (2012). Terf/TRIM17 Stimulates Degradation of Kinetochore Protein ZWINT and Regulates Cell Proliferation. *J. Biochem.* 151 (2), 139–144. doi:10.1093/jb/mvr128

Geismann, C., and Arlt, A. (2020). Coming in the Air: Hypoxia Meets Epigenetics in Pancreatic. *Can. Cells.* 9 (11), 2353. doi:10.3390/cells9112353

Gencel-Augusto, J., and Lozano, G. (2020). p53 Tetramerization: at the center of the Dominant-Negative Effect of Mutant P53. *Genes Dev.* 34 (17-18), 1128–1146. doi:10.1101/gad.340976.120

Karakostis, K., Lopez, I., Pena-Balderas, A. M., Fahareus, R., and Olivares-Illana, V. (2020). Molecular and Biochemical Techniques for Deciphering P53-MDM2 Regulatory Mechanisms. *Biomolecules.* 11 (1), 36. doi:10.3390/biom11010036

Kasuboski, J. M., Bader, J. R., Vaughan, P. S., Tauhata, S. B. F., Winding, M., Morrissey, M. A., et al. (2011). Zwint-1 Is a Novel Aurora B Substrate Required for the Assembly of a Dynein-Binding Platform on Kinetochores. *MBoC* 22 (18), 3318 3330. doi:10.1091/mbc.E11-03-0213

Kim, J. H., Youn, Y., Lee, J.-c., Kim, J., and Hwang, J.-H. (2020). Involvement of the NF-Kb Signaling Pathway in Proliferation and Invasion Inhibited by Zwint-1 Deficiency in Pancreatic Cancer Cells. *J. Cancer* 11 (19), 5601–5611. doi:10.7150/jca.46173

Lee, K. H., Chie, E. K., Im, S. A., Kim, J. H., Kwon, J., Han, S. W., et al. (2020). Phase II Trial of Postoperative Adjuvant Gemcitabine and Cisplatin Chemotherapy Followed by Chemoradiotherapy with Gemcitabine in Patients with Resected Pancreatic Cancer. *Cancer Res. Treat.* 53, 1096-1103. doi:10.4143/crt.2020.928

Leu, J. I.-J., Murphy, M. E., and George, D. L. (2020). Functional Interplay Among Thiol-Based Redox Signaling, Metabolism, and Ferroptosis Unveiled by a Genetic Variant of TP53. *Proc. Natl. Acad. Sci. USA* 117 (43), 26804–26811. doi:10.1073/pnas.2009943117

Mansilla, S. F., de la Vega, M. B., Calzetta, N. L., Siri, S. O., and Gottifredi, V. (2020). CDK-independent and PCNA-dependent Functions of P21 in DNA Replication. *Genes Basel* 11 (6), 593. doi:10.3390/genes11060593

Obuse, C., Iwasaki, O., Kiyomitsu, T., Goshima, G., Toyoda, Y., and Yanagida, M. (2004). A Conserved Mis12 Centromere Complex Is Linked to Heterochromatic HP1 and Outer Kinetochore Protein Zwint-1. *Nat. Cel Biol* 6 (11), 1135–1141. doi:10.1038/ncb1187

Peng, F., Li, Q., Niu, S.-Q., Shen, G.-P., Luo, Y., Chen, M., et al. (2019). ZWINT Is the Next Potential Target for Lung Cancer Therapy. *J. Cancer Res. Clin. Oncol.* 145 (3), 661–673. doi:10.1007/s00432-018-2823-1

Perri, G., and Katz, M. (2021). Neoadjuvant Chemotherapy in Pancreatic Cancer-Reply. *JAMA Surg* 156, 398. doi:10.1001/jamasurg.2020.6279

Qi, R., Wang, J., Jiang, Y., Qiu, Y., Xu, M., Rong, R., et al. (2021). Snail-induced Partial Epithelial-Mesenchymal Transition Orchestrates P53-P21-Mediated G2/M Arrest in the Progression of Renal Fibrosis via NF-Kb-Mediated Inflammation. *Cell Death Dis* 12 (1), 44. doi:10.1038/s41419-020-03322-y

Si, W., Zhou, B., Xie, W., Li, H., Li, K., Li, S., et al. (2021). Angiogenic Factor AGGF1 Acts as a Tumor Suppressor by Modulating P53 post-transcriptional Modifications and Stability via MDM2. *Cancer Lett.* 497, 28–40.

Siegel, R. L., Miller, K. D., and Jemal, A. (2020). Cancer Statistics, 2020. *CA A. Cancer J. Clin.* 70 (1), 7–30. doi:10.3322/caac.21590

Sun, X., Dyson, H. J., and Wright, P. E. (2021). A Phosphorylation-dependent Switch in the Disordered P53 Transactivation Domain Regulates DNA Binding. *Proc. Natl. Acad. Sci. U S A.* 118 (1). doi:10.1073/pnas.2021456118

Tao, J., Yang, G., Zhou, W., Qiu, J., Chen, G., Luo, W., et al. (2021). Targeting Hypoxic Tumor Microenvironment in Pancreatic Cancer. *J. Hematol. Oncol.* 14 (1), 14. doi:10.1186/s13045-020-01030-w

The Lancet Gastroenterology and Hepatology (2021). Pancreatic Cancer: a State of Emergency? *Lancet Gastroenterol. Hepatol.* 6 (2), 81. doi:10.1016/S2468-1253(20)30397-6

Woo Seo, D., Yeop You, S., Chung, W.-J., Cho, D.-H., Kim, J.-S., and Su Oh, J. (2015). Zwint-1 Is Required for Spindle Assembly Checkpoint Function and Kinetochore-Microtubule Attachment during Oocyte Meiosis. *Sci. Rep.* 5, 15431. doi:10.1038/srep15431

Xie, W., Wang, B., Wang, X., Hou, D., Su, H., and Huang, H. (2020). Nine Hub Genes Related to the Prognosis of HBV-Positive Hepatocellular Carcinoma Identified by Protein Interaction Analysis. *Ann. Transl Med.* 8 (7), 478. doi:10.21037/atm.2020.03.94

Xu, Z., Wu, W., Yan, H., Hu, Y., He, Q., and Luo, P. (2021). Regulation of P53 Stability as a Therapeutic Strategy for Cancer. *Biochem. Pharmacol.* 185, 114407. doi:10.1016/j.bcp.2021.114407

Yang, L., Han, N., Zhang, X., Zhou, Y., Chen, R., and Zhang, M. (2020). ZWINT: A Potential Therapeutic Biomarker in Patients with Glioblastoma Correlates with Cell Proliferation and Invasion. *Oncol. Rep.* 43 (6), 1831–1844. doi:10.3892/or.2020.7573

Yi, M., Li, T., Qin, S., Yu, S., Chu, Q., Li, A., et al. (2020). Identifying Tumorigenesis and Prognosis-Related Genes of Lung Adenocarcinoma: Based on Weighted Gene Coexpression Network Analysis. *Biomed. Res. Int.* 2020, 4169691. doi:10.1155/2020/4169691

Yogosawa, S., and Yoshida, K. (2018). Tumor Suppressive Role for Kinases Phosphorylating P53 in DNA Damage-induced Apoptosis. *Cancer Sci.* 109 (11), 3376–3382. doi:10.1111/cas.13792

Zhang, G., Lischetti, T., Hayward, D. G., and Nilsson, J. (2015). Distinct Domains in Bub1 Localize RZZ and BubR1 to Kinetochores to Regulate the Checkpoint. *Nat. Commun.* 6, 7162. doi:10.1038/ncomms8162

Zhao, S., and Yu, M. (2020). Identification ofMMP1as a Potential Prognostic Biomarker and Correlating with Immune Infiltrates in Cervical Squamous Cell Carcinoma. *DNA Cel Biol.* 39 (2), 255–272. doi:10.1089/dna.2019.5129

Zhou, G., Shen, M., and Zhang, Z. (2020a). ZW10 Binding Factor (ZWINT), a Direct Target of Mir-204, Predicts Poor Survival and Promotes Proliferation in Breast Cancer. *Med. Sci. Monit.* 26, e921659. doi:10.12659/MSM.921659

Zhou, Y., Chen, R., Luo, X., Zhang, W. D., and Qin, J. J.. (2020b). The E2 Ubiquitin-Conjugating Enzyme UbcH5c: an Emerging Target in Cancer and Immune Disorders. *Drug Discov. Today* 25, 1988-1997. doi:10.1016/j.drudis.2020.09.015

3

Quiescin Sulfhydryl Oxidase 2 Overexpression Predicts Poor Prognosis and Tumor Progression in Patients With Colorectal Cancer: A Study Based on Data Mining and Clinical Verification

Tao Jiang[1,2†], Li Zheng[3,4†], Xia Li[5†], Jia Liu[6], Hu Song[1,2], Yixin Xu[1,2], Chenhua Dong[1,5], Lianyu Liu[1,5], Hongyu Wang[1,5], Shuai Wang[7], Renhao Wang[1,2] and Jun Song[1,2*]*

[1] *Department of General Surgery, The Affiliated Hospital of Xuzhou Medical University, Xuzhou, China,* [2] *Institute of Digestive Diseases, Xuzhou Medical University, Xuzhou, China,* [3] *State Key Laboratory of Proteomics, Beijing Proteome Research Center, National Center for Protein Sciences, Beijing Institute of Lifeomics, Beijing, China,* [4] *State Key Laboratory of Food Nutrition and Safety, Tianjin University of Science and Technology, Tianjin, China,* [5] *The Graduate School, Xuzhou Medical University, Xuzhou, China,* [6] *Department of Pathology, The Affiliated Hospital of Xuzhou Medical University, Xuzhou, China,* [7] *School of Life Sciences, Xuzhou Medical University, Xuzhou, China*

***Correspondence:**
Jun Song
songjunwk@126.com
Renhao Wang
wangrenhao@xzhmu.edu.cn

† These authors have contributed equally to this work

Background: As a member of the atypical thiol oxidase family, quiescin sulfhydryl oxidase 2 (QSOX2) has been reported to play an important role in several biological processes, but the expression and function of QSOX2 in colorectal cancer (CRC) remains elusive.

Methods: The difference of QSOX2 expression, and its relationship with clinicopathological features and prognosis in CRC, was analyzed by bioinformatic analysis and validated by clinical CRC specimen cohort. The functional characterization of QSOX2 was detected via *in vitro* and *vivo* experiments in CRC cell lines, while the potential signaling pathways were predicted by Gene Set Enrichment Analysis (GSEA).

Results: Our data based on bioinformatical analysis and clinical validation demonstrated that the expression of QSOX2 in CRC tissues was significantly upregulated. Additionally, the chi-square test, logistic regression analysis, and Fisher's exact test showed that QSOX2 overexpression was significantly correlated with advanced clinicopathological parameters, such as pathological stage and lymph node metastasis. The Kaplan–Meier curves and univariate Cox regression model showed that QSOX2 overexpression predicts poor overall survival (OS) and disease-free survival (DFS) in CRC patients. More importantly, multivariate Cox regression model showed that QSOX2 overexpression could serve as an independent factor for CRC patients. *In vitro* and *vivo* data showed that the proliferation and metastasis ability of CRC cells were suppressed on condition of QSOX2 inhibition. In addition, GSEA showed that the QSOX2 high expression phenotype has enriched multiple potential cancer-related signaling pathways.

Conclusion: QSOX2 overexpression is strongly associated with malignant progression and poor oncological outcomes in CRC. QSOX2 might act as a novel biomarker for prognosis prediction and a new target for biotherapy in CRC.

Keywords: QSOX2, colorectal cancer, TCGA, TMAs, prognosis, GSEA

INTRODUCTION

Colorectal cancer, including colon cancer and rectal cancer, has leaped from the third leading cause of cancer death to the second cause in the world, which poses a more serious threat to the health of the people (Siegel et al., 2021). In the current clinical treatment, the standard therapy for CRC is surgery followed by chemotherapy or radiation (Provenzale et al., 2020). Due to the heterogeneity of CRC, patients may exhibit varied responses to the standard therapy (Zhai et al., 2017). Multistep and multifactorial process involved in several genetic alterations and biological pathway activation or inhibition may contribute to explain the mechanism of colorectal carcinogenesis and progression (Nguyen et al., 2020). In the past two decades, next-generation genome sequencing technology and numerous reports have identified some effective biomarkers, such as KRAS, SMAD2, BRAF, and PIK3CA/PIK3CB, which can assist doctors to predict the effect of adjuvant chemotherapy and the prognosis and recurrence of patients (De Roock et al., 2010; Sepulveda et al., 2017). Nevertheless, these findings are far from enough; more powerful and reliable biomarkers needs to be discovered, which will help doctors to develop new methods to improve clinical efficacy of CRC patients (Koncina et al., 2020).

Genes that contribute to oncogenicity has the potential to be explored for identifying cancer biomarkers and discovering new drug targets (Kamel and Al-Amodi, 2017). The atypical thiol oxidase family including two classes of QSOX transcript variants in vertebrates comprising, namely, QSOX1 and QSOX2, respectively (Codding et al., 2012; Israel et al., 2014). As the most wildly studied type, QSOX1 was observed to be upregulated and promote progression in multiple cancers, including prostate cancer, breast cancer, glioblastoma, lung cancer, pancreatic cancer, and malignant pleural mesothelioma (Katchman et al., 2011; Araujo et al., 2014; Knutsvik et al., 2016; Baek et al., 2018; Sung et al., 2018; Geng et al., 2020; Lacerenza et al., 2020). It is worth noting that upregulated QSOX1 expression was associated with features of poor outcomes in breast cancer, such as HER2 positivity and hormone receptor negativity (Knutsvik et al., 2016). As a highly homologous paralog of QSOX1, the human QSOX2 gene, chromosome 9q34.3, comprises 12 exons and encodes a putative protein of 698 amino acids (Hoober et al., 1999). A previous study has reported that the expression of QSOX2 appears to be lower than QSOX1 in most human normal tissues, such as the ovaries, prostate, and lung tissues (Coppock and Thorpe, 2006). Nevertheless, the exact expression and biological properties of QSOX2 in cancer remains to be elucidated. Given that QSOX2 and QSOX1 have 40% identity in the primary amino acid structure and higher identity in the functional domain, reaching 68% (Wang et al., 2018), we suspected that QSOX2 might also participate in the tumorigenesis and progression of cancers. However, the detailed expression status, prognostic role, and biological function of QSOX2 in human cancers, including CRC, remain unknown.

In this study, we first evaluate the mRNA and protein expression and asses the prognostic significance of QSXO2 in CRC based on bioinformatic analysis and clinical traits. In addition, experiments *in vitro* and *in vivo* were conducted to detect the biological function of QSOX2 in cell proliferation and metastasis of CRC. Furthermore, the QSOX2-related signaling pathways involved in CRC, which may support further investigation into the molecular mechanism underlying CRC, were analyzed by GSEA and verified by GEPIA correlation analysis and Western blotting analysis. Our results demonstrated that QSOX2 can be a promising biomarker for prognosis prediction in CRC.

MATERIALS AND METHODS

Publicly Available Database Analysis

Online public available databases, UALCAN[1] and TIMER2.0,[2] were used to observe the expression of QSOX2 in human pan-cancer in mRNA and protein level (Chandrashekar et al., 2017; Li et al., 2020). The correlation of mRNA level between QSOX2 and signaling pathway-related genes was analyzed by the online database Gene Expression Profiling Interactive Analysis (GEPIA)[3] (Tang et al., 2017).

Bioinformatics Analysis Based on TCGA Cohort

The original mRNA expression data of patients with COAD or READ, followed by corresponding basic information, such as gender, age, etc., and clinical information, such as tumor staging, etc., were downloaded from TCGA official website.[4] In total, the data of 452 COAD tissues, 41 adjacent normal tissues, 6 READ tissues, and 1 adjacent normal tissue were downloaded. The details of the COAD and READ patients are shown in **Table 1**. For further bioinformatic analysis, 314 COAD and READ cases were involved; those cases with expression or characteristic data

[1] http://ualcan.path.uab.edu/

[2] http://timer.cistrome.org/

[3] http://gepia.cancer-pku.cn/

[4] https://portal.gdc.cancer.gov/

TABLE 1 | Characteristics of patients with colorectal cancer (CRC) [colon adenocarcinoma (COAD) and rectum adenocarcinoma (READ)] in TCGA database.

Characteristics	Variable	Patients (458)	Percentages (%)
Age	<65 years	170	37.12
	≥65 years	288	62.88
Gender	Male	241	52.62
	Female	217	47.38
Pathological stage	I	78	17.03
	II	180	39.30
	III	125	27.29
	IV	64	13.97
	Unknown	11	2.40
T classification	Tis	1	0.22
	T1	11	2.40
	T2	78	17.03
	T3	311	67.90
	T4	57	12.45
N classification	N0	273	59.61
	N1	104	22.71
	N2	81	17.69
M classification	M0	338	73.80
	M1	64	13.97
	MX	49	10.70
	Unknown	7	1.53
Vital status	Alive	369	80.57
	Death	89	19.43

Data are presented as number (%).

that were incomplete and biased were excluded from further bioinformatic analysis. Then the original gene expression data were sorted and merged by the Perl programming language, while the QSOX2 expression was extracted by the limma package of R software. The extracted data were visualized by the limma package, while scatter difference diagrams were drawn by the beeswarm package. We use the R software to visualize the analysis results.

Verification of Quiescin Sulfhydryl Oxidase 2 Expression by the Gene Expression Omnibus Database

A search of RNA sequencing and the microarray data, which met the requirements from the Gene Expression Omnibus (GEO) dataset, was conducted, and a total of seven datasets (GSE106582, GSE37182, GSE83889, GSE21815, GSE21510, GSE9348, and GSE35279) were obtained, including 291 adjacent non-tumor tissues (adjacent NTTs), 661 CRC tissues, and original QSOX2 mRNA expression data (**Table 2**). The differences in QSOX2 expression were detected by the comprehensive meta-analysis via Review Manage 5.3. The combined value was calculated by standard mean difference (SMD) with a 95% confidence interval (CI). χ^2 and I^2 statistical tests were used to evaluate the heterogeneity between the included datasets. In condition of $p > 0.05$ or $I^2 < 50\%$, the fixed effect model was used for calculating the combined effect; otherwise ($p < 0.05$ or $I^2 > 50\%$), the random effect model was used. The results are visualized by forest plots.

Paraffin-Embedded and Fresh Frozen Tissue Specimen Cohort

A cohort of 568 formalin-fixed paraffin-embedded CRC cases was collected to conduct the tissue microarrays (TMAs) for IHC analysis. Details about the TMAs has been previously described (Jiang et al., 2018). The other cohort consists of 50 pairs of fresh frozen CRC tumor and adjacent NTTs ranging from September 2020 to January 2021 were collected at the same hospital and preserved at −80°C for qRT-PCR. The Ethics Committee of the Affiliated Hospital of Xuzhou Medical University approved the project, and the patients or their family members signed the informed consent form.

Immunohistochemistry Staining and Evaluation

IHC staining was performed on TMAs consisting of 568 formalin-fixed paraffin-embedded sections following a standard streptavidin–peroxidase (SP) method that has been previously described (Hou et al., 2018). Anti-QSOX2 antibodies were applied with 1:200 dilutions for primary antibody incubation (HPA012716, Sigma-Prestige, United States). The images of TMAs staining were obtained by an Olympus microscope (Tokyo, Japan).

The evaluation of the immunohistochemical reaction product has been previously described (Bai et al., 2019). The staining of QSOX2 was assessed blindly and independently by two pathologists, and all disagreements will be resolved through the participation of a third pathologist. Positive QSOX2 immunostaining signal was observed predominantly in the cytoplasm. The signals were quantified based on the intensity and percentage of positively stained cells. The QSOX2 staining intensity was scored 0–3 (0 = negative; 1 = weak; 2 = moderate; 3 = strong). The proportion of QSOX2-positive stained cells was

TABLE 2 | Information of GEO dataset involved in this study.

GEO dataset	Time	Country	GPL	Sample	N
GSE106582	2018	Germany	GPL10558	N	117
				T	77
GSE37182	2018	Italy	GPL6947	N	88
				T	84
GSE83889	2018	South Korea	GPL10558	N	35
				T	101
GSE21815	2019	Japan	GPL6480	N	9
				T	132
GSE21510	2019	Japan	GPL570	N	25
				T	123
GSE9348	2019	Singapore	GPL570	N	12
				T	70
GSE35279	2019	Japan	GPL6480	N	5
				T	74

GEO, Gene Expression Omnibus; N, normal; T, tumor; GPL, GEO platform.

scored as 1 (0–25%), 2 (26–50%), 3 (51–75%), and 4 (76–100%). The level of QSOX2 staining was evaluated by immunoreactivity score (IRS), which is calculated by multiplying the scores of staining intensity and percentage. According to IRS, the QSOX2 staining pattern was categorized as negative (IRS: 0), weak (IRS: 1–3), moderate (IRS: 4–6), and strong (IRS: 8–12). QSOX2 expression was classified as low (IRS: 0–4) or high (IRS: 6–12) group.

RNA Extraction and Quantitative Real-Time PCR

Trizol reagent (Invitrogen) was used to extract the total RNA from fresh frozen CRC tumor and adjacent NCTs according to the instructions of the manufacturer, and then the Trans Script one-step guide DNA removal and complementary DNA synthesis super mix (Trans Gen Biotech) was used for the reverse transcription reaction. The sequences of all the primers amplified for quantitative real-time PCR (qRT-PCR) were listed after: 5′-TCCCTTCTTGACAACCGTGG-3′ (forward) and 5′-AAATGCTTTGTCCCCGTCCA-3′ (reverse) for QSOX2; 5′-TTTCTCTCGGCTCCCCATGT-3′ (forward) and 5′-GCTGTATATTCAGCATTGTGGG-3′ (reverse) for p21; 5′-ACGGGAGCCCTAGCCTGGAGC-3′ (forward) and 5′-TGCCCTTCTCCACCTCTTGCC-3′ (reverse) for p27; 5′-TGAGGGACGCTTTGTCTGTC-3′ (forward) and 5′-CTTCTGCTGGAAACATGCCG-3′ (reverse) for cyclin D1; 5′-TAGCTGGTCTGGCGAGGTTT-3′ (forward) and 5′-ACAGGTGGCCAACAATTCCT-3′ (reverse) for cyclin E2; 5′-AAGGTCGGAGTCAACGGATTTG-3′ (forward) and 5′-CCATGGGTGGAATCATATTGGAA-3′ (reverse) for GAPDH; 5′-ATGGAGAACTTCCAAAAGGTGG-3′ (forward) and 5′-TCAGAGTCGAAGATGGGGTAC-3′ (reverse) for CDK2; 5′-ATGGCTACCTCTCGATATGAGC-3′ (forward) and 5′-CATTGGGGACTCTCACACTCT-3′ (reverse) for CDK4.

Colorectal Cancer Cell Culture and Transfection

HCT116 and LoVo, two types of human CRC cell lines, were gained from the Chinese Academy of Sciences Cell Bank. HCT116 and LoVo were cultured in DMEM Medium and RPMI 1640 medium, respectively, both supplemented with 10% fetal bovine serum (FBS) (Gibco, United States). All cell lines were incubated in a 37°C humidified incubator with 5% CO_2. The small interfering RNAs (siRNAs) against human QSOX2 and non-specific siRNA used as negative controls were gained from Gene pharma Technology (Shanghai, China) and transfected into the CRC cells by SilenFect reagent (Bio-Rad Laboratories, Inc.). All the experiments were performed according to the protocol of the manufacturer. The sequences of siRNAs were described as follows: siQSOX2#1 sense: GCAGCCAUUACGUGGCUAUTT; siQSOX2#2 sense: GGUACGUUCACACCUUCUUTT; siCtrl sense: UUCUCCGAACGUGUCACGUTT.

Transwell and Wounding Assay

Transwell filter inserts with a pore size of 8 μm (8.0 μm, Corning, NY, United States) were used to detect cell migration and invasion, which were carried out using invasion assay. The modified two-chamber plates were coated with Matrigel (BD Biosciences, Mississauga, Canada), while in the migration assay, they was not. After serum starvation overnight, cells were seeded in the top chamber accompanied by complete medium added to the bottom chambers. After incubation at 37°C with 5% CO_2 for 24–48 h, the migration and invasion cells were fixed and stained before calculation. In wound healing assay, CRC cells at a density of 1×10^6 cell/well were seeded onto six-well plates and cultured to a density of about 80%. Then artificial scratches were formed by sterile 10-μl pipette tips for each well. The suspended cells were cultured in a medium with 1% FBS after washing away with PBS. An inverted light microscope (IX71; Olympus, Tokyo, Japan) was used to photograph cell migration distance at 0 and 48 h.

Cell Counting Kit-8 and 5-Ethynyl-2′-Deoxyuridine Assay

HCT116 and LoVo cells were transfected with Ctrl siRNA or QSOX2 siRNA. For cell counting kit (CCK)-8 assay, the cells were counted before laying in a 96-well plate with 2,000 cells per well and continued to be cultured at 37°C in 5% CO_2 for 0, 24, 48, and 72 h. At specified time-points, the cells in each well will be added to 10 μl of cell counting kit (CCK)-8 solutions (Dojindo Molecular Technologies, Inc., Kumamoto, Japan) and continued to be cultured under the original conditions for 2 h. Absorbance was measured at 450 nm at the specified time-points. All experiments were performed in triplicate. For EdU (5-ethynyl-2′-deoxyuridine) assay, the cells were laid in a 96-well plate with 4,000 cells per well and cultured at 37°C in 5% CO_2 for 20 h. Then, the cells were treated with 50 μmol/L of EdU assay kit (RiboBio, Guangzhou, China) according to the protocol of the manufacturer and incubated at 37°C in 5% CO_2 for 2 h. Finally, 4% paraformaldehyde was used to fix the cells for 20 min, 0.5% Triton X-100 was used to permeabilize the cells for another 20 min, 100 μl of 1 × Apollo reaction cocktail was used to incubate the cells for 30 min at room temperature.

Gene Set Enrichment Analysis

As a computational method, the Gene Set Enrichment Analysis (GSEA) was performed to analyze the statistically significant and concordant differences between two different biological states based on *a priori* set of genes (Subramanian et al., 2007). According to the median value of QSOX2 expression, the CRC samples obtained from TCGA dataset were divided into the QSXO2 high and low groups, respectively. "c2.cp.kegg.v7.0.symbols.gmt," which was an annotated gene set, was finally selected as the reference gene set. In order to identify the significantly different signaling pathways, 1,000 times was set for analyzing the number of gene set permutations each time. The statistical significance and importance of the correlation between gene sets and signaling pathways were determined by nominal p-value, normalized enrichment score (NES), and false discovery rate (FDR) q-value.

Western Blot Analysis

Proteins were extracted from HCT116 and LoVo cells with RIPA buffer (Beyotime, Shanghai, China) supplemented with protease inhibitor cocktail and quantified by bicinchoninic acid (BCA) analysis (Beyotime, Shanghai, China). The prepared protein was loaded into a 10% SDS-PAGE gel with a content of 30 μg per well, then transferred to PVDF membranes, and blocked with 5% skimmed milk. Then, the PVDF membranes were incubated at 4° with antibodies against QSOX2 (1:1,000, Abcam, MA, United States), p21 (1:1,000, Cell Signaling Technology, MA, United States), p27 (1:1,000, Cell Signaling Technology, MA, United States), Cyclin D1 (1:1,000, Cell Signaling Technology, MA, United States), Notch1 (1:1,000, Cell Signaling Technology, MA, United States), GAPDH (1:5,000, Proteintech, Wuhan, China) for one night. The next day, the PVDF membranes were washed with TBST three times and then incubated with the secondary antibody for 2 h at room temperature. Finally, ECL substrate (Labgic Technology Co., Ltd., Beijing, China) was used to visualize the blots.

Xenograft Tumorigenesis Study

The ethical approval of animal experiments was approved by the Animal Care and Use Committee of Xuzhou Medical University. Four to 6-week-old BALB/c nude mice (female) were obtained from the Vital River Laboratory Animal Technology Co., Ltd. (Beijing, China) and housed under specific pathogen-free conditions. The lentiviral against human QSOX2 (shQSOX2 group) and non-specific lentiviral (shCtrl group) were transfected into HCT116 cells according to the instructions of the manufacturer. The stable HCT116 cell line including shCtrl and shQSOX2 groups were selected with puromycin and verified by Western blot. In order to construct models of xenograft tumor, 200 μl of serum-free DMEM containing groups of HCT116- shCtrl and HCT116–shQSOX2 cells (5×10^6) were injected subcutaneously into the flanks of mice. From the fifth day after the injection of cells, tumor volume (V) was calculated every 3 days by the following formula: $V = (\text{long axis} \times \text{short axis}^2)/2$. The mice were sacrificed at 24 days, and the tumors were used for HE and IHC staining after dissected and weighted.

Statistical Analysis

The difference in QSOX2 expression between non-paired cases was tested by Wilcoxon rank-sum test, while paired cases was tested by Wilcoxon matched-pairs signed-rank test. Kruskal-Wallis test was used to analyze the differences in QSOX2 expression among multiple clinical characteristic groups. Chi-square (χ^2) test was used to analyze the relationship between QSOX2 expression and clinicopathological parameters. The survival rate differences between QSOX2 high and low groups, including OS and DFS rates, was analyzed by Kaplan–Meier analysis and log rank test. The univariate Cox proportional hazard regression model combined with multivariate Cox proportional hazard regression model were used for determining the effects of QSOX2 or other clinicopathological parameters on survival. SPSS statistical software (version 23.0) and R software (version 2.15.3) were used for statistical analyses. For all tests, $p < 0.05$ was defined as statistically significance.

RESULTS

Quiescin Sulfhydryl Oxidase 2 Is Upregulated in Pan-Cancer and Colorectal Cancer

Given that QSOX2 has been poorly studied in human cancers, it is important to investigate whether QSOX2 is involved in human cancers. First, we analyzed the expression of QSOX2 in various cancer types using the public gene expression data available through TCGA and CPTAC. According to UALCAN analysis, compared with the corresponding normal tissue, the mRNA expression of QSOX2 was significantly upregulated in most human cancers (**Figures 1A,B**). Consistent with the analysis results of the UALCAN database, QSOX2 was also found to be upregulated in numerous human solid cancers according to the TIMER 2.0 online database, including COAD (colon adenocarcinoma) and READ (rectum adenocarcinoma) (**Figure 1C**). For further analysis, TCGA database was used to analyze the comprehensive expression of QSOX2 in CRC. The QSOX2 mRNA expression level in CRC tissues was significantly higher than that in the normal tissues (**Figure 1D**). Data from 41 tumors and paired adjacent NTTs of CRC patients in the TCGA database further corroborated these results (**Figure 1E**). The data from CPTAC database containing 97 CRC patients and 100 adjacent NTTs validated further the result of TCGA database (**Figure 1F**).

Validation of Quiescin Sulfhydryl Oxidase 2 Upregulation in Colorectal Cancer by Tissue Microarrays, Quantitative Real-Time PCR, and Standard Mean Difference

To characterize QSOX2 expression status in CRC, we first evaluated the endogenous QSOX2 expression in 568 CRC samples and adjacent NTTs in the TMAs using immunohistochemistry (IHC) (**Figure 2A**). Finally, 493 CRC specimens were included in the analysis, and the remaining samples were lost due to antigen retrieval. The paired Wilcoxon test showed that QSOX2 protein expression was significantly upregulated in cancerous tissues ($p < 0.001$) (**Figure 2B**). To further verify the difference in QSOX2 expression in the TCGA database, QSOX2 mRNA expression was validated in a small CRC cohort containing 50 pairs of fresh frozen tissue specimens. The results of qRT-PCR showed that that QSOX2 mRNA expression level was also upregulated in cancerous tissues relative to adjacent NTTs ($p < 0.001$) (**Figure 2C**). Additionally, the differences of QSOX2 expression in CRC were detected by the comprehensive meta-analysis in the GEO dataset (**Table 2**). The data showed that the I-square value was 94% ($p < 0.001$), according to the random effects model (95% CI:0.25–0.61), the final combined SMD of QSOX2 was 0.43. The data are

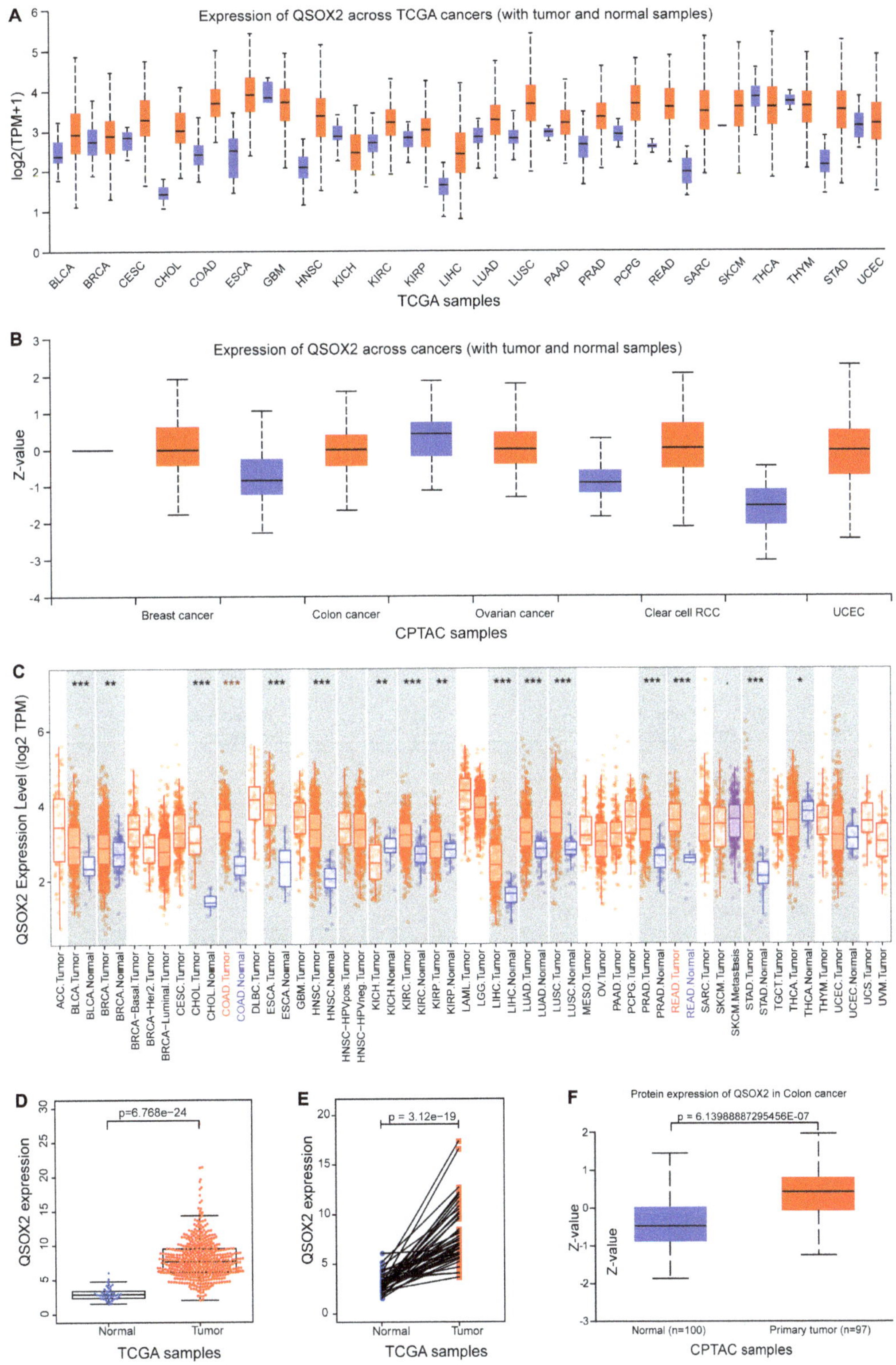

FIGURE 1 | Quiescin sulfhydryl oxidase 2 (QSOX2) expression in pan-cancer and in colorectal cancer (CRC). **(A,B)** The QSOX2 expression of mRNA level in multiple human cancers and corresponding normal tissues in the UALCAN database. **(C)** The QSOX2 expression of mRNA level in different human cancers and corresponding normal tissues in the TIMER database (*$p < 0.05$; **$p < 0.01$; ***$p < 0.001$). **(D)** The QSOX2 expression of mRNA level in CRC tumors and corresponding normal tissues from TCGA database. **(E)** QSOX2 mRNA expression in pairs of tumor and normal tissues of CRC patients from TCGA database. **(F)** QSOX2 protein expression in the primary tumors and normal tissues of CRC patients from CPTAC database.

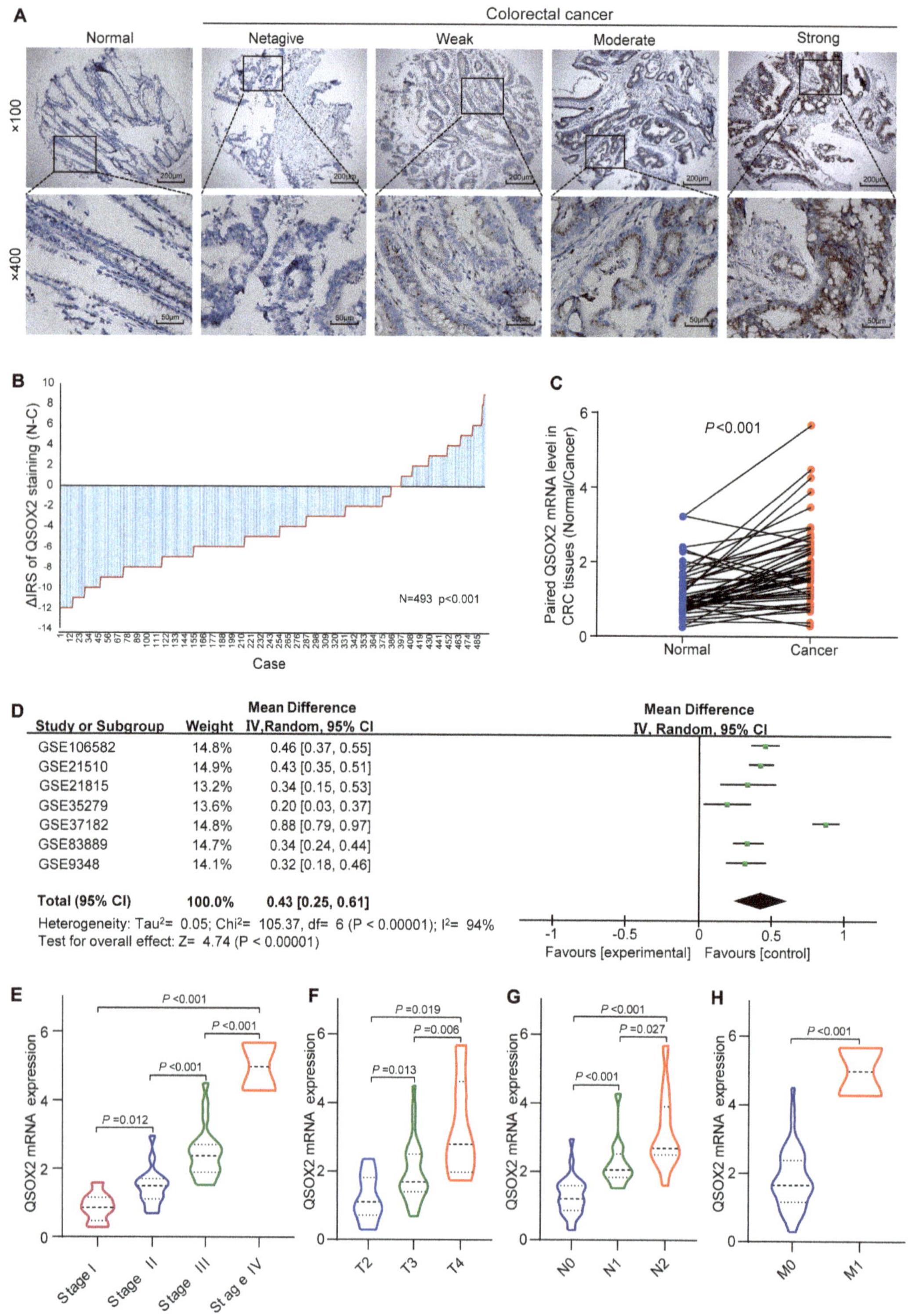

FIGURE 2 | Expression of QSOX2 is upregulated in clinical CRC patient specimens and GEO microarrays. **(A)** Representative images of QSOX2 expression in the tumor microarrays (TMAs) using immunohistochemistry (IHC) staining. **(B)** QSOX2 protein expression was significantly upregulated in cancerous tissues ($p < 0.001$, the paired Wilcoxon test). Note: N, paired adjacent non-tumor tissues (NTTs); C, CRC tissues. **(C)** The mRNA expression of QSOX2 in 50 cancerous tissues and corresponding non-tumor tissues were detected by quantitative real-time PCR (qRT-PCR) ($p < 0.001$). **(D)** Forest plot of QSOX2 expression data from GEO microarrays. Note: GEO, Gene Expression Omnibus; SMD, standard mean difference; CI, confidence interval. **(E–H)** Violin plot evaluating QSOX2 mRNA expression in different groups classified according to clinical characteristics. **(E)** TNM stage. **(F)** Depth of invasion. **(G)** Lymph node metastasis. **(H)** Distant metastasis.

statistically significant, thus, suggesting that QSOX2 expression was upregulated in CRC based on the GEO database (**Figure 2D**).

Quiescin Sulfhydryl Oxidase 2 Is Associated With Malignant Progression in Patients With Colorectal Cancer From TCGA Cohort

As we continue to explore the mRNA expression of QSOX2 in TCGA database, we were surprised to find that the expression of QSOX2 was different in groups classified by tumor pathological stage ($p = 0.004$), T classification ($p < 0.001$), N classification ($p = 0.009$), and M classification ($p < 0.001$) (**Supplementary Figures 1A–D**). To further analyze the relationship between QSOX2 expression and clinicopathological features, we collected original expression information and corresponding clinical data of 314 patients from TCGA database. As shown in **Table 3**, QSOX2 high expression was positively associated with pathological stage progression ($p = 0.003$) and lymph node metastasis ($p = 0.003$). Logistic regression analysis indicated that the QSOX2 overexpression was observed to be positively correlated with pathological stage (stage II vs. stage I, OR = 2.211, $p = 0.007$; stage III vs. stage I, OR = 5.049, $p < 0.001$; stage IV vs. stage I, OR = 3.088, $p = 0.007$), lymph node metastasis (N1/N2 vs. N0, OR = 2.239, $p = 0.001$) (**Table 4**).

High Quiescin Sulfhydryl Oxidase 2 Expression Is Associated With Advanced Clinicopathological Parameters in Patients With Colorectal Cancer During the Clinical Validation Phase

Consistent with the analysis results of TCGA cohort, QSOX2 mRNA expression in the CRC cohort containing 50 pairs of fresh frozen tissue specimens was also different in groups classified according to TNM stage, lymph node metastasis, depth of invasion, and distant metastasis (**Figures 2E–H**). To further understand the clinical significance of QSOX2 in the large CRC cohort containing 568 formalin-fixed paraffin-embedded CRC specimens, Fisher's exact test was used to analyze the relationship between QSOX2 expression and clinicopathological features. **Table 5** showed the relationship between QSOX2 expression and clinicopathological features of the CRC patients. QSOX2 overexpression was positively associated with aggressive features of CRC, such as tumor lymph node metastasis ($p = 0.048$), TNM stage progression ($p < 0.001$), tumor diameter ($p = 0.017$), and distant metastasis ($p = 0.008$). On the other hand, there was no striking relationship between QSOX2 expression and age, gender, differentiation, or depth of invasion.

High Quiescin Sulfhydryl Oxidase 2 Expression Is Related to Poor Survival in Patients With Colorectal Cancer Based on TCGA Cohort

The analysis of QSOX2 prognostic signature in CRC based on TCGA cohort was investigated by Kaplan–Meier risk estimates. The result showed that QSOX2 overexpression was positively associated with poor overall survival (**Figure 3A**). Besides, univariate and multivariate Cox proportional hazard regression models were conducted to assess the influence of QSOX2 expression and clinicopathological parameters on survival in CRC patients based on TCGA cohort. Univariate analysis revealed that QSOX2 expression (HR, 1.08; 95% CI, 1.02–1.14; $p = 0.006$), age (HR, 1.03; 95% CI, 1.01–1.05; $p = 0.008$), pathological stage (HR, 2.26; 95% CI, 1.73–2.94;

TABLE 3 | The relationship between quiescin sulfhydryl oxidase 2 (QSOX2) expression and CRC clinicopathological features based on TCGA cohort.

Variables	QSOX2 expression		Total	p-value
	High (n = 224)	Low (n = 90)		
Age				
<65 years	80 (70.2)	34 (29.8)	114	0.731
≥65 years	144 (72.0)	56 (28.0)	200	
Gender				
Male	119 (73.0)	44 (27.0)	163	0.497
Female	105 (69.5)	46 (30.5)	151	
Pathological stage				
I and II	96 (63.6)	55 (36.4)	151	0.003
III and IV	128 (78.5)	35 (21.5)	163	
T classification				
T1 and T2	34 (66.7)	17 (33.3)	51	0.420
T3 and T4	190 (72.2)	73 (27.8)	263	
Lymph node metastasis				
N0	103 (64.8)	56 (35.2)	159	0.003
N+	131 (79.4)	34 (20.6)	165	
Distant metastasis				
M0	176 (69.6)	77 (30.4)	253	0.157
M+	48 (78.7)	13 (21.3)	61	

TABLE 4 | QSOX2 expression correlated with clinicopathological features based on TCGA cohort.

Clinicopathological features	Total (N)	Odds ratio in QSOX2 expression	p-value
Age			
<65 vs. ≥ 65	447	1.135 (0.774–1,667)	0.517
Gender			
Male vs. female	447	0.829 (0.571–1.201)	0.321
Pathological stage			
Stage II vs. stage I	131	2.211 (1.077–4.654)	0.007
Stage III vs. stage I	129	5.049 (2.418–10.946)	0.000
Stage IV vs. stage I	104	3.088 (1.383–7.093)	0.007
T classification			
T2 vs. T1	59	1.500 (0.231–12.078)	0.670
T3 vs. T1	196	1.454 (0.236–11.221)	0.686
T4 vs. T1	50	1.714 (0.260–13.974)	0.575
Lymph node metastasis			
Yes vs. no	272	2.239 (1.382–3.654)	0.001
Distant metastasis			
Yes vs. no	367	1.226 (0.707–2.138)	0.469

TABLE 5 | Relationship between QSOX2 expression and clinicopathological features of CRC patients based on clinical CRC specimen cohort.

Variables	Cases	QSOX2 expression (*n* = 493 cases)		*p*-value
		Low	High	
All patients	493	164	329	
Age (years)[b]		62 ± 12	61 ± 13	0.531
≤60	211	72	139	
>60	282	92	190	
Gender[a]				0.923
Males	277	93	184	
Females	216	71	145	
Lymph node metastasis[a]				0.048
N0	309	113	196	
N1/N2/N3	184	51	133	
TNM stage[a]				<0.001
I/II	271	116	155	
III/IV	222	48	174	
Differentiation[a,c]				0.18
Poor	93	37	56	
Moderate/high	395	127	268	
Tumor diameter[a]				0.017
≤5 cm	260	99	161	
>5 cm	233	65	168	
Distant metastasis[a]				0.008
M0	433	153	280	
M1	60	11	49	
Depth of invasion[a]				0.663
T1/T2	128	45	83	
T3/T4	365	119	246	

[a] *Two-sided Fisher's exact tests.*
[b] *Two-sided Student's t-test.*
[c] *The type of differentiation of cancer in five patients cannot be assessed.*

$p < 0.001$), T classification (HR, 2.85; 95% CI, 1.80–4.52; $p < 0.001$), N classification (HR, 2.02; 95% CI, 1.54–2.65; $p < 0.001$), and M classification (HR, 4.45; 95% CI, 2.74–7.21; $p < 0.001$) were important risk factors for survival (**Table 6**). In addition, multivariate analysis showed that QSOX2 expression (HR, 1.06; 95% CI, 1.00–1.13; $p = 0.033$) was an independent risk factor for survival (**Figure 3B** and **Table 6**).

Upregulated Quiescin Sulfhydryl Oxidase 2 Expression Is a Predictor of Poor Prognosis in Colorectal Cancer During the Clinical Validation Phase

Similar results were observed during the clinical validation phase based on the survival follow-up information of 493 patients. Kaplan–Meier survival curves showed that the QSOX2 overexpression was positively associated with poor OS ($p < 0.001$) and DFS ($p < 0.001$) (**Figures 3C,D**). To further evaluate the prognostic significance of QSOX2 expression in CRC patients, univariate and multivariate Cox regression models were conducted in the 493 CRC specimens. Univariate Cox regression analysis suggested that QSOX2 expression, age, gender, TNM stage, LNM, tumor diameter, and distant metastasis were the significant risk factors for OS, while QSOX2 expression, depth of invasion, and TNM stage were the significant risk factors for DFS (**Table 7**). Finally, multivariate analysis showed that QSOX2 expression could serve as an independent prognostic biomarker for OS (HR, 2.512; 95% CI, 1.730–3.647; $p < 0.001$) and DFS (HR, 4.493; 95% CI, 2.640–7.649; $p < 0.001$) in CRC patients (**Table 8**).

Quiescin Sulfhydryl Oxidase 2 Promotes Colorectal Cell Proliferation, Migration, and Invasion *in vitro*

Since the results of bioinformatic analysis and clinical specimens showed that QSOX2 overexpression was associated with the malignant progression of CRC patients, we will focus on the biological function of QSOX2 in CRC. The expression of QSOX2 was reduced by small interfering RNAs (siRNAs) and detected by Western blotting and qRT-PCR analysis, respectively (**Figures 4A–C**). Given that QSOX2 overexpression was positively associated with tumor diameter and lymph node metastasis, we wanted to detect whether QSOX2 facilitates the ability of proliferation and metastasis in CRC cells. CCK-8 and EdU assays showed that inhibition of QSOX2 significantly reduced rates of cell proliferation in HCT116 and LoVo cells (**Figures 4D–G**). Transwell migration and invasion assays, and wound healing assays were used to estimate the influence of QSOX2 expression on CRC metastasis. The Transwell assays showed that QSOX2 inhibition reduced the ability of migration and invasion in HCT116 and LoVo cells (**Figures 4H,I**). Wound healing assays showed that QSOX2 inhibition reduced the speed of wound healing in HCT116 and LoVo cells (**Figures 4J,K**).

Identification of Quiescin Sulfhydryl Oxidase 2-Related Signaling Pathways by Gene Set Enrichment Analysis

GSEA was conducted to detect the potential molecular mechanism and signaling pathways involved in how QSOX2 promotes CRC progression. First, TCGA samples were classified into two groups according to the expression of QSOX2. Then, the significance of multiple functional sets of QSOX2 high and low groups was analyzed by GSEA (**Figure 5A**). In the comprehensive analysis of NES, normal *p*-value, and FDR *q*-value, 15 signaling pathways enriched in the QSOX2 high group were selected, including cell cycle, homologous recombination, pyrimidine metabolism, spliceosome, purine metabolism, nucleotide excision repair, notch signaling pathway, glyoxylate, dicarboxylate metabolism, ubiquitin-mediated proteolysis, DNA replication, mTOR signaling pathway, p53 signaling pathway, ERBB signaling pathway, threonine metabolism, glycine serine, and basal transcription factors (**Figure 5B** and **Table 9**). In addition, correlation analysis by the GEPIA database showed that the mRNA level of p21, p27, cyclin D1, Notch1, mTOR, PIK3CA, and ERBB3 were significantly associated with QSOX2, while p53 was not, indicating that

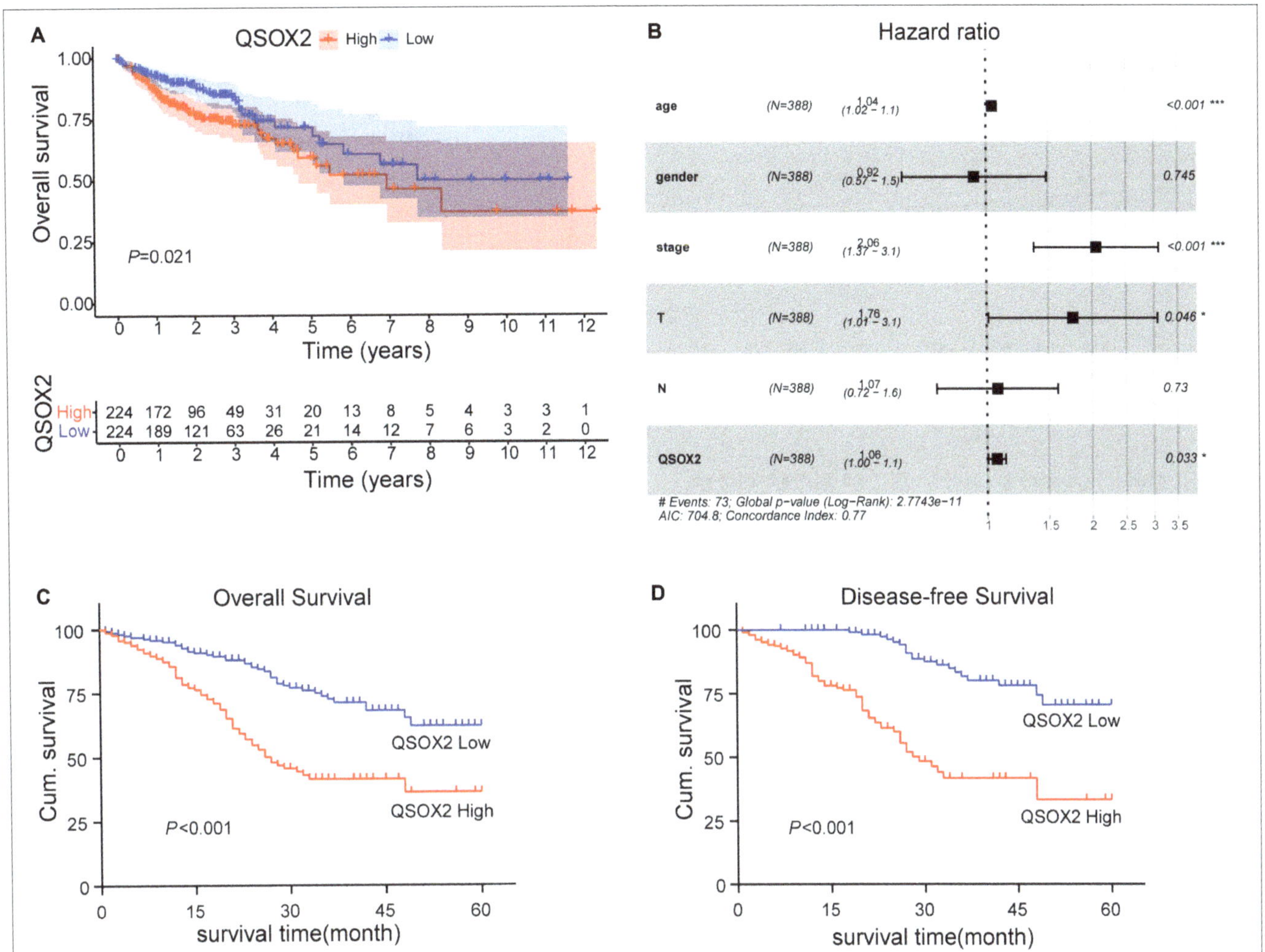

FIGURE 3 | Prognostic role of QSOX2 in CRC patients. **(A)** Kaplan–Meier survival curves show patients of CRC with high QSOX2 expression exhibited shorter overall survival (OS) (n = 224, p = 0.021) based on TCGA database. **(B)** Forest plot shows that QSOX2 expression was an independent risk factor for CRC based on TCGA data (HR, 1.06; 95% CI, 1.00–1.13; p = 0.033). HR, hazard ratio; CI, confidence interval; $^{*}p < 0.05$; $^{***}p < 0.001$. **(C,D)** Kaplan–Meier survival curves show that patients of CRC with high QSOX2 expression exhibited shorter OS (n = 493, $p < 0.001$) and disease-free survival (DFS) based on clinical specimen cohort.

QSOX2 may promote CRC cell proliferation and metastasis via some of these signaling pathways (**Figure 5C**). Intriguingly, cell cycle signaling pathway exhibited the most significant enrichment. Therefore, we focused on cell cycle signaling pathway for further detection. Furthermore, the expression of some cell cycle signaling pathway-related key regulators was detected by qRT-PCR. Consistent with our GEPIA analysis, the results of qRT-PCR analysis showed that QSOX2 knockdown significantly caused the accumulation of p21 and p27 in mRNA level, whereas it remarkably decreased the mRNA expression of cyclin D1, cyclin E2, CDK2, CDK4 (**Figure 5D**). The Western blot results showed that knockdown of QSOX2 in HCT116 and LoVo cells significantly increased the protein expression of p21 and p27, and reduced the protein expression of cyclinD1 and Notch1 (**Figure 5E**). More importantly, among these genes, p21 was significantly upregulated in mRNA and protein level after QSOX2 was knocked down. These results suggested that QSOX2 is very likely to promote the proliferation of colorectal cancer cells by regulating the cell cycle progression mediated by p21.

Quiescin Sulfhydryl Oxidase 2 Promotes Colorectal Cancer Cell Proliferation *in vivo*

Xenograft tumorigenesis model was conducted to detect the effect of QSOX2 on proliferation of CRC cell in *in vivo*. The protein expression of QSOX2 in HCT116 stable transfected cell line was confirmed by Western blot assay (**Figure 6A**). The mice were sacrificed at 24 days, and the subcutaneous tumor in mice was dissected. The results showed that the xenograft tumors formed by shCtrl cells were significantly heavier and larger than that of shQSOX2 cells (**Figures 6B–D**). H&E staining was performed to confirm the xenograft tumors (**Figure 6E**). Furthermore, immunohistochemistry staining was performed to detect the expression of QSOX2, p21, and the cancer cell

TABLE 6 | Univariate and multivariate Cox proportional hazards analysis of overall survival (OS) in CRC patients based on TCGA cohort.

Parameters	Univariate analysis		Multivariate analysis	
	HR (95% CI)	*p*-value	HR (95% CI)	*p*-value
QSOX2	1.08 (1.02–1.14)	0.006	1.06 (1.00–1.13)	0.033
Age	1.03 (1.01–1.05)	0.008	1.04 (1.02–1.06)	<0.001
Gender	1.11 (0.70–1.77)	0.653	0.92 (0.57–1.49)	0.745
Pathological stage	2.26 (1.73–2.94)	<0.001	2.06 (1.37–3.09)	<0.001
T	2.85 (1.80–4.52)	<0.001	1.76 (1.01–3.07)	0.046
N	2.02 (1.54–2.65)	<0.001	1.07 (0.72–1.60)	0.730
M	4.45 (2.74–7.21)	<0.001		

HR, hazard ratio; CI, confidence interval.

TABLE 7 | Univariate Cox regression analysis on OS and disease-free survival (DFS) in CRC based on clinical specimen cohort.

Variables[a]	Overall survival		Disease-specific survival	
	HR (95% CI)	*p*-value	HR (95% CI)	*p*-value
QSOX2	2.866 (1.989–4.128)	<0.001	5.149 (3.069–8.636)	<0.001
Age	1.424 (1.031–1.965)	0.032	1.008 (0.991–1.025)	0.359
Gender	1.294 (0.949–1.765)	0.103	1.456 (0.965–2.197)	0.074
Differentiate	0.865 (0.593–1.262)	0.451	0.789 (0.551–1.129)	0.194
Depth of invasion	1.260 (0.866–1.834)	0.227	1.266 (1.033–1.552)	0.023
TNM stage	1.781 (1.305–2.432)	<0.001	2.224 (1.448–3.418)	<0.001
LNM	1.344 (0.982–1.839)	0.065	1.408 (0.857–2.313)	0.177
Tumor diameter	1.455 (1.065–1.987)	0.019	1.300 (0.927–1.822)	0.128
Distant metastasis	2.719 (1.703–4.343)	<0.001		

HR, hazard ratio; CI, confidence interval; LNM, lymph node metastasis.
[a]QSOX2: low vs. high; age: ≤ 60 vs. >60; gender: male vs. female; differentiate: poor vs. moderate and high; depth of invasion: T1 and T2 vs. T3 and T4; TNM stage was ranked as I and II vs. III and IV; LNM, N0 vs. N+; tumor diameter: ≤ 5 vs. >5; distant metastasis: M0 vs. M+.

TABLE 8 | Multivariate Cox regression analysis on OS and DFS in CRC based on clinical specimen cohort.

Variables[a]	Overall survival		Disease-free survival	
	HR (95% CI)	*p*-value	HR (95% CI)	*p*-value
QSOX2	2.512 (1.730–3.647)	<0.001	4.493 (2.640–7.649)	<0.001
Age	1.423 (1.024–1.977)	0.036	1.677 (1.067–2.634)	0.025
Gender	1.357 (0.979–1.879)	0.067	1.301 (0.826–2.047)	0.256
Tumor diameter	1.352 (0.986–1.853)	0.061	1.244 (0.811–1.909)	0.318
TNM stage	1.667 (1.201–2.314)	0.002	1.955 (1.207–3.166)	0.006
Differentiate	0.752 (0.514–1.101)	0.143	0.846 (0.526–1.361)	0.491

HR, hazard ratio; CI, confidence interval; LNM, lymph node metastasis.
[a]QSOX2: low vs. high; age: ≤ 60 vs. >60; gender: male vs. female; differentiate: poor vs. moderate and high; depth of invasion: T1 and T2 vs. T3 and T4; TNM stage was ranked as I and II vs. III and IV; LNM: N0 vs. N+; tumor diameter: ≤ 5 vs. >5; distant metastasis: M0 vs. M+.

proliferation marker Ki67 in shQSOX2 and shCtrl groups. The staining results showed that QSOX2 stable knockdown resulted in weaker staining intensity of QSOX2 and Ki67 in the tumor sections but a stronger staining intensity of p21 (**Figure 6F**).

DISCUSSION

The increasing disease burden caused by CRC has become one of the major global threats to human health, with about 1.88 million new cases and 900,000 death cases annually (Sung et al., 2021). Although CRC has been extensively studied, more powerful and reliable biomarkers used to predict CRC progression and prognosis are still required for providing clinical significance. In the past years, with the growing development of next-generation genome sequencing technology, various data of gene expression level in CRC samples were uploaded to the public database, such as TCGA and GEO, which provides chances for biomarker discovery and validation (Long et al., 2019; Liu et al., 2020). The quiescin sulfhydryl oxidase family consists of QSOX1 and QSOX2; unlike QSOX1, which has been wildly studied in tumors, the expression and function of QSOX2 in tumors is largely unclear. With this in mind, in this study, the expression of QSOX2 in various human tumors was first analyzed via the publicly available databases TIMER2.0 and UALCAN. The results indicated that QSOX2 gene expression was upregulated in multiple solid tumors, such as colorectal cancer, bladder cancer, breast cancer, clear cell renal cell cancer, esophageal cancer, stomach cancer, and others than in their matched adjacent NTTs. Then, we focused on the expression of QSOX2 in colorectal cancer.

In the present study, we purposed to detect the expression and function of QSOX2 in CRC progression, especially its role as a prognostic biomarker. Moreover, we also tried to identify the potential signaling pathways involved in the regulation of CRC development by QSOX2. First, we evaluated the expression of QSOX2 in CRC by bioinformatic analysis based on TCGA cohort. Compared with adjacent NTTs, QSOX2 expression level was significantly upregulated in patients with CRC, and the results have been verified both in mRNA and protein level by qRT-PCR and IHC based on our paraffin-embedded and fresh frozen tissue specimen cohort. The results of meta-analysis based on GEO database are consistent with those of bioinformatics analysis and clinical trials. These results indicate that QSOX2 may act as an oncogene and play an important role in CRC initiation and progression. More specifically, QSOX2 mRNA expression was different in the clinical characteristic groups classified by pathological stage, T, N, and M stages, and these results were confirmed by frozen tissue specimen cohort. Based on this, the relationship between QSOX2 expression and clinicopathological parameters was analyzed in TCGA cohort and validated in our well-characterized clinical cohort. We demonstrated that high QSOX2 expression is closely associated with various malignant clinicopathological factors such as TNM stage, tumor diameter, lymph node metastasis, and so on. These findings may accelerate early risk recognition and precise management of CRC patients.

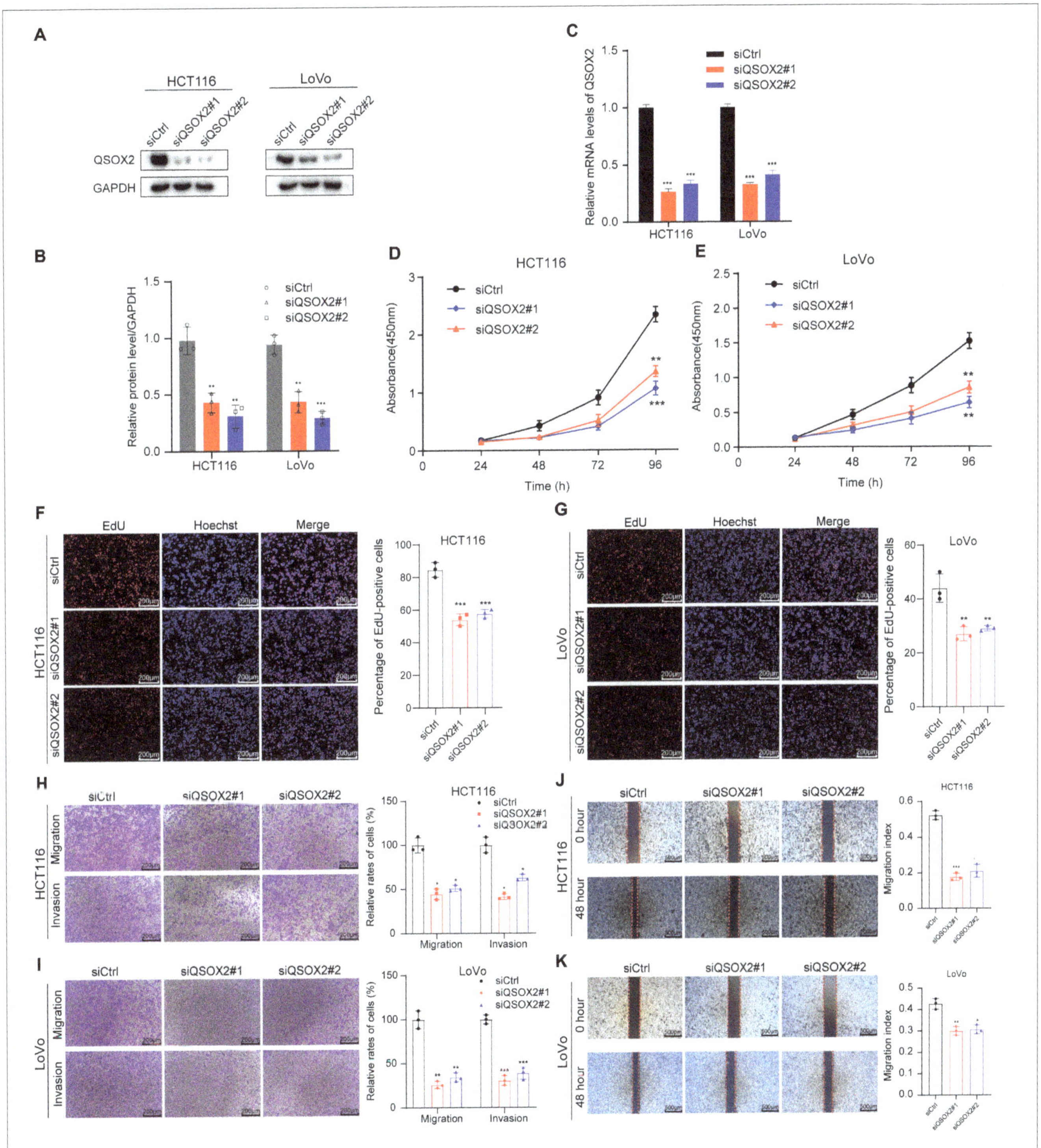

FIGURE 4 | QSOX2 promotes CRC cell proliferation, migration, and invasion *in vitro*. **(A–C)** The inhibition of QSOX2 protein and mRNA expression was confirmed in HCT116 and LoVo cells by Western blotting and qRT-PCR, respectively. Densitometry values of QSOX2 normalized to GAPDH. **(D,E)** QSOX2 inhibition significantly reduced ability of proliferation in HCT116 and LoVo cells via cell counting kit 8 (CCK-8) assay. **(F,G)** QSOX2 inhibition significantly reduced ability of proliferation in HCT116 and LoVo cells via 5-ethynyl-2′-deoxyuridine (EdU) incorporation assay. **(H,I)** Inhibition of QSOX2 significantly suppressed the ability of migration and invasion in HCT116 and LoVo cells via Transwell assay. **(J,K)** Inhibition of QSOX2 significantly inhibited the wound healing speed in HCT116 and LoVo cells by wound healing assay. All experiments were repeated three times, and the final data are shown as mean ± standard deviations. *$p < 0.05$; **$p < 0.01$; ***$p < 0.001$.

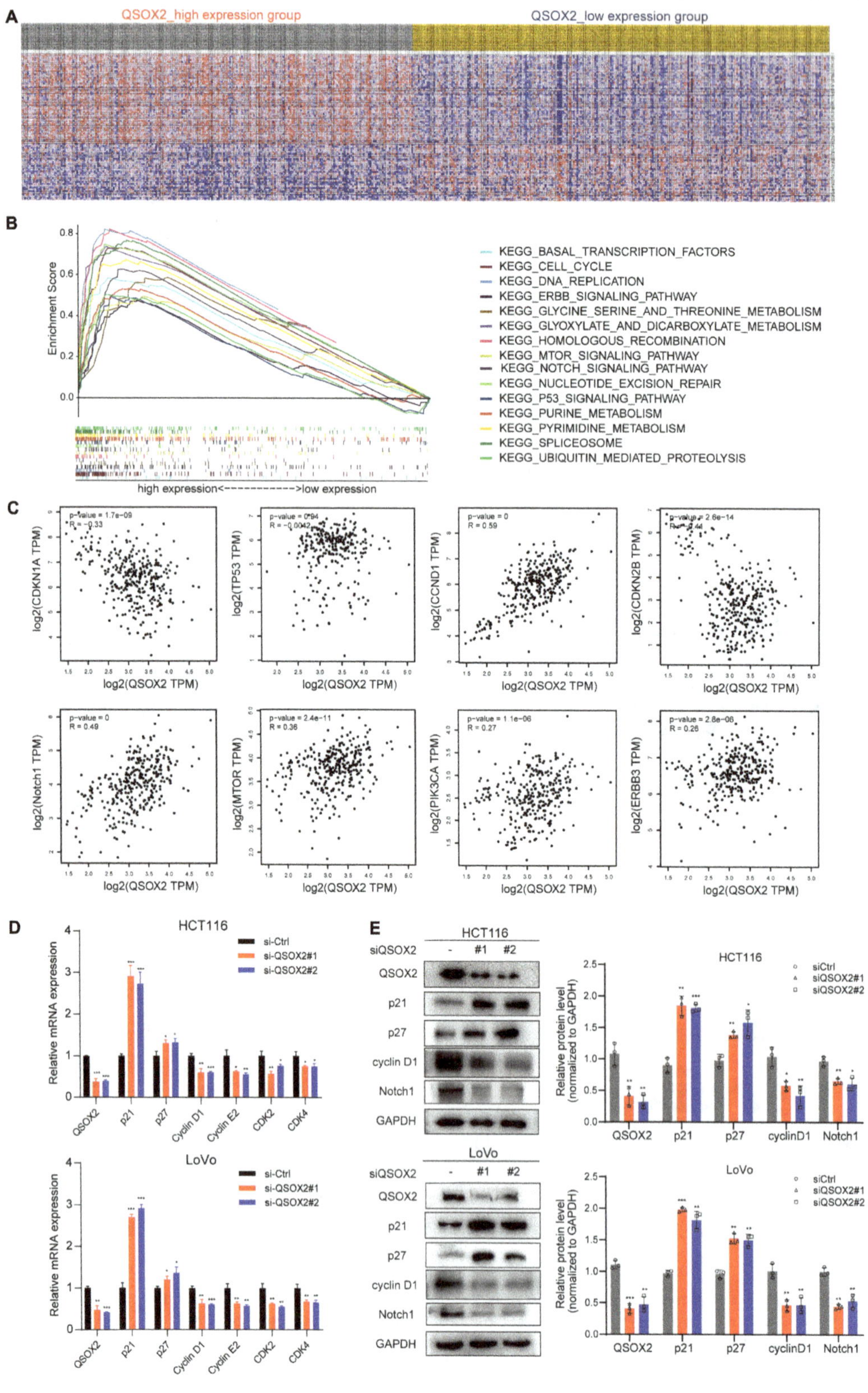

FIGURE 5 | Mechanistic investigation into how QSOX2 promotes CRC progression. **(A)** The heat map generated based on genes enriched in QSOX2 high and low in TCGA database. **(B)** Enrichment plots from Gene Set Enrichment Analysis (GSEA) including enrichment score and gene sets. **(C)** Correlation between QSOX2 and signaling pathway-related genes, including p21, p27, cyclin D1, p53, Notch1, mTOR, PIK3CA, and ERBB3. **(D)** The mRNA expression of cell cycle signaling pathway genes in CRC with knockdown of QSOX2 were determined by qRT-PCR. **(E)** The expression of QSOX2 and signaling pathway-related genes were detected by Western blotting, and GAPDH was used as a reference control. $^{*}p < 0.05$; $^{**}p < 0.01$; $^{***}p < 0.001$.

Prognostic biomarkers are applied to monitor postoperative treatments, evaluate the level of cancer, and predict remission or recurrence in individual patients (Nair et al., 2014). In addition, on the basis of TCGA database, Kaplan–Meier survival analysis demonstrated that the group of QSOX2 high expression exhibited poor OS than the group of QSOX2 low expression. Importantly, Cox regression analyses showed that QSOX2 expression could serve as an independent prognostic biomarker for survival in CRC patients. These results are supported by the data of clinical validation. At this point, in our research, QSOX2 was found to be not only a factor of tumor progression in CRC but also a biomarker of prognosis. The results of bioinformatics analysis and clinical verification suggest that QSOX2 overexpression was closely related to the malignant progression of CRC patients, such as the ability of proliferation and metastasis, which is also an important feature of malignant tumors. To further detect the biological function of QSOX2 in colorectal cancer cells, we performed experiments *in vitro*, such as Transwell, wounding healing, CCK-8, and EdU assays, and xenograft tumorigenesis model *in vivo*. The results showed that the proliferation and metastasis ability of HCT116 and LoVo is reduced by inhibition of QSOX2.

The QSOX2-related potential signaling pathways in CRC was analyzed by the GSEA. Of note, 15 significantly enriched signaling pathways were selected; among them, cell cycle, notch, mTOR, p53, and ERBB signaling pathway were closely related to the progression of CRC. Intriguingly, cell cycle signaling pathway exhibited the most significant enrichment. Accumulating evidence has showed that cell cycle disorders may lead to enhanced tumor cell proliferation (Otto and Sicinski, 2017). Cyclin D1, p21, and p27 were the key regulators associated with the G1 phase (Chen et al., 2019). As a well–known tumor suppressor, activation of the transcription factor p53 plays a central role in cell cycle arrest (Engeland, 2018). P53 regulates cell cycle progression by regulating some key genes, including p21 (Vogelstein et al., 2000). Correlation analysis shows that QOSX2 is negatively correlated with p21 and p27, and positively correlated with cyclin D1, but not p53, and the results of qRT-PCR showed that QSOX2 knockdown significantly caused the accumulation of p21 and p27 mRNA and the decrease in the mRNA expression of cyclin D1, cyclin E2, CDK2, CDK4, which suggests that QSOX2 may promote the proliferation of colorectal cancer by partially regulating G1/S phase transition independent of p53. The Notch signaling pathway is activated in primary colorectal cancer and plays an important part in the initiation and progression process (Tyagi et al., 2020). Notch receptors have been reported to take part in several functions of CRC cells, such as apoptosis, proliferation, angiogenesis, and cell migration (Jackstadt et al., 2019). What is also worth noticing is that the abnormal activation of Notch1 is closely related to the severity of CRC (Vinson et al., 2016). The results of GEPIA showed that QSOX2 was positively correlated with Notch1 in mRNA level, and our Western blotting results showed that knockdown of QSOX2 remarkably decreased the expression of Notch1 protein. We estimate that QSOX2 may promote the migration and proliferation by activation of Notch signaling pathway. The constituents of tumor extracellular matrix (ECM) secreted by tumor cells and non-malignant stroma are a critical factor for cancer invasion and metastasis. Since proteins in the ECM contains disulfide bonds, QSOX2, as an enzyme that generates disulfide bonds in substrate proteins, may also promote cancer cell growth, adherence, and invasion by regulating the ECM. The mechanistic target of rapamycin (mTOR) is a highly conserved kinase, and the activation of mTOR signaling pathway is closely related to CRC cell autophagy, differentiation, apoptosis, proliferation, angiogenesis, and metastasis (Wang and Zhang, 2014). Experimental and preclinical studies have proven that mTOR is an effective target for colorectal cancer

TABLE 9 | Signaling pathways enriched in the QSOX2 high group.

Gene sets	NES	NOM *p*-value	FDR *q*-value
KEGG_CELL_CYCLE	2.435	0.000	0.000
KEGG_HOMOLOGOUS_RECOMBINATION	2.319	0.000	0.000
KEGG_PYRIMIDINE_METABOLISM	2.255	0.000	0.003
KEGG_SPLICEOSOME	2.209	0.000	0.004
KEGG_PURINE_METABOLISM	2.197	0.000	0.003
KEGG_NUCLEOTIDE_EXCISION_REPAIR	2.156	0.000	0.006
KEGG_NOTCH_SIGNALING_PATHWAY	2.029	0.006	0.010
KEGG_GLYOXYLATE_AND_ DICARBOXYLATE_METABOLISM	1.955	0.000	0.018
KEGG_UBIQUITIN_MEDIATED_ PROTEOLYSIS	1.952	0.006	0.017
KEGG_DNA_REPLICATION	1.951	0.002	0.017
KEGG_MTOR_SIGNALING_PATHWAY	1.902	0.002	0.023
KEGG_P53_SIGNALING_PATHWAY	1.856	0.020	0.032
KEGG_ERBB_SIGNALING_PATHWAY	1.855	0.006	0.031
KEGG_GLYCINE_SERINE_AND_THREONINE_METABOLISM	1.852	0.008	0.031
KEGG_BASAL_TRANSCRIPTION_FACTORS	1.829	0.016	0.037

NES, normalized enrichment score; NOM, nominal; FDR, false discovery rate.

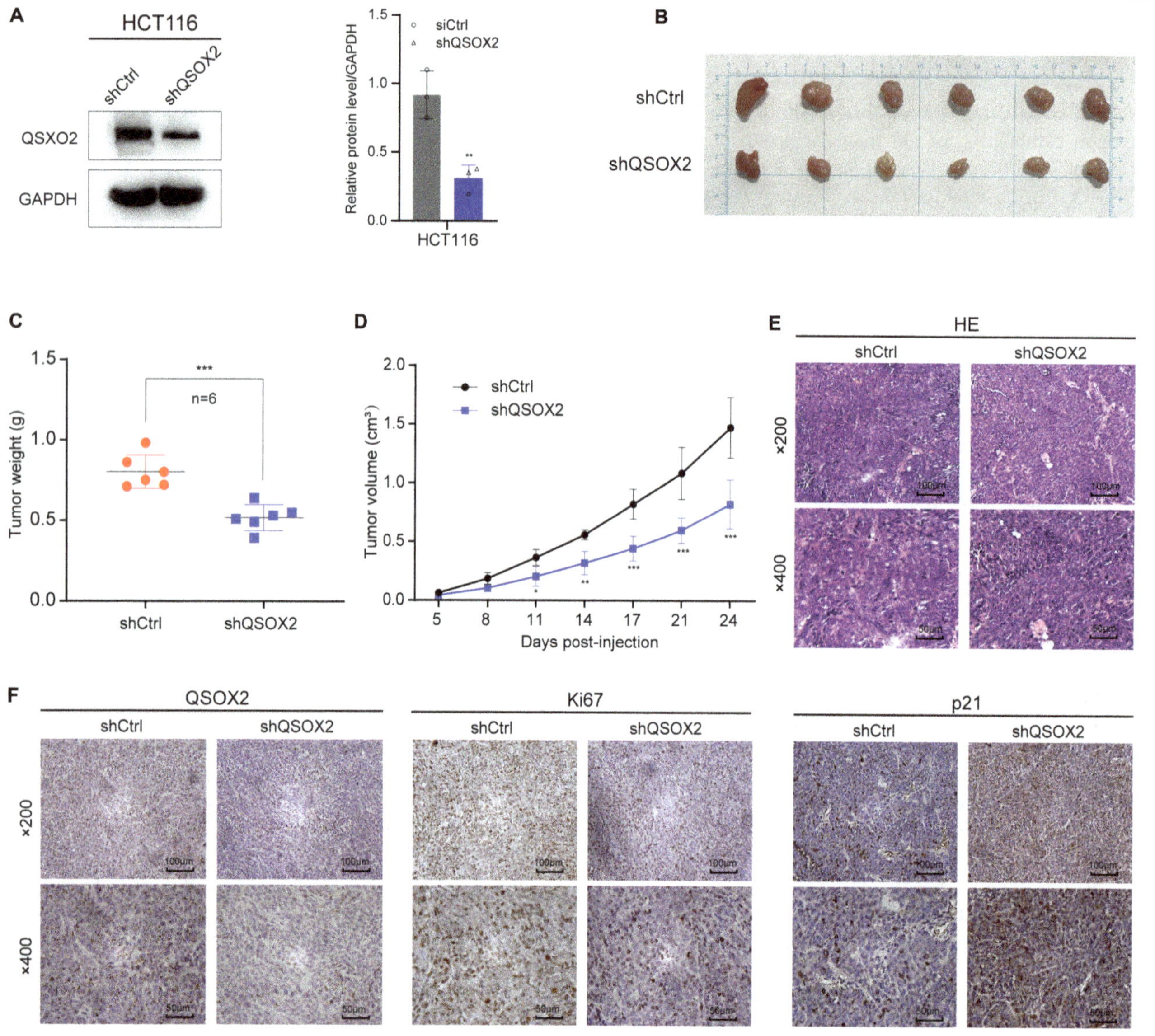

FIGURE 6 | QSOX2 promotes CRC cell proliferation *in vivo*. **(A)** The protein expression of QSOX2 in HCT116 stable transfected cell line was confirmed by Western blot assay **(Left)**. Densitometry values of QSOX2 normalized to GAPDH **(Right)**. **(B)** The dissected subcutaneous tumor in mice formed by the shCtrl and shQSOX2 groups (n = 6 in each group). **(C)** Analysis of the weight of dissected xenograft tumors. **(D)** The growth curve of xenograft tumors in mice. **(E)** The sections of xenograft tumors were stained by H&E and IHC using QSOX2, Ki67, and p21 antibodies.

therapy, and considering the close correlation between QSOX2 and mTOR, QSOX2 also may provide promising perspectives for CRC therapy.

Although our study investigated the expression and prognostic value of QSOX2 in CRC by a variety of methods and a large number of clinical samples, there are still some limitations. First, there is a lack of some specific clinical information involved in analysis, such as microsatellite instability (MSI) and surgical methods. Second, the specimens used in this study were limited to one hospital, and lack of multicenter research. Finally, the deeper molecular mechanisms of QSOX2 in CRC are not detected by experiments *in vitro* and *in vivo*. Thus, more clinical specimens and cell biology experiments are required for further investigation in the future.

In summary, based on bioinformatics analysis and clinical verification, our study demonstrated that QSOX2 is upregulated in CRC, and the upregulation of QSOX2 is closely correlated with clinical aggressive progression and poor survival in TCGA clinical and two independent specimen cohorts. We also found that QSOX2 facilitates the proliferation and metastasis ability of CRC cells, and these results suggest that QSOX2 plays a vital part in the initiation and progression of CRC. In conclusion, QSOX2 might act as a novel biomarker for prognosis prediction and a new target for biotherapy in CRC.

ETHICS STATEMENT

The studies involving human participants were reviewed and approved by the Ethnic Committee of the Affiliated Hospital of Xuzhou Medical University. The patients/participants provided their written informed consent to participate in this study. The animal study was reviewed and approved by the Animal Care and Use Committee of Xuzhou Medical University. All standard biosecurity and institutional safety procedures have been adhered to in all the experiment procedures in this study.

AUTHOR CONTRIBUTIONS

TJ, JS, and RW designed the study and drafted the manuscript. LZ and XL analyzed the data, prepared the figures, and they contributed equally with TJ. HS and YX collected the surgical specimens and associated clinical data. JL assisted in the IHC staining and assessment. HW and SW helped to downloading the database from TCGA and GEO. CD and LL performed the experiments *in vitro*. All authors have read and discussed the manuscript and agreed with the final manuscript.

ACKNOWLEDGMENTS

We would like to thank Qiuwen Sun for her assistance in bioinformatics analysis.

REFERENCES

Araujo, D. G., Nakao, L., Gozzo, P., Souza, C. D., Balderrama, V., Gugelmin, E. S., et al. (2014). Expression level of quiescin sulfhydryl oxidase 1 (QSOX1) in neuroblastomas. *Eur. J. Histochem.* 58:2228. doi: 10.4081/ejh.2014.2228

Baek, J. A., Song, P. H., Ko, Y., and Gu, M. J. (2018). High expression of QSOX1 is associated with tumor invasiveness and high grades groups in prostate cancer. *Pathol. Res. Pract.* 214, 964–967. doi: 10.1016/j.prp.2018.05.019

Bai, J., Wu, K., Cao, M. H., Yang, Y., Pan, Y., Liu, H., et al. (2019). SCF(FBXO22) targets HDM2 for degradation and modulates breast cancer cell invasion and metastasis. *Proc. Natl. Acad. Sci. U.S.A.* 116, 11754–11763. doi: 10.1073/pnas.1820990116

Chandrashekar, D. S., Bashel, B., Balasubramanya, S. A. H., Creighton, C. J., Ponce-Rodriguez, I., Chakravarthi, B., et al. (2017). UALCAN: a portal for facilitating tumor subgroup gene expression and survival analyses. *Neoplasia* 19, 649–658. doi: 10.1016/j.neo.2017.05.002

Chen, Y., Liu, X., Wang, H., Liu, S., Hu, N., and Li, X. (2019). Akt regulated phosphorylation of GSK-3beta/Cyclin D1, p21 and p27 contributes to cell proliferation through cell cycle progression from G1 to S/G2M phase in low-dose arsenite exposed HaCat cells. *Front. Pharmacol.* 10:1176. doi: 10.3389/fphar.2019.01176

Codding, J. A., Israel, B. A., and Thorpe, C. (2012). Protein substrate discrimination in the quiescin sulfhydryl oxidase (QSOX) family. *Biochemistry* 51, 4226–4235. doi: 10.1021/bi300394w

Coppock, D. L., and Thorpe, C. (2006). Multidomain flavin-dependent sulfhydryl oxidases. *Antioxid. Redox Signal.* 8, 300–311. doi: 10.1089/ars.2006.8.300

De Roock, W., Claes, B., Bernasconi, D., De Schutter, J., Biesmans, B., Fountzilas, G., et al. (2010). Effects of KRAS, BRAF, NRAS, and PIK3CA mutations on the efficacy of cetuximab plus chemotherapy in chemotherapy-refractory metastatic colorectal cancer: a retrospective consortium analysis. *Lancet Oncol.* 11, 753–762. doi: 10.1016/S1470-2045(10)70130-3

Engeland, K. (2018). Cell cycle arrest through indirect transcriptional repression by p53: i have a DREAM. *Cell Death Differ.* 25, 114–132. doi: 10.1038/cdd.2017.172

Geng, Y., Xu, C., Wang, Y., and Zhang, L. (2020). Quiescin sulfhydryl oxidase 1 regulates the proliferation, migration and invasion of human glioblastoma cells via PI3K/Akt pathway. *Onco Targets Ther.* 13, 5721–5729. doi: 10.2147/OTT.S255941

Hoober, K. L., Glynn, N. M., Burnside, J., Coppock, D. L., and Thorpe, C. (1999). Homology between egg white sulfhydryl oxidase and quiescin Q6 defines a new class of flavin-linked sulfhydryl oxidases. *J. Biol. Chem.* 274, 31759–31762. doi: 10.1074/jbc.274.45.31759

Hou, P. F., Jiang, T., Chen, F., Shi, P. C., Li, H. Q., Bai, J., et al. (2018). KIF4A facilitates cell proliferation via induction of p21-mediated cell cycle progression and promotes metastasis in colorectal cancer. *Cell Death Dis.* 9:477. doi: 10.1038/s41419-018-0550-9

Israel, B. A., Jiang, L., Gannon, S. A., and Thorpe, C. (2014). Disulfide bond generation in mammalian blood serum: detection and purification of quiescin-sulfhydryl oxidase. *Free Radic. Biol. Med.* 69, 129–135. doi: 10.1016/j.freeradbiomed.2014.01.020

Jackstadt, R., van Hooff, S. R., Leach, J. D., Cortes-Lavaud, X., Lohuis, J. O., Ridgway, R. A., et al. (2019). Epithelial NOTCH signaling rewires the tumor microenvironment of colorectal cancer to drive poor-prognosis subtypes and metastasis. *Cancer Cell* 36, 319–336.e7. doi: 10.1016/j.ccell.2019.08.003

Jiang, T., Li, H., Jiang, R., Li, H., Hou, P., Chen, Y., et al. (2018). Pin2/TRF1binding protein X1 inhibits colorectal cancer cell migration and invasion in vitro and metastasis in vivo via the nuclear factorkappaB signaling pathway. *Oncol. Rep.* 40, 1533–1544. doi: 10.3892/or.2018.6570

Kamel, H. F. M., and Al-Amodi, H. (2017). Exploitation of gene expression and cancer biomarkers in paving the path to era of personalized medicine. *Genomics Proteomics Bioinformatics* 15, 220–235. doi: 10.1016/j.gpb.2016.11.005

Katchman, B. A., Antwi, K., Hostetter, G., Demeure, M. J., Watanabe, A., Decker, G. A., et al. (2011). Quiescin sulfhydryl oxidase 1 promotes invasion of pancreatic tumor cells mediated by matrix metalloproteinases. *Mol. Cancer Res.* 9, 1621–1631. doi: 10.1158/1541-7786.MCR-11-0018

Knutsvik, G., Collett, K., Arnes, J., Akslen, L. A., and Stefansson, I. M. (2016). QSOX1 expression is associated with aggressive tumor features and reduced survival in breast carcinomas. *Mod. Pathol.* 29, 1485–1491. doi: 10.1038/modpathol.2016.148

Koncina, E., Haan, S., Rauh, S., and Letellier, E. (2020). Prognostic and predictive molecular biomarkers for colorectal cancer: updates and challenges. *Cancers (Basel)* 12:319. doi: 10.3390/cancers12020319

Lacerenza, S., Ciregia, F., Giusti, L., Bonotti, A., Greco, V., Giannaccini, G., et al. (2020). Putative biomarkers for malignant pleural mesothelioma suggested by proteomic analysis of cell secretome. *Cancer Genomics Proteomics* 17, 225–236. doi: 10.21873/cgp.20183

Li, T., Fu, J., Zeng, Z., Cohen, D., Li, J., Chen, Q., et al. (2020). TIMER2.0 for analysis of tumor-infiltrating immune cells. *Nucleic Acids Res.* 48, W509–W514. doi: 10.1093/nar/gkaa407

Liu, X., Bing, Z., Wu, J., Zhang, J., Zhou, W., Ni, M., et al. (2020). Integrative gene expression profiling analysis to investigate potential prognostic biomarkers for colorectal cancer. *Med. Sci. Monit.* 26:e918906. doi: 10.12659/MSM.918906

Long, N. P., Park, S., Anh, N. H., Nghi, T. D., Yoon, S. J., Park, J. H., et al. (2019). High-throughput omics and statistical learning integration for the discovery and validation of novel diagnostic signatures in colorectal cancer. *Int. J. Mol. Sci.* 20:296. doi: 10.3390/ijms20020296

Nair, M., Sandhu, S. S., and Sharma, A. K. (2014). Prognostic and predictive biomarkers in cancer. *Curr. Cancer Drug Targets* 14, 477–504. doi: 10.2174/1568009614666140506111118

Nguyen, L. H., Goel, A., and Chung, D. C. (2020). Pathways of colorectal carcinogenesis. *Gastroenterology* 158, 291–302. doi: 10.1053/j.gastro.2019.08.059

Otto, T., and Sicinski, P. (2017). Cell cycle proteins as promising targets in cancer therapy. *Nat. Rev. Cancer* 17, 93–115. doi: 10.1038/nrc.2016.138

Provenzale, D., Ness, R. M., Llor, X., Weiss, J. M., Abbadessa, B., Cooper, G., et al. (2020). NCCN guidelines insights: colorectal cancer screening, version 2.2020. *J. Natl. Compr. Canc. Netw.* 18, 1312–1320. doi: 10.6004/jnccn.2020.0048

Sepulveda, A. R., Hamilton, S. R., Allegra, C. J., Grody, W., Cushman-Vokoun, A. M., Funkhouser, W. K., et al. (2017). Molecular biomarkers for the evaluation of colorectal cancer: guideline from the American Society for Clinical Pathology, College of American Pathologists, Association for Molecular Pathology, and American Society of Clinical Oncology. *J. Mol. Diagn.* 19, 187–225. doi: 10.1016/j.jmoldx.2016.11.001

Siegel, R. L., Miller, K. D., Fuchs, H. E., and Jemal, A. (2021). Cancer statistics, 2021. *CA Cancer J. Clin.* 71, 7–33. doi: 10.3322/caac.21654

Subramanian, A., Kuehn, H., Gould, J., Tamayo, P., and Mesirov, J. P. (2007). GSEA-P: a desktop application for gene set enrichment analysis. *Bioinformatics* 23, 3251–3253. doi: 10.1093/bioinformatics/btm369

Sung, H. J., Ahn, J. M., Yoon, Y. H., Na, S. S., Choi, Y. J., Kim, Y. I., et al. (2018). Quiescin sulfhydryl oxidase 1 (QSOX1) secreted by lung cancer cells promotes cancer metastasis. *Int. J. Mol. Sci.* 19:3213. doi: 10.3390/ijms19103213

Sung, H., Ferlay, J., Siegel, R. L., Laversanne, M., Soerjomataram, I., Jemal, A., et al. (2021). Global cancer statistics 2020: GLOBOCAN estimates of incidence and mortality worldwide for 36 cancers in 185 countries. *CA Cancer J. Clin.* 71, 209–249. doi: 10.3322/caac.21660

Tang, Z., Li, C., Kang, B., Gao, G., Li, C., and Zhang, Z. (2017). GEPIA: a web server for cancer and normal gene expression profiling and interactive analyses. *Nucleic Acids Res.* 45, W98–W102. doi: 10.1093/nar/gkx247

Tyagi, A., Sharma, A. K., and Damodaran, C. (2020). A review on notch signaling and colorectal cancer. *Cells* 9:1549. doi: 10.3390/cells9061549

Vinson, K. E., George, D. C., Fender, A. W., Bertrand, F. E., and Sigounas, G. (2016). The Notch pathway in colorectal cancer. *Int. J. Cancer* 138, 1835–1842. doi: 10.1002/ijc.29800

Vogelstein, B., Lane, D., and Levine, A. J. (2000). Surfing the p53 network. *Nature* 408, 307–310. doi: 10.1038/35042675

Wang, T. E., Li, S. H., Minabe, S., Anderson, A. L., Dun, M. D., Maeda, K. I., et al. (2018). Mouse quiescin sulfhydryl oxidases exhibit distinct epididymal luminal distribution with segment-specific sperm surface associations. *Biol. Reprod.* 99, 1022–1033. doi: 10.1093/biolre/ioy125

Wang, X. W., and Zhang, Y. J. (2014). Targeting mTOR network in colorectal cancer therapy. *World J. Gastroenterol.* 20, 4178–4188. doi: 10.3748/wjg.v20.i15.4178

Zhai, Z., Yu, X., Yang, B., Zhang, Y., Zhang, L., Li, X., et al. (2017). Colorectal cancer heterogeneity and targeted therapy: clinical implications, challenges and solutions for treatment resistance. *Semin. Cell Dev. Biol.* 64, 107–115. doi: 10.1016/j.semcdb.2016.08.033

4

Overexpression of PLXDC2 in Stromal Cell-Associated M2 Macrophages is Related to EMT and the Progression of Gastric Cancer

Yiming Guan[1†], Yuzhang Du[1†], Guanzheng Wang[1], Hongquan Gou[1], Yilun Xue[1], Jingsong Xu[1], Enhao Li[1], David W. Chan[2], Di Wu[1], Peiqing Xu[1], Peihua Ni[1], Dakang Xu[1] and Yiqun Hu[1*]*

[1] Faculty of Medical Laboratory Science, Ruijin Hospital, School of Medicine, Shanghai Jiao Tong University, Shanghai, China,
[2] Department of Obstetrics and Gynaecology, LKS Faculty of Medicine, The University of Hong Kong, Hong Kong, China

***Correspondence:**
Yiqun Hu
ichunhu@126.com
Dakang Xu
dakang_xu@163.com

† These authors have contributed equally to this work

The tumor microenvironment (TME) comprises distinct cell types, including stromal types such as fibroblast cells and macrophage cells, which have recently become a critical factor in tumor development and progression. Here, we identified the TME-related gene, plexin domain containing 2 (PLXDC2), in a high-stromal-score population. And we revealed that this gene was related to poor survival and advanced (tumor-node-metastasis) stage in gastric cancer (GC) patients from The Cancer Genome Atlas database. An integrated gene profile and functional analysis of the proportions of tumor-infiltrating immune cells revealed that the expression of the M2 macrophages cell marker CD163 was positively correlated with PLXDC2 expression. In addition, the M2 macrophages gene signature and high PLXDC2 expression were associated with the inflammatory signaling pathway and the epithelial-to-mesenchymal transition (EMT)-related gene signature. Single-cell study of GC identified PLXDC2 was enriched specifically in fibroblasts and monocytes/macrophages populations, which supported its important role in the stroma. Furthermore, according to a tissue microarray immunohistochemistry analysis, the expression of PLXDC2 elevated in human GC stromal specimens compared to tumor tissue specimens. Moreover, PLXDC2 overexpression in the stromal compartment was associated with CD163-positive regulatory M2 macrophages, and its functions were related to the pathogenesis of GC. Multiplexed immunohistochemistry verified PLXDC2's correlation with EMT markers. Our data suggested that PLXDC2 was expressed in stromal cells and that its crosstalk with tumor-associated macrophages could contribute to cancer biology by inducing the EMT process.

Keywords: tumor-associated M2 macrophages, gastric cancer, plexin domain containing 2 (PLXDC2), stroma, EMT

INTRODUCTION

Gastric cancer (GC) is one of the major causes of cancer-related mortality worldwide. It has been reported that 1.0337 million new GC cases and approximately 783,000 GC- related deaths occurred in 2018 (Bray et al., 2018; Siegel et al., 2021). This may be attributed to the high *Helicobacter pylori* (HP) infection rate (Hatakeyama, 2019; Kotilea et al., 2019). In total, around 679,000 new GC cases and 498,000 GC-related deaths occur each year in China; these values are second only to those of lung cancer, indicating that GC is a major health issue (Chen et al., 2016; Zong et al., 2016). Although recent studies have proposed new treatment strategies based on disease risk stratification [tumor-node-metastasis (TNM) stage] and histological grade according to tumor size, lymph node or distant metastasis (also AJCC system, *T* describes the size of the original tumor and whether it has invaded nearby tissue, *N* describes nearby lymph nodes that are involved, and *M* describes distant metastasis; Edge and Compton, 2010), the ability of these strategies to improve the prognosis of GC patients has been widely questioned. Further studies on the diagnosis and treatment of this type of malignancy are required. Molecular diagnosis has been previously proven to be effective. Discoveries of biomarkers, such as ERBB2 and EGFR, aid in informed treatment decision making by medical oncologists (Yasui et al., 2001). Innovations related to molecular biomarkers are likely to improve the prognosis and treatment response of GC patients. Thus, a study seeking novel GC molecular biomarkers might offer a solution to our current challenges.

Alteration of the tumor microenvironment (TME) has been proven to be a pivotal strategy for improving GC prognosis (Wu and Dai, 2017). Studies have shown that TME influences the therapeutic response and clinical outcome. A recent comprehensive analysis of the TME of GC, comprising 1524 GC samples, depicted the landscape of GC's TME characteristics. The results proved that the TME of GC patients could help predict the response to immunotherapies and provide new strategies for treating GC (Zeng et al., 2019). The non-tumor components of TME, including borders, extracellular matrix (ECM), stromal cells, blood vessels, lymph vessels, and immune/inflammatory cells, have been recognized as affecting GC patients' prognosis. By dynamically interacting with tumor cells, stromal cells participate in all stages of tumorigenesis, progression, metastasis, recurrence and drug response, thereby affecting the fate of patients. In the process of tumor evolution and metastasis, the stromal cells in TME have also undergone some changes and played a role in the inhibition and promotion of metastasis, and the overall function of stromal cells is conducive to survival and migration of cancer cells. Immune-related cells also play a decisive role in cell fate. Tumor suppressive immune cells, such as $CD8^+$ T cells, and tumor progressive immune cells, such as regulatory T cells, are directly connected to tumor growth. Among all types of immune cells of different functions, T cells and macrophages, are most abundant in the TME. T cells' mechanisms of cytotoxicity have been explored in numerous studies, whereas the behavior patterns of macrophages are less well understood. Therefore, a macrophages- related TME study of GC has the potential to provide novel insight into this malignancy.

Macrophages, which are believed to be an essential type of immune cell during inflammation, can both promote and suppress tumor growth (Lewis and Pollard, 2006; Szebeni et al., 2017). M1 macrophages have been labeled as antitumor factors, whereas M2 macrophages have been identified as protumor factors (Yunna et al., 2020). Persuasive evidence at both clinical and experimental levels indicates that M2 macrophages can promote cancer initiation and malignant progression (Jackaman et al., 2017). Nevertheless, the complexity of immune cell behaviors led us to ambiguity in macrophages M2-related characteristics. Although previous studies have explored the immune-related functions of M2 macrophages, few explorations have tried to determine whether M2 macrophages can affect tumor growth by other crucial mechanisms, including Epithelial-to-mesenchymal transition (EMT) or angiogenesis. Clarifying this particular immune cell type's behaviors might aid in improving the prognosis of tumors such as GC.

Epithelial-to-mesenchymal transition has been proven to be a survival-related program (Zhang and Weinberg, 2018). Its function of increasing the motility or invasiveness of cancer cells suggests its involvement in metastasis, which contributes to high mortality rates among cancer patients (Pastushenko and Blanpain, 2019). EMT is a cell biological program that transforms epithelial cells to more mesenchymal cell-like cells. In a sense, the occurrence of EMT indicates the malignant process of tumors. Decreased expression of E-cadherin and cytokeratin and increased expression of N-cadherin, Twist and Zeb1 is a common EMT program signature (Krebs et al., 2017). Studies on EMT are required to better understand cancer metastasis and to gain control over this process that increases malignant potential.

Plexin domain containing 2 (PLXDC2), also known as TEM7R, is a member of the tumor endothelial marker (TEM) family, which is associated with tumor-specific angiogenesis. PLXDC2 has been identified as a regulator of several brain activities, including the coordinated control of proliferation and cell fate specification along and across the neuroaxis (Miller-Delaney et al., 2011). Studies of PLXDC2 and its closest homolog, PLXDC1, have been conducted in cancers, including breast cancer, colorectal cancer, and typical liver cancer types. They are recognized as possible targets of treatment and have certain prognostic value (Nanda et al., 2004; Rmali et al., 2005; Yamamoto et al., 2020). However, none of the previous studies examined the linkage between PLXDC2 and GC. While PLXDC2 demonstrates a clear linkage with stroma-related behaviors, the relationship between PLXDC2 and the EMT program remains unknown; however, clarification of this relationship could provide a potential breakthrough in terms of GC prognosis.

In the current study, we utilized the accessible GC patient data from The Cancer Genome Atlas (TCGA) stomach adenocarcinoma (STAD) dataset alongside an additional Gene Expression Omnibus (GEO) GSE84437 GC dataset. The ESTIMATE algorithm was used to explore stromal and immune characteristics, and PLXDC2, a gene not previously studied in the context of GC, was identified to be related to the disease. Further studies on this gene were conducted. Gene Set Enrichment Analysis (GSEA) and the novel tool CIBERSORTx provided clear evidence that PLXDC2 affects the EMT program and inflammatory response and is linked to protumor M2 macrophages. An integration of Single-cell analysis and IHC study provided solid evidence that PLXDC2 upregulation in stroma-related cells contribute to poor survival. The utilization of multiplexed immunohistochemistry (mIHC) verified PLXDC2's correlation with EMT markers. Thus, the PLXDC2/EMT/M2 macrophages axis was established.

MATERIALS AND METHODS

Data Acquisition

RNA-seq data of 375 GC samples and 32 matched non-cancerous samples were downloaded from TCGA. Clinical data, including age, sex, tumor grade, clinical stage, TNM stage, and survival time, were also downloaded. Data extraction was conducted with R software 4.0.3 (R Foundation for Statistical Computing, Vienna, Austria). A subsidiary GC tissue dataset was downloaded from the GEO. The GSE84437 dataset (Yoon et al., 2020), containing Illumina HumanHT-12 V3.0 beadchip microarray expression series matrix files based on the GPL6947 platform, was selected. The Single-Cell RNA samples used in this study were from a previous single cell analysis study of GC[1] (Sathe et al., 2020).

Analysis of the Immune Score and Stromal Score of the TME

ESTIMATE[2] (Yoshihara et al., 2013) is a well-established algorithm that generates immune and stromal scores based on RNA-seq data. A high score indicates a large proportion of the corresponding component in the TME. In this research, the ESTIMATE algorithm was employed via the "estimate" package 1.0.13 of R software.

Analysis of the Correlation Between Survival and Immune/Stromal Score

A total of 371 TCGA tumor samples and 433 GEO tumor samples were adequate for survival analysis. Kaplan–Meier plots of patients from datasets grouped by both stromal score and immune score were generated via GraphPad Prism 8.0 software with log-rank $p < 0.05$ as the indicator of statistical significance.

Identifying Differentially Expressed Genes Between High- and Low-Immune/Stromal Score Groups

Samples from the TCGA and GEO datasets were sorted into high score groups and low score groups according to the median immune score and stromal score. "limma" package 3.44.3 (Ritchie et al., 2015) of the Bioconductor project (Huber et al., 2015) was then utilized to determine the differences in gene expression between the high score group and the low score group. Genes with a $|\log2(\text{fold change})| > 1$ and a false discovery rate (FDR) < 0.05 were considered significantly differentially expressed and were selected for subsequent analysis. Heatmaps of differentially expressed genes (DEGs) were then generated via the "pheatmap" package 1.0.12.

Analysis of the Correlation of Stromal Score With Clinical Stage

The correlation of the stromal score with the clinicopathological characteristics in the TCGA dataset was explored via GraphPad Prism software. One-way ANOVA (Analysis of Variance) was conducted, and statistical significance was indicated by a p value less than 0.05.

Cox Regression Analysis

The "survival" package 3.2-7 of R software was used for univariate Cox regression analysis of the TCGA samples. Genes that passed the univariate Cox test are shown in the plot.

Exploring DEGs and Their Correlations With Survival

The second version of Gene Expression Profiling Interactive Analysis (GEPIA2)[3] (Tang et al., 2019) was utilized to determine the differences in expression between tumor samples and normal gastric samples from the TCGA and Genotype-Tissue Expression (GTEx) databases. A Kaplan–Meier survival plot was also generated via Kaplan–Meier Plotter[4] (Szasz et al., 2016) using GC gene chip data. A receiver operating characteristic (ROC) curve was generated via the "survival ROC" R package 1.0.3.

Gene Set Enrichment Analysis

Gene Set Enrichment Analysis was performed to investigate whether there were significant differences in the expression of the identified genes between the two groups. Hallmark gene sets v7.2 were downloaded as the target sets, and GSEA (Subramanian et al., 2005) was performed using GSEA_4.0.3 software. The nominal (NOM) p value, FDR and normalized enrichment score (NES) were used to identify the pathways enriched in each phenotype. Gene sets with NOM $p < 0.05$ and FDR $q < 0.06$ were considered significant.

Identifying Immune Cell Profiles

The novel CIBERSORTx[5](Steen et al., 2020) computational method was applied to estimate all tumor samples' tumor-infiltrating immune cells (TICs) abundance profiles. In total, 289 samples passed the significance test. Survival and correlation analysis were conducted via TIMER 2.0[6].

Single-Cell Analysis

The Single-Cell RNA Sequencing (scRNA-seq) samples in this study were downloaded from https://dna-discovery.stanford.edu/research/datasets/. We used filtered output of Cellranger from scRNA-seq of GC, which consists of 8 patients' cells from GC, paired normal tissue, and PBMCs (Sathe et al., 2020). All samples were input in Seurat V3, and a total of (43147/56167) cells were obtained after a restrict quality control (number of detected gene > 200, log10 Gene per nUMI > 0.8, percentage of mitochondrial genes $< 20\%$; Stuart et al., 2019). We removed potential doublets cells by

[1]https://dna-discovery.stanford.edu/research/datasets/

[2]https://bioinformatics.mdanderson.org/estimate/

[3]http://gepia2.cancer-pku.cn/#index

[4]http://www.kmplot.com/analysis/

[5]https://cibersortx.stanford.edu

[6]http://timer.cistrome.org

DoubletFinder in default, and assuming doublet formation rate was based on Single Cell 3' Reagent Kits v2 User Guide[7] (McGinnis et al., 2019). After "NormalizeData," different samples were merged by "IntegrateData" workflow and IKAP were used to scale (batch, nUMI and percentage of mitochondrial genes), to determine nPCs (PC18K11) and to visualize in UMAP (Chen et al., 2019). NK cells and B cells were next distinguished from first determined immune cells. "FindAllMarkers" function was set (min.pct = 0.25, logfc.threshold = 1, and tes.use = "wilcox") to find markers of all cell types. Dot plot were plotted by "Dotplot" function, and Violin plot were plotted by "Vlnplot" function.

Pathology Analysis

Tissue microarrays (TMAs) containing 90 human GC and adjacent non-tumorous specimens were obtained from the Ruijin Hospital, School of Medicine, Shanghai Jiao Tong University from April 2008 to October 2009. All the protocols using human specimens were approved by the Ethics Committee of Shanghai Jiao Tong University. The slide was deparaffinized, rehydrated and microwaved-heated. Primary antibody, CD163, was incubated at RT for 30 min. Nuclei were stained with hematoxylin, cytoplasm with eosin. A pathologist identified the interface of tumor and stromal tissue. Image recognition for tissue-component segmentation of tumor cells and stroma regions based on spectral channel was conducted with inForm (Akoya Biosciences, Marlborough, United States). The expression levels of target proteins in tissue were examined by a pathologist blinded to the patients' clinical characteristics. According to the fluorescence intensity threshold, the positive degree was divided into 0 (negative), 1, 2, and 3 (threshold criteria: 0.0625, 0.1250, 0.1875, and 0.2500). Images were acquired with a Vectra microscope.

Multiplexed Immunohistochemistry and Immunofluorescence Analysis

Paraffin sections were dewaxed with xylene and gradient ethanol solution. Endogenous peroxidase blocking solution (Beyotime, Shanghai, China) was used for peroxidase blocking, and the blocking/antibody (Panovue, Beijing, China) was used for unrelated antibody blocking. The primary antibodies included anti-PLXDC2 (12285-1-AP, Proteintech, Chicago, United States), anti-E-Cadherin (ab76011, Abcam, Cambridge, United Kingdom), and anti-Vimentin (ab92547, Abcam, Cambridge, United Kingdom). Opal 4-color manual IHC kit (Akoya biosciences, MA, United States) was used for mIHC. The Vectra Polaris (PerkinElmer, Spokane, WA, United States) was used to capture the staining image. The inform software (Akoya Biosciences, Marlborough, United States) was used for data analyzing. PLXDC2 High Expression Region was defined as the region which had at least 95 percent of PLXDC2 positive cells. PLXDC2 Low Expression Region was defined as the region which has at most 5 percent of PLXDC2 positive cells. The percentage of PLXDC2, E-Cadherin and Vimentin positive cells was calculated as the number of positive cells divided by the total number of DAPI-positive cells. To quantify the expression levels, ten different fields were selected for the calculation.

Statistical Analyses

All statistical analyses were performed in R software (version 4.0.3) and GraphPad Prism 8 software. The threshold for statistical significance for all statistical tests was $p < 0.05$. The log-rank test was utilized to assess significance for Kaplan–Meier survival analysis.

RESULTS

Identification of Key Regulated Genes in GC Through the ESTIMATE Algorithm

In hopes of discovering novel regulators in GC, data including 407 samples from the TCGA STAD dataset and 433 samples from the GSE84437 dataset were downloaded and organized into two files. The ESTIMATE algorithm was conducted, and independent stromal scores and immune scores were generated. Common DEGs from the high/low immune score and stromal score comparisons were then analyzed with univariate Cox regression. Survival-related genes that were expressed differently in tumor and stromal samples were then discovered. We focused on PLXDC2, a gene that was not previously linked with GC. GSEA and CIBERSORTx analysis were conducted sequentially and proved that PLXDC2 was associated with immunity and the EMT process. Our results were ultimately confirmed with Single-Cell analysis and TMA study. The analytical procedure for the study is shown in **Supplementary Figure 1**.

An Elevated Stromal Score Is Significantly Correlated With Advanced Clinicopathological Indicators and a Poor Prognosis

To establish the linkage between estimated scores and the overall survival rate, Kaplan–Meier plots were generated. Higher respective scores indicated larger amounts of the immune or stromal components in the TME. Both datasets' plots suggested a favorable prognosis for patients with low stromal scores, as shown in **Figures 1A–D**, which implied that GC stromal score is an independent prognostic indicator. A further linkage between stromal scores and the clinicopathological characteristics of GC patients was then explored. As the GEO dataset GSE84437 included limited clinicopathological data, analyses were only conducted with TCGA STAD samples. As shown in **Figures 1E–H**, the GC stromal score was positively correlated with several GC classifications, including tumor grade ($p < 0.0001$), clinical stage ($p = 0.0009$), and T classification of the TNM stage ($p < 0.0001$), which implied that stromal scores are associated with GC progression. The results above suggested that a high stromal score is correlated with advanced

[7] https://www.10xgenomics.com/products/single-cell-gene-expression

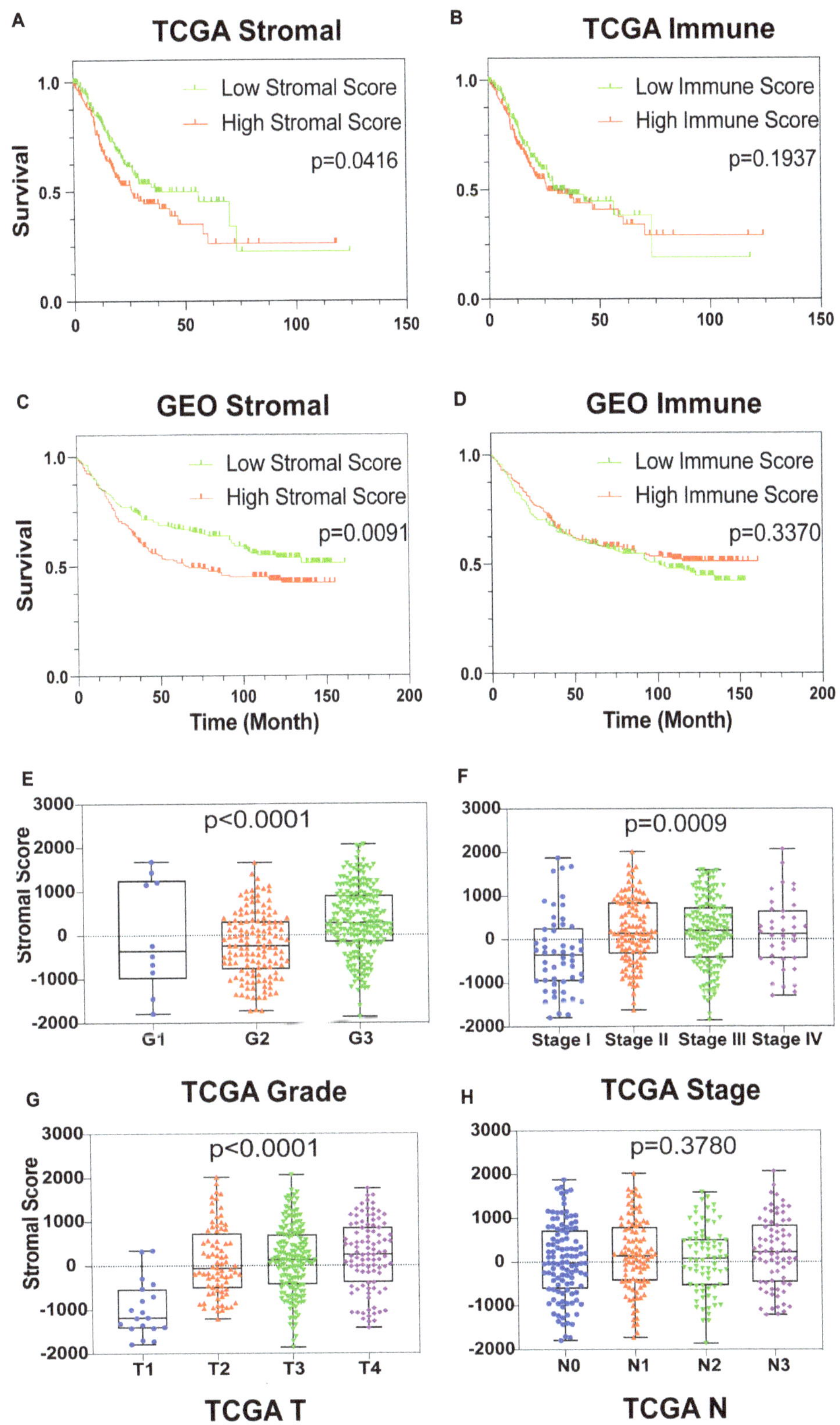

FIGURE 1 | Identification of GC Stromal Scores' linkage with prognosis and clinicopathology. **(A–D)** Kaplan–Meier survival analysis of TCGA STAD patients and GEO GSE84437 patients grouped by immune score and stromal score. The red line indicates the high ESTIMATE score group, and the green line indicates the low ESTIMATE score group. **(E–H)** The relationship between the TCGA ESTIMATE stromal score and tumor grade, clinical stage, *T* stage and *N* stage. Each dot signifies the stromal score in a sample.

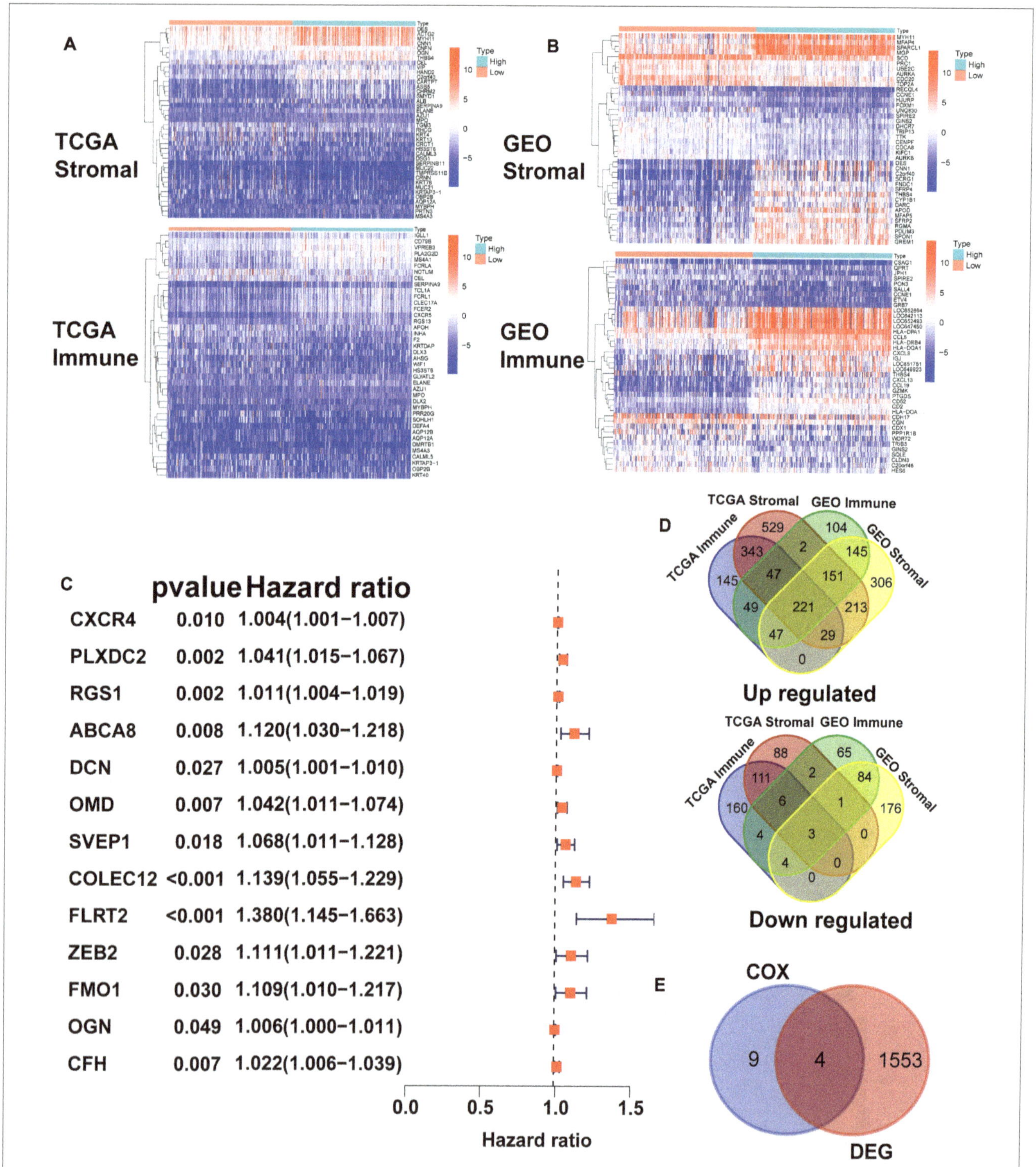

FIGURE 2 | Identification of prognostic gene markers according to patients' stromal and immune scores. **(A)** Heatmaps of the top 20 DEGs generated by comparing the high stromal/immune score group and the low stromal/immune score groups of TCGA STAD patients. The heatmaps' row name is the gene name, and the ID of the samples is the column name, which is not shown in the plot. DEGs were determined by the Wilcoxon rank sum test with $q = 0.05$ and | fold change| (FC) > 1 after $\log_2$ transformation as the thresholds for significance. **(B)** Heatmaps of DEGs in GEO patients, similar to **(A)**. **(C)** Venn plots generated via an online tool (http://bioinformatics.psb.ugent.be/webtools/Venn/) depicting the up-regulated and down-regulated DEGs shared by the TCGA STAD and GEO datasets. **(D)** Forest plot of Cox regression (with 95% confidence interval), which was conducted with the 224 DEGs. **(E)** Venn plot depicting genes that were both related to survival and differentially expressed between tumor samples and normal samples.

clinicopathological indicators and therefore is an adverse prognostic factor.

Identification of PLXDC2 as a Key Regulator That Promotes GC Progression

After identifying the prognostic value of the stromal scores, key genes of TME associated with survival were selected. A comparison analysis between the high score group and low score group of both datasets was first carried out. A total of 224 DEGs were screened out, including 221 up-regulated and 3 down-regulated genes. Heatmaps and Venn plots were generated to demonstrate the process (**Figures 2A,B,D**). The selected 224 genes were then assessed by univariate Cox regression analysis, which identified 13 genes related to survival (**Figure 2C**). The genes finally overlapped with genes that exhibited expression differences in STAD tumor samples and normal samples. The genes with an absolute log2(fold change) value threshold of 1.6, calculated with the limma plot, were selected. This method identified four genes, namely, CXCR4, PLXDC2, ABCA8, and RGS1, identified by this method (**Figure 2E**). Although ABCA8 is a DEG with survival correlation, its connection was not coordinative with survival rates, as it suggests higher expression in cancer than normal while indicating better prognosis, the gene was eliminated. The three genes screened above were then examined via different methods. Given that previous studies have recognized CXCR4 and RGS1 as prognostic markers of GC, we focused our research on PLXDC2, a gene that was not previously discovered as a GC marker. Differential expression of PLXDC2 in tumor and normal samples were first demonstrated in **Figure 3A**, using the GEPIA2 webtool, which combined the TCGA STAD samples with the GTEx normal samples. The Kaplan–Meier survival plot is presented in **Figure 3B** ($p = 0.0373$). An additional Kaplan–Meier plot of patient survival based on PLXDC2 expression was then generated via the Kaplan–Meier Plotter webtool (see text footnote 4) using the mRNA gene chip data of GC ($p < 0.0001$), and the results supported the prognostic value of PLXDC2 (**Figure 3C**). A ROC curve for PLXDC2 was obtained (**Figure 3D**). The area under the curve (AUC) represents the set of all possible statistical tests of the microarray data with equal probability for a true positive and a false positive result based on each decision threshold value. The plot suggested PLXDC2 as a preferrable gene marker for indicating GC prognosis. Further correlations between PLXDC2 expression and the clinicopathological characteristics of GC patients are shown in **Figures 3E–H**, indicating that PLXDC2 was positively correlated with several GC classifications, namely, tumor grade ($p < 0.0001$), clinical stage ($p = 0.0370$), and T classification of TNM stages ($p = 0.0018$). These results

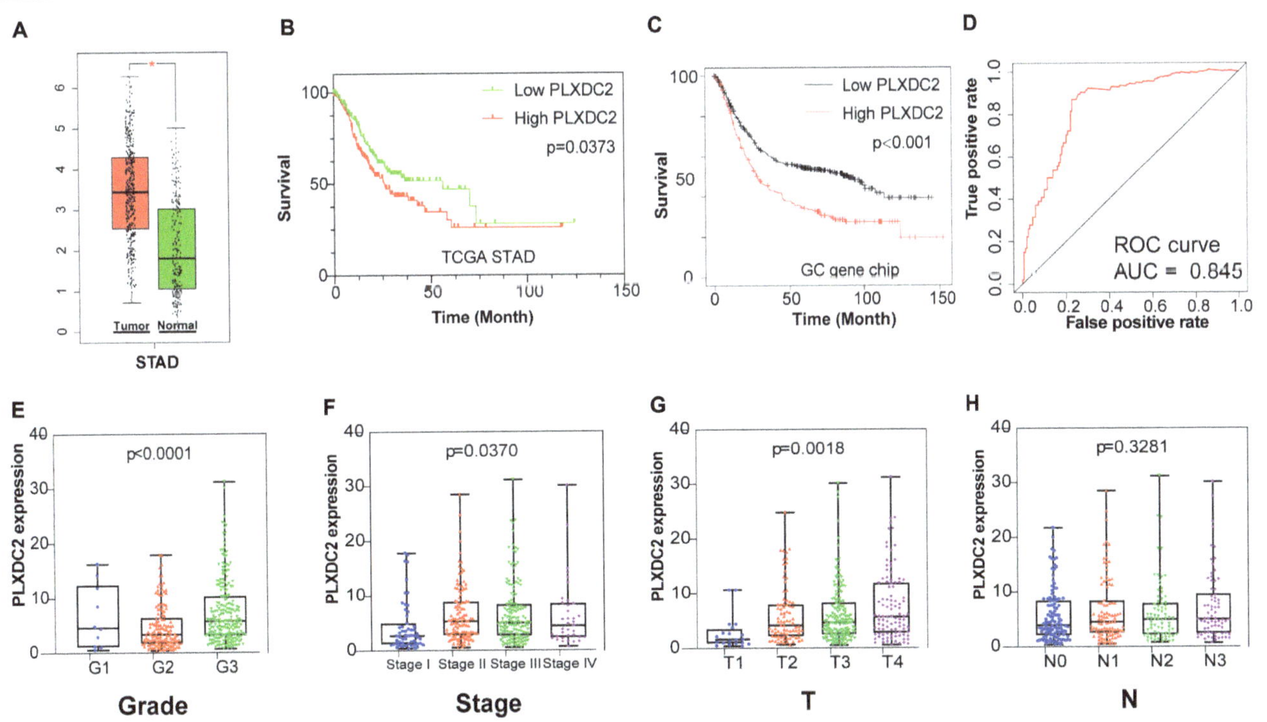

FIGURE 3 | PLXDC2 is a DEG capable of propelling GC progress. **(A)** Differential expression of PLXDC2 in normal and tumor samples generated by GEPIA2. Analyses were performed across normal and tumor samples of TCGA STAD alongside GTEx normal samples. **(B)** Survival analysis of TCGA STAD patients with different PLXDC2 expression levels. Patients were sorted into high expression or low expression groups according to the median expression level ($p = 0.0373$ by log-rank test). **(C)** Survival curves of GC patients generated by Kaplan–Meier Plotter ($p < 0.0001$ by log-rank test). **(D)** ROC curve for PLXDC2. An AUC close to 1 suggests high reliability. **(E–H)** The relationship between PLXDC2 expression and tumor grade, clinical stage, *T* stage and *N* stage. Each dot signifies the PLXDC2 expression level in a sample.

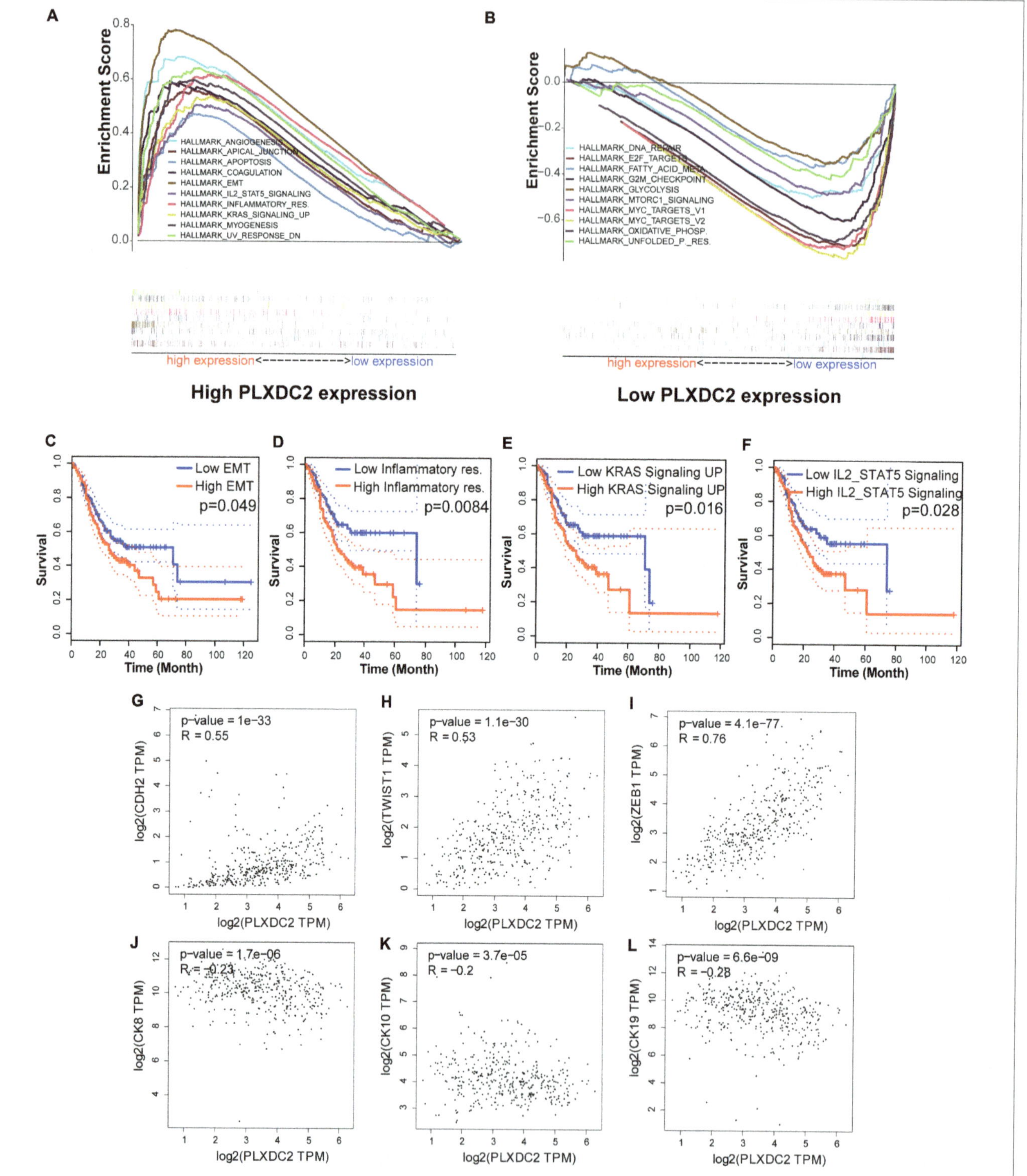

FIGURE 4 | PLXDC2 is relevant to EMT and several immune-related pathways. **(A)** Up-regulated HALLMARK pathways in samples with high PLXDC2 expression. Particular gene sets are represented with lines of unique color, and up-regulated genes are located on the left approaching the origin of the coordinates, while the down-regulated genes are on the right of the *x*-axis. Only gene sets with NOM $p < 0.05$ and FDR $q < 0.06$ were considered significant. Several leading gene sets are displayed in the plot. **(B)** Down-regulated HALLMARK pathways in samples with low PLXDC2 expression, similar to **(A)**. **(C–F)** Kaplan–Meier plots according to the expression of DEGs within the top 10 up-regulated pathways. EMT and 3 other pathways, namely, inflammatory response, IL2-STAT5 signaling and KRAS signaling (up), were proven to be related to survival. **(G–L)** The correlation scatterplots of PLXDC2 and EMT markers. CDH2 (N-cadherin), TWIST1 and ZEB1 are up-regulated EMT markers, while CK8, CK10, and CK19 (three E- cadherin genes) are down-regulated EMT markers.

provide solid evidence that PLXDC2 acts as a key regulator and stimulates GC progression.

PLXDC2 Expression Was Correlated With EMT and Inflammatory Signaling Pathways

As the PLXDC2 expression level was correlated with survival time and clinicopathological characteristics, an additional GSEA was conducted to explore its relationship with HALLMARK pathways to reveal the cellular functions of PLXDC2. The samples were separates into a high expression group and a low expression group according to the median expression level of PLXDC2. 10 up-regulated pathways and 10 down-regulated pathways were then obtained. Among them, EMT was the most correlated pathway (**Figures 4A,B**). Survival analyses were then conducted according to the expression of DEGs in the top 10 up-regulated pathways. EMT along with three correlated immune pathways, namely, inflammatory response, IL2-STAT5 signaling and KRAS signaling (up), were identified to be survival related (**Figures 4C–F**), which supported the role of PLXDC2 as a gene affecting inflammatory signaling. Additional analysis was performed to study the correlation of PLXDC2 and classic EMT markers by generating correlation scatterplots, and the results were coordinate with GSEA results. The up-regulated EMT markers displayed positive correlation with PLXDC2, while its down-regulated counterpart exhibited otherwise, with a negative correlation (**Figures 4G–L**). These results confirmed the function of PLXDC2 in regulating EMT and inflammation.

M2 Macrophages Gene Signatures Were Positively Associated With PLXDC2 Expression

We explored the correlation of PLXDC2 expression with the proportion of TICs subsets. The novel CIBERSORTx algorithm was applied to generate the profiles of 22 kinds of immune cells in STAD samples. STAD samples were grouped according to the median PLXDC2 expression level, and a violin plot was generated (**Figure 5A**). Within the 22 kinds of TICs, 5 of them were discovered as most differentially expressed ($p < 0.001$). According to the result of CIBERSORTx, the cell fractions of both T cells CD8 and Tregs are more pronounced in low PLXDC2 expression group compared to high PLXDC2 expression group, which might suggest that patients with high PLXDC2 have some suppress function to the subset T cell competent. Those results are consistent with our finding of PLXDC2 promoted CD163 M2 macrophages and our GSEA results. Those subset macrophages might trigger inflammation resolution and suppress T cell population or activation via several mechanisms (Noy and Pollard, 2014). The Tumor Immune Estimation Resource (TIMER)[8] web tool was utilized for further exploration of the correlation between PLXDC2 and GC patients' immune cells (Li et al., 2016, 2020). The results demonstrated that macrophages exhibited the highest correlation with PLXDC2 expression and survival rate among the cell types (**Figure 5B** and **Supplementary Figure 2**). The correlations between PLXDC2 and macrophages subtypes were also assessed (**Figure 5C**). Among the subtypes, M2 macrophages had the highest correlation, with a larger R value and a smaller p value. The correlation of PLXDC2 with macrophages M2 immune markers was demonstrated using the data of the "Gene-Corr" module of TIMER 2.0 (see text footnote 6; **Figure 5D**). These results provide solid evidence proving that the PLXDC2 expression level was closely associated with a particular immune cell type (M2 macrophages).

Identification of PLXDC2 Upregulation in Fibroblasts and Macrophages

New efforts in single-cell profiling will enable a better understanding of the microenvironment composition in GC development. To better understand PLXDC2 expression pattern in the TME, we utilized a single-cell RNA sequence of GC. The process of the single cell analysis was demonstrated in **Figures 6A,B** with a Uniform Manifold Approximation and Projection (UMAP) and a bubble blot that displayed the cell markers of each cell type. The expression level of PLXDC2 in a single cell study is illustrated in **Figures 6C,D**. The UMAP and violin plots indicated that PLXDC2 upregulates in fibroblasts and monocytes/macrophages via unique gene markers of each cell type. Comparison of PLXDC2 expression level in different samples (metaplasia, normal, PBMC, and tumor) was established, and the result showed that PLXDC2 scarcely express in the normal sample, while upregulating in PBMC and tumor samples in both macrophages and fibroblasts, and metaplasia in macrophages (**Figures 6E,F**). The results revealed that PLXDC2 might be of certain significance inside a stromal environment and contribute to metaplasia in macrophages.

Validation of the Correlations of PLXDC2 Expression and Metastatic Index and Its Prognostic Value

To further study the potential clinical relevance of PLXDC2 expression in tumor progression, we made use of 67 TMA with adequate PLXDC2 and CD163 staining effect of GC patient samples to compare the expression of PLXDC2 between GC tumor tissues and stromal tissues. PLXDC2 staining was more intense in the cytoplasm than in the nucleus. The whole slide photo of the TMA and staining of CD163 is attached in **Supplementary Figures 3**, **4**. Higher PLXDC2 expression was observed in GC stromal tissues than in tumor tissues within 52 cases, the number of which is after the removal of films with poor dyeing quality (**Figures 7A–C**). The comparisons of PLXDC2 expression of lymphatic metastasis (high vs. low, N1-N3b of AJCC are considered to have metastasis, N0 is considered to have no metastasis) and proportion of positive lymph node (>50% vs. <50%, within the total lymph nodes removed during operation), according to the unpaired t test results, showed no significant difference (**Figures 7D,E**). The level of tumor invasion (T4-T4b of AJCC was considered to be of level of invasion, and T0-T3 was considered to be of low level of invasion, T4 is the demarcation point between whether the tumor invades the

[8]https://cistrome.shinyapps.io/timer/

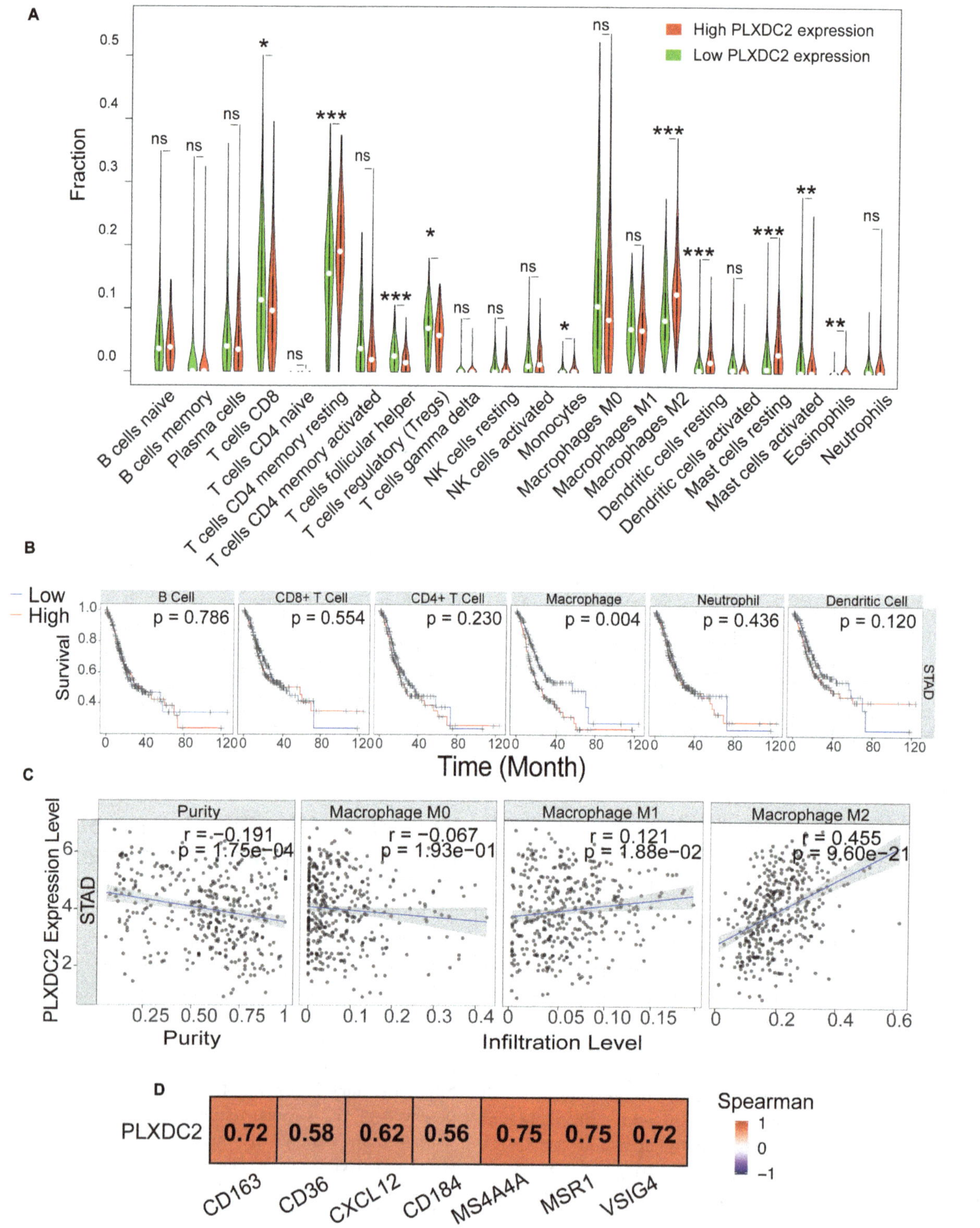

FIGURE 5 | The correlation of PLXDC2 correlation with M2 macrophages and gene markers. **(A)** The ratio differentiation of 22 kinds of immune cells between TCGA STAD tumor samples with high or low PLXDC2 expression relative to the median PLXDC2 expression level; the Wilcoxon rank sum test was used as the significance test. "ns" represents $p > 0.05$, * represents $0.05 > p > 0.01$, ** represents $0.01 > p > 0.001$, and *** represents $p < 0.001$. **(B)** Kaplan–Meier plots according to the proportions of 6 general types of immune cells (macrophages $p = 0.004$ by the log-rank test). **(C)** Scatter plot showing the correlation of M0, M1, and M2 macrophages proportions with PLXDC2 expression ($p < 0.05$) generated by TIMER 2. The blue line in each plot was a fitted linear model that indicates the proportion of immune cells and the expression of PLXDC2; the Pearson coefficient was used for the correlation test. **(D)** The relationship between PLXDC2 and the immune markers of M2 macrophages. A redder color suggests a better correlation according to the Spearman test generated by TIMER 2.

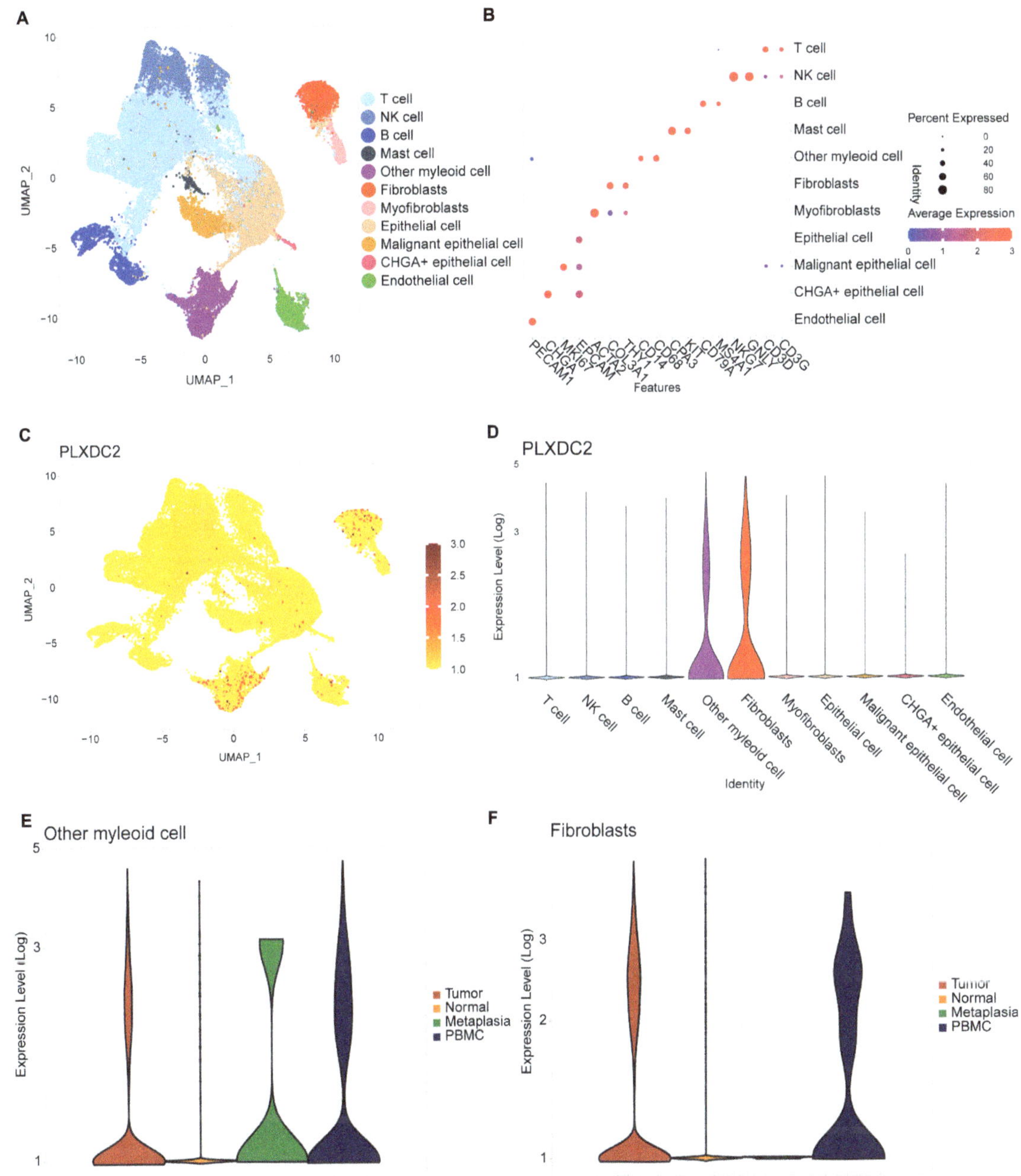

FIGURE 6 | PLXDC2 expression level ascend in Fibroblasts and Macrophages. **(A)** Uniform manifold approximation and projection (UMAP) dimensionality reduction analysis. 11 cell types were identified with its unique gene marker. Other myeloid cell represents monocytes and macrophages. **(B)** Bubble plot demonstrating each cell type and its gene marker. **(C)** UMAP revealing the expression level of PLXDC2. Higher expression is indicated with a redder color. **(D)** Violin plot showing the expression of PLXDC2 in each cell type. **(E)** Violin plot showing the expression level of PLXDC2 in other myeloid cell of Metaplasia, Normal, PBMC and Tumor samples, metaplasia represents the transformation of one differentiated cell type to another differentiated cell type, and PBMC resembles peripheral blood mononuclear cell. **(F)** Violin plot showing the expression level of PLXDC2 in fibroblasts of Metaplasia, Normal, PBMC and Tumor samples, similar to **(E)**.

serosa and adjacent organs) of PLXDC2 high staining score group was significantly stronger than that of PLXDC2 low staining score group (**Figure 7F**). The data above might lead us to the conclusion that PLXDC2 affects tumor metastasis in a non-lymphatic manner. Afterward, we studied the correlation of PLXDC2 and M2 macrophages' gene marker of CD163. The correlation plot indicated that PLXDC2 score in stromal is linked to $CD163^{+}$ cell density in GC, therefore correlated with M2 macrophages (**Figure 7G**). The information of GC patients suitable for study was demonstrated in **Table 1**. To test whether PLXDC2 expression could be a potential prognostic predictor in GC, a Kaplan Meier plot comparing high and low PLXDC2 score

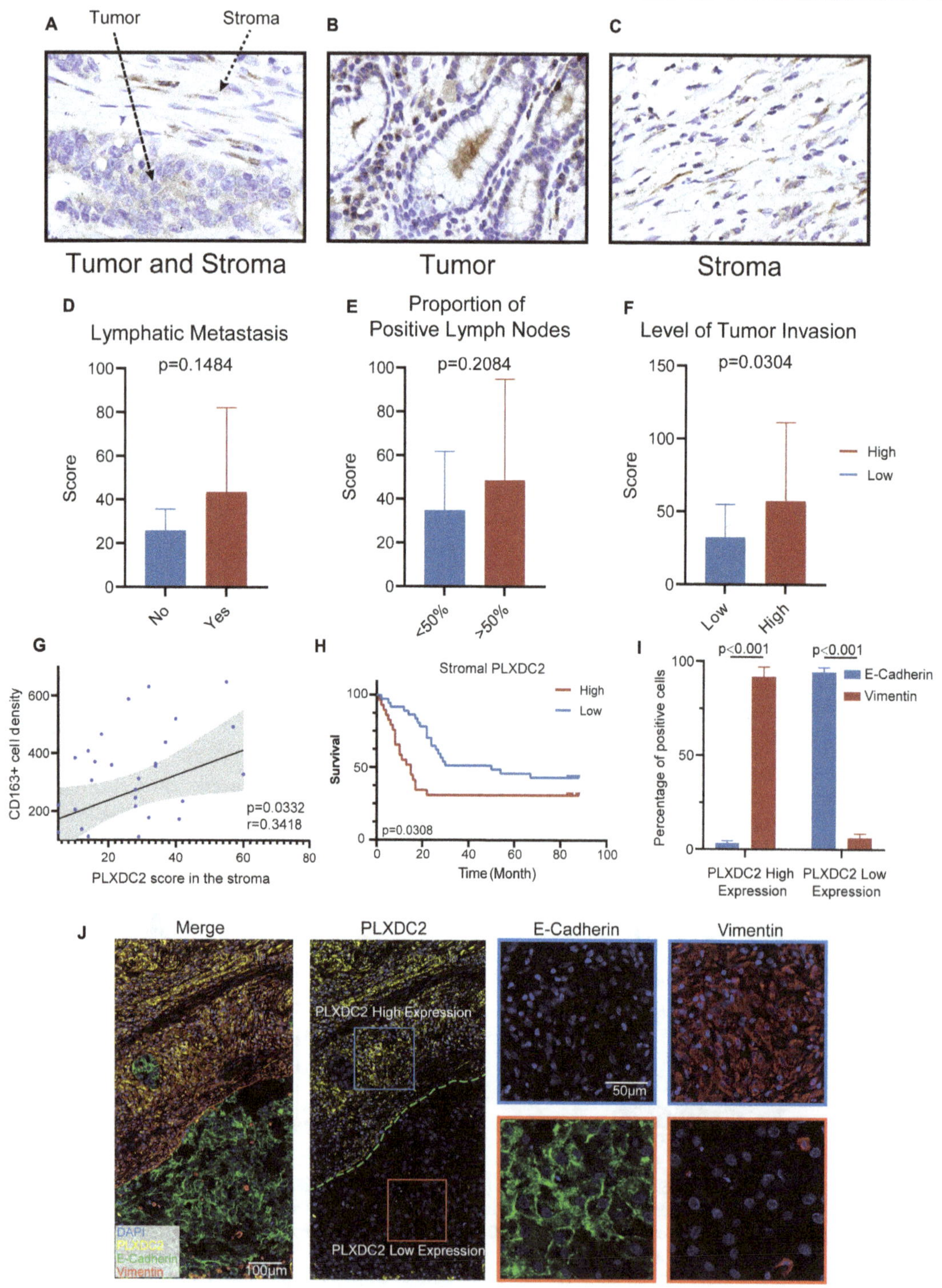

FIGURE 7 | PLXDC2 upregulation in Stroma indicates poor survival and high tumor invasion level. **(A)** PLXDC2 IHC staining images of GC tumor and stromal tissues (20x). **(B)** PLXDC2 IHC staining images of GC stromal tissues (20x). **(C)** PLXDC2 IHC staining images of GC tumor tissues [20x; **(D)**] PLXDC2 staining scores of GC tumor tissues in samples group by whether lymphatic metastasis exist. Lymphatic Metastasis is consistent with N in AJCC standard. A paired *t* test was used for analysis. **(E)** PLXDC2 staining scores of GC tumor tissues in the samples group by comparing with 50% of the positive lymph nodes. The proportion of Positive Lymph Nodes refers to the proportion of positive lymph nodes in lymph nodes removed during operation. A paired *t* test was used for analysis. **(F)** PLXDC2 staining scores of GC tumor tissues in samples group by level of tumor invasion (high vs. low). Level of Tumor Invasion is consistent with T in AJCC standard. A paired *t* test was used for analysis. **(G)** Scatter plot showing the correlation of PLXDC2 score in the stroma and $CD163^+$ cell density ($p = 0.0332$, $r = 0.3418$). **(H)** Kaplan–Meier plot assessing survival according to High and Low PLXDC2 score in the stroma. $p = 0.0308$ by log-rank test. **(I)** mIHC staining scores exhibiting the percentage of positive cells of GC tumor tissues group by PLXDC2 expression level [high vs. low, $p < 0.001$; **(J)**] mIHC staining images of GC section (Merge and PLXDC2-10x, E-Cadherin and Vimentin-40x).

in stromal according to the medium was generated (**Figure 7H**). The result of the plot confirmed PLXDC2 capability to assess survival of GC patients. Immunohistochemistry method verified our *in silico* result that PLXDC2 is a vital metastatic related gene that effect within the stroma of cancer patients. The results above approved PLXDC2's important role of promoting cancer metastasis in the stroma.

To further confirm the association between PLXDC2 and EMT process, mIHC was used to demonstrate the markers associated with EMT, including epithelial marker E-cadherin and mesenchymal marker Vimentin (**Figures 7I,J**). The staining results showed that E-cadherin was hardly expressed in the regions with high expression of PLXDC2, while Vimentin was strongly expressed. The opposite result was found in the region with low expression of PLXDC2. The mIHC results demonstrated that the overexpression of PLXDC2 was strongly correlated with the progression of EMT.

DISCUSSION

Gastric cancer is one of the most lethal malignancies, partly for lack of knowledge regarding the molecular patterns of GC subtypes in different stages of disease progression. Thus, this study embarked on an exploration of the TME in GC patients. Identification of PLXDC2 as a key gene was enabled with TME features of both stromal and immune domains, along with survival-related analysis. Further inquiry linked PLXDC2 with multiple clinicopathological characteristics and EMT/inflammatory signaling pathways, which implied a connection between the gene and vital clinical function. In addition, with the aid of CIBERSORTx, we discovered the linkage between PLXDC2 and a particular subtype of macrophages, M2 macrophages, which were recognized as protumor cells.

TABLE 1 | Patients' information.

Parameter	Stratification	Number of patients
Gender	Male	44
	Female	23
Age	<67	28
	≥67	39
Status	Deceased	42
	Survival	25
Clinical stage	1	3
	2	24
	3–4	40
PLXDC2 score	Low	17
	Medium	31
	High	19
CD163	Positive	44
	Negative	23

Note: The information of gastric cancer patients that participated in the tissue microarray study. Gender, age, status, clinical stage, PLXDC2 score, and CD163 available.

The TME comprises multiple complex components capable of suppressing and promoting tumor growth and metastasis. The TME has been identified to contribute to cell growth in several tumors, as it protects tumor cells from the attack of tumor-infiltrating lymphocytes (TILs; Peranzoni et al., 2018). In our study, we assessed TME characteristics via ESTIMATE and CIBERSORTx. The former computed the ratio of immune and stromal components, which was utilized to screen and identify key genes. The latter calculated the TICs proportions, which contributed to exploring key genes linked with M2 macrophages. More recent study reported that scRNA-seq highlights the role of inflammatory cancer-associated fibroblasts in bladder urothelial carcinoma (Chen et al., 2020). TME study based on single-cell RNA sequence also aided us in exploring GC TME. Based on the given estimations, we discovered that a high stromal score could be a potential indicator of a poor prognosis in GC patients.

Furthermore, with the novel CIBERSORTx tool, we identified the close correlation between our key gene (PLXDC2) and a particular subtype of immune cells (M2 macrophages). Consistent with previous studies, a high proportion of M2 macrophages in the TME of GC was an unfavorable prognostic factor, which matched the influence of PLXDC2 on survival. Our study demonstrated the linkage of PLXDC2 and M2 macrophages and may encourage PLXDC2 and M2 macrophages markers' clinical application in prognosis evaluation.

Plexin domain containing 2 is a vital member of the TEM family and is associated with tumor-specific angiogenesis. It encodes a type I transmembrane protein with some homology to nidogen and to plexins. Previous studies implied that it is an additional component in the network of proteins regulating proliferation and differentiation in the developing nervous system. While the functions of PLXDC2 in some tumors have been explored and demonstrated to have potential significance in the progression and molecular targeting of cancers such as colorectal cancer, few studies have focused on the behavior of PLXDC2 in GC, and our study addressed this gap (Rmali et al., 2005). Our TME-based study revealed the potential prognostic value of PLXDC2 in GC stroma as an indicator of poor outcomes, which may provide a novel line of thinking around GC prognosis evaluation. Despite the fact that PLXDC2 demonstrated a correlation with several clinicopathological characteristics and was revealed as a key regulator that promotes GC progression, the gene was discovered to have a low correlation with previously identified immune checkpoints, such as PD-L1, which may indicate that PLXDC2 acts independently of well-known immune regulatory genes, such as PD-L1. Previous studies concluded that deficiency of PLXDC2 is associated with increased inflammation, but our study shows otherwise. GSEA results in our study indicated that elevation of PLXDC2 in a GC cohort was linked with increased inflammation. Our results challenge the previous belief and may enable us to comprehend the role of PLXDC2 in inflammatory signaling while provoking further studies on this topic. The function of PLXDC2 in promoting angiogenesis has recently been discovered. Our study confirmed this previous finding and identified a new EMT-related function for PLXDC2. Epithelial-mesenchymal transition in GC have been discussed in previous studies of our lab, and this study extended our understanding of EMT in GC (Liu et al., 2021). The function of our key gene in EMT may indicate that PLXDC2 is a regulator of tumor metastasis. It has also been reported that deficiency of PLXDC2 suppresses the bacterial colonization of HP infection (Tubau-Juni et al., 2020). In our studies, however, we discovered no clear evidence that the expression level of PLXDC2 may influence HP infection in GC (**Supplementary Figure 2**). The relationship between PLXDC2 and HP infection could be a topic requiring further exploration. In contrast to a recent study, despite being the closest homolog of PLXDC2, PLXDC1 was not significantly differentially expressed between tumor samples and normal samples at the gene level, leaving PLXDC2 as the only TEM suitable for predicting the survival outcomes of GC (Zhang et al., 2015).

As a major component of innate immune cells, macrophages exert great influence in the TME (Davies et al., 2013). The accumulation of certain types of macrophages can indicate poor outcomes, as they hinder $CD8^+$ T lymphocytes' function. M2 macrophages, or alternatively activated macrophages, have been confirmed by multiple studies to play a decisive role in promoting tumor growth and cancer development. Tumor associated macrophages' behavior pattern is a topic that our group previously looked into (Wu et al., 2020). As a portion of our study, we confirmed the protumor function of M2 macrophages and linked this particular type of macrophages with the expression of our key gene PLXDC2. The gene exhibited a strong correlation with M2 macrophages and their markers, such as CD163. In addition to the fact that PLXDC2 gene expression shows a strong correlation with cytokines' expression levels, such as IL10, the linkage of PLXDC2 and macrophages demonstrated in this study might suggest that PLXDC2 plays some role in recruiting M2 macrophages. Single-cell analysis of our study confirmed PLXDC2's upregulation in Macrophages. On the other hand, the phenotype of M2 macrophages was not enough to explain the function of our key gene PLXDC2 in GC samples. M2 macrophages have been well recognized as anti-inflammatory components, whereas our gene PLXDC2 demonstrated proinflammatory behaviors according to GSEA (Orecchioni et al., 2019). This might bring us to the conclusion that our gene does not influence the phenotype of M2 macrophages in an inflammatory form. Further exploration of the inflammatory function of PLXDC2 will be needed for a rigorous conclusion. Both our TCGA study and IHC study found significance in comparison of high and low levels of tumor invasion but not in metastasis through lymph nodes. Along with single-cell study's result that PLXDC2 is an important stromal related cell and the GSEA result that PLXDC2 affects EMT, our results point to the fact that PLXDC2 supports tumor invasion via a non-lymphatic, EMT related method.

CONCLUSION

Our study identified the TME-related gene PLXDC2 in a high-stromal population and had a prognostic signature correlated to the CD163 M2 macrophages, further promoting EMT markers. Similar to the previous reporting that stromal EMT gene signature affects GC prognosis and immunotherapy responsiveness (Zheng and Li, 2020; Liu et al., 2021). The combined PLXDC2/EMT/M2 macrophages axis may affect GC outcome and immunotherapy responsiveness. The crosstalk between PLXDC2 expressed tumor stroma and CD163 macrophages and with tumor cell's EMT process is extricate and interesting. Further study of stromal PLXDC2, CD163 related EMT, and their targeted genes will help provide potential novel targets for GC.

ETHICS STATEMENT

The studies involving human participants were reviewed and approved by Ethics Committee of Shanghai Jiao Tong University. The patients/participants provided their written informed consent to participate in this study.

AUTHOR CONTRIBUTIONS

YH and DX contributed to the conception and design of the research work. YG, YD, GW, HG, YX, EL, and JX performed the experiments and performed data acquisition and analysis and interpretation. YG, YH, and DX drafted the article. PX, PN, DW, DX, and YH provided critical reagents and supervised the research. All authors have read and agreed to the published version of the manuscript.

REFERENCES

Bray, F., Ferlay, J., Soerjomataram, I., Siegel, R. L., Torre, L. A., and Jemal, A. (2018). Global cancer statistics 2018: GLOBOCAN estimates of incidence and mortality worldwide for 36 cancers in 185 countries. *CA Cancer J. Clin.* 68, 394–424. doi: 10.3322/caac.21492

Chen, W., Zheng, R., Baade, P. D., Zhang, S., Zeng, H., Bray, F., et al. (2016). Cancer statistics in China, 2015. *CA Cancer J. Clin.* 66, 115–132. doi: 10.3322/caac.21338

Chen, Y. C., Suresh, A., Underbayev, C., Sun, C., Singh, K., Seifuddin, F., et al. (2019). IKAP-Identifying K mAjor cell population groups in single-cell RNA-sequencing analysis. *Gigascience* 8:giz121.

Chen, Z., Zhou, L., Liu, L., Hou, Y., Xiong, M., Yang, Y., et al. (2020). Single-cell RNA sequencing highlights the role of inflammatory cancer-associated fibroblasts in bladder urothelial carcinoma. *Nat. Commun.* 11: 5077.

Davies, L. C., Jenkins, S. J., Allen, J. E., and Taylor, P. R. (2013). Tissue-resident macrophages. *Nat. Immunol.* 14, 986–995.

Edge, S. B., and Compton, C. C. (2010). The American joint committee on cancer: the 7th edition of the AJCC cancer staging manual and the future of TNM. *Ann. Surg. Oncol.* 17, 1471–1474.

Hatakeyama, M. (2019). Malignant *Helicobacter pylori*-associated diseases: gastric cancer and MALT Lymphoma. *Adv. Exp. Med. Biol.* 1149, 135–149. doi: 10.1007/5584_2019_363

Huber, W., Carey, V. J., Gentleman, R., Anders, S., Carlson, M., Carvalho, B. S., et al. (2015). Orchestrating high-throughput genomic analysis with Bioconductor. *Nat. Methods* 12, 115–121. doi: 10.1038/nmeth.3252

Jackaman, C., Tomay, F., Duong, L., Abdol Razak, N. B., Pixley, F. J., Metharom, P., et al. (2017). Aging and cancer: the role of macrophages and neutrophils. *Age. Res. Rev.* 36, 105–116. doi: 10.1016/j.arr.2017.03.008

Kotilea, K., Bontems, P., and Touati, E. (2019). Epidemiology, diagnosis and risk factors of *Helicobacter pylori* infection. *Adv. Exp. Med. Biol.* 1149, 17–33. doi: 10.1007/5584_2019_357

Krebs, A. M., Mitschke, J., Lasierra Losada, M., Schmalhofer, O., Boerries, M., Busch, H., et al. (2017). The EMT-activator Zeb1 is a key factor for cell plasticity and promotes metastasis in pancreatic cancer. *Nat. Cell Biol.* 19, 518–529. doi: 10.1038/ncb3513

Lewis, C. E., and Pollard, J. W. (2006). Distinct role of macrophages in different tumor microenvironments. *Cancer Res.* 66, 605–612. doi: 10.1158/0008-5472.can-05-4005

Li, B., Severson, E., Pignon, J. C., Zhao, H., Li, T., Novak, J., et al. (2016). Comprehensive analyses of tumor immunity: implications for cancer immunotherapy. *Genome Biol.* 17:174.

Li, T., Fu, J., Zeng, Z., Cohen, D., Li, J., Chen, Q., et al. (2020). TIMER2.0 for analysis of tumor-infiltrating immune cells. *Nucleic Acids Res.* 48, W509–W514.

Liu, C., Deng, L., Lin, J., Zhang, J., Huang, S., Zhao, J., et al. (2021). Zinc finger protein CTCF Regulates Extracellular Matrix (ECM)-related gene expression associated with the Wnt signaling pathway in gastric cancer. *Front. Oncol.* 10:625633. doi: 10.3389/fonc.2020.625633

McGinnis, C. S., Murrow, L. M., and Gartner, Z. J. (2019). DoubletFinder: doublet detection in single-cell RNA sequencing data using artificial nearest neighbors. *Cell Syst.* 8, 329–337.e4.

Miller-Delaney, S. F., Lieberam, I., Murphy, P., and Mitchell, K. J. (2011). Plxdc2 is a mitogen for neural progenitors. *PLoS One* 6:e14565. doi: 10.1371/journal.pone.0014565

Nanda, A., Buckhaults, P., Seaman, S., Agrawal, N., Boutin, P., Shankara, S., et al. (2004). Identification of a binding partner for the endothelial cell surface proteins TEM7 and TEM7R. *Cancer Res.* 64, 8507–8511. doi: 10.1158/0008-5472.can-04-2716

Noy, R., and Pollard, J. W. (2014). Tumor-associated macrophages: from mechanisms to therapy. *Immunity* 41, 49–61. doi: 10.1016/j.immuni.2014.06.010

Orecchioni, M., Ghosheh, Y., Pramod, A. B., and Ley, K. (2019). Macrophage polarization: different gene signatures in M1(LPS+) vs. Classically and M2(LPS-) vs. alternatively activated macrophages. *Front Immunol.* 10.1084. doi: 10.3389/fimmu.2019.01084

Pastushenko, I., and Blanpain, C. E. M. T. (2019). Transition states during tumor progression and metastasis. *Trends Cell Biol.* 29, 212–226. doi: 10.1016/j.tcb.2018.12.001

Peranzoni, E., Lemoine, J., Vimeux, L., Feuillet, V., Barrin, S., Kantari-Mimoun, C., et al. (2018). Macrophages impede CD8 T cells from reaching tumor cells and limit the efficacy of anti-PD-1 treatment. *Proc. Natl. Acad. Sci. U.S.A.* 115, E4041–E4050.

Ritchie, M. E., Phipson, B., Wu, D., Hu, Y., Law, C. W., Shi, W., et al. (2015). limma powers differential expression analyses for RNA-sequencing and microarray studies. *Nucleic Acids Res.* 43:e47. doi: 10.1093/nar/gkv007

Rmali, K. A., Puntis, M. C., and Jiang, W. G. (2005). Prognostic values of tumor endothelial markers in patients with colorectal cancer. *World J. Gastroenterol.* 11, 1283–1286. doi: 10.3748/wjg.v11.i9.1283

Sathe, A., Grimes, S. M., Lau, B. T., Chen, J., Suarez, C., Huang, R. J., et al. (2020). Single-Cell genomic characterization reveals the cellular reprogramming of the gastric tumor microenvironment. *Clin. Cancer Res.* 26, 2640–2653. doi: 10.1158/1078-0432.ccr-19-3231

Siegel, R. L., Miller, K. D., Fuchs, H. E., and Jemal, A. (2021). Cancer statistics, 2021. *CA Cancer J. Clin.* 71, 7–33.

Steen, C. B., Liu, C. L., Alizadeh, A. A., and Newman, A. M. (2020). Profiling cell type abundance and expression in bulk tissues with CIBERSORTx. *Methods Mol. Biol.* 2117, 135–157. doi: 10.1007/978-1-0716-0301-7_7

Stuart, T., Butler, A., Hoffman, P., Hafemeister, C., Papalexi, E., Mauck, W. M. III, et al. (2019). Comprehensive integration of single-cell data. *Cell* 177, 1888–1902.e21.

Subramanian, A., Tamayo, P., Mootha, V. K., Mukherjee, S., Ebert, B. L., Gillette, M. A., et al. (2005). Gene set enrichment analysis: a knowledge-based approach for interpreting genome-wide expression profiles. *Proc. Natl. Acad. Sci. U.S.A.* 102, 15545–15550. doi: 10.1073/pnas.0506580102

Szasz, A. M., Lanczky, A., Nagy, A., Forster, S., Hark, K., Green, J. E., et al. (2016). Cross-validation of survival associated biomarkers in gastric cancer using transcriptomic data of 1,065 patients. *Oncotarget* 7, 49322–49333. doi: 10.18632/oncotarget.10337

Szebeni, G. J., Vizler, C., Kitajka, K., and Puskas, L. G. (2017). Inflammation and cancer: extra- and intracellular determinants of tumor-associated macrophages as tumor promoters. *Med. Inflamm.* 2017:9294018.

Tang, Z., Kang, B., Li, C., Chen, T., and Zhang, Z. (2019). GEPIA2: an enhanced web server for large-scale expression profiling and interactive analysis. *Nucleic Acids Res.* 47, W556–W560.

Tubau-Juni, N., Bassaganya-Riera, J., Leber, A., Zoccoli-Rodriguez, V., Kronsteiner, B., Viladomiu, M., et al. (2020). Identification of new regulatory genes through expression pattern analysis of a global RNA-seq dataset from a *Helicobacter pylori* co-culture system. *Sci. Rep.* 10:11506.

Wu, K., Lin, K., Li, X., Yuan, X., Xu, P., Ni, P., et al. (2020). Redefining tumor-associated macrophage subpopulations and functions in the tumor microenvironment. *Front. Immunol.* 11:1731. doi: 10.3389/fimmu.2020.01731

Wu, T., and Dai, Y. (2017). Tumor microenvironment and therapeutic response. *Cancer Lett.* 387, 61–68. doi: 10.1016/j.canlet.2016.01.043

Yamamoto, N., Eguchi, A., Hirokawa, Y., Ogura, S., Sugimoto, K., Iwasa, M., et al. (2020). Expression pattern of plexin domain containing 2 in human hepatocellular carcinoma. *Monoclon. Antib. Immunodiagn. Immunother.* 39, 57–60. doi: 10.1089/mab.2019.0050

Yasui, W., Oue, N., Kuniyasu, H., Ito, R., Tahara, E., and Yokozaki, H. (2001). Molecular diagnosis of gastric cancer: present and future. *Gastr. Cancer* 4, 113–121. doi: 10.1007/pl00011733

Yoon, S. J., Park, J., Shin, Y., Choi, Y., Park, S. W., Kang, S. G., et al. (2020). Deconvolution of diffuse gastric cancer and the suppression of CD34 on the BALB/c nude mice model. *BMC Cancer* 20:314. doi: 10.1186/s12885-020-06814-4

Yoshihara, K., Shahmoradgoli, M., Martinez, E., Vegesna, R., Kim, H., Torres-Garcia, W., et al. (2013). Inferring tumour purity and stromal and immune cell admixture from expression data. *Nat. Commun.* 4:2612.

Yunna, C., Mengru, H., Lei, W., and Weidong, C. (2020). Macrophage M1/M2 polarization. *Eur. J. Pharmacol.* 877:173090. doi: 10.1016/j.ejphar.2020.173090

Zeng, D., Li, M., Zhou, R., Zhang, J., Sun, H., Shi, M., et al. (2019). Tumor microenvironment characterization in gastric cancer identifies prognostic and immunotherapeutically relevant gene signatures. *Cancer Immunol. Res.* 7, 737–750. doi: 10.1158/2326-6066.cir-18-0436

Zhang, Y., and Weinberg, R. A. (2018). Epithelial-to-mesenchymal transition in cancer: complexity and opportunities. *Front. Med.* 12, 361–373. doi: 10.1007/s11684-018-0656-6

Zhang, Z. Z., Hua, R., Zhang, J. F., Zhao, W. Y., Zhao, E. H., Tu, L., et al. (2015). TEM7 (PLXDC1), a key prognostic predictor for resectable gastric cancer, promotes cancer cell migration and invasion. *Am. J. Cancer Res.* 5, 772–781.

Zheng, P., and Li, W. (2020). Crosstalk between mesenchymal stromal cells and tumor-associated macrophages in gastric cancer. *Front. Oncol.* 10:571516. doi: 10.3389/fonc.2020.571516

Zong, L., Abe, M., Seto, Y., and Ji, J. (2016). The challenge of screening for early gastric cancer in China. *Lancet* 388:2606. doi: 10.1016/s0140-6736(16)32226-7

5

CBX4 Provides an Alternate Mode of Colon Cancer Development *via* Potential Influences on Circadian Rhythm and Immune Infiltration

*Wangzhi Wei, Wei Zhao and Yu Zhang**

Life Science Institute of Jinzhou Medical University, Jinzhou, China

***Correspondence:**
Yu Zhang
zhangyu007@bjmu.edu.cn

The circadian machinery is critical for the normal physiological functions and cellular processes. Circadian rhythm disruption has been associated with immune suppression which leads to higher cancer risk, suggesting a putative tumor protective role of circadian clock homeostasis. CBX4, as an epigenetic regulator, has been explored for its involvement in tumorigenesis. However, little is known about the correlation between CBX4 and circadian rhythm disruption in colon cancer as well as the potential impact on the tumor immunity. A significant upregulation of CBX4 was identified in the TCGA colon adenocarcinoma (COAD) samples when compared with the normal controls ($p < 0.001$). This differential expression was confirmed at the protein level using colon adenocarcinoma tissue array ($p < 0.01$). CBX4 was up-regulated in the recurred/progressed colon cancer cases compared with the disease-free samples ($p < 0.01$), suggesting CBX4 as a potential predictor for poor prognosis. With regard to nodular metastasis, CBX4 was found to be associated with early onset of metastatic diseases but not late progression. The circadian rhythm is orchestrated by the alternating activation and suppression of the CLOCK/ARNTL-driven positive loop and the PER/CRY-controlled negative loop. In COAD, CBX4 was negatively correlated with CLOCK ($p < 0.001$), and positively correlated with PER1 ($p < 0.001$), PER3 ($p < 0.01$), and CRY2 ($p < 0.001$) as well as NR1D1 ($p < 0.001$), a critical negative regulator of the circadian clock. These interactions consistently impacted on patient survival based on the colorectal cancer cohorts GSE17536 and GSE14333 of PrognoScan. CBX4 showed significant negative correlations with infiltrating B cells ($p < 0.05$) and $CD4^+$ T cells ($p < 0.01$), and positive correlations with myeloid derived suppressor cells (MDSCs) ($p < 0.05$) and cancer associated fibroblast (CAFs) ($p < 0.001$), as well as a low immunoscore. Moreover, CBX4 displayed significant correlations with diverse immune metagenes. PER1 and PER3, consistent with their coordinated expression with CBX4, also had strong correlations with these gene representatives in COAD, suggesting a potential interaction of CBX4 with the circadian machinery. Our studies implicate that CBX4 may contribute to colon cancer development via potential influence on circadian rhythm and immune infiltration. These findings provide new insights into deciphering the function of CBX4, and may contribute to the development of new targeting strategies.

Keywords: chromobox 4 (CBX4), circadian rhythm, circadian clock gene, colon cancer, immune infiltration

INTRODUCTION

Colorectal carcinoma (CRC) is one of the leading causes of morbidity and mortality worldwide. It accounted for 9.2% of total cancer deaths in 2018 (Bray et al., 2018). For incidence, it is the second frequent burden of cancer among females, and the third of that among males (Bray et al., 2018). Screening has been demonstrated to reduce both incidence and mortality of CRC (Zauber, 2015), and targeting of essential oncogenes represents an effective way for the therapies. Although numerous potential targets have been identified in CRC, the biological and molecular mechanisms underlying CRC development and progression are still far from being fully understood (Malki et al., 2020).

Polycomb group (PcG) proteins act as important transcriptional repressors that mediate epigenetic gene silencing through histone modification (Simon and Kingston, 2009). Two distinct polycomb repressive complexes (PRC), PRC1 and PRC2, play a critical role in regulation of cellular functions (Sauvageau and Sauvageau, 2010). Several polycomb chromobox (CBX) proteins including CBX2, CBX4, CBX6, CBX7, and CBX8, interact with the core PRC1 complex (Vandamme et al., 2011). The chromodomain in the N terminus and two SUMO-interacting motifs (SIMs) of CBX4 protein contribute to its polycomb- and SUMO E3 ligase-dependent functions, respectively (Luis et al., 2011). CBX4 plays oncogenic or tumor suppressive effects in a cell type dependent manner (Li et al., 2014; Wang et al., 2016; Meng et al., 2018). Despite extensive characterization of the potential mechanisms of CBX4-mediated tumorigenesis, additional partners engaged by CBX4 remain to be explored. When we focused on in-depth exploration of CBX4's functional panorama, an interesting potential connection between CBX4 and circadian rhythm attracted our attention.

The 2017 Nobel Prize in Physiology or Medicine was awarded to Jeffrey C. Hall, Michael Rosbash and Michael W. Young for their leading discoveries of the molecular mechanisms controlling the circadian rhythm (Burki, 2017). The circadian machinery governs a remarkable variety of physiological functions and cellular processes. It is orchestrated by the regulatory feedback loops of core clock genes, which are comprised of bHLH-PAS transcription factors CLOCK (Circadian Locomoter Output Cycles Kaput) and ARNTL (Aryl Hydrocarbon Receptor Nuclear Translocator Like), as well as their downstream clock-controlled targets including Period (*Per1, Per2, Per3*) and Cryptochrome (*Cry1 and Cry2*). In the morning, the CLOCK:ARNTL heterodimer activates the transcription of PER, CRY and other Clock controlled genes (CCGs). Late in the day, PER and CRY proteins accumulate and translocate from the cytoplasm to the nucleus, where they associate and negatively regulate the circadian machinery by inhibiting the CLOCK:ARNTL complex. The alternating activation and suppression of the CLOCK:ARNT -driven positive loop and the PER/CRY-controlled negative loop result in a circadian oscillation of the molecular clock (Kettner et al., 2016; Papagiannakopoulos et al., 2016). Several studies in line with the epidemiological studies have documented the association of dysregulated circadian rhythms and increased susceptibility for developing multiple malignancies including breast (Lesicka et al., 2018; Lin and Farkas, 2018), colon (Innominato et al., 2009; Fuhr et al., 2019), prostate (Flynn-Evans et al., 2013; Wendeu-Foyet and Menegaux, 2017), lung (Papagiannakopoulos et al., 2016) cancers and hepatocellular carcinoma (Kettner et al., 2016). For example, the expression of the *Per* genes was deregulated in breast cancer and non-small lung cancer cells (Chen et al., 2005; Gery et al., 2007). Mice lacking the circadian genes were reported to be cancer prone (Lee et al., 2010). In addition, the rhythmic control of cell fate was found to affect cancer therapies (Dallmann et al., 2016; Lesicka et al., 2018).

The immune system imposes a profound impact on tumor progression through infiltration of both innate and adaptive immune cells into tumor microenvironment. Interactions between tumor cells and neighboring infiltrating cells affect cancer cell phenotype as well as neoplastic outcome (Colangelo et al., 2017). Immune functions are subject to the regulation of circadian rhythm. For example, leukocyte trafficking occurs in a circadian manner, and the cyclical recruitment of immune cells to tissues is critical for immune responses (Scheiermann et al., 2013). Perturbation of circadian clock can cause immune suppression and increased cancer risk, supporting a putative tumor protective role of circadian clock homeostasis (Savvidis and Koutsilieris, 2012; Labrecque and Cermakian, 2015).

Despite still a preliminary stage of this study, we anticipate to provide a new functional implication of CBX4 and direct more researchers toward the delineation of the mechanisms linking circadian rhythm disruption to cancers, which is a major public health issue that has yet to receive the recognition it deserves.

MATERIALS AND METHODS

Tumor IMmune Estimation Resource (TIMER) Analyses

Tumor IMmune Estimation Resource (TIMER) is a comprehensive resource for analysis of molecular characterization of tumor-immune interactions (Li et al., 2016, 2017). Human CBX4 expression was screened via the DiffExp module of TIMER. Distributions of the CBX4 expression levels were displayed in the box plots and the statistical significance was evaluated by Wilcoxon test. Up- or down- regulation of CBX4 in the tumors was compared to normal tissues for each cancer type.

Correlations between CBX4 expression and abundance of the immune infiltrates were investigated via the Gene module of TIMER2.0, which integrates multiple algorithms for immune infiltration estimation instead of only using one algorithm in the original TIMER (Li et al., 2020). The partial Spearman's correlation was performed by selecting the "Purity Adjustment" option. Genes highly expressed in tumor microenvironment intend to have negative associations with tumor purity, while those with positive associations are expected to be highly expressed in tumor cells (Aran et al., 2015; Li et al., 2017).

Correlations between CBX4 and the related markers were explored via the gene correlation module of TIMER2. The scatter plots were generated using CBX4 expression as the Y-axis and the related makers as the X-axis, together with the partial

Spearman's rho coefficient and the statistical significance. The gene expression levels were displayed with log2 TPM.

Influences of the immune infiltrating subsets on the clinical outcome of colon adenocarcinoma (COAD) were evaluated by the Survival module. The Kaplan-Meier plots were output for B cells, CD4 + Th2 cells, MDSC, and CAFs to visualize the survival differences between the high and low infiltration levels. The hazard ratio and p value for Cox model and the log-rank p value for Kaplan-Meier curve were shown.

Queries of TCGA Data *via* Cbioportal and UALCAN Web Portals

Influences of CBX4 on clinicopathologic features of colon cancer were evaluated by UALCAN[1], an interactive web tool not only to compare primary tumor with normal tissue samples, but also to analyze different tumor subgroups as defined by individual cancer stages, histological subtypes, nodular metastasis status, and other clinical parameters based on TCGA level 3 RNA-seq and clinical data from 31 cancer types (Chandrashekar et al., 2017). The individual cancer stages are categorized into Stage I (T1 or T2 N0 M0); Stage II (T3 or T4 N0 M0); Stage III (Tx N1 or N2 M0); Stage IV(Tx Nx M1) (Chandrashekar et al., 2017). The histological subtypes are divided into adenocarcinoma and mucus adenocarcinoma, and the nodular metastasis status is grouped into N0 (No regional lymph node metastasis); N1 (Metastases in 1 to 3 axillary lymph nodes); N2 (Metastases in 4 to 9 axillary lymph nodes) (Chandrashekar et al., 2017).

The cBioPortal for Cancer Genomics[2] provides a web resource for integrative analysis of cancer genomics and clinical profiles (Cerami et al., 2012; Gao et al., 2013). A histogram of alteration frequencies of CBX4 across cancers, including mutations, amplifications and deletions, was summarized based on TCGA Pan Cancer Atlas studies in which 594 of the colorectal carcinoma cases were included. A frequently mutated gene (FMG) is defined as a mutation frequency greater than 5% in a type of cancer. Using the "*Co-expression*," the correlations between CBX4 expression (log RNA Seq V2 RSEM) and the circadian clock genes (log RNA Seq V2 RSEM) were displayed in the scatter plots. Spearman's and Pearson's coefficients were indicated with significance. Using the "*Plot*," levels of CBX4 mRNA expression (z scores relative to normal samples) (n = 222) were compared between the recurred/progressed colon cancer cases (n = 29) and the disease-free samples (n = 193). The data were collected from the clinical attribute of the study.

Tissue Array Immunohistochemistry

Formalin-fixed paraffin-embedded tissue array sections including a total of 101 cases of primary colon adenocarcinoma (Catalog# HColA180Su17) were obtained from Outdo Biotech (Shanghai, China). The sections were dewaxed in five changes of xylene, rehydrated through graded alcohols, and heat treated in Tris-EDTA buffer at pH 9.0 for antigen retrieval. Endogenous peroxidase activity was blocked using 3% hydrogen peroxide. After blocking with 2.5% normal serum for 20 min, the sections were then incubated with 1:200 diluted CBX4 antibody (Abcam) for 1hr at RT, followed by incubation with ImmPRESS horse anti-rabbit IgG polymer reagent for 30 min as per kit instructions (Vector Laboratory). After wash in Tris buffered saline for 2 × 5 min, the reaction was visualized with DAB (DAKO). The sections were counterstained with Mayer's hematoxylin, dehydrated in alcohols, cleared in xylene, and mounted with MM24 Leica mounting medium (VWR).

Each patient was represented by one core of adenocarcinoma sample (n = 93), and the majority contained one core of non-neoplastic colon tissue control (n = 71). The evaluation of CBX4 expression levels was based on a staining intensity score (i) and a distribution score (Pi). The staining intensity was classified into four levels, namely 0, 1+, 2+, and 3+, which were designated as negative, weakly positive, moderately positive, and strongly positive signals, respectively; The percentage of stained cells was categorized as 0 (0%), 1(< 25%), 2 (25–50%), 3 (50–75%), and 4 (>75%), respectively. The total score Pi* (i + 1) was calculated by multiplying the intensity score by the corresponding distribution score. A total score of eight was used as a cutoff to compare the dichotomized cases with high and low expression of CBX4.

STRING Database

STRING database provides access to predict functional protein-protein interactions (PPI) (von Mering et al., 2003; Szklarczyk et al., 2019). The associated PPI network of CBX4 pertaining to Homo sapiens was constructed by STRING v11.0 based on a highest confidence coefficient defined by a minimum interaction score >0.9. All the active interaction parameters were selected, including text-mining, experiments, databases, co-expression, neighborhood, gene fusion, and co-occurrence. 16 of STRING interactants for CBX4 was summarized with PPI enrichment p-value: $<1.0 \times 10^{-16}$.

PrognoScan Survival Analysis

PrognoScan evaluates prognostic value of potential tumor makers or therapeutic targets using minimum P-value approach to find optimal cutpoints (Mizuno et al., 2009). Relationships between gene expression and patient endpoints, such as overall survival (OS) and disease-free survival (DFS) are analyzed according to a collection of public cancer microarray datasets with clinical annotation (Mizuno et al., 2009). For each optimal cutpoint, patients are dichotomized and survival difference between high and low expression groups is calculated by log-rank test. Here, Kaplan-Meier survival curves comparing the high and low expression of CBX4 as well as the circadian rhythm genes in colorectal carcinoma, were generated based on two colorectal cancer cohorts GSE17536 (Probe ID: 227558_at CBX4; 217563 at CLOCK; 202861 at PER1; 212695_at CRY2) and GSE14333 (Probe ID: 206724_at CBX4, 1569701_at PER3). The threshold was adjusted to a Cox P-value. 95% confidence intervals (CI) for each group were indicated by dotted lines in each plot.

Gene Correlation Analysis in GEPIA

GEPIA (Gene Expression Profiling Interactive Analysis) includes 9,736 tumors and 8,587 normal samples from TCGA and the GTEx projects. It can be divided into

[1] http://ualcan.path.uab.edu

[2] http://cbioportal.org

several major functions including pairwise gene correlation analysis (Tang et al., 2017). Correlations between CBX4 and the related markers were explored, and the Spearman's and Pearson's correlation coefficients were indicated. The COAD tumor and normal colon tissue data sets were used for the analysis.

Estimation of Infiltrating Immune Cells by ESTIMATE Algorithm

ESTIMATE (Estimation of STromal and Immune cells in MAlignant Tumor tissues using Expression data) is used as an algorithm to calculate stromal and immune scores to infer the levels of infiltrating stromal and immune cells which are major non-tumor constituents of tumor samples (Yoshihara et al., 2013). 210 of TCGA samples were divided into two groups based on CBX4 mRNA expression levels (FPKM). The corresponding immune scores were profiled from the RNA-seq-V2 platform of the ESTIMATE database and analyzed based on the dichotomized cases with high and low expression of CBX4.

Statistical Analyses

Distributions of the CBX4 expression levels were evaluated by the Wilcoxon test (**Figure 1A**); The comparisons were determined by *T*-test in **Figures 1B, 3B,C, 4F**; Chi-square and Fisher's exact test were used for the tissue array analysis in **Figure 1C**; Spearman's and/or Pearson's correlation analysis were performed in **Figures 2, 4, Tables 1–3** as well as **Supplementary Figures 2, 3**; Log-rank test and Kaplan-Meier estimators were implemented for survival analysis in **Figures 3A, 4G**. Significance was shown as $^{*}P < 0.05$, $^{**}P < 0.01$, $^{***}P < 0.001$.

TABLE 1 | Correlations between CBX4 and gene representatives of various functional cell subsets in COAD determined by TIMER2.0.

Cell type	Gene marker	Colon adenocarcinoma (COAD) CBX4 Correlation (TIMER 2.0) Purity-adjusted partial spearman's rho value	P Value
T cell exhaustion	PD-1(PDCD1)	0.152	**
	CTLA4	0.093	0.062
	LAG3	0.138	**
	TIM-3 (HAVCR2)	0.066	0.182
Regulatory T cells	FOXP3	0.127	*
	TGFβ (TGFB1)	0.225	***
	L1CAM	0.469	***
	PTGIR	0.238	***
	ITGA4	0.016	0.743
Th1 cells	T-bet (TBX21)	0.119	*
	STAT1	0.197	***
	STAT4	0.02	0.687
	IFN-γ (IFNG)	0.076	0.126
Th2 cells	GATA3	0.197	***
	STAT6	0.253	***
Th17 cells	IL-6R	0.203	***
	STAT3	0.221	***
	RORγt (RORC)	-0.035	0.479
	IL-17A	-0.071	0.154
Macrophage	CD68	0.174	***
MDSC	CD11b (ITGAM)	0.139	**
	IL-4R	0.286	***
	CD33	−0.006	0.902
	CD14	0.126	*
	S100A9	−0.007	0.881

$^{*}P < 0.05$, $^{**}P < 0.01$, and $^{***}P < 0.001$.

RESULTS

CBX4 Is Preferentially Expressed in Human Colon Adenocarcinoma

Elusive documentations and paradoxical effects of CBX4 in colon cancer provoked our further investigations on its actions. Since CBX4 plays a critical role for physiological functioning, we thus analyzed the potential molecular alterations of this gene during colorectal carcinogenesis. As shown in **Supplementary Figure 1**, CBX4 gene alteration frequencies varied notably among cancers. In colorectal carcinoma, the mutation frequency was lower than 5%, a threshold usually used to define a FMG. As much as the copy number variation was concerned, amplification or deletion was rarely observed in colorectal carcinoma. Hence, CBX4 appears to be relatively stable at the genomic level.

The low frequencies of the genomic alterations in CBX4 indicated that the abnormalities might be regulated at the expression level. Therefore, we performed a pan-cancer screening of CBX4 expression via the DiffExp module of TIMER which allows to compare differential expression of a gene of interest between tumors and adjacent normal tissues across the TCGA malignancies. A significant up-regulation of CBX4 was identified in COAD when compared with normal controls ($p < 0.001$) (**Figure 1A**). UALCAN analysis confirmed the up-regulation of CBX4 in primary COAD tumor ($n = 286$) versus normal tissue samples ($n = 41$) ($p < 0.001$). Of note, the increased expression was seen in both colon adenocarcinoma ($n = 243$) and colon mucinous adenocarcinoma ($n = 37$) ($p < 0.001$) (**Figure 1B**).

Next, we explored CBX4 protein expression using a tissue array composed of 71 normal colon tissues and 93 cancer samples. CBX4 was found to be preferentially expressed in glandular cells with intracellular localization (**Figure 1C**). By taking into consideration of staining intensity and the percentage of stained cells, a score was assigned for each sample. Using a score of 8 as cutoff, 53.8% of the adenocarcinoma samples demonstrated a high level of CBX4 protein, whereas only 14.1% of the non-neoplastic colon tissues showed high expression ($p < 0.01$). Taken together, these data support a significant up-regulation of CBX4 gene expression in colon adenocarcinoma.

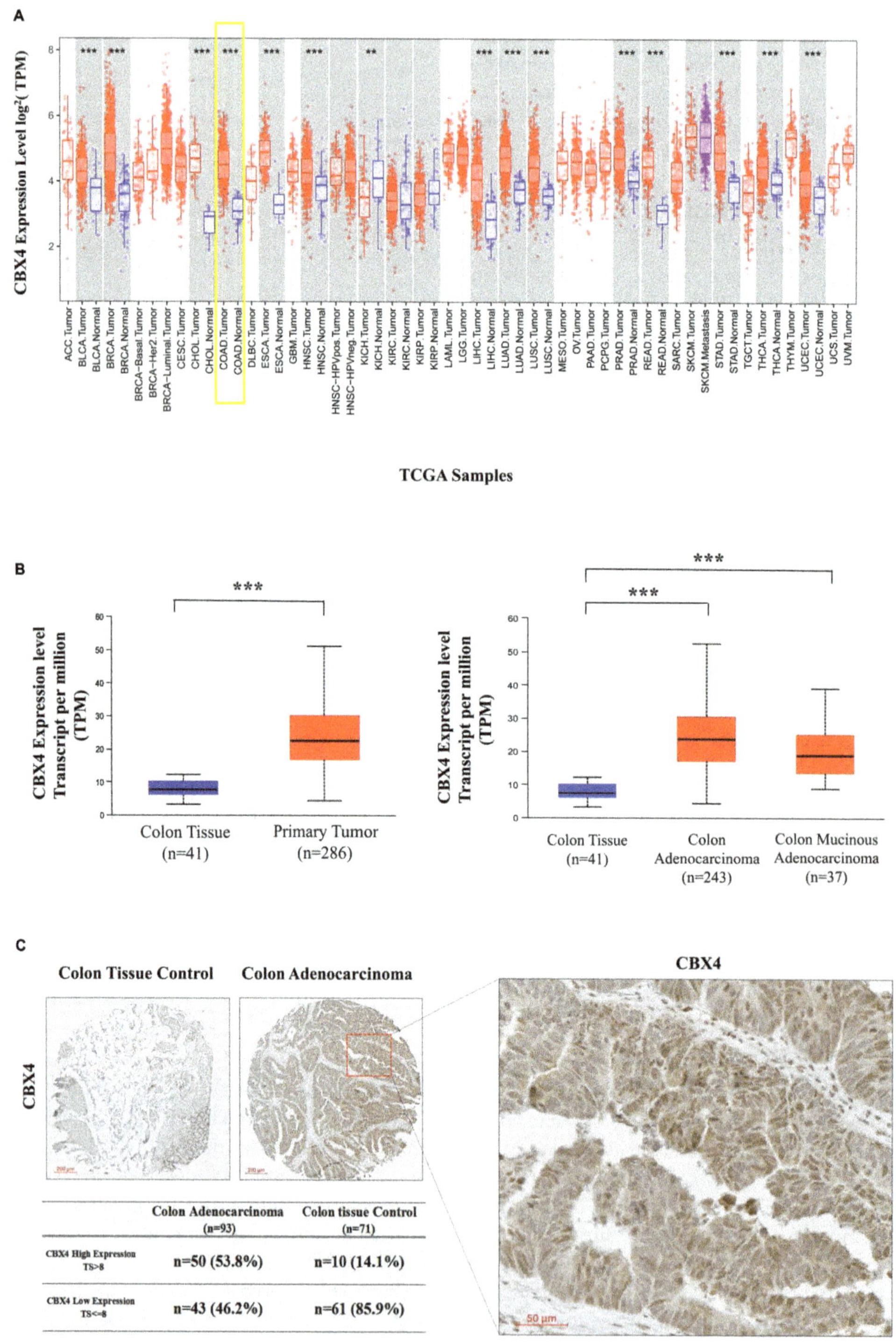

	Colon Adenocarcinoma (n=93)	Colon tissue Control (n=71)
CBX4 High Expression TS>8	n=50 (53.8%)	n=10 (14.1%)
CBX4 Low Expression TS<=8	n=43 (46.2%)	n=61 (85.9%)

FIGURE 1 | CBX4 is Preferentially Expressed in Human Colon Adenocarcinoma (COAD). **(A)** Human CBX4 expression levels in different tumor types derived from TCGA were determined by the Diff Exp module of TIMER. Red bars represent tumor tissues and blue bars are adjacent normal tissues. The gray columns here mean "normal control data are available". The significant up- or down- regulation of CBX4 in the tumors, when compared to normal tissues, was indicated with the symbols (**P* < 0.05, ***P* < 0.01, and ****P* < 0.001). **(B)** CBX4 expression levels in COAD were analyzed by UALCAN, box plots (left) showing the levels of CBX4 in normal (*n* = 41) and colon cancer samples (*n* = 286), and box plots (right) showing those of CBX4 in normal (*n* = 41), colon adenocarcinoma (*n* = 243) and colon mucinous adenocarcinoma (*n* = 37). The read counts were normalized in TPM (Transcripts Per Kilobase Million). **(C)** Immunohistochemitry on a total of 93 cases of primary colon adenocarcinoma. Each patient was represented by one core of adenocarcinoma sample (*n* = 93), and the majority contained one core of non-neoplastic colon tissue control (*n* = 71). By taking into consideration of a intensity score (i) and a distribution score (Pi), a total score (TS) = Pi* (i + 1) was assigned for each sample using a score of 8 as a cutoff to compare the dichotomized cases with high and low expression of CBX4.

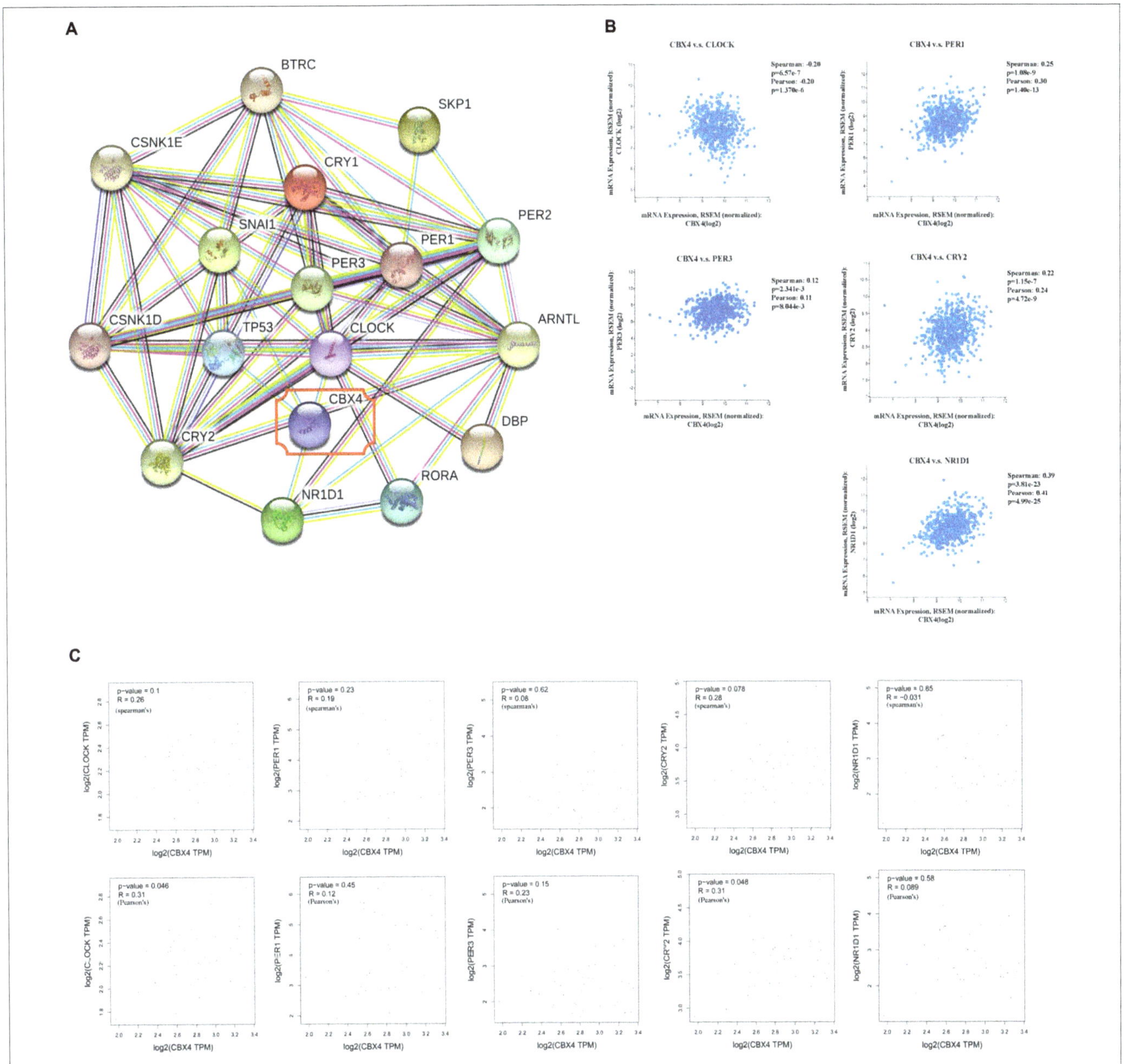

FIGURE 2 | CBX4 Expression Correlates with That of Circadian Clock Genes in Colon Adenocarcinoma. **(A)** The associated PPI network of CBX4 pertaining to Homo sapiens was constructed by STRING v11.0 based on a highest confidence coefficient defined by a minimum interaction score >0.9. 16 of STRING interactants for CBX4 were summarized, PPI enrichment p-value: $<1.0 \times 10^{-16}$. **(B)** The correlations between CBX4 and the circadian clock genes including CLOCK, PER1, PER3, CRY2, NR1D1 in COAD samples were determined by cBioportal. Levels of the mRNA expression were normalized in Log2 RSEM. The correlation coefficients and the significance were indicated. **(C)** The correlations between CBX4 and the circadian genes in normal colon tissue samples were examined by GEPIA database. The gene expression levels were shown in TPM. Spearman's (upper) and Pearson's (lower) R and the significance were indicated.

CBX4 Expression Correlates With That of Circadian Clock Genes in Colon Adenocarcinoma

To understand the underlying molecular mechanisms and actions of CBX4 in colon cancer, functional protein-protein interaction (PPI) predictions by STRING were performed. The associated PPI network of CBX4 pertaining to Homo sapiens was constructed based on a highest confidence coefficient defined by a minimum interaction score >0.9. Notably, several components of the network were associated with circadian clock genes (**Figure 2A**). To further explore the connection between CBX4 and the circadian machinery, 594 of colorectal adenocarcinoma samples from TCGA were accessed to perform a query for CBX4 via cBioportal. Coordinated expression of CBX4 was revealed with several circadian clock genes (**Figure 2B**).

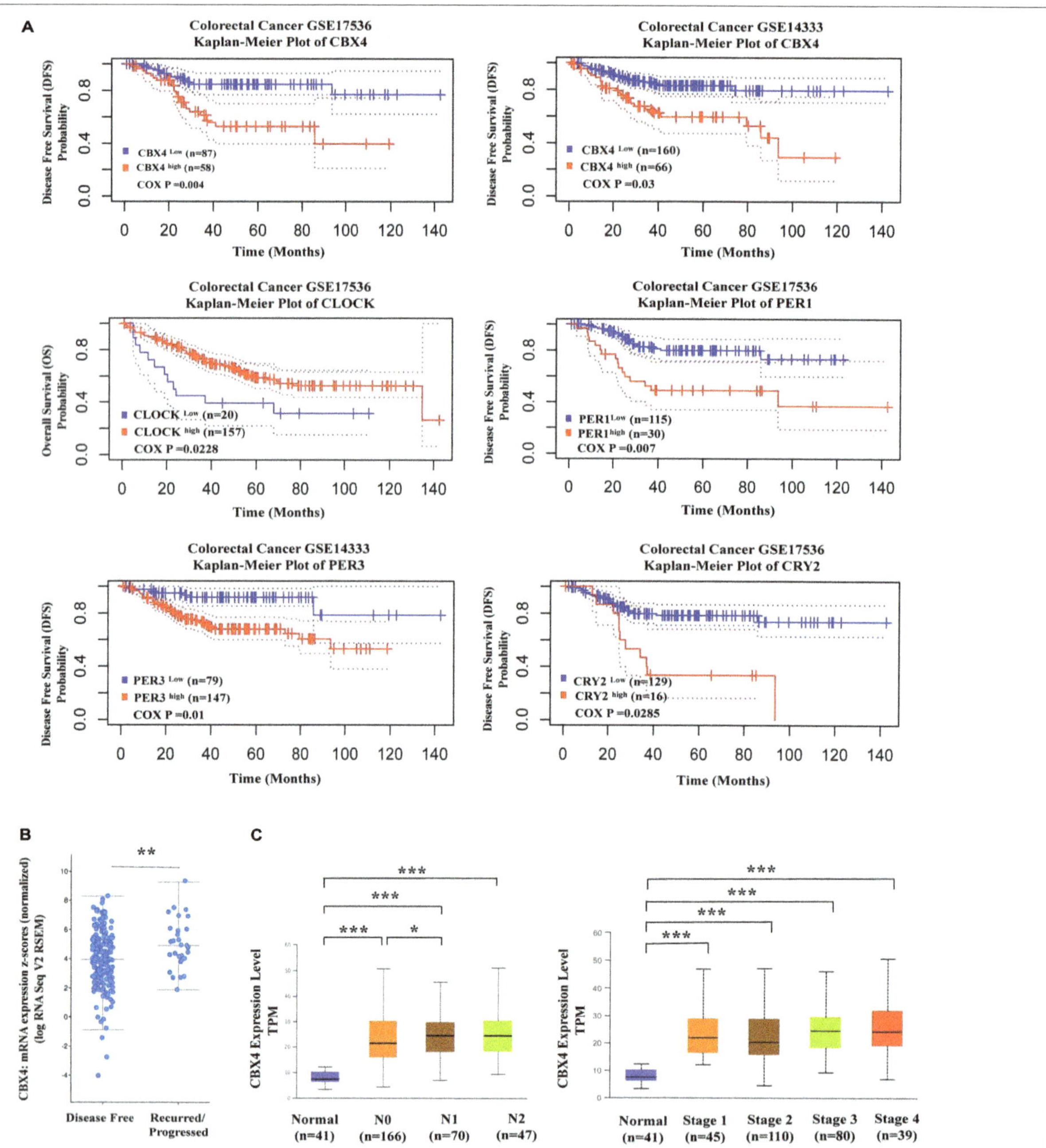

FIGURE 3 | Elevated CBX4 expression predicts poor prognosis in Colon Carcinoma. **(A)** Shown (upper) are the Kaplan-Meier survival curves comparing the high and low expression of CBX4 in colorectal carcinoma generated by the PrognoScan database. Disease Free Survival (DFS) in two colorectal cancer cohorts GSE17536 (n = 145) and GSE14333 (n = 226) was analyzed. Shown (lower) are the Kaplan-Meier survival curves comparing the high and low expression of the core clock gene PER1, PER3, CLOCK, and CRY2. DFS or Overall survival (OS) in two colorectal cancer cohorts GSE17536 and GSE14333 was analyzed. The X-axis represents months to follow-up and the Y axis is survival rate, 95% confidence intervals for each group are indicated by dotted lines. **(B)** Based on the study of Colorectal Adenocarcinoma (TCGA, PanCancer Atlas), levels of CBX4 mRNA expression (log RNA Seq V2 RSEM) (n = 222) were compared between the recurred/progressed colon cancer cases (n = 29) and the disease-free samples (n = 193). The data were collected from the clinical attribute of the study. The vertical axis represents CBX4 mRNA expression (z scores relative to normal samples), and the horizontal axis is the categories of disease free status. **(C)** The correlation of CBX4 expression with colon adenocarcinma metastasis was analyzed using UALCAN. Levels of CBX4 expression was normalized in TPM. For the nodular metastasis status, N0 is no regional lymph node metastasis; N1 is Metastases in 1 to 3 axillary lymph nodes; N2 is Metastases in 4 to 9 axillary lymph nodes. For the cancer stages, Stage I: T1 or T2 N0 M0; Stage II – T3 or T4 N0 M0; Stage III – Tx N1 or N2 M0; Stage IV – Tx Nx M1. * $P < 0.05$, ** $P < 0.01$, *** $P < 0.001$.

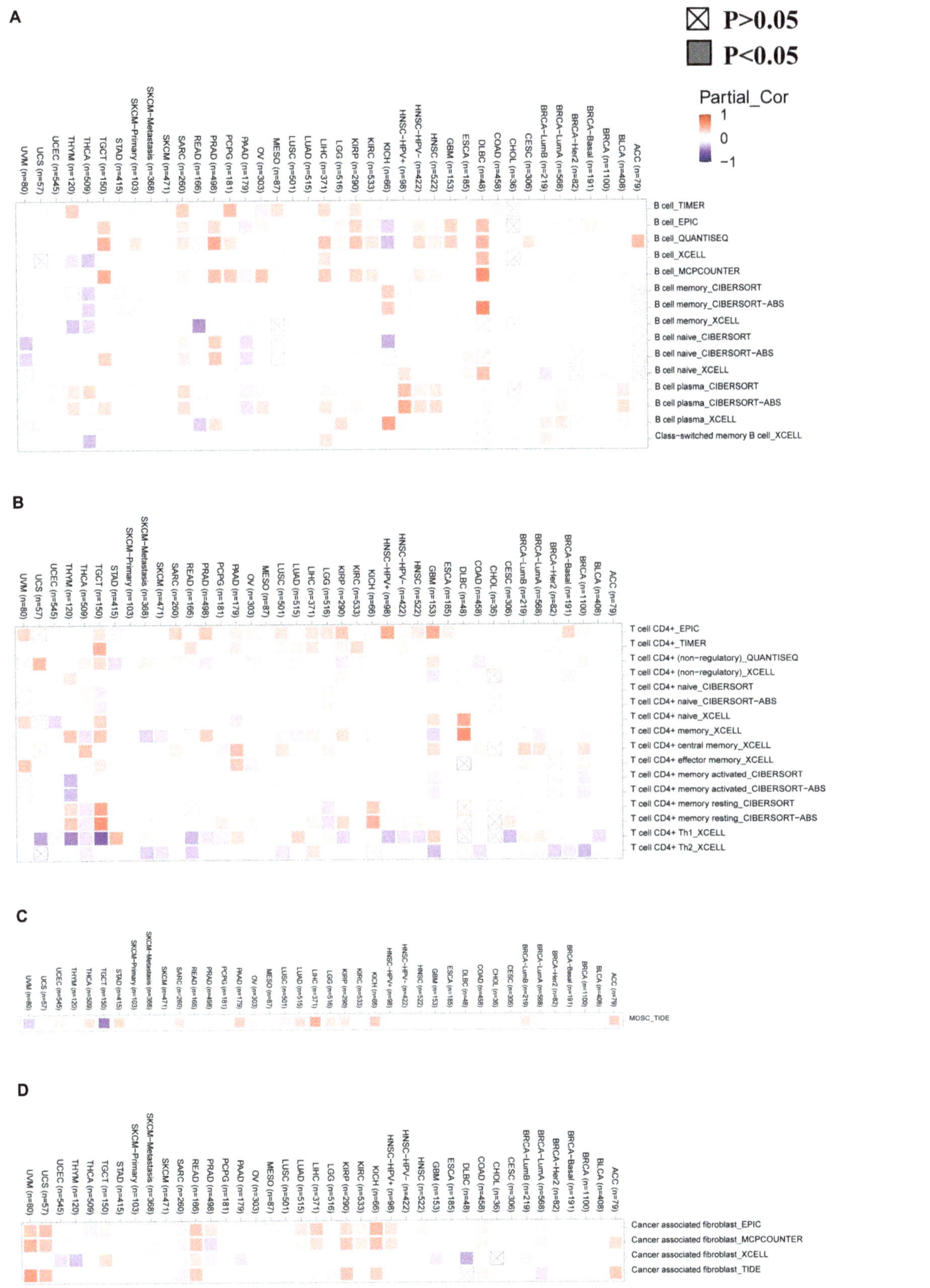

FIGURE 4 | Continued

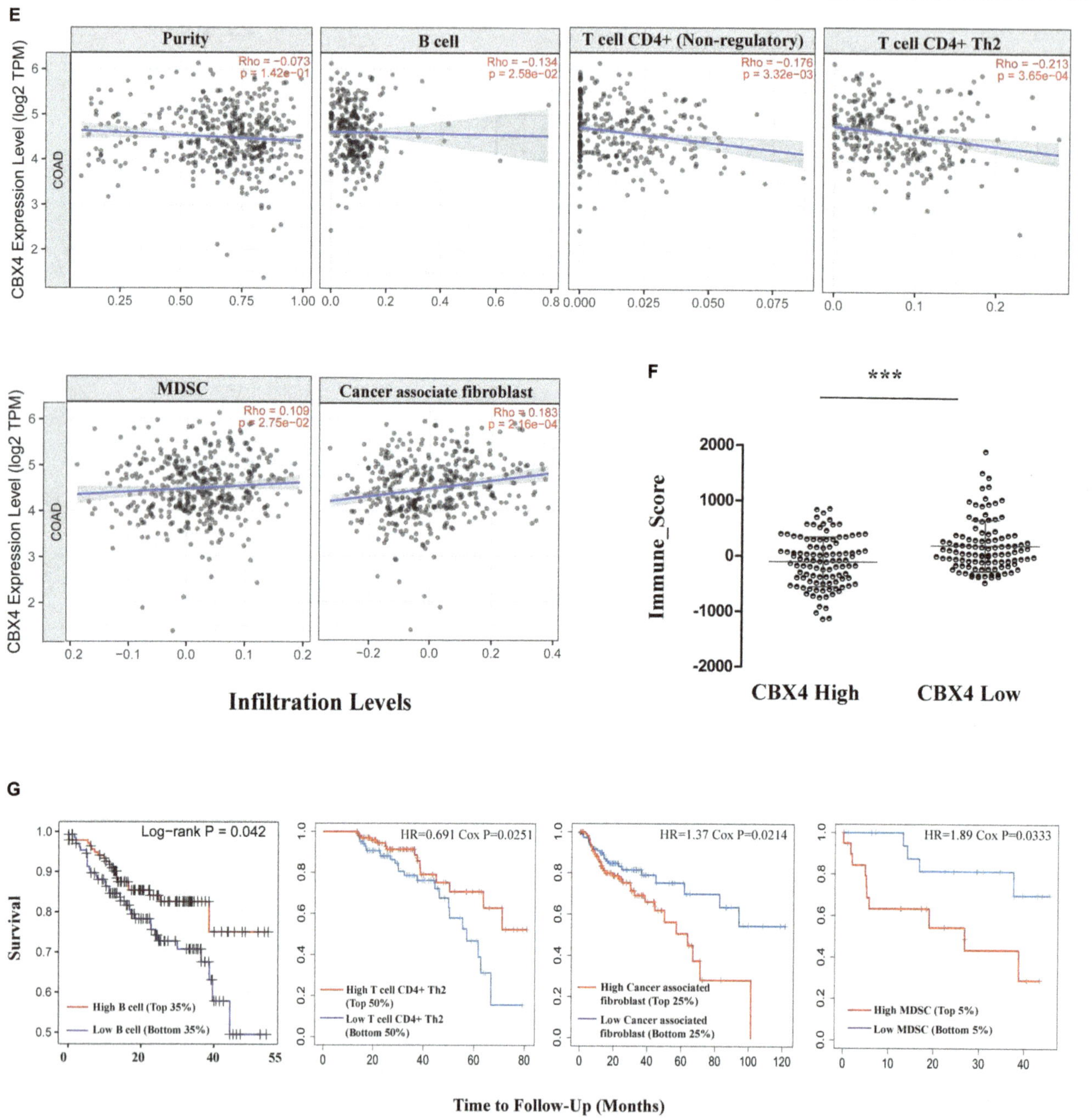

FIGURE 4 | CBX4 Impacts Immunophenotype in Colon Cancer. Correlations between CBX4 expression and the infiltration abundance of B cells **(A)**, CD4 + T cells **(B)**, myeloid derived suppressor cells (MDSCs) **(C)** and cancer associated fibroblast (CAFs) **(D)** were assessed in the 40 cancer types from the Gene module of TIMER2.0. The heat maps integrated multiple algorithms for immune infiltration estimation and showed the purity-adjusted partial spearman's rho across various cancer types. Positive correlations (rho > 0) are red and negative correlations (rho < 0) are blue. The significance of these correlations was classified into $P < 0.05$, shown in solid squares and $P > 0.05$, shown in hollow squares. **(E)** In COAD ($n = 458$), scatter plots showed the relationship between CBX4 expression in log2 TPM and levels of tumor purity, infiltrating B cells, CD4 + T cells, MDSCs, and CAFs. Spearman's rho and statistical significance were shown. **(F)** The immune score of ESTIMATE algorithm representing the overall infiltration levels of the immune cells in COAD. 210 of TCGA samples were divided into two groups based on the FPKM levels of CBX4. The immune scores for these samples were collected from the RNAseq V2 platform of the ESTIMATE database, and analyzed based on the dichotomized cases with high and low expression of CBX4. * $P < 0.05$, ** $P < 0.01$, *** $P < 0.001$ **(G)** Influences of the above immune infiltrating subsets on the clinical outcome of COAD were evaluated by the Survival module of TIMER. The Kaplan-Meier plots visualized the survival differences between the high and low infiltration levels of B cells, CD4 + Th2 cells, MDSCs and CAFs. The hazard ratio and p value for Cox model and the log-rank p value for Kaplan-Meier curve were shown.

CLOCK, one of the major activators that drive the positive regulatory loop of circadian rhythm, was negatively correlated with CBX4 ($p < 0.001$). On the contrary, PER1 ($p < 0.001$), PER3 ($p < 0.01$), and CRY2 ($p < 0.001$), members of the PER/CRY-controlled negative loop of the circadian clock, were positively correlated with CBX4. A positive correlation was also identified with NR1D1 ($p < 0.001$), a critical negative regulator of circadian rhythm directly repressing the core clock components (Polidarova et al., 2017). These results suggested such a possibility that up-regulated CBX4 expression in COAD might be cooperated with altered circadian clock gene actions. Furthermore, the relationship between CBX4 and the circadian regulators was tested in normal colon tissues via GEPIA. None of the significant correlations described above was observed in normal tissues (**Figure 2C**), suggesting that these interactive events may be specifically involved, and represent functional significance in tumor environment.

Elevated CBX4 Expression Predicts Poor Prognosis in Colon Carcinoma

To reveal the prognostic potential of CBX4 in colon cancer, DFS in two colorectal cancer cohorts GSE17536 ($n = 145$) and GSE14333 ($n = 226$) was analyzed, comparing the dichotomized cases with high and low expression of CBX4. In both cohorts, increased expression of CBX4 was associated with significant poor DFS (**Figure 3A** upper). In line with these findings, cBioportal analysis demonstrated that cancer samples from the recurred/progressed patients had higher CBX4 mRNA levels than those from the disease-free patients (**Figure 3B**). Furthermore, we interrogated the correlation of CBX4 expression with cancer metastasis using UALCAN. The nodular metastasis status was grouped into N0 ($n = 166$), N1 ($n = 70$) and N2 ($n = 47$). CBX4 expression levels were compared among differential groups and the statistical significance was shown as follows: $P_{\text{Normal-vs-N0}} < 0.001$; $P_{\text{Normal-vs-N1}} < 0.001$; $P_{\text{Normal-vs-N2}} < 0.001$; $P_{\text{N0-vs-N1}} < 0.05$; $P_{\text{N0-vs-N2}} = 0.12$; $P_{\text{N1-vs-N2}} = 0.876$ (**Figure 3C** left). It is interesting to note that altered CBX4 expression primarily occurred during the early onset instead of the progressive stages. Similarly, CBX4 expression levels were evaluated against cancer stages which are categorized into normal (n=41), stage I (n=45), stage II (n=110), stage III (n= 80), and stage IV ($n = 39$), and the statistical significance was shown as follows: $P_{\text{Normal-vs-Stage1}} < 0.001$; $P_{\text{Normal-vs-Stage2}} < 0.001$; $P_{\text{Normal-vs-Stage3}} < 0.001$; $P_{\text{Normal-vs-Stage4}} < 0.001$; $P_{\text{Stage1-vs-Stage2}} = 0.73$; $P_{\text{Stage1-vs-Stage3}} = 0.053$; $P_{\text{Stage1-vs-Stage4}} = 0.087$; $P_{\text{Stage2-vs-Stage3}} = 0.0786$; $P_{\text{Stage2-vs-Stage4}} = 0.1$; $P_{\text{Stage3-vs-Stage4}} = 0.794$ (**Figure 3C** right). Again, CBX4 tended to be associated with colon cancer early development instead of its late progression. Together, all these data suggested a role of CBX4 as a predictor for poor prognosis.

Given the potential interaction of CBX4 with the circadian clock core genes, we further explored the correlation between the patient survival and the clock gene expression in COAD. While higher level of CLOCK was associated with improved overall survival (Cox $p < 0.05$), increased expression of PER1 (Cox $p < 0.01$), PER3 (Cox $p < 0.05$), and CRY2 (Cox $p < 0.05$) predicted poor prognosis (**Figure 3A** lower). These results were consistent with their coordinated expression with CBX4.

CBX4 Impacts Immunophenotype in Colon Cancer

Tumor infiltrating lymphocytes (TILs) are recognized to predict lymphatic metastasis and survival in cancers (Azimi et al., 2012). We next investigated how immune infiltration levels were affected by CBX4 expression. We assessed the correlations of CBX4 expression with tumor immune infiltration abundance in the 40 cancer types from the Gene module of TIMER2.0. Among the diverse infiltrates, we found that CBX4 expression was shown to have significant correlations with infiltrating B cells in 33 types (**Figure 4A**), infiltrating $CD4^+$ T cells in 36 types (**Figure 4B**), myeloid derived suppressor cells (MDSCs) in 17 types (**Figure 4C**) and cancer associated fibroblast (CAFs) in 28 types of the 40 cancers (**Figure 4D**) ($p < 0.05$). Given the multiple potential correlations of CBX4 expression with the infiltration levels in diverse types of tumors, we next focused on colon adenocarcinoma for further investigations. As shown in **Figure 4E**, CBX4 was negatively correlated with infiltrating B cells (Spearman's rho = −0.134, $p < 0.05$) and CD4 + T cells (Spearman's rho = −0.176, $p < 0.01$) including CD4 + Th2 cells (Spearman's rho = −0.213, $p < 0.001$). Conversely, significant positive correlations were observed with MDSC (Spearman's rho = 0.109, $p < 0.05$) and CAFs (Spearman's rho = 0.183, $p < 0.001$). In view of the potential interactions between CBX4 and these immune infiltrates in COAD, we further evaluated the association of these tumor immune subsets with the clinical outcome via the Survival module of TIMER. The Kaplan-Meier plots were output to visualize the survival differences between high and low levels of infiltrating B cells, CD4 + Th2 cells, MDSC and CAFs. Infiltrating B cells ($p < 0.05$) and CD4 + Th2 cells ($p < 0.05$) were both significantly associated with increased survival rate, while MDSC ($p < 0.05$) and CAFs ($p < 0.05$) predicted poor prognosis in COAD (**Figure 4G**). Furthermore, the COAD patients were dichotomized based on the CBX4 mRNA expression levels (FPKM) of the TCGA cases listed in **Supplementary Table 1**. The corresponding immune scores were profiled on the RNA-seq-V2 platform of the ESTIMATE algorithm. We found that CBX4 expression levels were associated with relatively low immune scores (**Figure 4F**).

In addition to the major cellular composition of the immune infiltrates, we investigated the relationship of CBX4 expression and a compendium of gene representatives of various $CD4^+$ T cell subsets, including Th1, Th2, Th17, and regulatory T cells, as proposed by Charoentong and colleagues (Charoentong et al., 2017). As illustrated in **Tables 1**, **2**, CBX4 was partially associated with some gene markers of Th1 and Th17 cells, whereas it is worth noting that its expression level was strong-positively correlated with Th2 – associated transcriptional factor GATA-3 ($p < 0.001$) and STAT6 ($p < 0.001$) which function to stably commit differentiating cells toward the Th2 phenotype. In addition, CBX4 showed significant positive correlations with

TABLE 2 | Correlations between CBX4 and gene representatives of various functional cell subsets in COAD determined by GEPIA.

Immune markers	CBX4 Correlation (GEPIA)							
	COAD Tumor				COAD Normal			
	Spearman's	*p* value	Pearson's	*p* value	Spearman's	*p* value	Pearson's	*p* value
PD-1(PDCD1)	0.17	**	0.17	**	0.28	0.079	0.38	0.015
LAG3	0.15	*	0.21	***	0.15	0.34	0.19	0.24
FOXP3	0.12	*	0.12	*	0.2	0.21	0.27	0.089
TGFβ (TGFB1)	0.27	***	0.33	***	0.65	***	0.71	***
L1CAM	0.44	***	0.32	***	0.15	0.37	0.24	0.14
PTGIR	0.25	***	0.14	*	0.16	0.32	0.25	0.11
T-bet (TBX21)	0.15	*	0.15	*	0.16	0.32	0.2	0.2
STAT1	0.24	***	0.3	***	0.096	0.55	−0.09	0.58
GATA3	0.19	**	0.15	*	0.36	*	0.41	**
STAT6	0.23	***	0.19	**	0.42	**	0.44	**
IL-6R	0.22	***	0.13	*	−0.22	0.18	−0.16	0.33
STAT3	0.27	***	0.25	***	0.37	*	0.25	0.11
CD68	0.18	**	0.22	***	0.097	0.55	0.068	0.67
CD11b (ITGAM)	0.2	***	0.13	*	0.51	***	0.4	**
IL-4R	0.27	***	0.21	***	0.2	0.2	0.29	0.064

$^{*}P < 0.05$, $^{**}P < 0.01$, and $^{***}P < 0.001$.

those T cell exhaustion and Treg-associated parameters, such as PD-1 ($p < 0.01$), TGFβ ($p < 0.001$), Foxp3 ($p < 0.05$), L1CAM ($p < 0.001$) and PTGIR ($p < 0.001$), as well as the markers of MDSC, such as CD11b ($p < 0.01$) (Charoentong et al., 2017) (**Table 1** and **Supplementary Figure 2**). These interactions were further confirmed by using the GEPIA database (**Table 2** and **Supplementary Figure 3**). Consistent with their coordinated expression with CBX4, PER1, and PER3, the key members of the PER/CRY-controlled negative loop of the circadian clock, showed strong positive correlations with these gene representatives in COAD (**Table 3**). These data suggested a potential role of CBX4 and deregulated circadian rhythm in immune escape in the colon cancer microenvironment.

DISCUSSION

Here we demonstrate that CBX4 may contribute to colon cancer development via the potential interactions with the circadian rhythm genes. As illustrated in **Figure 2**, CBX4 expression is negatively correlated with that of CLOCK. At the first glance, this result may be interpreted as the transcriptional repression of CLOCK imposed by CBX4, a key component of the PRC1 repressor complex. In such a scenario, one would expect the accompanied down-regulation of downstream clock controlled genes, which is contradictory to the observation of positive correlation of PER1, PER3, CRY2, and NR1D1. As such, we speculate that there is another possibility that the interactions are more likely dependent on the SUMO E3 ligase activity of CBX4. Previous studies have reported that the two SUMO-interacting motifs (SIMs) of CBX4 protein contribute to its SUMO E3 ligase-dependent functions (Luis et al., 2011). SUMO E3 ligases mainly act as adapters to recruit the E2 to the substrates (Kagey et al., 2003). Here, whether CBX4 may directly or indirectly function to bridge E2 and SUMO isoforms to the CLOCK/ARNTL substrates and initiate dynamic post-translational regulation has become our concern.

Heterodimers of CLOCK/ARNTL drive rhythmic expression of clock-controlled genes, thereby mediating circadian physiological behaviors. Colon function is controlled and optimized by endogenous circadian clock, allowing the anticipation of the chyme appearance at certain time (Polidarova et al., 2017). Interventions to the key regulators of the circadian rhythm feedback loops are associated with disorders in colon function, leading to increased susceptibility for developing colon cancer. Numerous studies have emphasized the role of post-translational modifications of the circadian rhythm components in regulating the molecular circadian machinery (Lee et al., 2008). CLOCK has been identified to be a substrate of SUMO, and the sumoylation sites of CLOCK are the highly conserved lysine residues K67 and K851 which are located in the bHLH/PAS and C-terminal regions, respectively (Li et al., 2013). K67 is essential for the associations of CLOCK with other proteins, such as ARNTL, PER1, and CRY1. K851 also exerts regulatory effects on CLOCK activity (Li et al., 2013). These SUMO modifications are found to potentiate the transcriptional activity of the CLOCK/ARNTL complex by stimulating its E-box binding activity (Lee et al., 2008; Li et al., 2013). Thus this might suggest such an interpretation of our observations that up-regulated CBX4 in COAD might directly or indirectly enhance the transcriptional activity of the CLOCK/ARNTL complex through SUMO modification, which in turn activates the downstream clock controlled genes. Accumulation of PERs and CRYs exerts a feedback inhibition to the CLOCK/ARNTL complex. Therefore, the level of CLOCK might be determined by the enhanced inhibitory

TABLE 3 | Correlations between PER1, PER3, and gene representatives of various functional cell subsets in COAD determined by TIMER2.0.

		Colon Adenocarcinoma (COAD)			
Cell type	**Gene marker**	**PER1**		**PER3**	
		spearman's rho	***P* Value**	**spearman's rho**	***P* Value**
T cell exhaustion	PD-1(PDCD1)	0.272	***	0.246	***
	CTLA4	0.305	***	0.259	***
	LAG3	0.309	***	0.257	***
	TIM-3 (HAVCR2)	0.258	***	0.255	***
Regulatory T cells	FOXP3	0.269	***	0.286	***
	TGFβ (TGFB1)	0.34	***	0.231	***
	L1CAM	0.189	***	0.147	**
	PTGIR	0.315	***	0.214	***
	ITGA4	0.205	***	0.342	***
Th1 cells	T-bet (TBX21)	0.303	***	0.287	***
	STAT1	0.308	***	0.351	***
	STAT4	0.224	***	0.305	***
	IFN-γ (IFNG)	0.122	*	0.209	***
Th2 cells	GATA3	0.245	***	0.282	***
	STAT6	0.195	***	0.229	***
Th17 cells	IL-6R	0.209	***	0.395	***
	STAT3	0.282	***	0.406	***
	RORγt (RORC)	−0.087	0.08	0.145	**
	IL-17A	−0.231	***	−0.072	0.15
Macrophage	CD68	0.254	***	0.277	***
MDSC	CD11b (ITGAM)	0.232	***	0.244	***
	IL-4R	0.413	***	0.354	***
	CD33	0.146	**	0.223	***
	CD14	0.239	***	0.228	***
	S100A9	0.01	0.834	−0.031	0.539

$^{*}P < 0.05$, $^{**}P < 0.01$, and $^{***}P < 0.001$.

feedback effect of the downstream clock controlled genes, rather than direct transcriptional suppression induced by CBX4. Although further delineation is needed to support such a mechanism, this scenario will provide an alternate functional avenue of CBX4.

CBX4 was associated with a poor prognosis in COAD, whereas the circadian clock genes correlated with differential clinical outcomes as illustrated in **Figure 3**. CLOCK, negatively correlated with CBX4, was associated with good overall survival. On the other hand, PER1, PER3, CRY2 which were positively correlated with CBX4, were associated with poor prognosis. Circadian clock homeostasis is believed to have a tumor protective role (Savvidis and Koutsilieris, 2012; Labrecque and Cermakian, 2015). When each circadian clock core gene is subject to aberrant regulation, they might perform differential actions in certain context of tumor microenvironment. Interventions to the key regulators of molecular circadian clock may contribute to disorders in circadian homeostasis, which eventually lead to changes in cellular functions.

As an immunogenic tumor, colon adenocarcinoma is characterized by a strong intrinsic immune suppressive microenvironment as well as a high immune evasion, which may represent a major impediment for effective immune responses against tumor (Zhang et al., 2020). Therefore, we next unmask a landscape of infiltrating lymphocytes in COAD engaged by CBX4. As illustrated in **Figure 4**, levels of CBX4 were significantly negatively correlated with infiltrating B cells and $CD4^{+}$ T cells, while positively correlated with MDSCs and CAFs. The role of TILs is highly content and stage dependent. In colon cancer, B cells constitute a significant proportion of the tumor immune infiltrates, characterized by accumulation of terminally memory B cells or plasma cells suggestive of a specific anti-tumor immune response (Shimabukuro-Vornhagen et al., 2014). The abundance of infiltrating B appears to have a beneficial impact on the patient's clinical outcome as illustrated in **Figure 4G**. CD4 + Th cells target tumor cells either directly through cytolytic mechanisms or indirectly by modulating the tumor microenvironment (TME) (Borst et al., 2018). CD4 + Th1 and Th17 cells have been well documented to activate cytotoxic T lymphocytes, whereas Tregs inhibit efficacious anti-tumor responses (Sun et al., 2002). Here, CD4 + Th2 infiltration also appeared to have a favorable prognosis in COAD when the follow-up time was started from 13months (**Figure 4G**), and the infiltration level was negatively correlated with CBX4 (**Figure 4E**). As inhibitory regulatory cells, MDSCs attenuate antitumor immunity by suppressing T cell activation and perturbing innate immune cells (Zhang et al., 2020). By secreting growth factors, cytokines, and chemokines, CAFs in TME facilitate cancer cell proliferation, metastasis, angiogenesis and drug resistance, and shield tumor cells from immune surveillance by enhancing key immune checkpoints (Zhang et al., 2020). The significant positive correlations of CBX4 with these two immune subsets suggested a possible role of CBX4 in immune escape in the colon cancer microenvironment.

The implication of CBX4 in the regulation of tumor immunity was further supported by analyzing the correlations between CBX4 expression and the gene representatives of various functional T cell and MDSC subsets in COAD. Strikingly, we noticed that CBX4 showed strong positive correlations with a variety of parameters characteristic of T cell exhaustion, regulatory T cells and MDSCs (**Tables 1**, **2**), which supported a potential involvement of CBX4 in immuno-suppression. Furthermore, significant positive correlations of CBX4 with STAT1 and IL-6R/STAT3 were observed, and the activation of STAT1 and IL-6/STAT3 signaling has been reported to promote immunosuppression in the TME of colon cancer (Zhang et al., 2020). However, pivotal Th1 regulatory cytokine IFN-γ and another key Th17 -associated transcriptional factor RORγt were not affected by CBX4. In addition, we note that CBX4 was strongly correlated with Th2 – associated transcriptional factor GATA-3 and STAT6 which function to stably commit differentiating cells toward the Th2 phenotype. Therefore, CBX4-expressing tumors appear to be featured by an immune response biased toward type 2. Again, it is interesting to note that PER1 and PER3, consistent with their coordinated expression with CBX4, showed strong positive correlations with these immune metagenes as well, suggesting a possible interaction between CBX4 and the circadian machinery.

CONCLUSION

Despite extensive studies on potential mechanisms of CBX4-mediated tumorigenesis, CBX4's functional panorama remains to be explored. Circadian rhythm disruption is associated with higher cancer risk, whereas delineation of the mechanisms linking circadian rhythm disruption to cancers has yet to be elaborated. Little is known about the relationship between CBX4 and circadian rhythm genes in colon cancer as well as the potential impacts on the tumor immunity. Despite still a preliminary stage of this study, our data suggest that CBX4 is up-regulated and associated with poor clinical outcome in COAD. It is significantly correlated with the circadian clock core genes, and impacts tumor immune infiltration, supporting a potential involvement in immune escape in the colon tumor microenvironment. We anticipate our findings will provide a framework for future studies that will further elucidate in-depth molecular mechanism of CBX4-mediated circadian disruption, which may provide better insights for development of new targeting strategies.

AUTHOR CONTRIBUTIONS

WW designed the experiments, collected the data, and wrote the manuscript. WZ contributed to data organization and technical assistance. YZ supervised the project, edited the manuscript, and provided overall guidance. All authors approved the submitted version.

ACKNOWLEDGMENT

We thank Jinyi Zhang and the UHN Pathology Research Program for technical assistance.

SUPPLEMENTARY MATERIAL

Supplementary Figure 1 | The Genomic Alterations of CBX4 across Cancers. Proportions of CBX4 mutations and somatic copy number alterations including amplification and deletion in TCGA samples were analyzed via cBioportal, based on TCGA Pan Cancer Atlas studies in which 594 of colorectal carcinoma cases were included. The Green bars indicate non-synonymous mutations, red bars are gene amplifications, blue bars are deep deletions, and gray bars indicate multiple alterations.

Supplementary Figure 2 | Correlations between CBX4 and immune marker sets of various functional immune cells in COAD determined by TIMER2.0. The purity-adjusted partial spearman's rho value represents the degree of the correlation, and the significance was indicated.

Supplementary Figure 3 | Correlations between CBX4 and gene representatives of various functional cell subsets in COAD determined by GEPIA. COAD tumor: colon adenocarcinoma tissue in TCGA; COAD normal: adjacent normal tissues in TCGA. Spearman's and Pearson's R and the significance were indicated.

REFERENCES

Aran, D., Sirota, M., and Butte, A. J. (2015). Systematic pan-cancer analysis of tumour purity. *Nat. Commun.* 6:8971. doi: 10.1038/ncomms9971

Azimi, F., Scolyer, R. A., Rumcheva, P., Moncrieff, M., Murali, R., McCarthy, S. W., et al. (2012). Tumor-infiltrating lymphocyte grade is an independent predictor of sentinel lymph node status and survival in patients with cutaneous melanoma. *J. Clin. Oncol.* 30, 2678–2683. doi: 10.1200/jco.2011.37.8539

Borst, J., Ahrends, T., Babala, N., Melief, C. J. M., and Kastenmuller, W. (2018). CD4(+) T cell help in cancer immunology and immunotherapy. *Nat. Rev. Immunol.* 18, 635–647. doi: 10.1038/s41577-018-0044-0

Bray, F., Ferlay, J., Soerjomataram, I., Siegel, R. L., Torre, L. A., and Jemal, A. (2018). Global cancer statistics 2018: GLOBOCAN estimates of incidence and mortality worldwide for 36 cancers in 185 countries. *CA Cancer J. Clin.* 68, 394–424. doi: 10.3322/caac.21492

Burki, T. (2017). Nobel Prize awarded for discoveries in circadian rhythm. *Lancet* 390:e25. doi: 10.1016/S0140-6736(17)32661-2

Cerami, E., Gao, J., Dogrusoz, U., Gross, B. E., Sumer, S. O., Aksoy, B. A., et al. (2012). The cBio cancer genomics portal: an open platform for exploring multidimensional cancer genomics data. *Cancer Discov.* 2, 401–404. doi: 10.1158/2159-8290.cd-12-0095

Chandrashekar, D. S., Bashel, B., Balasubramanya, S. A. H., Creighton, C. J., Ponce-Rodriguez, I., Chakravarthi, B., et al. (2017). UALCAN: a portal for facilitating tumor subgroup gene expression and survival analyses. *Neoplasia* 19, 649–658. doi: 10.1016/j.neo.2017.05.002

Charoentong, P., Finotello, F., Angelova, M., Mayer, C., Efremova, M., Rieder, D., et al. (2017). Pan-cancer immunogenomic analyses reveal genotype-immunophenotype relationships and predictors of response to checkpoint blockade. *Cell Rep.* 18, 248–262. doi: 10.1016/j.celrep.2016.12.019

Chen, S. T., Choo, K. B., Hou, M. F., Yeh, K. T., Kuo, S. J., and Chang, J. G. (2005). Deregulated expression of the PER1, PER2 and PER3 genes in breast cancers. *Carcinogenesis* 26, 1241–1246. doi: 10.1093/carcin/bgi075

Colangelo, T., Polcaro, G., Muccillo, L., D'Agostino, G., Rosato, V., Ziccardi, P., et al. (2017). Friend or foe? The tumour microenvironment dilemma in colorectal cancer. *Biochim. Biophys. Acta Rev. Cancer* 1867, 1–18. doi: 10.1016/j.bbcan.2016.11.001

Dallmann, R., Okyar, A., and Levi, F. (2016). Dosing-time makes the poison: circadian regulation and pharmacotherapy. *Trends Mol. Med.* 22, 430–445. doi: 10.1016/j.molmed.2016.03.004

Flynn-Evans, E. E., Mucci, L., Stevens, R. G., and Lockley, S. W. (2013). Shiftwork and prostate-specific antigen in the National Health and Nutrition Examination Survey. *J. Natl. Cancer Inst.* 105, 1292–1297. doi: 10.1093/jnci/djt169

Fuhr, L., Abreu, M., Carbone, A., El-Athman, R., Bianchi, F., Laukkanen, M. O., et al. (2019). The interplay between colon cancer cells and tumour-associated stromal cells impacts the biological clock and enhances malignant phenotypes. *Cancers (Basel)* 11:988. doi: 10.3390/cancers11070988

Gao, J., Aksoy, B. A., Dogrusoz, U., Dresdner, G., Gross, B., Sumer, S. O., et al. (2013). Integrative analysis of complex cancer genomics and clinical profiles using the cBioPortal. *Sci. Signal.* 6:l1. doi: 10.1126/scisignal.2004088

Gery, S., Komatsu, N., Kawamata, N., Miller, C. W., Desmond, J., Virk, R. K., et al. (2007). Epigenetic silencing of the candidate tumor suppressor gene Per1 in non-small cell lung cancer. *Clin. Cancer Res.* 13, 1399–1404. doi: 10.1158/1078-0432.ccr-06-1730

Innominato, P. F., Focan, C., Gorlia, T., Moreau, T., Garufi, C., Waterhouse, J., et al. (2009). Circadian rhythm in rest and activity: a biological correlate of quality of life and a predictor of survival in patients with metastatic colorectal cancer. *Cancer Res.* 69, 4700–4707. doi: 10.1158/0008-5472.can-08-4747

Kagey, M. H., Melhuish, T. A., and Wotton, D. (2003). The polycomb protein Pc2 is a SUMO E3. *Cell* 113, 127–137. doi: 10.1016/s0092-8674(03)00159-4

Kettner, N. M., Voicu, H., Finegold, M. J., Coarfa, C., Sreekumar, A., Putluri, N., et al. (2016). Circadian homeostasis of liver metabolism suppresses hepatocarcinogenesis. *Cancer Cell* 30, 909–924. doi: 10.1016/j.ccell.2016.10.007

Labrecque, N., and Cermakian, N. (2015). Circadian clocks in the immune system. *J. Biol. Rhythms* 30, 277–290. doi: 10.1177/0748730415577723

Lee, J., Lee, Y., Lee, M. J., Park, E., Kang, S. H., Chung, C. H., et al. (2008). Dual modification of BMAL1 by SUMO2/3 and ubiquitin promotes circadian activation of the CLOCK/BMAL1 complex. *Mol. Cell Biol.* 28, 6056–6065. doi: 10.1128/mcb.00583-08

Lee, S., Donehower, L. A., Herron, A. J., Moore, D. D., and Fu, L. (2010). Disrupting circadian homeostasis of sympathetic signaling promotes tumor development in mice. *PLoS One* 5:e10995. doi: 10.1371/journal.pone.0010995

Lesicka, M., Jablonska, E., Wieczorek, E., Seroczynska, B., Siekierzycka, A., Skokowski, J., et al. (2018). Altered circadian genes expression in breast cancer tissue according to the clinical characteristics. *PLoS One* 13:e0199622. doi: 10.1371/journal.pone.0199622

Li, B., Severson, E., Pignon, J. C., Zhao, H., Li, T., Novak, J., et al. (2016). Comprehensive analyses of tumor immunity: implications for cancer immunotherapy. *Genome Biol.* 17:174. doi: 10.1186/s13059-016-1028-7

Li, J., Xu, Y., Long, X. D., Wang, W., Jiao, H. K., Mei, Z., et al. (2014). Cbx4 governs HIF-1alpha to potentiate angiogenesis of hepatocellular carcinoma by its SUMO E3 ligase activity. *Cancer Cell.* 25, 118–131. doi: 10.1016/j.ccr.2013.12.008

Li, S., Wang, M., Ao, X., Chang, A. K., Yang, C., Zhao, F., et al. (2013). CLOCK is a substrate of SUMO and sumoylation of CLOCK upregulates the transcriptional activity of estrogen receptor-alpha. *Oncogene* 32, 4883–4891. doi: 10.1038/onc.2012.518

Li, T., Fan, J., Wang, B., Traugh, N., Chen, Q., Liu, J. S., et al. (2017). TIMER: a web server for comprehensive analysis of tumor-infiltrating immune cells. *Cancer Res.* 77, e108–e110. doi: 10.1158/0008-5472.can-17-0307

Li, T., Fu, J., Zeng, Z., Cohen, D., Li, J., Chen, Q., et al. (2020). TIMER2.0 for analysis of tumor-infiltrating immune cells. *Nucleic Acids Res.* 48, W509–W514. doi: 10.1093/nar/gkaa407

Lin, H. H., and Farkas, M. E. (2018). Altered circadian rhythms and breast cancer: from the human to the molecular level. *Front. Endocrinol.* 9:219. doi: 10.3389/fendo.2018.00219

Luis, N. M., Morey, L., Mejetta, S., Pascual, G., Janich, P., Kuebler, B., et al. (2011). Regulation of human epidermal stem cell proliferation and senescence requires polycomb- dependent and -independent functions of Cbx4. *Cell Stem Cell.* 9, 233–246. doi: 10.1016/j.stem.2011.07.013

Malki, A., ElRuz, R. A., Gupta, I., Allouch, A., Vranic, S., and Al Moustafa, A. E. (2020). Molecular mechanisms of colon cancer progression and metastasis: recent insights and advancements. *Int. J. Mol. Sci.* 22:130. doi: 10.3390/ijms22010130

Meng, R., Fang, J., Yu, Y., Hou, L. K., Chi, J. R., Chen, A. X., et al. (2018). miR-129-5p suppresses breast cancer proliferation by targeting CBX4. *Neoplasma* 65, 572–578. doi: 10.4149/neo_2018_170814N530

Mizuno, H., Kitada, K., Nakai, K., and Sarai, A. (2009). PrognoScan: a new database for meta-analysis of the prognostic value of genes. *BMC Med. Genomics* 2:18. doi: 10.1186/1755-8794-2-18

Papagiannakopoulos, T., Bauer, M. R., Davidson, S. M., Heimann, M., Subbaraj, L., Bhutkar, A., et al. (2016). Circadian rhythm disruption promotes lung tumorigenesis. *Cell Metab.* 24, 324–331. doi: 10.1016/j.cmet.2016.07.001

Polidarova, L., Houdek, P., Sladek, M., Novosadova, Z., Pacha, J., and Sumova, A. (2017). Mechanisms of hormonal regulation of the peripheral circadian clock in the colon. *Chronobiol. Int.* 34, 1–16. doi: 10.1080/07420528.2016.1231198

Sauvageau, M., and Sauvageau, G. (2010). Polycomb group proteins: multi-faceted regulators of somatic stem cells and cancer. *Cell Stem Cell.* 7, 299–313. doi: 10.1016/j.stem.2010.08.002

Savvidis, C., and Koutsilieris, M. (2012). Circadian rhythm disruption in cancer biology. *Mol. Med.* 18, 1249–1260. doi: 10.2119/molmed.2012.00077

Scheiermann, C., Kunisaki, Y., and Frenette, P. S. (2013). Circadian control of the immune system. *Nat. Rev. Immunol.* 13, 190–198. doi: 10.1038/nri3386

Shimabukuro-Vornhagen, A., Schlosser, H. A., Gryschok, L., Malcher, J., Wennhold, K., Garcia-Marquez, M., et al. (2014). Characterization of tumor-associated B-cell subsets in patients with colorectal cancer. *Oncotarget* 5, 4651–4664. doi: 10.18632/oncotarget.1701

Simon, J. A., and Kingston, R. E. (2009). Mechanisms of polycomb gene silencing: knowns and unknowns. *Nat. Rev. Mol. Cell Biol.* 10, 697–708. doi: 10.1038/nrm2763

Sun, Q., Burton, R. L., and Lucas, K. G. (2002). Cytokine production and cytolytic mechanism of CD4(+) cytotoxic T lymphocytes in ex vivo expanded therapeutic Epstein-Barr virus-specific T-cell cultures. *Blood* 99, 3302–3309. doi: 10.1182/blood.v99.9.3302

Szklarczyk, D., Gable, A. L., Lyon, D., Junge, A., Wyder, S., Huerta-Cepas, J., et al. (2019). STRING v11: protein-protein association networks with increased coverage, supporting functional discovery in genome-wide experimental datasets. *Nucleic Acids Res.* 47, D607–D613. doi: 10.1093/nar/gky1131

Tang, Z., Li, C., Kang, B., Gao, G., Li, C., and Zhang, Z. (2017). GEPIA: a web server for cancer and normal gene expression profiling and interactive analyses. *Nucleic Acids Res.* 45, W98–W102. doi: 10.1093/nar/gkx247

Vandamme, J., Volkel, P., Rosnoblet, C., Le Faou, P., and Angrand, P. O. (2011). Interaction proteomics analysis of polycomb proteins defines distinct PRC1 complexes in mammalian cells. *Mol. Cell Proteomics* 10:M110.002642. doi: 10.1074/mcp.M110.002642

von Mering, C., Huynen, M., Jaeggi, D., Schmidt, S., Bork, P., and Snel, B. (2003). STRING: a database of predicted functional associations between proteins. *Nucleic Acids Res.* 31, 258–261. doi: 10.1093/nar/gkg034

Wang, X., Li, L., Wu, Y., Zhang, R., Zhang, M., Liao, D., et al. (2016). CBX4 suppresses metastasis via recruitment of HDAC3 to the Runx2 promoter in colorectal carcinoma. *Cancer Res.* 76, 7277–7289. doi: 10.1158/0008-5472.can-16-2100

Wendeu-Foyet, M. G., and Menegaux, F. (2017). Circadian disruption and prostate cancer risk: an updated review of epidemiological evidences. *Cancer Epidemiol. Biomarkers Prev.* 26, 985–991. doi: 10.1158/1055-9965.epi-16-1030

Yoshihara, K., Shahmoradgoli, M., Martinez, E., Vegesna, R., Kim, H., Torres-Garcia, W., et al. (2013). Inferring tumour purity and stromal and immune cell admixture from expression data. *Nat. Commun.* 4:2612. doi: 10.1038/ncomms3612

Zauber, A. G. (2015). The impact of screening on colorectal cancer mortality and incidence: has it really made a difference? *Dig. Dis. Sci.* 60, 681–691. doi: 10.1007/s10620-015-3600-5

Zhang, Y., Rajput, A., Jin, N., and Wang, J. (2020). Mechanisms of immunosuppression in colorectal cancer. *Cancers (Basel)* 12:3850. doi: 10.3390/cancers12123850

6

The CAGE–MiR-181b-5p–S1PR1 Axis Regulates Anticancer Drug Resistance and Autophagy in Gastric Cancer Cells

Minjeong Yeon[1], Youngmi Kim[2], Deepak Pathak[3], Eunju Kwon[3], Dong Young Kim[3], Myeong Seon Jeong[1,4], Hyun Suk Jung[1] and Dooil Jeoung[1]*

[1] Department of Biochemistry, College of Natural Sciences, Kangwon National University, Chuncheon, South Korea, [2] Institute of New Frontier Research, College of Medicine, Hallym University, Chuncheon, South Korea, [3] College of Pharmacy, Yeungnam University, Gyeongsan, South Korea, [4] Chuncheon Center, Korea Basic Science Institute, Chuncheon, South Korea

***Correspondence:**
Dooil Jeoung
jeoungd@kangwon.ac.kr

Cancer-associated gene (CAGE), a cancer/testis antigen, has been known to promote anticancer drug resistance. Since the underlying mechanisms of CAGE-promoted anticancer drug resistance are poorly understood, we established Anticancer drug-resistant gastric cancer cells (AGS^R) to better elucidate possible mechanisms. AGS^R showed an increased expression level of CAGE and autophagic flux compared with anticancer drug-sensitive parental gastric cancer cells (AGS cells). AGS^R cells showed higher invasion potential, growth rate, tumor spheroid formation, and angiogenic potential than AGS cells. CAGE exerted effects on the response to anticancer drugs and autophagic flux. CAGE was shown to bind to Beclin1, a mediator of autophagy. Overexpression of CAGE increased autophagic flux and invasion potential but inhibited the cleavage of PARP in response to anticancer drugs in CAGE CRISPR–Cas9 cell lines. TargetScan analysis was utilized to predict the binding of miR-302b-5p to the promoter sequences of CAGE, and the results show that miR-302b-5p directly regulated CAGE expression as illustrated by luciferase activity. MiR-302b-5p regulated autophagic flux and the response to anticancer drugs. CAGE was shown to bind the promoter sequences of miR-302b-5p. The culture medium of AGS^R cells increased CAGE expression and autophagic flux in AGS cells. ImmunoEM showed CAGE was present in the exosomes of AGS^R cells; exosomes of AGS^R cells and human recombinant CAGE protein increased CAGE expression, autophagic flux, and resistance to anticancer drugs in AGS cells. MicroRNA array revealed miR-181b-5p as a potential negative regulator of CAGE. MiR-181b-5p inhibitor increased the expression of CAGE and autophagic flux in addition to preventing anticancer drugs from cleaving poly(ADP-ribose) polymerase (PARP) in AGS cells. TargetScan analysis predicted sphingosine 1-phosphate receptor 1 (SIPR1) as a potential target for miR-181b-5p. CAGE showed binding to the promoter sequences of S1PR1. The downregulation or inhibition of S1PR1 led to decreased autophagic flux but enhanced the sensitivity to anticancer drugs in AGS^R cells. This study presents a novel role of the CAGE–miR-181b-5p–S1PR1 axis in anticancer drug resistance and autophagy.

Keywords: anticancer drug resistance, autophagic flux, cancer-associated gene, miR-181b-5p, sphingosine 1-phosphate receptor

INTRODUCTION

Cancer-associated gene (CAGE), a cancer/testis gene, was initially discovered in the sera of patients with gastric cancers (Cho et al., 2002). The expression level of CAGE was closely related to the methylation status of CAGE promoter sequences (Cho et al., 2003). Anti-CAGE antibody was shown to be present in 7 of 13 (53.8%) patients with microsatellite instability-positive endometrial cancer and in 1 of 3 patients with atypical endometrial hyperplasia (Iwata et al., 2005). This suggests that CAGE could be utilized as a marker for the detection of microsatellite instability-positive endometrial cancers. There was the presence of CAGE in the sera of 12% of early-stage gastric cancer patients (Hurtado López et al., 2020). In addition, CAGE shows promise as an immunotherapeutic target in chronic myelomonocytic leukemia (Hurtado López et al., 2020).

Cancer-associated gene also enhances cellular proliferation by increasing the expression of cyclinD1 in an AP-1-dependent manner (Por et al., 2010). CAGE induces anticancer drug resistance by decreasing the expression of p53 (Kim et al., 2010). MiR-200b enhances the sensitivity of anticancer drugs by decreasing the expression of CAGE (Kim et al., 2013). CAGE is crucial to confer resistance to Taxol in cervical cancer cells (Park et al., 2018). CAGE increases cyclin D1 expression and enhances resistance to anticancer drugs through binding to glycogen synthase kinase 3 β (GSK3β) (Kim et al., 2017a). CAGE enhances the self-renewal and tumorigenic potential of anticancer drug-sensitive melanoma cells (Kim et al., 2017b).

Autophagy is closely associated with the response to anticancer drugs in many types of cancer. UTI (ulinastatin) inhibits EPI (epirubicin)-induced autophagy, promotes apoptosis, and enhances sensitivity to EPI in hepatic cancer cells (Song et al., 2015). Autophagy inhibition sensitizes breast cancer cells to paclitaxel (Wang et al., 2017). Autophagy is induced by chemotherapy and is associated with chemoresistance (Belounis et al., 2016). The inhibition of autophagy significantly enhanced AGEs (advanced glycation end products) and induced cell apoptosis (Xu et al., 2016). Thus, CAGE may play a role in autophagy.

Cancer-associated gene binds to epidermal growth factor receptor (EGFR) and increases self-renewal, in addition to increasing autophagic flux (Kim et al., 2016). The CAGE–miR-140-5p–proto-oncogene Wnt1 axis regulates autophagic flux in colon cancer cells (Yeon et al., 2019). CAGE promotes cellular interactions mediated by exosomes (Yeon et al., 2019). These reports suggest that CAGE may regulate anticancer drug resistance and autophagic flux by mediating cellular interactions.

MiR-300 activates protein phosphatase 2A (PP2A) and is necessary for anticancer drug resistance conferred by leukemic stem cells (Silvestri et al., 2020). *TUG1* long noncoding RNA is necessary for the survival of these leukemic stem cells by regulating the apoptotic function of miR-300 function (Silvestri et al., 2020). MiR-200b negatively regulates CAGE expression and enhances sensitivity to anticancer drugs in melanoma cells (Kim et al., 2013). MiR-217 enhances anticancer drug sensitivity by regulating CAGE expression and the interaction between CAGE and EGFR (Kim et al., 2016). These reports imply the roles of miRNAs in anticancer drug resistance and autophagy.

In this study, we found that both anticancer drug resistance and autophagic flux were regulated by a CAGE–miR-302b-5p negative feedback loop and displayed a close relationship. We showed that CAGE regulated anticancer drug resistance and was present in the exosomes of anticancer drug-resistant gastric cancer cells (AGS^R). The miR-181b-5p–S1PR1 axis acts as a negative regulator of anticancer drug resistance and autophagic flux. CAGE was shown to act as a direct regulator of sphingosine 1-phosphate receptor 1 (S1PR1) expression. Taking our data as a whole, we clearly demonstrate that the CAGE–miR-181b-5p–S1PR1 axis can be utilized as a target for the development of anticancer therapeutics.

MATERIALS AND METHODS

Materials

We purchased chemicals from Sigma Chemical Company. We purchased anti-mouse and anti-rabbit IgG-horseradish peroxidase conjugate antibody from Pierce Company (Rockford, IL, United States). Lipofectamine and PLUS™ reagent for transfection were purchased from Invitrogen (San Diego, CA, United States). Oligonucleotides, miRNA mimic, miR inhibitors, and siRNAs used in this study were purchased from Bioneer Company (Daejeon, Korea). We purchased tissue microarray from Signosis (California, United States).

Cell Lines and Cell Culture

Cancer cell lines were cultured in Dulbecco's modified minimal essential medium (Invitrogen) supplemented with heat-inactivated 10% fetal bovine serum (Invitrogen) and antibiotics. Cells were maintained at 37°C in 5% CO_2. Anticancer drug-resistant cancer cell lines were established as described (Kim et al., 2010).

Generation of Knockout Cell Line With the CRISPR/Cas9 System

To generate CAGE-deficient AGS^R cells, CRISPR/Cas9-mediated gene editing was performed. A plasmid encoding Cas9 was purchased from ToolGen. For sgRNA expression, the hU6-sgRNA plasmid that targeted CAGE (5′-AGGCTAATCCAAGAGACCTTGGG-3′) was used (ToolGen). AGS^R cells were transfected with Cas9, hU6-sgRNA, and hygromycin B-resistant reporter plasmid (ToolGen). After 48 h of transfection, cells were treated with hygromycin B (150 µg/ml) three times a week. Hygromycin-resistant colonies were isolated and subjected to immunoblot.

Colony Formation

Colonies were stained with 0.01% crystal violet and counted.

Cell Viability Determination

MTT assays were employed to determine the response to anticancer drugs. Viable cell number counting was carried out by trypan blue exclusion assays.

Matrigel Plug Assays

BALB/C mice (Nara Biotech) were given a subcutaneous injection with 0.1 ml of Matrigel containing culture medium and 10 units of heparin (Sigma). Hemoglobin (Hb) content in the Matrigel plugs was measured using Drabkin's reagent (Sigma, United States).

Chemo Invasion Assays

A transwell chamber system with 8-µm pore polycarbonate filter inserts (CoSTAR, Acton, MA, United States) was employed. Trypsinized cells (5×10^3) in the serum-free RPMI 1,640 medium containing 0.1% bovine serum albumin were added to each upper chamber of the transwell. RPMI 1,640 medium supplemented with 10% fetal bovine serum was placed in the lower chamber and cells were incubated at 37°C for 16 h. The invaded cells were stained and counted as described (Kim et al., 2017a). Differences were considered significant when $p < 0.05$.

Tumor Spheroid-Forming Potential

Cells were plated (5×10^4 cells/well) in ultralow attachment plates (Corning Inc.) in DMEM/F12 stem cell medium. Cells were fed with 0.2 ml of fresh stem cell medium on days 2, 4, and 6. The total number of spheres was counted after 7 days by inverted microscopy (Olympus).

RNA Extraction and Quantitative Real-Time PCR

Total miRNA was isolated using the *mir*Vana miRNA isolation kit (Ambion) and was extended by a poly(A) tailing reaction using the A-Plus poly(A) polymerase tailing kit (CellScript). CDNA was synthesized according to the manual provided by the manufacturer (Quanta Biogenesis). Levels of miRNAs were determined by a SYBR Green qRT-PCR kit (Ambion). The expression of miR-302b-5p was defined based on the threshold (C_t), and relative expression levels were determined as $2^{-((Ct\ of miR302b-5p) - (Ct\ of U6))}$ after normalization to the expression of U6 small nuclear RNA. Primer sequences are listed in the **Supplementary Tables**.

MiRNA Target Analysis

Genes that contain the miRNA-binding site(s) in the UTR were obtained using the http://TargetScan program[1], Diana laboratory[2], and miRDB[3].

Transfection

Cells were transiently transfected with the miRNA inhibitor, miRNA mimic, or siRNA (each at 10 nM) with jetPRIME® (Polyplus, cat. 114–15). The sequences of miR mimic, miR inhibitors, and siRNAs are listed in the **Supplementary Tables**.

Luciferase Activity Assays

PCR-amplified 3′ UTR of S1PR1 (381 bp) was cloned into the *Xba*I site of pGL3 luciferase plasmid. The mutant pGL3-3′ UTR–S1PR1 construct was made with the QuikChange site-directed mutagenesis kit (Stratagene). Luciferase activity assay was performed as described (Kim et al., 2019).

Immunofluorescence Staining

Cells were washed and fixed with 4% paraformaldehyde before permeabilization with Triton X-100. After blocked with goat serum (10%) in 0.1% BSA/PBS, cells were incubated with anti-LC3 or anti-CAGE at 4°C overnight and then incubated with anti-rabbit Alexa Fluor 488 (for LC3 and CAGE) secondary antibody. After removal of antibodies, cells were stained with DAPI and mounted with mounting medium. The immune fluorescent images were observed and captured using a confocal laser scanning microscope.

Immunoblot and Immunoprecipitation

Immunoblot and immunoprecipitation were performed as described (Yeon et al., 2019). Cell lysates were prepared using lysis buffer [62.5 mM Tris–HCl, pH 6.8, 2% (w/v) SDS, 10% (v/v) glycerol, 50 mM dithiothreitol, 0.01% (w/v) bromphenol blue, 10 mM NaF, 1% (v/v) protease inhibitor mixture (Roche), 1 mM sodium orthovanadate]. The denatured cell lysates (20 µg/well) were analyzed on a 10% SDS-PAGE and were transferred onto PVDF membrane and subjected to immunoblotting. The following primary antibodies were used in this study: CAGE (MBS2524843, MyBioSource); AMPKα (AF3194, R&D Systems); pAMPKα^{Thr172} (2535S, Cell Signaling), PARP (9542S, Cell Signaling), pBeclin1^{Ser15} (84966S, Cell Signaling), LC3 (12741S, Cell Signaling), Bcl-2 (3498S, Cell Signaling), E-cadherin (3195S, Cell Signaling), vimentin (5741S, Cell Signaling), mTOR (2972S, Cell Signaling), pmTOR^{Ser2448} (2971S, Cell Signaling), Alix (2171S, Cell Signaling), and p53 (2524S, Cell Signaling); Beclin1

[1] http://www.targetscan.org
[2] http://diana.imis.athena-innovation.gr
[3] http://mirdb.org

(sc-48341, Santa Cruz), IgG (sc-2025, Santa Cruz), SNAIL (sc-271977, Santa Cruz), ATG5 (sc-133158, Santa Cruz), PAI-1 (sc-5297, Santa Cruz), biotin (sc-101339, Santa Cruz), TSG101 (sc-7964, Santa Cruz), FAK (sc-558, Santa Cruz), and CD81 (sc-166029, Santa Cruz); actin (A2228, Sigma) and FLAG (F3166, Sigma); caspase-3 (PA05689A0Rb, Cusabio); p62 (ab56416, Abcam); and S1PR1 (55133-I-AP, Proteintech).

The following secondary antibodies were used in this study: anti-mouse HRP secondary antibody (31430, Invitrogen), anti-goat HRP secondary antibody (31402, Invitrogen), anti-rabbit HRP secondary antibody (ADI-SAB-300-J, Enzo), and anti-rabbit Alexa Fluor 488 secondary antibody (A11008, Invitrogen).

Chromatin Immunoprecipitation Assays

Assays were performed using a kit from Upstate Company. For detection of the binding of CAGE to miR-302b-5p promoter sequences, specific primers of miR-302b-5p promoter-1 sequences [5′-TCTGTTTCATTTCTGACTCT-3′ (sense) and 5′-CCAAGTCATTGTGAATGTAT-3′ (antisense)], miR-302b-5p promoter-2 sequences [5′-GCCAATTAAATTTTTGAGTGT CTG-3′ (sense) and 5′-ACGGGGTGTTTTGTTCTACT-3′ (antisense)], and miR-302b-5p promoter-3 sequences [5′-CCACCCAGGATCATACATTC-3′ (sense) and 5′-AAAGATTC GTGTTCTCCTCC-3′ (antisense)] were used. For binding of CAGE to S1PR1 promoter sequences, specific primers of S1PR1 promoter-1 sequences [5′-TGGCGGGGGGAG TACAGGAA-3′ (sense) and 5′-TCAGCACACCGATCCTCC TAGGG-3′ (antisense)], S1PR1 promoter-2 sequences [5′-GGCCGTCCTCTGCCTCCTC-3′ (sense) and 5′-TTTGTTG TTTGGGGAGGAGGGGT-3′ (antisense)], and S1PR1 promoter-3 sequences [5′-GCTTCTGCCCCAGATCTTTC CTGG-3′ (sense) and 5′-GGCCATTGGAGTGCTCCGC-3′ (antisense)] were used.

Electron Microscopic Observation of the Autophagic Process

Cells were treated with the fixation solution [2.5% glutaraldehyde in 0.1 M cacodylate solution (pH 7.0) for 1 h] and then mixed with 2% osmium tetroxide for 2 h at 4°C. The samples were dehydrated with a graded acetone series and embedded into a Spurr medium (Electron Microscopy System). The samples were sectioned (60 nm) by using an ultra-microtome (RMC MTXL, Arizona, United States). The section was stained with 2% uranyl acetate (for 20 min) followed by staining of lead citrate (for 10 min). The sections were viewed under a transmission electron microscope (JEM-2100F, Japan) at 200 kV.

Isolation of Exosomes

Cells were cultured under serum-free medium (Invitrogen, Carlsbad, CA, United States) and the culture medium was harvested after 48 h of incubation. Isolation of exosomes was carried out by using ExoQuick-TC reagent (System Biosciences, Mountain View, CA, United States). Exosomes were observed under a transmission electron microscope (JEM-2100F, Japan) at 200 kV.

Size Distribution Analysis of Exosomes

Exosomes were incubated on the ExoView chip (ExoView, United States) for 16 h. The chips were then washed three times in PBS with 0.05% Tween-20 (PBST) and then imaged with the ExoView R100 reader (ExoView, United States) using the ExoScan (ExoView, United States) acquisition software.

Internalization of Exosomes

Exosomes prepared from AGS^R cells were labeled with PKH67 Fluorescent Cell Linker kits (Sigma-Aldrich, St. Louis, MO, United States). In order to examine the internalization of exosomes, AGS cells were plated out onto a coverslip (2×10^4 cells). The following day, each medium containing PKH67-labeled exosomes or PKH67-unlabeled exosomes was added into each well for 24 h. After incubation, the coverslips were washed with PBS, and 4% paraformaldehyde solution was then added to the slides and incubated for 15 min. Cells were visualized under a confocal laser scanning microscope LX70 FV300 05-LPG-193 (Olympus, Japan).

The Presence of CAGE in the Exosomes

Exosomes extracted from AGS^R cells (REF, KIT model) were subjected to centrifugation at $60{,}000 \times g$ for 30 min to precipitate extracellular vesicles. Collected vesicles were prefixed with 0.1% glutaraldehyde and 2% paraformaldehyde in phosphate buffer (pH 7.4) for 1 h at 4°C and then postfixed in 2% osmium tetroxide for 30 min at 4°C. Samples were dehydrated with a graded series of ethanol and then treated with graded propylene oxide series. Dehydrated samples were embedded into epoxy resin (PELCO, United States). Preparation of ultrathin sections (~80 nm) was carried out with Ultracut UCT (Leica, Germany). Sections were mounted on copper grids and stained with 1% uranyl acetate and lead citrate (for 10 min) for the subsequent observations. For immunogold labeling electron microscopy, sections (~80 nm) on the grids were treated with 0.02 M glycine for 10 min. Sections were then washed in deionized water, floated for 1 h in PBS containing 1% BSA, and incubated with the primary rabbit or mouse antibody (anti-CAGE or/and anti-TSG101 antibodies, respectively) at 1:20 dilutions overnight at 4°C. The grids were washed with 0.1% BSA in PBS (five times) and incubated in secondary antibody, anti-rabbit IgG conjugated to 10 nm or anti-mouse IgG conjugated to 25 nm (AURION, Holland) diluted 1:20 in 0.1% BSA–PBS. The sample grids were stained with uranyl acetate and lead citrate. The sectioned and immunogold-labeled grids were examined using a JEOL-2100F transmission electron microscope (JEOL, United States) operated at 200 kV.

Expression and Purification of CAGE Protein

Full-length CAGE gene (residues 1–631) was inserted into pETDuet-1 vector (Merck Millipore, Billerica, MA, United States) expressing N-terminal 6_XHis and thioredoxin followed by TEV protease cleavage site, and then the plasmid was transformed into *Escherichia coli* strain BL21 Star (DE3) (Thermo Fischer Scientific, United States). Transformed cells were grown in LB media at 37°C. The media were cooled when OD_{600} (optical density at 600 nm) reached 0.6~0.7 and 0.4 mM IPTG was then added into the culture media to induce CAGE expression. After overnight incubation at 15°C, the cells were harvested by using centrifugation at 3,000 × *g* (for 10 min). The cells were resuspended in buffer A (20 mM HEPES pH 7.5, 0.5 m NaCl, 0.2 mM TCEP, and 5% glycerol), lysed by sonication, and clarified by centrifugation at 20,000 × *g* for 30 min after the addition of DNase I and RNase A. CAGE was then purified by IMAC (immobilized metal affinity chromatography) and SEC (size exclusion chromatography). The clarified cell lysate was loaded onto a 5-ml HisTrap nickel chelating column (GE Healthcare Bio-Sciences, Uppsala, Sweden), and the resin was washed with buffer A containing 40 mM imidazole. Proteins bound to the resin were eluted by an imidazole gradient. Fractions that contain CAGE were pooled and treated with TEV protease overnight at 4°C. After complete cleavage, the protein solution was dialyzed against buffer A and passed through the Ni-NTA resin (Thermo Scientific, United States). CAGE was further purified by SEC using Superdex 200 preparatory grade column (GE Healthcare Biosciences, United States) pre-equilibrated with buffer A.

Tissue Microarray and Immunohistochemical Staining

Immunohistochemical staining of tissue microarray was performed using an avidin–biotin detection method (Vectastain ABC kit, Vector Laboratories Inc., Burlingame, CA, United States). The tissue microarray contains gastric tumor tissues and adjacent nontumor gastric tissues from 40 gastric cancer patients. The anti-S1PR1 antibody (55133-I-AP, Proteintech) was used at 1:500 dilution. After washing, biotinylated secondary antibody (MP-7500, Vector Inc.) was applied at 1:100 or 1:200 dilutions for 1 h. Color was developed with diaminobenzidine (SK-4100, Vector Inc.). Sections were counterstained with Mayer's hematoxylin. IHC staining intensity was determined by using Celleste™ Image Analysis Software. Staining intensity was scored as follows: 1 = weak staining, 2 = medium staining, and 3 = strong staining. The IHC staining score was determined by measuring both the percentage of cells that stained positive for S1PR1 and the staining intensity.

Statistical Analysis

Statistical analysis was performed using the GraphPad Prism Statistics Program (Version 7, GraphPad Prism Software). All the data were obtained from experiments with adequate sample size and presented as means ± SE. Student's *t*-tests were performed for comparisons between two groups. One-way ANOVA was carried out for comparisons among three or more groups and was followed by Tukey's *post hoc* test. Values were considered to be significant at $p < 0.05$.

RESULTS

Anticancer Drug-Resistant Gastric Cancer Cells Show Enhanced Autophagic Process and Antiapoptotic Effects

To better understand the mechanism of anticancer drug resistance, AGS^R (cells) were established. AGS^R cells showed higher resistance to various anticancer drugs compared with parental AGS cells (**Table 1**). AGS^R cells showed increased autophagic flux, including AMP-activated protein kinase ($pAMPKa^{T172}$), $pBeclin1^{Ser15}$, and LC3-II formation in comparison with AGS cells (**Figure 1A**). The increased LC3-II formation is a hallmark of autophagy (Klionsky et al., 2021). AGS^R cells showed an increased expression of CAGE compared with AGS cells (**Figure 1A**). AGS^R cells showed decreased levels of $pAKt^{Ser473}$ and p62 compared with AGS cells (**Figure 1A**). CAGE was shown to confer anticancer drug resistance in melanoma cells (Kim et al., 2017a). In AGS^R cells, CAGE was shown to bind to Beclin1 (**Figure 1A**). AGS^R cells displayed an increased number of LC3 puncta (**Figure 1B**). CAGE showed localization in the nucleus and nuclear membrane (**Figure 1C**). AGS^R cells displayed an enhanced autophagic process when compared with AGS cells (**Figure 1D**). AGS cells, but not AGS^R cells, showed the cleavage of PARP and caspase-3 in response to various anticancer drugs (**Figure 1E**). Anticancer drug-resistant melanoma cells ($Malme3M^R$) showed a higher expression of CAGE than the anticancer drug-sensitive Malme3M cells (Kim et al., 2017a). $Malme3M^R$ cells, but not Malme3M cells, showed an increased expression of $pBeclin1^{Ser15}$ and binding of CAGE to Beclin1 (**Supplementary Figure 1A**). CAGE induced the binding of CAGE to Beclin1 and inhibited the binding of Beclin1 to Bcl-2, an inhibitor of autophagy (**Supplementary Figure 1B**). $Malme3M^R$ cells also displayed an enhanced autophagic process compared with Malme3M cells (**Supplementary Figure 1C**). Therefore, anticancer drug resistance is closely associated with antiapoptotic effects and autophagic flux.

CAGE Regulates the Response to Anticancer Drugs and Autophagic Flux

The decreased expression of CAGE decreased autophagic flux (**Figure 2A**) and the number of LC3 puncta (**Figure 2C**). The

TABLE 1 | Anticancer drug resistance of AGS^R cells.

	IC_{50} (μ M)	
	AGS	**AGS^R**
Celastrol	0.94 ± 0.09	1.96 ± 0.53
Taxol	0.29 ± 0.019	0.81 ± 0.03
Doxorubicin	0.05 ± 0.1	0.18 ± 0.09
Docetaxel	8.17 ± 0.76	10.06 ± 2.4

The indicated cancer cell line was treated with the indicated drugs for 48 h. The cell viability was analyzed by an MTT assay. The IC_{50} value of each cell line was determined from the concentration–response curves. All values indicate the mean ± SD.

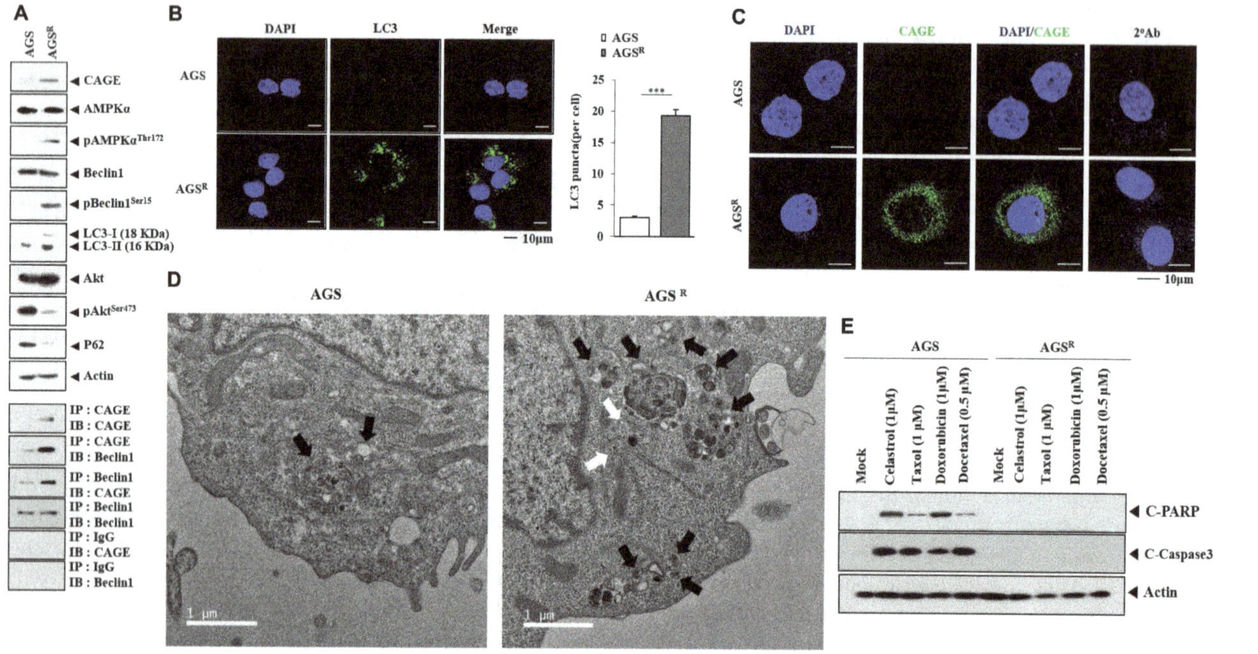

FIGURE 1 | Anticancer drug resistance is correlated with enhanced autophagy and antiapoptotic effects. **(A)** Cell lysates were subjected to immunoblot and immunoprecipitation. Representative blots of three independent experiments are shown. Immunofluorescence staining of LC3 **(B)** and cancer-associated gene (CAGE) **(C)** was performed. ***, $p < 0.001$. **(D)** Representative electron micrograph of AGS cells and AGS^R cells is shown. The black arrows indicate autolysosomes. The white arrows indicate multivesicular bodies. **(E)** After 48 h of treatment, immunoblot was performed. C-PARP denotes cleaved PARP. Representative blots of three independent experiments are shown.

downregulation of CAGE enhanced the effects of anticancer drugs on the cleavage of PARP in AGS^R cells (**Figure 2B**). CAGE increased the expression of pBeclin1^{Ser15} and LC3-II formation but decreased the level of p62, a selective receptor of autophagy, in AGS cells (**Figure 2D**). CAGE inhibited the effects of anticancer drugs on the cleavage of PARP (**Figure 2E**) but increased the number of LC3 puncta in AGS cells (**Figure 2F**). CRISPR/Cas9 KO cell lines were established to further determine the role of CAGE in relation to autophagy and anticancer drug resistance. AGS$^{R\Delta\ CAGE\#5}$ and AGS$^{R\Delta\ CAGE\#7}$ cell lines showed decreased expression of CAGE, autophagic flux (**Supplementary Figure 2A**), and LC3 puncta compared with AGS^R cells (**Supplementary Figure 2B**). AGS$^{R\Delta\ CAGE\#5}$ and AGS$^{R\Delta\ CAGE\#7}$ cell lines showed a lower invasion potential than AGS^R cells (**Supplementary Figure 2C**). AGS$^{R\Delta\ CAGE\#5}$ and AGS$^{R\Delta\ CAGE\#7}$ cell lines showed decreased expression levels of SNAIL and vimentin compared with AGS^R cells (**Supplementary Figure 2C**). AGS$^{R\Delta\ CAGE\#5}$ and AGS$^{R\Delta\ CAGE\#7}$ cell lines showed enhanced sensitivity to anticancer drugs compared with AGS^R cells (**Supplementary Figure 2D**). AGS$^{R\Delta\ CAGE\#5}$ and AGS$^{R\Delta\ CAGE\#7}$ cell lines showed lower tumor spheroid-forming potential (**Supplementary Figure 2E**) and proliferation potential than AGS^R cells (**Figure 2F**). Overexpression of CAGE increased autophagic flux (**Supplementary Figure 3A**), invasion potential (**Supplementary Figure 3B**), proliferation potential (**Supplementary Figure 3C**), tumor spheroid-forming potential, and the expression of SRY-Box Transcription Factor 2 (SOX2), an indicator of cancer stemness (**Supplementary Figure 3D**); however, it decreased the apoptotic effects of anticancer drugs in AGS$^{R\Delta\ CAGE\#5}$ and AGS$^{R\Delta\ CAGE\#7}$ cell lines (**Supplementary Figure 3E**). Thus, CAGE regulates both anticancer drug resistance and autophagic flux.

Autophagy Is Accompanied by Anticancer Drug Resistance and Binding of CAGE to Beclin1

Rapamycin, an autophagy inducer, increased CAGE expression and autophagic flux but decreased p62 expression in AGS cells (**Figure 3A**). Rapamycin induced the binding of CAGE to Beclin1 (**Figure 3A**) and increased the number of LC3 puncta (**Figure 3B**). Rapamycin inhibited the effects of anticancer drugs on the cleavage of PARP (**Figure 3C**). Chloroquine (CQ), an inhibitor of autophagy, decreased the expression of CAGE, pBeclin1^{Ser15}, and autophagy-related-5 (ATG5), but increased LC3-II formation in AGS^R cells (**Figure 3D**). CQ inhibited the interaction between CAGE and Beclin1 (**Figure 3D**). Additionally, CQ enhanced the effects of anticancer drugs on the cleavage of PARP (**Figure 3E**). Thus, increased autophagic flux is accompanied by the increased expression of CAGE.

MiR-302b-5p Targets CAGE

MiR-302b-5p was predicted to bind to the 3′ UTR of CAGE (**Figure 4A**). The miR-302b-5p mimic decreased the luciferase activity of wild-type CAGE 3′ UTR, but not the luciferase activity of the mutant CAGE 3′ UTR (**Figure 4B**). AGS^R

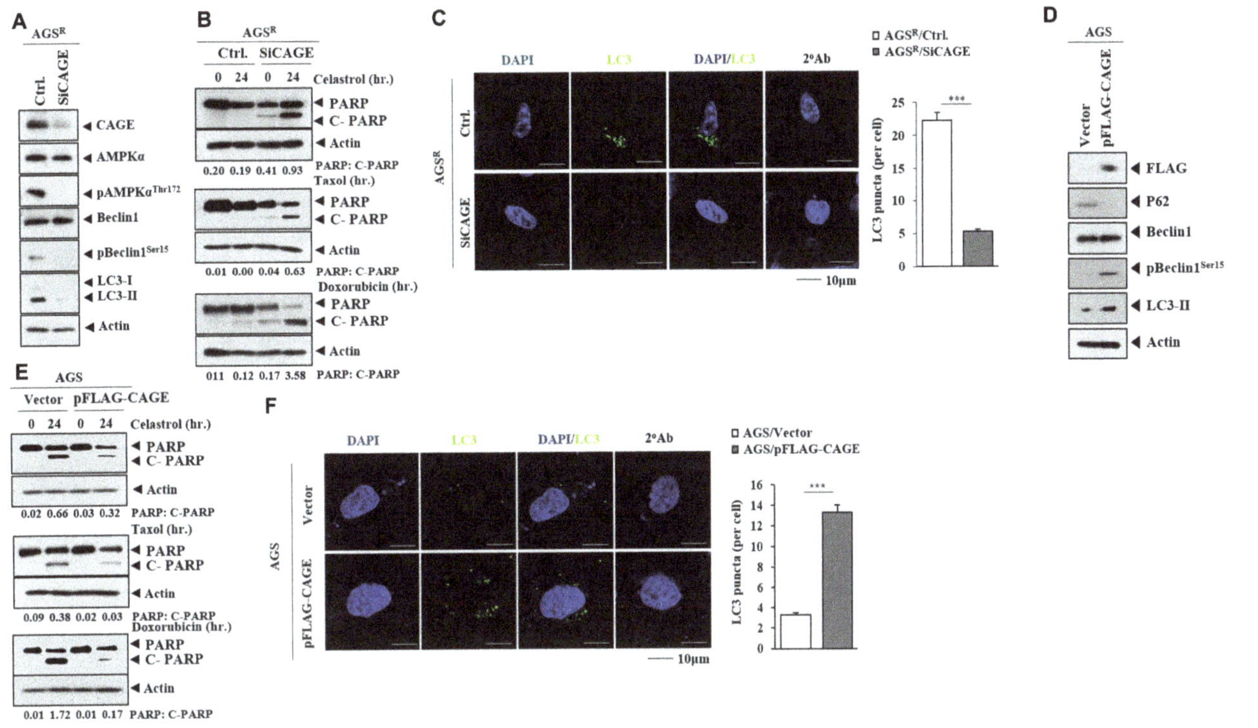

FIGURE 2 | CAGE regulates anticancer drug resistance and autophagic flux. **(A)** After 48 h of transfection with the indicated siRNA (each at 10 nM), immunoblot was performed. Representative blots of three independent experiments are shown. Ctrl. denotes control siRNA. **(B)** After 24 h of transfection, cells were treated with the indicated anticancer drug for 24 h. Quantification of band intensity was represented by the ratio of cleaved/full-length PARP normalized to actin. **(C)** Same as **(A)** except that immunofluorescence staining was performed. ***, $p < 0.001$. **(D)** After 48 h of transfection with the indicated construct, immunoblot was performed. Representative blots of three independent experiments are shown. **(E)** After 24 h of transfection, the cells were treated with the indicated anticancer drug (each at 1 μM) for 24 h. **(F)** Same as **(D)** except for the immunofluorescence staining.

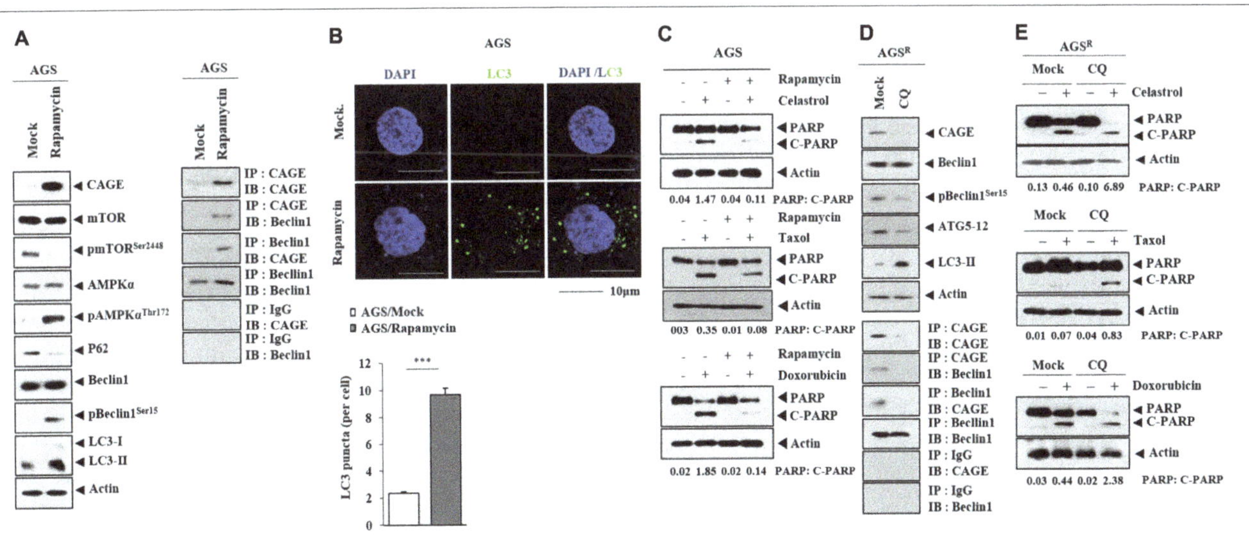

FIGURE 3 | CAGE expression is regulated by autophagy regulators. **(A)** AGS cells were treated with or without rapamycin for 24 h. Representative blots of three independent experiments are shown. **(B)** AGS cells were treated with or without rapamycin for 24 h, followed by immunofluorescence staining. ***, $p < 0.001$. **(C)** AGS cells were treated with or without rapamycin (5 μM) for 24 h, followed by treatment with celastrol (1 μM), Taxol (1 μM), or doxorubicin (1 μM) for 24 h. Representative blots of three independent experiments are shown. **(D)** AGS^R cells were treated with or without chloroquine (CQ) (100 μM) for 24 h. Representative blots of three independent experiments are shown. **(E)** AGS^R cells were treated with or without CQ (100 μM) for 24 h, followed by treatment with the indicated anticancer drug for 24 h. Representative blots of three independent experiments are shown.

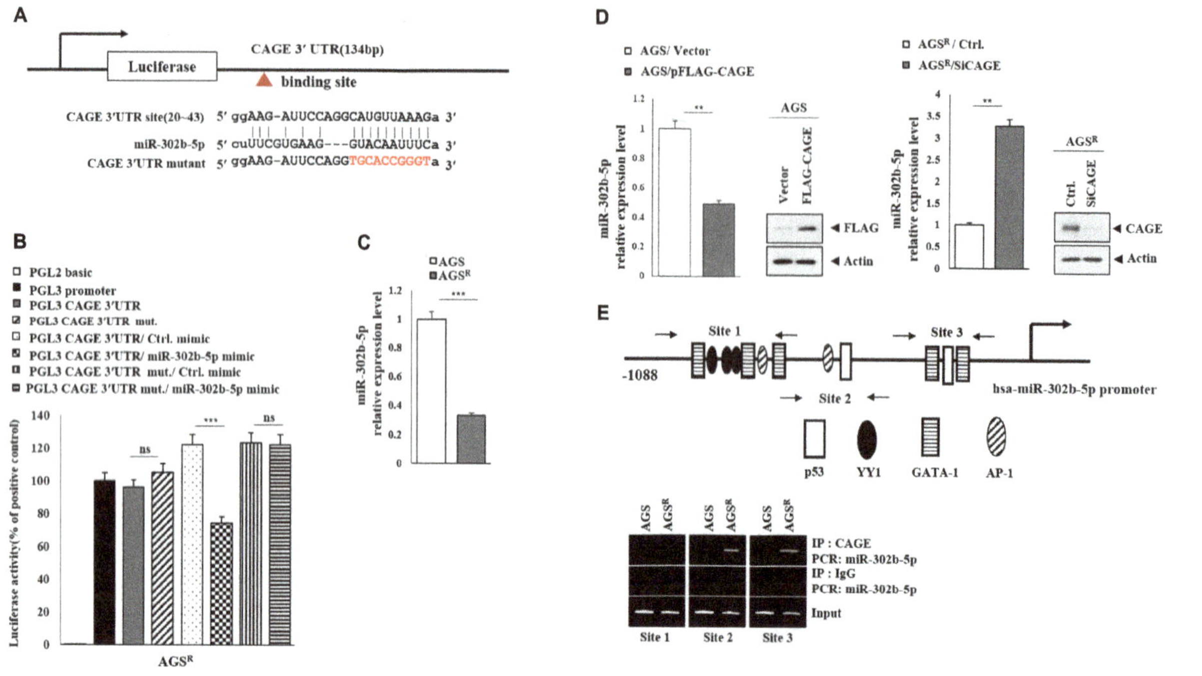

FIGURE 4 | CAGE and miR-302b-5p form a negative feedback loop. **(A)** Shows the binding site for miR-302b-5p in the 3′ UTR of CAGE. **(B)** After 48 h of transfection, luciferase activity assays were performed as described. ***, $p < 0.001$. Average values of three independent experiments are shown. Ns denotes not significant. **(C)** qRT-PCR analysis was performed. ***, $p < 0.001$. Average values of three independent experiments are shown. **(D)** After 48 h of transfection, qRT-PCR and immunoblot were performed. **, $p < 0.01$. Average values of three independent experiments are shown. **(E)** ChIP assays were performed as described.

cells showed a lower expression of miR-302b-5p compared with AGS cells (**Figure 4C**). CAGE decreased miR-302b-5p expression level in AGS cells (**Figure 4D**), while the decreased expression of CAGE increased miR-302b-5p expression in AGS^R cells (**Figure 4D**). MiR-302b-5p promoter displays the potential binding sites for p53, AP1, YY1, and GATA-1 (**Figure 4E**). CAGE was shown to bind to the promoter sequences of miR-302b-5p in chromatin immunoprecipitation (ChIP) assays (**Figure 4E**). Thus, CAGE and miR-302b-5p cross-regulate each other. It is likely that miR-302b-5p may regulate autophagic flux.

MiR-302b-5p Regulates Autophagic Flux

The miR-302b-5p inhibitor increased the expression of CAGE, autophagic flux, the binding of CAGE to Beclin1 (**Figure 5A**), and the number of LC3 puncta (**Figure 5B**). The miR-302b-5p inhibitor decreased miR-302b-5p expression in AGS cells (**Figure 5C**). The miR-302b-5p inhibitor inhibited the effects of anticancer drugs on the cleavage of PARP (**Figure 5D**). The miR-302b-5p mimic decreased CAGE expression and autophagic flux but increased p62 level (**Figure 5E**). In AGS^R cells, the miR-302b-5p mimic inhibited CAGE binding to Beclin1 (**Figure 5E**). MiR-302b-5p mimic decreased the number of LC3 puncta in AGS^R cells (**Figure 5F**). Transfection of miR-302b-5p mimic increased miR-302b-5p expression in AGSR cells (**Figure 5G**). MiR-302b-5p mimic enhanced the effects of anticancer drugs on the cleavage of PARP (**Figure 5H**). Thus, miR-302b-5p regulates autophagic flux and anticancer drug resistance through a negative feedback loop with CAGE.

Soluble Factors Regulate Autophagic Flux

Next, we examined whether anticancer drug resistance could be transferred. The culture medium from AGS^R cells increased the expression of CAGE and autophagic flux and induced CAGE binding to Beclin1 in AGS cells (**Figure 6A**). The culture medium from AGS^R cells, but not from AGS cells, increased the number of LC3 puncta in AGS cells (**Figure 6B**). The culture medium of AGS^R cells showed a higher expression of PAI-1 than that of AGS cells (**Figure 6C**). PAI-1 has been shown to promote angiogenesis (Park et al., 2014). The culture medium from AGS^R also showed an enhanced angiogenic potential compared with the AGS cell culture medium based on Matrigel plug assays (**Figure 6D**). AGS^R cells displayed a higher expression of PAI-1 than AGS cells (**Figure 6E**). The downregulation of CAGE led to decreased expression of PAI-1 in AGS^R cells (**Figure 6E**). PAI-1 was necessary for increased CAGE expression and autophagic flux in AGS cells by culture medium of AGS^R cells (**Figure 6F**). The culture medium from AGS^R cells increased autophagic flux in CAGE CRISPR–Cas9 cell lines (**Figure 6G**). The CAGE-derived AQTGTGKT peptide inhibited CAGE binding to Beclin1 and enhanced the sensitivity to anticancer drugs in nonsmall cell lung cancer cells and melanoma cells, respectively (Kim et al., 2017a; Yeon et al., 2018). The AQTGTGKT negatively

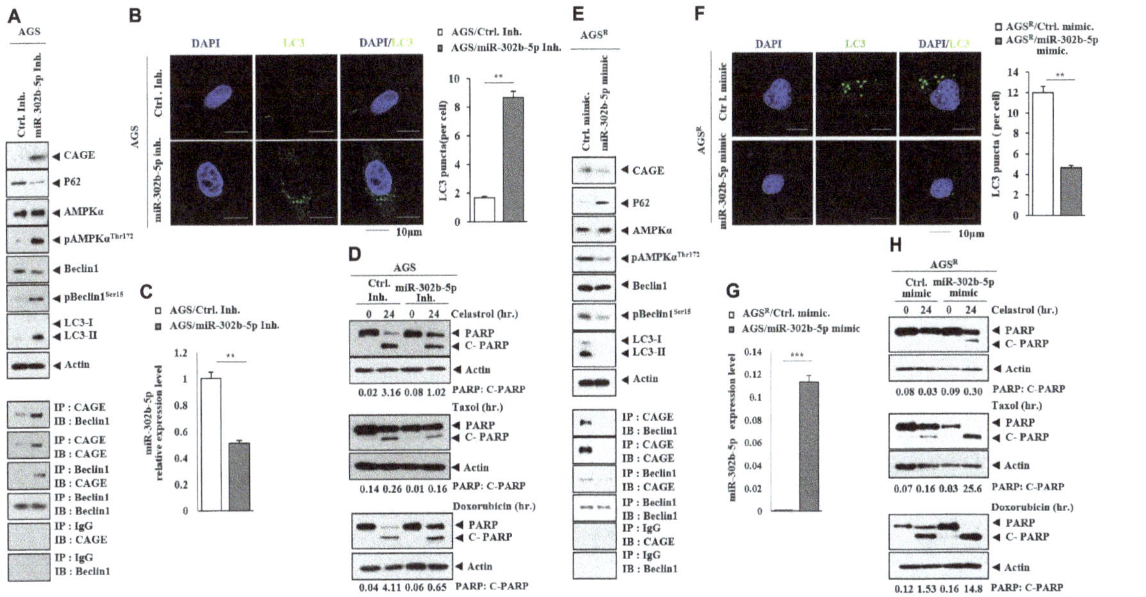

FIGURE 5 | MiR-302b-5p regulates autophagic flux and anticancer drug resistance. **(A)** After 48 h of transfection with the indicated inhibitor (each at 10 nM), immunoblot and immunoprecipitation were performed. Representative blots of three independent experiments are shown. **(B)** Same as **(A)** except that immunofluorescence staining was performed. **, $p < 0.01$. **(C)** qRT-PCR was performed. **, $p < 0.01$. Average values of three independent experiments are shown. **(D)** AGS cells were transfected with the indicated inhibitor (each at 10 nM). The following day, cells were then treated with or without celastrol (1 μM), Taxol (1 μM), or doxorubicin (1 μM) for 24 h. Representative blots of three independent experiments are shown. **(E)** After 48 h of transfection with the indicated mimic (each at 10 nM), immunoblot and immunoprecipitation were performed. Representative blots of three independent experiments are shown. **(F)** Same as **(E)** except that the number of LC3 puncta was determined. **, $p < 0.01$. **(G)** qRT-PCR analysis was performed. ***, $p < 0.001$. Average values of three independent experiments are shown. **(H)** AGS^R cells were transfected with the indicated mimic (each at 10 nM). The next day, cells were then treated with or without celastrol (1 μM), Taxol (1 μM), or doxorubicin (1 μM) for 24 h. Representative blots of three independent experiments are shown.

regulated autophagic flux and inhibited CAGE binding to Beclin1 in AGS^R cells (**Supplementary Figure 4A**) and was shown to bind to CAGE in AGS^R cells (**Supplementary Figure 4B**) and decreased the number of LC3 puncta (**Supplementary Figure 4C**). The culture medium from AGS^R cells that were treated with the AQTGTGKT peptide did not increase the autophagic flux in AGS cells (**Supplementary Figure 4D**). GW4869, an inhibitor of exosome formation, inhibited the effect of the culture medium of AGS^R cells on autophagic flux in AGS cells (**Supplementary Figure 5A**). Also, GW4869 inhibited the effect of the culture medium of AGS^R cells on the number of LC3 puncta (**Supplementary Figure 5B**). These results suggest that soluble factors may regulate autophagic flux and anticancer drug resistance.

Exosomes Regulate Autophagic Flux and the Response to Anticancer Drugs

CAGE was shown to be present in the sera of various cancer patients (Cho et al., 2003). This implies the presence of CAGE in exosomes. Immunoblot and ImmunoEM revealed the presence of CAGE in the exosomes of AGS^R cells (**Figure 7A**). **Figure 7B** shows the size distribution of exosomes. Exosomes from AGS^R cells increased CAGE expression and autophagic flux and induced the CAGE binding to Beclin1 in AGS cells (**Figure 7C**). Exosomes from AGS^R cells inhibited the effects of anticancer drugs on the cleavage of PARP (**Figure 7D**). PKH labeling showed the internalization of the exosomes from AGS^R cells into AGS cells (**Figure 7E**). GW4869 inhibited the effects of the culture medium from Malme3M^R cells on the expression of CAGE expression and autophagic flux in Malme3M cells (**Supplementary Figure 6A**). GW4869 inhibited the effects of the culture medium of Malme3M^R cells on the cleavage of PARP and FAK in Malme3M cells (**Supplementary Figure 6B**). ImmunoEM (**Supplementary Figure 6C**) and immunoblot (**Supplementary Figure 6D**) analyses revealed the presence of CAGE within the exosomes. Human recombinant CAGE protein increased autophagic flux and induced CAGE binding to Beclin1 in AGS cells (**Supplementary Figure 7A**) and enhanced the invasion potential of AGS cells (**Supplementary Figure 7B**), in addition to increasing the number of LC3 puncta (**Supplementary Figure 7C**). Human recombinant CAGE protein prevented CQ from decreasing autophagic flux (**Supplementary Figure 7D**). Human recombinant CAGE protein inhibited the effects of anticancer drugs on the PARP cleavage in AGS cells (**Supplementary Figure 7E**). Thus, CAGE may act as a soluble mediator of anticancer drug resistance.

MiR-181-5p Negatively Regulates the Expression of CAGE and Autophagic Flux

MiRNAs that were differentially expressed between AGS and AGS^R cells were identified by miRNA array analysis **Figure 8A**). MiR-181-b-5p was one of those miRNAs that could act as a

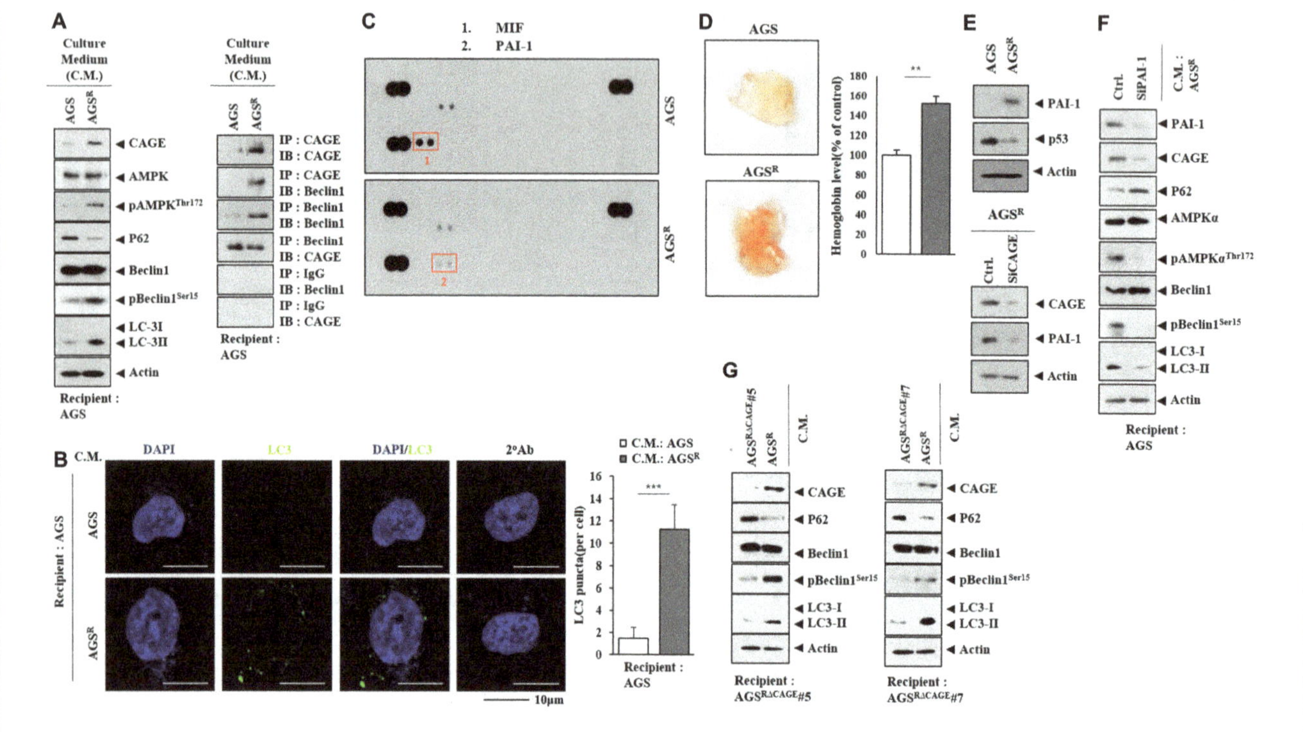

FIGURE 6 | Soluble factors regulate autophagic flux. **(A)** Culture medium of AGS^R cells were added to AGS cells for 24 h. Representative blots of three independent experiments are shown. **(B)** Same as **(A)** except that the number of LC3 puncta was determined. ***, $p < 0.001$. **(C)** Cytokine array analysis was performed. **(D)** Matrigel plug assays using culture medium were performed. **(E)** Immunoblot was performed. Representative blots of three independent experiments are shown. **(F)** After 48 h of transfection with the indicated siRNA (each at 10 nM), culture medium was added to AGS cells for 24 h. Representative blots of three independent experiments are shown. **(G)** Culture medium of the indicated cancer cells was added to the CAGE CRISPR–Cas9 cell line for 24 h. Representative blots of three independent experiments are shown.

negative regulator of anticancer drug resistance (**Figure 8A**). qRT-PCR showed a higher expression of miR-181b-5p in AGS cells in comparison with AGS^R cells (**Figure 8B**). The miR-181b-5p inhibitor increased CAGE expression and pBeclin1^{Ser15} but decreased p62 level (**Figure 8C**). The miR-181b-5p inhibitor negatively regulated the effects of anticancer drugs on the cleavage of PARP in response to anticancer drugs in AGS cells (**Figure 8D**).

S1PR1 Serves as a Target of MiR-181b-5p

S1PR1 was predicted as a potential target of miR-181b-5p in TargetScan analysis. The miR-181-b-5p mimic decreased the luciferase activity of the wild-type 3′ UTR of S1PR1, but not the luciferase activity of the mutant 3′ UTR of S1PR1 (**Figure 9A**). AGS^R cells showed a higher expression of S1PR1 compared with AGS cells (**Figure 9B**). S1PR1 was localized in the cytoplasm of AGS^R cells (**Figure 9C**). Rapamycin increased S1PR1 expression in AGS cells, while CQ decreased S1PR1 expression in AGS^R cells (**Figure 9D**). CAGE (**Figure 9E**), miR-181b-5p inhibitor (**Figure 9F**), and miR-181b-5p mimic (**Figure 9G**) regulated S1PR1 expression. CAGE was shown to bind to the promoter sequences of S1PR1 in ChIP assays (**Figure 9H**). Thus, the CAGE–miR-181b-5p–S1PR1 axis and autophagy cross-regulate each other.

S1PR1 Regulates Autophagic Flux and the Response to Anticancer Drugs

The expression of S1PR1 in nontumor gastric tissues and gastric cancer tissues was examined. The GEPIA database showed that gastric cancer tissues had a higher expression of *SIPR1* mRNA than nontumor gastric tissues (**Supplementary Figure 8A**). Gastric cancer tissues showed higher expression of SIPR1 compared with other nontumor gastric tissues (**Supplementary Figures 8B,C**). A high expression level of S1PR1 was correlated with low survival rates in gastric cancer patients (**Supplementary Figure 8D**). The downregulation of S1PR1 decreased CAGE expression and autophagic flux but increased p62 level in AGS^R cells (**Figure 10A**). The downregulation of S1PR1 resulted in a decreased number of LC3 puncta (**Figure 10B**), while the effects of anticancer drugs on the cleavage of PARP were enhanced (**Figure 10C**). The inhibition of S1PR1 by FTY720 decreased the expressions of CAGE and pBeclin1^{Ser15}, but increased p62 level and LC3-II formation in AGS^R cells (**Figure 10D**). FTY720 increased the number of LC3 puncta in AGS^R cells (**Figure 10E**). Just like CQ, FTY720 may inhibit the fusion of autophagosomes and lysosomes. FTY enhanced the effects of anticancer drugs on the cleavage of PARP (**Figure 10F**). FTY720 decreased the colony-forming potential of AGS^R cells (**Figure 10G**). These results indicate that CAGE and S1PR1 form a positive feedback loop to regulate anticancer drug resistance and autophagic flux.

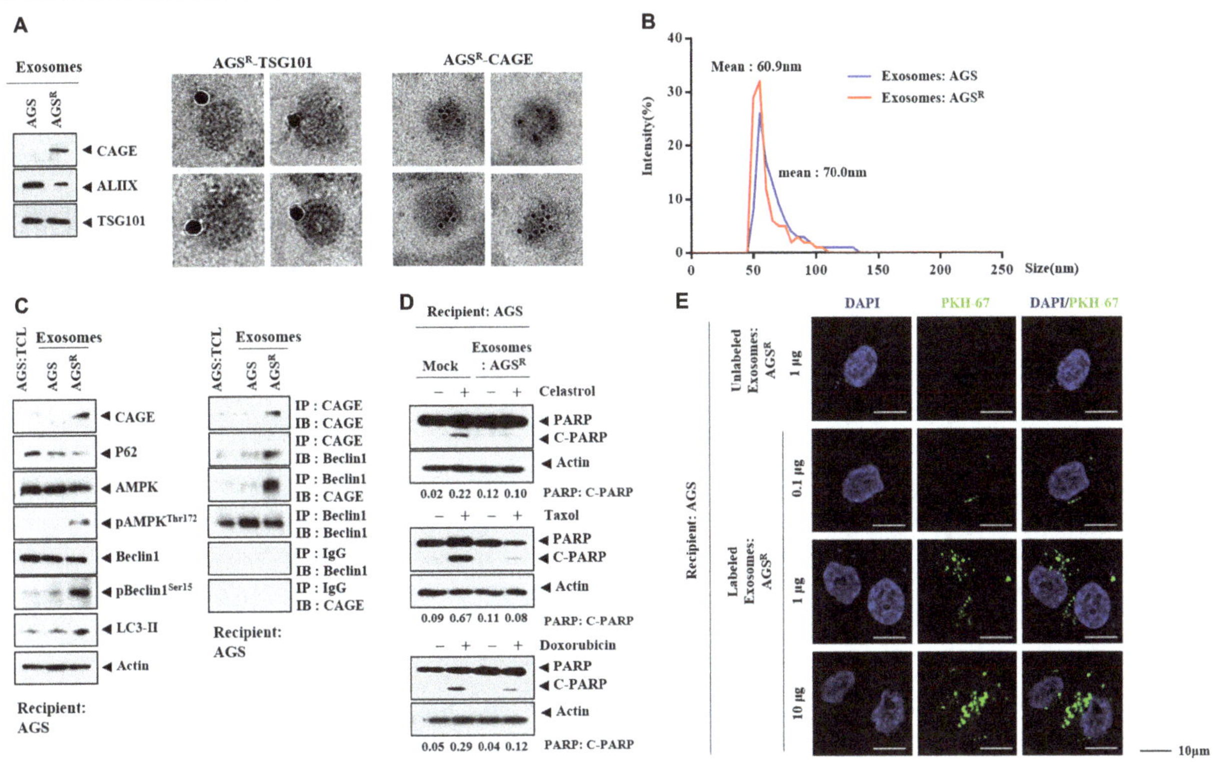

FIGURE 7 | Exosomes of AGS^R cells enhance autophagic flux and decrease the PARP cleavage. **(A)** Immunoblot (left) and ImmunoEM (left) show the presence of CAGE in the exosomes. Immunogold staining images using anti-TSG101 and anti-CAGE antibody are shown. Twenty-five and 10 nm gold particles are used to indicate the localization of TSG 101 and CAGE, respectively. CAGE is present in the lumen of the exosomes. **(B)** Size distribution of exosomes is shown. **(C)** Exosomes (10 μg/ml) of the indicated cancer cells were added to AGS cells for 24 h. TCL denotes total cell lysates. Representative blots of three independent experiments are shown. **(D)** AGS cells were treated with or without exosomes (10 μg/ml) of AGS^R cells for 24 h, followed by treatment with the indicated anticancer drug for 24 h. Representative blots of three independent experiments are shown. **(E)** Exosomes (10 μg/ml) of AGS^R cells were labeled with or without PKH67. Exosomes were then added to AGS cells for 24 h.

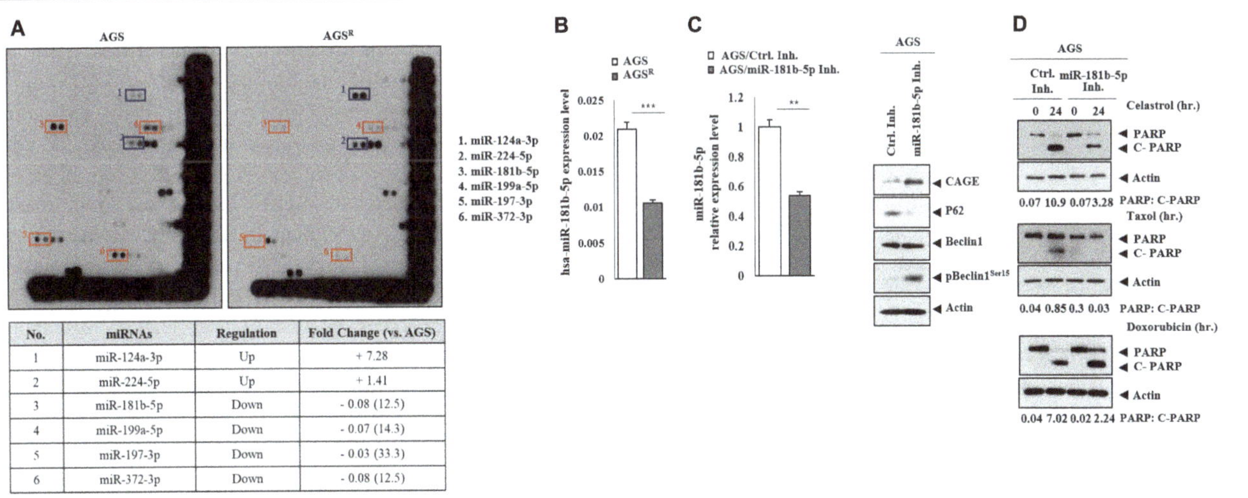

No.	miRNAs	Regulation	Fold Change (vs. AGS)
1	miR-124a-3p	Up	+ 7.28
2	miR-224-5p	Up	+ 1.41
3	miR-181b-5p	Down	- 0.08 (12.5)
4	miR-199a-5p	Down	- 0.07 (14.3)
5	miR-197-3p	Down	- 0.03 (33.3)
6	miR-372-3p	Down	- 0.08 (12.5)

FIGURE 8 | MiR-181b-5p negatively regulates the expression of CAGE, autophagic flux. **(A)** MicroRNA array analysis was performed. The red rectangles show miRNAs expressed highly in AGS cells. The blue rectangles show miRNAs expressed highly in AGS^R cells. **(B)** qRT-PCR analysis was performed. ***, $p < 0.001$. Average values of three independent experiments are shown. **(C)** After 48 h of transfection with the indicated inhibitor (each at 10 nM), qRT-PCR and immunoblot were performed. **, $p < 0.01$. Average values of three independent experiments are shown. **(D)** AGS cells were transfected with the indicated inhibitor (each at 10 nM). The following day, the cells were then treated with or without celastrol (1 μM) or Taxol (1 μM) for 24 h, followed by immunoblot. Representative blots of three independent experiments are shown.

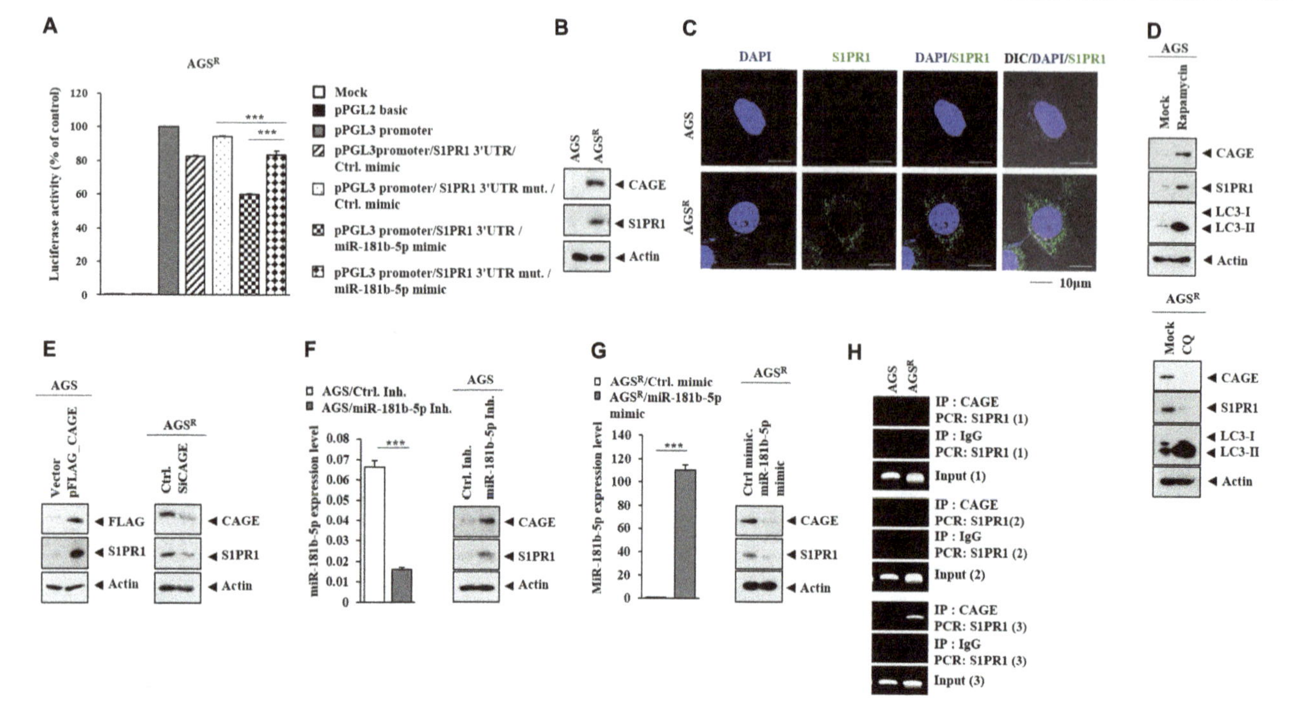

FIGURE 9 | SIPR1 serves as a target of miR-181b-5p. **(A)** After 48 h of transfection with the indicated construct (each at 1 μg) and/or mimic (each at 10 nM), luciferase activity assays were performed. ***, $p < 0.001$. Average values of three independent experiments are shown. **(B)** Immunoblot was performed. Representative blots of three independent experiments are shown. **(C)** Cytoplasmic localization of S1PR1 is shown. **(D)** The indicated cancer cells were treated with or without rapamycin (5 μM) or CQ (100 μM) for 24 h. Representative blots of three independent experiments are shown. **(E)** After 48 h of transfection, immunoblot was performed. Representative blots of three independent experiments are shown. **(F)** After 48 h of transfection, qRT-PCR and immunoblot were performed. ***, $p < 0.001$. Average values of three independent experiments are shown. **(G)** After 48 h of transfection, qRT-PCR and immunoblot were performed. ***, $p < 0.001$. Average values of three independent experiments are shown. **(H)** ChIP assays were performed as described.

DISCUSSION

Anticancer drug-resistant gastric cancer cells cells displayed an increased expression of CAGE and autophagic flux compared with AGS cells (**Figure 1A**). Autophagy may protect tumor cells from chemotherapeutic drugs by inhibiting apoptotic cell death (Liu et al., 2018). The inhibition of autophagy by CQ enhances apoptosis (Pan et al., 2019). CAGE regulated autophagic flux (**Figures 2A,D**). CAGE has been shown to regulate autophagic flux in nonsmall cell lung cancer cells (Yeon et al., 2018). The downregulation of CAGE enhanced the effects of anticancer drugs on the cleavage of PARP in AGS^R cells (**Figure 2B**). This suggests that CAGE may affect the response to anticancer drugs by regulating autophagic flux. MAPK activation results in the increased autophagic flux in EGFR tyrosine kinase inhibitor-resistant nonsmall cell lung cancer cells (Lotsberg et al., 2020). MAPK activation may lead to increased CAGE expression in AGS^R cells. In future studies, it may be necessary to identify downstream targets of CAGE.

CAGE enhances the self-renewal activity of breast cancer cells (Kim et al., 2017c). Also, CAGE enhances the self-renewal and tumorigenic potential of Malme3M^R cells through interaction with SOX2 (Kim et al., 2017b). AGS^R cells displayed more enhanced tumor spheroid-forming potential compared with AGS cells (**Supplementary Figure 2E**). The binding of CAGE to SOX2 may lead to enhanced tumor spheroid-forming potential in AGS^R cells.

Luciferase activity assays demonstrate that miR-302b-5p acts as a negative regulator of CAGE (**Figure 4B**). MiR-302b-5p regulated both the autophagic flux (**Figures 5A,E**) and the response to anticancer drugs (**Figures 5D,H**). MiR-302 members enhance the chemosensitivity of breast cancer cells by decreasing breast cancer resistance protein (BCRP) expression and may cooperatively downregulate BCRP expression to increase the chemosensitivity of breast cancer cells (Wang et al., 2016). MiR-302b suppresses gastric cancer cell tumorigenesis and metastasis by regulating the EphA2/Wnt/β-catenin/EMT pathway (Huang et al., 2017). Overexpression of CAGE activates Wnt1 signaling in colon cells (Yeon et al., 2019). MiR-302b suppresses cell proliferation by inhibiting the effects on the increased expression levels of TGFβRII, phosphorylated ERK1/2, and MMP9 by TGF-β1 (Li et al., 2016). MiR-302b-3p targets IGF-1R and decreases the expression of cell cycle regulators such as cyclin D1 and CDK6 (Guo et al., 2017). MiR-302-367 cell-to-cell transfer decreases the expression levels of CXCR4/SDF1, SHH, cyclin D, cyclin A, and E2F1 to inhibit glioblastoma growth (Fareh et al., 2017). MiR-302 directly represses cyclin D1 and suppresses the proliferation of glioblastoma cells (Debruyne et al., 2018). Other downstream targets of miR-302b may regulate autophagic flux and anticancer drug resistance.

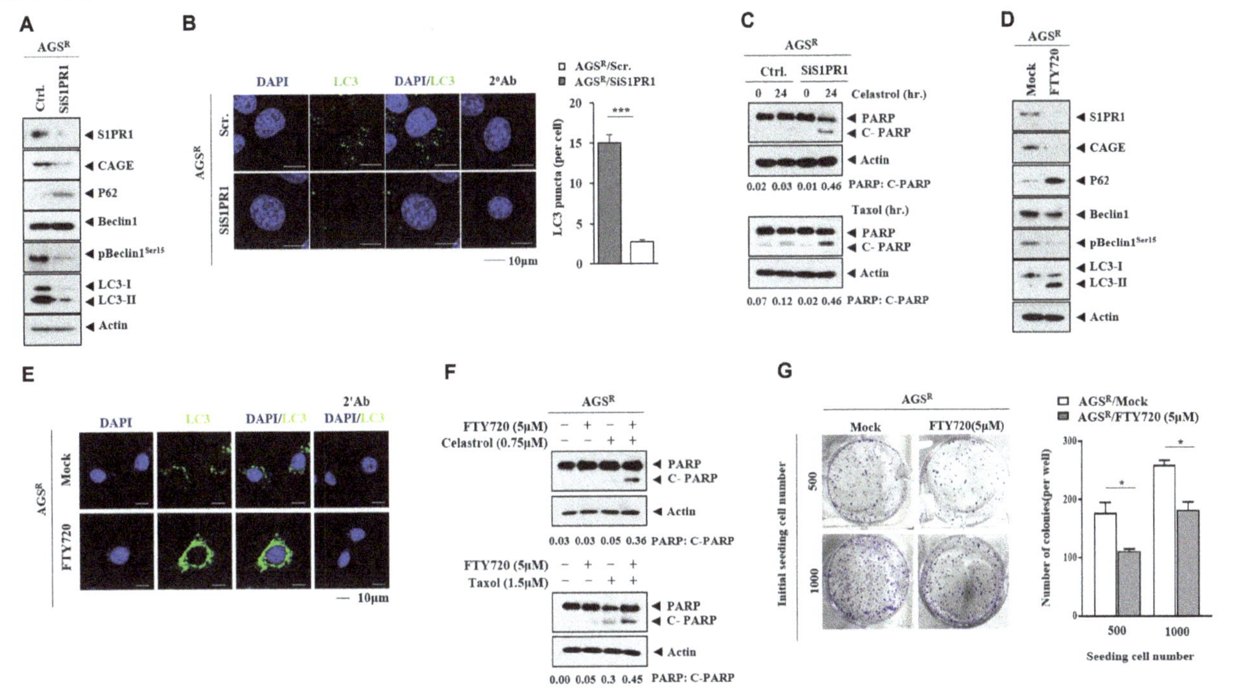

FIGURE 10 | S1PR1 regulates autophagic flux and anticancer drug resistance. **(A)** After 48 h of transfection, immunoblot was performed. Representative blots of three independent experiments are shown. **(B)** The number of LC3 puncta was determined. ***, $p < 0.001$. **(C)** After 24 h of transfection, cells were then treated with or without the indicated anticancer drug for 24 h. Representative blots of three independent experiments are shown. **(D)** The indicated cancer cells were treated with or without FTY720 (5 μM) for 24 h. Representative blots of three independent experiments are shown. **(E)** Immunofluorescence staining was performed. **(F)** AGS^R cells were treated with or without FTY720 (5 μM) for 24 h. Cells were then treated with the anticancer drug for 24 h. Representative blots of three independent experiments are shown. **(G)** Colony-forming potential was determined. *, $p < 0.05$. Average values of three independent experiments are shown.

AGS^R cells revealed an increased expression of PAI-1 compared with AGS cells (**Figure 6D**). PAI-1 mediates pyruvate-induced angiogenesis (Jung et al., 2011) and serves as a target of HDAC3, thereby acting as an angiogenic factor (Park et al., 2014). AGS^R cells displayed a lower expression of HDAC3 than AGS cells (personal observations). The downregulation of PAI-1 decreased the expression levels of LC3 and Beclin1 (Wang et al., 2014). The culture medium of AGS^R cells increased autophagic flux in AGS cells in a PAI-1-dependent manner (**Figure 6F**). PAI-1 promotes the proliferation of head and neck cancer tumor-initiating cells (TICs) by increasing SOX2 expression (Lee et al., 2016). The effects of PAI-1 on the cancer stem cell-like properties of gastric cancer cells call for further investigation.

Soluble factors may regulate autophagic flux and anticancer drug resistance (**Figure 6A**). The AQTGTGKT peptide inactivates CAGE and prevents the culture medium of AGS^R cells from enhancing the autophagic flux in AGS cells (Figure S4D). This suggests that soluble factors may regulate autophagic flux in a CAGE-dependent manner. Exosomes promote autophagic flux in an AMPK-dependent manner (Zeng et al., 2020) and also confer resistance to anticancer drugs (Chinnappan et al., 2020). Gastric cancer-derived exosomes remodel the tumor microenvironment and affect anticancer drug resistance (Huang et al., 2019). Next, we examined the presence of CAGE in the exosomes. CAGE was found to be present in the exosomes of AGS^R cells (**Figure 7A**) and Malme3M^R cells (**Supplementary Figure 6C**). Exosomes from AGS^R cells increased autophagic flux (**Figure 7C**) and exerted antiapoptotic effects (**Figure 7C**). Thus, exosomal CAGE protein may confer resistance to anticancer drugs and further enhance autophagic flux. Exosomes from Taxol-resistant nasopharyngeal cancer cells show the presence of CAGE (Yuan and Zhou, 2021). In future studies, identification of miRNAs and soluble factors that could present differential expression in exosomes of AGS and AGS^R cells will be necessary.

A high miR-181b level results in an improved prognosis of human lung adenocarcinomas (Tan et al., 2018). The miR-181 family regulates VCAM-1 expression, and a low level of miR-181b is observed in high-grade glioma patients (Liu et al., 2017). MiR-181b-5p inhibits cellular invasion by regulating the expression of S1PR1 (Miao et al., 2020). AGS^R cells showed a lower expression of miR-181b-5p compared with AGS cells (**Figures 8A,B**). The miR-181b-5p inhibitor increased CAGE expression and autophagic flux in AGS cells (**Figure 8C**). CAGE did not affect the expression of miR-181b-5p (personal observations), implying that CAGE functions downstream of miR-181b-5p. It is possible that miR-181b-5p can predict the survival rate of gastric cancer patients.

MiR-181b-5p directly regulated the expression of S1PR1 (**Figure 9A**). FTY720, an inhibitor of S1PR1, overcomes resistance to ErbB inhibitors, such as afatinib (Booth et al., 2019). A high expression of S1PR1 predicts poor prognosis in breast cancer patients (Pyne et al., 2016) and gastric cancer patients

(**Supplementary Figure 7D**). FTY720 decreased the expression of CAGE and autophagic flux (**Figure 10D**). It is necessary to examine the effect of sphingosine 1-phosphate on autophagic flux and identify additional targets of S1PR1. Sphingosine 1-phosphate may regulate autophagic flux and the identification of additional targets of S1PR1 is necessary.

In this study, we investigated the mechanism of CAGE-promoted anticancer drug resistance. Most importantly, we identified a novel role of the CAGE–miR-181b-5p–S1PR1 axis in the anticancer drug resistance and autophagic process. We show that CAGE can be employed as a target for the development of anticancer drugs.

ETHICS STATEMENT

The animal study was reviewed and approved by the Institutional Animal Care and Use Committee (IACUC) of Kangwon National University. Written informed consent was obtained from the owners for the participation of their animals in this study.

AUTHOR CONTRIBUTIONS

DJ and YK provided the idea. DJ wrote the manuscript. MY performed most of the experiments in this study. DP, EK, and DK performed the expression and purification of CAGE protein. MJ and HJ performed the electron microscopy experiments. All authors contributed to the article and approved the submitted version.

REFERENCES

Belounis, A., Nyalendo, C., Le Gall, R., Imbriglio, T. V., Mahma, M., Teira, P., et al. (2016). Autophagy is associated with chemoresistance in neuroblastoma. *BMC Cancer* 16:891. doi: 10.1186/s12885-016-2906-9

Booth, L., Roberts, J. L., Spiegel, S., Poklepovic, A., and Dent, P. (2019). Fingolimod augments Pemetrexed killing of non-small cell lung cancer and overcomes resistance to ERBB inhibition. *Cancer Biol. Ther.* 20, 597–607. doi: 10.1080/15384047.2018.1538616

Chinnappan, M., Srivastava, A., Amreddy, N., Razaq, M., Pareek, V., Ahmed, R., et al. (2020). Exosomes as drug delivery vehicle and contributor of resistance to anticancer drugs. *Cancer Lett.* 486, 18–28. doi: 10.1016/j.canlet.2020.05.004

Cho, B., Lee, H., Jeong, S., Bang, Y. J., Lee, H. J., Hwang, K. S., et al. (2003). Promoter hypomethylation of a novel cancer/testis antigen gene CAGE is correlated with its aberrant expression and is seen in premalignant stage of gastric carcinoma. *Biochem. Biophys. Res. Commun.* 307, 52–63. doi: 10.1016/s0006-291x(03)01121-5

Cho, B., Lim, Y., Lee, D. Y., Park, S. Y., Lee, H., Kim, W. H., et al. (2002). Identification and characterization of a novel cancer/testis antigen gene CAGE. *Biochem. Biophys. Res. Commun.* 292, 715–726. doi: 10.1006/bbrc.2002.6701

Debruyne, D. N., Turchi, L., Burel-Vandenbos, F., Fareh, M., Almairac, F., Virolle, V., et al. (2018). DOCK4 promotes loss of proliferation in glioblastoma progenitor cells through nuclear beta-catenin accumulation and subsequent miR-302-367 cluster expression. *Oncogene* 37, 241–254. doi: 10.1038/onc.2017.323

Fareh, M., Almairac, F., Turchi, L., Burel-Vandenbos, F., Paquis, P., Fontaine, D., et al. (2017). Cell-based therapy using miR-302-367 expressing cells represses glioblastoma growth. *Cell Death Dis.* 8:e2713. doi: 10.1038/cddis.2017.117

Guo, B., Zhao, Z., Wang, Z., Li, Q., Wang, X., Wang, W., et al. (2017). MicroRNA-302b-3p suppresses cell proliferation through AKT pathway by targeting IGF-1R in human gastric cancer. *Cell Physiol. Biochem.* 42, 1701–1711. doi: 10.1159/000479419

Huang, J., He, Y., McLeod, H. L., Xie, Y., Xiao, D., Hu, H., et al. (2017). miR-302b inhibits tumorigenesis by targeting EphA2 via Wnt/ beta-catenin/EMT signaling cascade in gastric cancer. *BMC Cancer* 17:886. doi: 10.1186/s12885-017-3875-3

Huang, T., Song, C., Zheng, L., Xia, L., Li, Y., and Zhou, Y. (2019). The roles of extracellular vesicles in gastric cancer development, microenvironment, anti-cancer drug resistance, and therapy. *Mol. Cancer* 18:62. doi: 10.1186/s12943-019-0967-5

Hurtado López, A. M., Chen-Liang, T. H., Zurdo, M., Carrillo-Tornel, S., Panadero, J., Salido, E. J., et al. (2020). Cancer testis antigens in myelodysplastic syndromes revisited: a targeted RNA-seq approach. *Oncoimmunology* 9:1824642. doi: 10.1080/2162402X.2020.1824642

Iwata, T., Fujita, T., Hirao, N., Matsuzaki, Y., Okada, T., Mochimaru, H., et al. (2005). Frequent immune responses to a cancer/testis antigen, CAGE, in patients with microsatellite instability-positive endometrial cancer. *Clin. Cancer Res.* 11, 3949–3957. doi: 10.1158/1078-0432.CCR-04-1702

Jung, S. Y., Song, H. S., Park, S. Y., Chung, S. H., and Kim, Y. J. (2011). Pyruvate promotes tumor angiogenesis through HIF-1-dependent PAI-1 expression. *Int. J. Oncol.* 38, 571–576. doi: 10.3892/ijo.2010.859

Kim, H., Kim, Y., and Jeoung, D. (2017c). DDX53 promotes cancer stem cell-like properties and autophagy. *Mol. Cells* 40, 54–65. doi: 10.14348/molcells.2017.2258

Kim, M., Park, Y., Kwon, Y., Kim, Y., Byun, J., Jeong, M. S., et al. (2019). MiR-135-5p-p62 axis regulates autophagic flux, tumorigenic potential, and cellular interactions mediated by extracellular vesicles during allergic inflammation. *Front. Immunol.* 10:738. doi: 10.3389/fimmu.2019.00738

Kim, Y., Kim, H., Park, D., Han, M., Lee, H., Lee, Y. S., et al. (2016). miR-217 and CAGE form feedback loop and regulates the response to anti-cancer drugs through EGFR and HER2. *Oncotarget* 7, 10297–10321. doi: 10.18632/oncotarget.7185

Kim, Y., Kim, H., Park, D., Lee, H., Lee, Y. S., Choe, J., et al. (2017a). The pentapeptide Gly-Thr-Gly-Lys-Thr confers sensitivity to anti-cancer drugs by inhibition of CAGE binding to GSK3beta and decreasing the expression of cyclinD1. *Oncotarget* 8, 13632–13651. doi: 10.18632/oncotarget.14621

Kim, Y., Park, D., Kim, H., Choi, M., Lee, H., Lee, Y. S., et al. (2013). miR-200b and cancer/testis antigen CAGE form a feedback loop to regulate the invasion and tumorigenic and angiogenic responses of a cancer cell line to microtubule-targeting drugs. *J. Biol. Chem.* 288, 36502–36518. doi: 10.1074/jbc.M113.502047

Kim, Y., Park, H., Park, D., Lee, Y. S., Choe, J., Hahn, J. H., et al. (2010). Cancer/testis antigen CAGE exerts negative regulation on p53 expression through HDAC2 and confers resistance to anti-cancer drugs. *J. Biol. Chem.* 285, 25957–25968. doi: 10.1074/jbc.M109.095950

Kim, Y., Yeon, M., and Jeoung, D. (2017b). DDX53 regulates cancer stem cell-like properties by binding to SOX-2. *Mol. Cells* 40, 322–330. doi: 10.14348/molcells.2017.0001

Klionsky, D. J., Abdel-Aziz, A. K., Abdelfatah, S., Abdellatif, M., Abdoli, A., Abel, S., et al. (2021). Guidelines for the use and interpretation of assays for monitoring autophagy (4th edition)(1). *Autophagy* 17, 1–382. doi: 10.1080/15548627.2020.1797280

Lee, Y. C., Yu, C. C., Lan, C., Lee, C. H., Lee, H. T., Kuo, Y. L., et al. (2016). Plasminogen activator inhibitor-1 as regulator of tumor-initiating cell properties in head and neck cancers. *Head Neck* 38(Suppl. 1), E895–E904. doi: 10.1002/hed.24124

Li, J., Yu, J., Zhang, H., Wang, B., Guo, H., Bai, J., et al. (2016). Exosomes-derived MiR-302b suppresses lung cancer cell proliferation and migration via TGFbetaRII inhibition. *Cell Physiol. Biochem.* 38, 1715–1726. doi: 10.1159/000443111

Liu, Y., Tang, J., Liu, D., Zhang, L., He, Y., Li, J., et al. (2018). Increased autophagy in EOC re-ascites cells can inhibit cell death and promote drug resistance. *Cell Death Dis.* 9:419. doi: 10.1038/s41419-018-0449-5

Liu, Y. S., Lin, H. Y., Lai, S. W., Huang, C. Y., Huang, B. R., Chen, P. Y., et al. (2017). MiR-181b modulates EGFR-dependent VCAM-1 expression and monocyte adhesion in glioblastoma. *Oncogene* 36, 5006–5022. doi: 10.1038/onc.2017.129

Lotsberg, M. L., Wnuk-Lipinska, K., Terry, S., Tan, T. Z., Lu, N., Trachsel-Moncho, L., et al. (2020). AXL targeting abrogates autophagic flux and induces immunogenic cell death in drug-resistant cancer cells. *J. Thorac. Oncol.* 15, 973–999. doi: 10.1016/j.jtho.2020.01.015

Miao, J., Zhu, Y., Xu, L., Huang, X., and Zhou, X. (2020). miR181b5p inhibits trophoblast cell migration and invasion through targeting S1PR1 in multiple abnormal trophoblast invasionrelated events. *Mol. Med. Rep.* 22, 4442–4451. doi: 10.3892/mmr.2020.11515

Pan, H., Wang, Y., Na, K., Wang, Y., Wang, L., Li, Z., et al. (2019). Autophagic flux disruption contributes to Ganoderma lucidum polysaccharide-induced apoptosis in human colorectal cancer cells via MAPK/ERK activation. *Cell Death Dis.* 10:456. doi: 10.1038/s41419-019-1653-7

Park, D., Park, H., Kim, Y., Kim, H., and Jeoung, D. (2014). HDAC3 acts as a negative regulator of angiogenesis. *BMB Rep.* 47, 227–232. doi: 10.5483/bmbrep.2014.47.4.128

Park, S. Y., Kim, W. J., Byun, J. H., Lee, J. J., Jeoung, D., Park, S. T., et al. (2018). Role of DDX53 in taxol-resistance of cervix cancer cells in vitro. *Biochem. Biophys. Res. Commun.* 506, 641–647. doi: 10.1016/j.bbrc.2018.10.145

Por, E., Byun, H. J., Lee, E. J., Lim, J. H., Jung, S. Y., Park, I., et al. (2010). The cancer/testis antigen CAGE with oncogenic potential stimulates cell proliferation by up-regulating cyclins D1 and E in an AP-1- and E2F-dependent manner. *J. Biol. Chem.* 285, 14475–14485. doi: 10.1074/jbc.M109.084400

Pyne, N. J., McNaughton, M., Boomkamp, S., MacRitchie, N., Evangelisti, C., Martelli, A. M., et al. (2016). Role of sphingosine 1-phosphate receptors, sphingosine kinases and sphingosine in cancer and inflammation. *Adv. Biol. Regul.* 60, 151–159. doi: 10.1016/j.jbior.2015.09.001

Silvestri, G., Trotta, R., Stramucci, L., Ellis, J. J., Harb, J. G., Neviani, P., et al. (2020). Persistence of drug-resistant leukemic stem cells and impaired NK cell immunity in CML patients depend on MIR300 antiproliferative and PP2A-activating functions. *Blood Cancer Discov.* 1, 48–67. doi: 10.1158/0008-5472.BCD-19-0039

Song, B., Bian, Q., Shao, C. H., Li, G., Liu, A. A., Jing, W., et al. (2015). Ulinastatin reduces the resistance of liver cancer cells to epirubicin by inhibiting autophagy. *PLoS One* 10:e0120694. doi: 10.1371/journal.pone.0120694

Tan, X., Banerjee, P., Liu, X., Yu, J., Gibbons, D. L., Wu, P., et al. (2018). The epithelial-to-mesenchymal transition activator ZEB1 initiates a prometastatic competing endogenous RNA network. *J. Clin. Invest.* 128:3198. doi: 10.1172/JCI122740

Wang, M., Liao, C., Hu, Y., Qinwen, P., and Jiang, J. (2017). Sensitization of breast cancer cells to paclitaxel by dichloroacetate through inhibiting autophagy. *Biochem. Biophys. Res. Commun.* 489, 103–108. doi: 10.1016/j.bbrc.2017.05.097

Wang, Y., Zhao, L., Xiao, Q., Jiang, L., He, M., Bai, X., et al. (2016). miR-302a/b/c/d cooperatively inhibit BCRP expression to increase drug sensitivity in breast cancer cells. *Gynecol. Oncol.* 141, 592–601. doi: 10.1016/j.ygyno.2015.11.034

Wang, Z. H., Ren, W. Y., Zhu, L., and Hu, L. J. (2014). Plasminogen activator inhibitor-1 regulates LPS induced inflammation in rat macrophages through autophagy activation. *ScientificWorldJournal* 2014:189168. doi: 10.1155/2014/189168

Xu, L., Fan, Q., Wang, X., Zhao, X., and Wang, L. (2016). Inhibition of autophagy increased AGE/ROS-mediated apoptosis in mesangial cells. *Cell Death Dis.* 7:e2445. doi: 10.1038/cddis.2016.322

Yeon, M., Byun, J., Kim, H., Kim, M., Jung, H. S., Jeon, D., et al. (2018). CAGE Binds to Beclin1, regulates autophagic flux and CAGE-derived peptide confers sensitivity to anti-cancer drugs in non-small cell lung cancer cells. *Front. Oncol.* 8:599. doi: 10.3389/fonc.2018.00599

Yeon, M., Lee, S., Lee, J. E., Jung, H. S., Kim, Y., and Jeoung, D. (2019). CAGE-miR-140-5p-Wnt1 axis regulates autophagic flux, tumorigenic potential of mouse colon cancer cells and cellular interactions mediated by exosomes. *Front. Oncol.* 9:1240. doi: 10.3389/fonc.2019.01240

Yuan, F., and Zhou, Z. F. (2021). Exosomes derived from Taxol-resistant nasopharyngeal carcinoma (NPC) cells transferred DDX53 to NPC cells and promoted cancer resistance to Taxol. *Eur. Rev. Med. Pharmacol. Sci.* 25, 127–138. doi: 10.26355/eurrev_202101_24375

Zeng, Q., Zhou, Y., Liang, D., He, H., Liu, X., Zhu, R., et al. (2020). Exosomes secreted from bone marrow mesenchymal stem cells attenuate oxygen-glucose deprivation/reoxygenation-induced pyroptosis in PC12 cells by promoting AMPK-dependent autophagic flux. *Front. Cell Neurosci.* 14:182. doi: 10.3389/fncel.2020.00182

7

Follistatin-Like 3 Enhances Invasion and Metastasis via β-Catenin-Mediated EMT and Aerobic Glycolysis in Colorectal Cancer

Yuqiang Li[1,2,3], Mengxiang Tian[1,2], Wenxue Liu[2,4], Dan Wang[1,2], Zhongyi Zhou[1,2], Qian Pei[1,2], Yan Huang[5,6,7], Fengbo Tan[1,2] and Cenap Güngör[3]*

[1] *Department of General Surgery, Xiangya Hospital, Central South University, Changsha, China,* [2] *National Clinical Research Center for Geriatric Disorders, Xiangya Hospital, Central South University, Changsha, China,* [3] *Department of General, Visceral and Thoracic Surgery, University Medical Center Hamburg-Eppendorf, Hamburg, Germany,* [4] *Department of Cardiology, Xiangya Hospital, Central South University, Changsha, China,* [5] *Key Laboratory of Protein Chemistry and Developmental Biology of Ministry of Education, College of Life Sciences, Hunan Normal University, Changsha, China,* [6] *Department of Neurosurgery, Second Affiliated Hospital of Hunan Normal University, Changsha, China,* [7] *Hunan Provincial Key Laboratory of Neurorestoration, Changsha, China*

***Correspondence:**
Fengbo Tan
fengbotan@csu.edu.cn

Previous studies reported that Follistatin-like 3 (FSTL3) is abundantly expressed in several solid tumors and participate in the regulation of cell metabolism. However, the clinico-pathological significance, biological role and molecular mechanism of FSTL3 in colorectal cancer (CRC) is still unclear. Here we report that the expression level of FSTL3 in colon cancer specimens was significantly higher, compared to normal tissue and interestingly, the expression of FSTL3 was related to lymph node metastasis, tumor stage, tumor size, and intravascular emboli (IVE). As an upstream molecular event, we found that transcriptional regulation of FSTL3 was highly dependent on YAP1 de-phosphorylation events and that increased FSTL3 expression readily activated the β-Catenin pathway, which is a well-known signaling hub that promotes EMT processes and aerobic glycolysis in cancer cells. We found that elevated FSTL3 expression strongly promotes migration, invasion and metastatic formation of CRC cells by directly activating β-Catenin -mediated EMT and aerobic glycolysis. In the xenograft mouse model, FSTL3 expression was linked to increased metastatic formation of CRC cells. Together, the activation of YAP1 induces FSTL3 expression. FSTL3-mediated β-Catenin pathway activation promotes EMT and aerobic glycolysis and therefore affecting the invasive and metastatic capacity of CRC cells. The abundant FSTL3 expression is a poor prognostic factor and pharmacological targeting of YAP1 can counteract FSTL3 expression, suggesting a promising therapeutic target for anti-metastatic strategies in patients suffering from CRC.

Keywords: FSTL3, β-Catenin, colorectal cancer, EMT, aerobic glycolysis, metastasis

HIGHLIGHTS

- The high expression of FSTL3 is a poor prognostic factor for patients with CRC.
- The activation of YAP1 can induce FSTL3 expression, which then promotes EMT and enhances aerobic glycolysis to affect invasion and metastasis formation of CRC cells by activating the β-Catenin pathway.
- This study provides a new crosstalk mechanism between Hippo/YAP and Wnt/β-Catenin pathways, which suggests a new strategy for colorectal cancer treatment.

INTRODUCTION

Colorectal cancer (CRC) is the third most frequent cancer which results in the 2nd cancer-related mortality worldwide (Siegel et al., 2020). Treatment modalities for CRC includes surgical resection, chemotherapy, and/or radiation therapy. In recent years, the prognosis of patients with CRC has been significantly improved due to advances in surgery combined with adjuvant therapy in the past decades (Li Y. et al., 2019). However, invasion and metastatic formation of tumor cells are still the main causes of death in patients suffering from CRC (Siegel et al., 2020). Hence, the exploration of key molecules and their related molecular mechanisms regulating invasion and metastasis can provide prognostic markers and potentially new therapeutic targets for the treatment course of CRC in future settings.

Epithelial-mesenchymal transition (EMT) is a process in which cells gradually loses their epithelial phenotype and transforms into a mesenchymal phenotype. EM-transitioned cells are linked to: (i) enhanced cell motility, (ii) promotes transition from *carcinoma in situ* to an invasive carcinoma, (iii) enables tumor cells to invade into neighboring tissues (vascular/lymphatic) and promoting the metastatic cascade (Sánchez-Tilló et al., 2011). Increasing evidences demonstrate that EMT can also initiate the metastatic progression of CRC (Thiery et al., 2009; Sleeman and Thiery, 2011; Dongre and Weinberg, 2019). The molecular characteristics of EMT contain the suppression of epithelial markers (e.g., *E*-cadherin) and the concomitant promotion of mesenchymal markers such as *N*-cadherin, Fibronectin1, and Vimentin (Kalluri and Weinberg, 2009). Therefore, exploration of the role and molecular mechanism of key genes that regulate EMT can provide a basis for controlling the invasion and metastatic formation of CRC cells.

Moreover, cancer cells rewire their metabolism and breakdown glucose to lactate in the presence of oxygen (aerobic glycolysis), a phenomenon known as the Warburg effect (Vander Heiden et al., 2009; Lunt and Vander Heiden, 2011). The alteration of metabolism endues cancer cells the ability to survive and grow in a nutrient-deficient and highly hypoxic tumor microenvironment (Binnewies et al., 2018; Sullivan, 2018). This metabolic re-programming involves altered expression and post-translational modification of several key metabolic enzymes. However, the molecular mechanisms underlying the altered expression or post-translational modifications of key metabolic proteins in CRC tumors are still not fully understood. Much attention has been paid to the glucometabolic re-programming of tumor cells in recent years. Drugs targeting key regulators of aerobic glycolysis effectively inhibit tumor progression *in vitro* and *in vivo* (Ganapathy-Kanniappan and Geschwind, 2013). Therefore, it is still necessary to further investigate key genes of aerobic glycolysis in CRC.

Follistatin-like 3 (FSTL3) is expressed in various normal human tissues (Tsuchida et al., 2000). Increasing evidences indicated that FSTL3 plays an important role in regulating embryonic development, osteogenesis, glucose, and lipid metabolism (Mukherjee et al., 2007). Moreover, FSTL3 was recently found abundantly expressed in non-small cell lung cancer (Gao et al., 2020) and breast cancer (Couto et al., 2017), and participates in tumor progression including invasion and metastasis. FSTL3 is an independent risk factor and is linked with poor prognosis within various cancers. However, the molecular mechanisms and impact of FSTL3 on CRC progression is still unclear.

YAP1, a key molecule in the HIPPO pathway, can translocate into the nucleus upon dephosphorylation where it functions to regulate and maintain cancer stem cell properties as well as the invasion and metastatic ability of CRC cells (Tan et al., 2018). Meanwhile, β-Catenin, the rate-limiting molecule of Wnt pathway, is involved in the regulation of various physiological events in CRC cells. Recent studies indicated that the crosstalk between the HIPPO/YAP1 and Wnt/β-Catenin signaling pathways can play a key role in the progression of CRC (Konsavage et al., 2012; Jiao et al., 2017). Various clinical trials with HIPPO/YAP1-inhibitors or Wnt/β-Catenin-inhibitors have already been started in solid tumors[1]. However, therapeutical targets inhibiting the crosstalk between the two signal pathways still needs to be discovered.

Our study revealed that increased FSTL3 expression is a poor prognostic factor in CRC patients and that transcriptional activation of FSTL3 is strongly induced following YAP1 activation. Additionally, abundant FSTL3 expression promotes EMT and enhances aerobic glycolysis to positively affect the invasive and metastatic capacity of CRC cells by activating the β-Catenin pathway. Our findings illustrate that FSTL3 could serve as a bridging molecule in the crosstalk between HIPPO/YAP1 and Wnt/β-Catenin pathways and that FSTL3 is a crucial regulatory factor of the β-Catenin molecular mechanisms in CRC. Therefore, therapeutically targeting of either FSTL3 and/or YAP1 is may be a promising anti-metastatic strategy in CRC patients.

MATERIALS AND METHODS

Patients and Specimens

Tumor and matched para-carcinoma tissues were removed by radical resection from 130 stage III CRC patients without preoperative chemotherapy or radiotherapy at the Xiangya Hospital of Central South University (Changsha, China) randomly. The samples were then embedded in paraffin.

[1]www.clinicaltrials.gov

Follow-up of patients was terminated on September 1st, 2018. Disease-free survival (DFS) was defined as the time to any event, irrespective of cause, except for any second primary cancers. Recurrence of or death from the same cancer and all treatment-related deaths or deaths from other causes are events. Second primary same cancers and other primary cancers were ignored, and loss to follow-up is censored. Overall survival (OS) was defined as the time to death, irrespective of cause. Local recurrence, distant metastases, second primary CRCs, and second other primary cancers were ignored. Loss to follow-up is censored. All procedures were in compliance with the ethical guidelines of the Xiangya Hospital. The normal mucosa was excised 5cm away from the tumor and was confirmed by pathologists for absence of tumor cells. Tumor stage was classified according to the 7th edition of the AJCC TNM staging system for CRC.

Cell Culture and Reagents

The CRC cell lines [HT-29 (RRID: CVCL_0320), SW480 (RRID: CVCL_0546), SW620 (RRID: CVCL_0547), LOVO (CVCL_0399), HCT116 (RRID: CVCL_0291), DLD1 (RRID: CVCL_0248), and RKO (RRID: CVCL_0504)] were purchased from American Type Culture Collection (ATCC, United States). The cell lines were incubated in a humidified atmosphere with 5% CO_2 at 37°C and cultivated in the recommended growth medium, supplemented with 10% FBS, 100 mg/ml streptomycin and 100 U/mL penicillin (Sigma-Aldrich, United States). The YAP inhibitor, Verteporfin (VP) was purchased from Selleck Chemicals (Houston, TX, United States).

Western Blotting (WB)

The WB assay was performed as previously described (Tan et al., 2015). CRC cells were homogenized and lysed in RIPA buffer supplemented with protease inhibitors. Equal amounts of proteins were loaded and separated on 6% SDS-PAGE gel. Following electrophoresis, proteins were transferred to a PVDF membrane (Millipore, United States), the membrane was blocked in 5% (w/v) non-fat milk and incubated with the primary antibodies overnight, and followed by secondary antibody incubation (1:2000 dilution, CST, United States) for 1 h. Bands were visualized and quantitated using the ECL Advance Detection System (Millipore, United States). The primary antibodies used for WB analysis are listed in **Supplementary Table 1**.

Quantitative Real-Time Polymerase Chain Reaction (qRT-PCR)

The qRT-PCR assay was performed as previously described (Tan et al., 2015). Total RNA was extracted from cells and tissues using TRIzol Reagent (TAKARA, Japan), and equal amounts of RNA were used for real-time qRT-PCR analysis (TAKARA, Japan) according to the manufacturer's instructions. GAPDH was used as loading control. Primers are listed in **Supplementary Table 2**. The mRNA expression was quantitated using the $2\text{-}(^{\Delta\ Ct}$ sample$-^{\Delta\ Ct}$ control) method.

Wound-Healing/Scratch Assay

The wound-healing assay was performed as previously described (Li C. et al., 2019). The transfected cells were cultured in 6-well plates. After the cells reached 90–95% confluence, a standard 200 μl pipette tip was subsequently utilized to scratch linear wounds. In addition, cell monolayers were cultivated in FBS-free medium. After scratching, the images of the wound closure were captured at 0 and 36 h.

Transwell Migration and Invasion Assay

The Transwell migration and invasion assay was performed as previously described (Li C. et al., 2019). 8×10^4 cells, suspended in medium without FBS, were seeded into Transwell chambers (Costar Corning, United States), with or without Matrigel (Sigma-Aldrich, United States) coating. The lower chamber contained medium with 10% FBS. After 24 h, the migratory/invasive cells on the lower surface of the chamber were photographed and counted in 10 randomly selected microscopic fields after crystal violet staining.

Immunofluorescence (IF)

The IF assay was performed as previously described (Tan et al., 2015). Cells cultured in 24-well chamber slides were washed twice with cold PBS, fixed with 4% paraformaldehyde for 10 min, permeabilized with 0.1% Triton-X for 5 min, blocked with 5% BSA, and incubated with primary antibodies at 4°C overnight. The cells were then stained with secondary antibodies and DAPI (4,6-diamidino-2-phenylindole) to visualize the nuclei. Images were acquired using a confocal microscope (Leica, Germany). The primary antibodies used for IF analysis are listed in **Supplementary Table 1**.

Immunohistochemistry (IHC)

The protocol for IHC staining was performed as previously published (Davidson et al., 2013). The IHC staining results were evaluated by two independent pathologists (double-blinded). Briefly, the percentage of stained tumor cells (0: 0–5%; 1: 6–25%; 2: 26–50%; 3: 50–100%) and staining intensity scores (0: negative; 1: weak; 2: moderate; 3: strong) were summed. The CRC tissues were categorized into four groups: negative: $\leq$5% cells stained, regardless of intensity; weak expression: 1–2 points; moderate expression: 3–4 points; and strong expression: 5–6 points. The total score $\geq$ 3 was classified as significant overexpression and was considered as positive expression. Antibodies used for the IHC analysis are listed in **Supplementary Table 1**.

Transduction/Transfection

Different lentiviral vectors with FSTL3-shRNA and negative-control shRNA were purchased from GENECHEM (Shanghai, China). HCT-116 and DLD-1 cells were transduced with FSTL3-shRNA and control-shRNA. Scrambled control-siRNA (siScr) and si-YAP1 were purchased from RiboBio (Guangzhou, China). HCT-116 cells were transduced using lentiviral vectors with siRNA targeting YAP1. For YAP1 overexpression, DLD-1 cells were transduced using lentiviral vectors carrying either full-length YAP1 cDNA or control sequences, respectively (GENECHEM, Shanghai, China). DLD-1 cells were transduced with lentiviral vectors containing shRNA-sequences targeting β-Catenin or control-shRNA, which were purchased from GENECHEM (Shanghai, China). Efficient knockdown and overexpression were detected by WB and qRT-PCR analysis.

Luciferase Reporter Assay

Luciferase reporter assay was performed in HCT-116 and DLD-1 cell lines stably harboring luciferase reporter plasmids fused to the promoter region of human FSTL3 (**Supplementary Figure 1**). Cells were collected and cell extracts were prepared. Luciferase activity was measured using Luciferase assay kit (Promega, China) according to the manufacturer's instructions.

CRC – Mice Model

Female BABL/c athymic nude mice purchased from Hunan SJA Laboratory Animal Co., Ltd (Changsha, Hunan, China). Aged 5–6 weeks were used. Ethical statement was approved by the Ethics Committee of XiangYa Hospital Central South University (Changsha, China). All animal care and procedures were performed according to the guidelines on treating experimental animals well formulated by the ministry of science and technology of China. The capacity to metastasize to the liver was determined following a previously described method (Gavert et al., 2007). Briefly, all mice were anesthetized by inhalation of isoflurane (0.5–1.0%) and oxygen. Through a 1-cm incision in the upper left lateral abdomen, the spleen was exposed and 10^6 cells suspended in 20 μL phosphate-buffered saline (PBS) were injected into the distal tip of the spleen using a Hamilton syringe. Following injection, the spleen was replaced in the abdomen and the incision was closed with staples. The animals were sacrificed after 5–6 weeks and spleen and liver were isolated and paraffin embedded.

ATP Assay/Metabolism

Intracellular ATP production was measured using an ATP Assay Kit (Abcam, United States). Lactate production were measured using L-Lactate Assay Kit (Abcam, United States) and glucose uptake were measured using a Glucose Uptake Assay Kit (Abnova, China) according to the manufacturers' instructions, respectively.

Statistical Analysis

The data analysis was conducted using a Student's *t*-test for the comparison between groups. The χ^2 test was utilized to evaluate the association between protein levels and clinical characteristics. The correlations in gene expression levels were analyzed by Spearman's rank correlation coefficients. Differences were thought to be significant at $^{*}p < 0.05$, $^{**}p < 0.01$, $^{***}p < 0.001$, and $^{****}p < 0.0001$. n.s, no significance. The results were analyzed with SPSS 19.0 software (SPSS Inc., United States). All *in vitro* experiments were repeated at least three times.

RESULTS

FSTL3 Is Frequently Overexpressed in CRC Tissues

The data from the GEPIA database[2] illustrated that FSTL3 was significantly overexpressed in CRC specimens (T) relative to the adjacent normal colonic mucosa (NT) (**Figure 1A**). The mRNA expression levels of FSTL3 were correlated with the AJCC staging of CRC (**Figure 1B**). Moreover, the survival curves demonstrated that FSTL3 was obviously related to disease-free survival (DFS) ($p = 0.0087$) and overall survival (OS) ($p = 0.0052$) in GEPIA database (**Figure 1C**). In addition, the data from other databases, including the Human Protein Atlas project[3], OncoLnc[4], GSE17536 and GSE41258, further displayed that abundant FSTL3 expression was a poor prognostic factor in CRC patients (**Supplementary Figure 2**). Then, 130 CRC tumor and matched para-carcinoma tissues were randomly collected from the Xiangya Hospital of Central South University (Changsha, China). The correlation between FSTL3 expression and clinico-pathological characters of 130 CRC patients was summarized in **Table 1**. The expression of FSTL3 significantly correlated to lymph node metastasis, staging, tumor size and intravascular emboli (IVE). The immunohistochemistry images indicated low- or negative expression levels of FSTL3 in the paired normal tissues (NT) and high-expression in tumor (T), metastatic lymph node (LN), and IVE tissues (**Figure 1D**). Moreover, there were significant differences regarding sub-staging in stage III CRC ($p = 0.045$) and formation of IVE ($p = 0.008$) between the FSTL3 high and low expression groups (**Figure 1E**). Our data also confirmed that expression of FSTL3 was obviously related to DFS ($p < 0.0001$) and OS ($p < 0.0001$) (**Figure 1F** and **Table 2**). Collectively, our data suggest that elevated FSTL3 expression is associated with a worse outcome in CRC patients.

FSTL3 Promotes Migration and Invasion of CRC Cells *in vitro*

FSTL3 protein expression levels were investigated in CRC cell lines and SW480, SW620, HCT-116, and RKO exhibited high-expression of FSTL3, whereas HT-29, Lovo and DLD-1 cells showed low-expression of FSTL3 (**Figure 2A**). HCT-116 and DLD-1 cell lines were selected for further investigations because of their invasive and migrative capabilities. Stable FSTL3-knockdown (HCT-116) and FSTL3-overexpression (DLD-1) cell lines were then established to examine the molecular function of FSTL3 (**Figure 2B**). The effect of FSTL3 on migration capacity in CRC cells was detected using the wound-healing/scratch and transwell assays. These results demonstrated that CRC cells with elevated FSTL3 expression have enhanced migrative ability, compared to their respective control cells (**Figure 2C**). One disadvantage of the scratch assay is, that it is not quantitative. Therefore, we also performed transwell assays (with and without matrigel) and confirmed that elevated FSTL3 expression was

[2]http://gepia.cancer-pku.cn/
[3]http://www.proteinatlas.org
[4]http://www.oncolnc.org

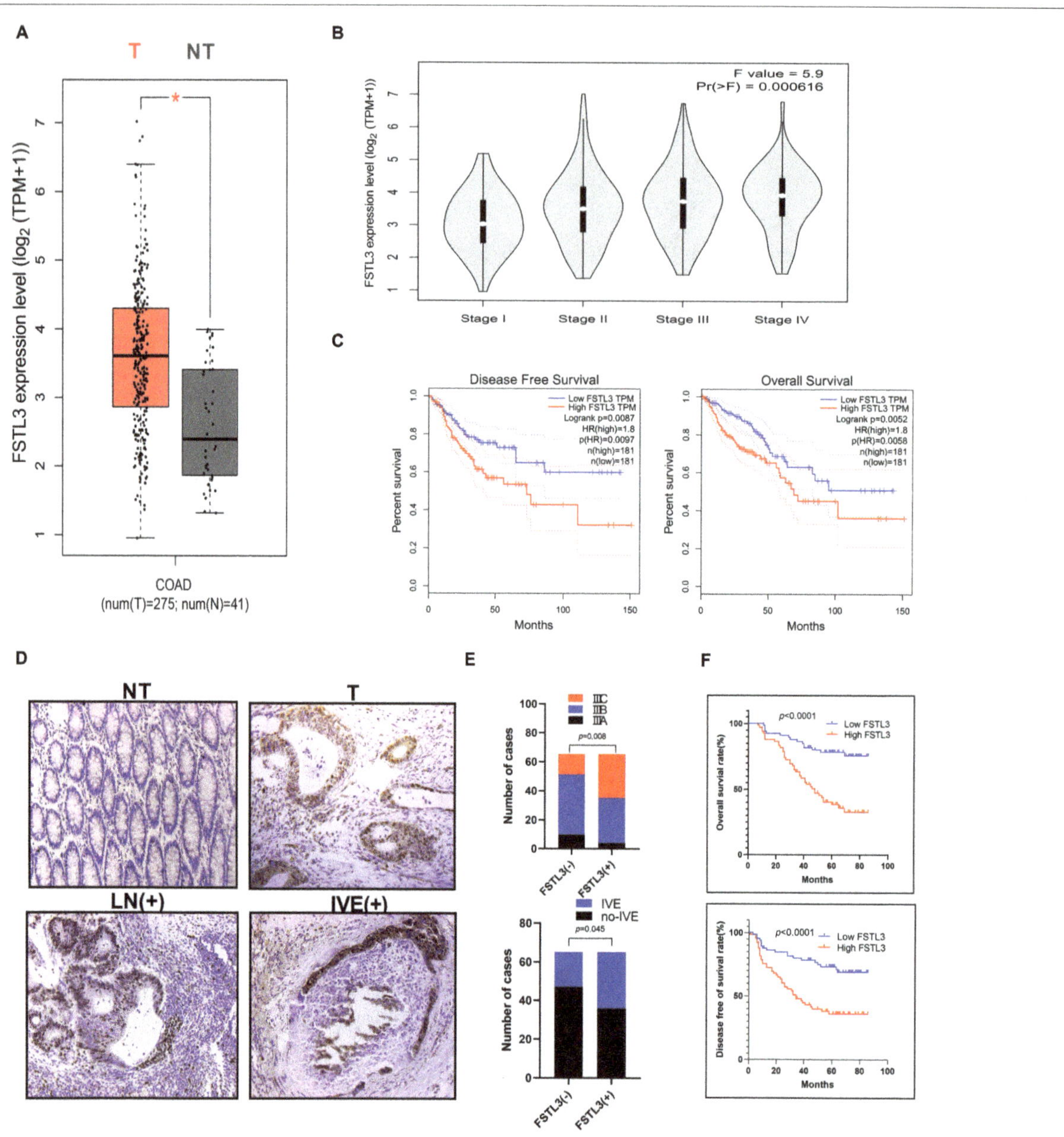

FIGURE 1 | FSTL3 is in CRC. **(A)** The box plots indicated differential FSTL3 expression between CRC specimens (T) and paired normal tissues (NT), analyzed within the GEPIA database. *Differences were thought to be significant. **(B)** The pathological stage plot compared FSTL3 expression in different CRC stages, analyzed within the GEPIA database. **(C)** The survival plots demonstrated that FSTL3 is obviously related to DFS (p = 0.0087) and OS (p = 0.0052), analyzed within the GEPIA database. **(D)** Representative immunohistochemistry images of FSTL3 expression levels in NT, T, LN (metastatic lymph node tissue), and IVE (intravascular emboli). **(E)** The histogram indicates that FSTL3 expression correlates with tumor stage and IVE. **(F)** Survival plots were obtained to verify that FSTL3 expression is obviously related to DFS and OS (p < 0.0001).

able to strengthen the migrative and invasive capacity of CRC cells *in vitro* (**Figures 2D,E**). In sum, elevated FSTL3 expression promoted migration and invasion of CRC cells *in vitro*.

FSTL3 Expression Is Regulated by YAP1 in CRC Cells

As a transcriptional cofactor, Yes-associated protein-1 (YAP1) is known to modulate the transcriptional activity of various transcription factors to regulate and maintain cancer stem cell properties and organ size during embryonic development (Tan et al., 2018). A recent study indicated that the mRNA expression of YAP1 is correlated with that of FSTL3 (Lee et al., 2017). We therefore hypothesized that YAP1 is able to modulate FSTL3 gene expression in CRC cells. Initially, we found a significant correlation between FSTL3 and YAP1 expression in CRC using the GEPIA database (see footnote 2) (**Figure 3A**). To pinpoint whether YAP1 is responsible for increased FSTL3

TABLE 1 | Correlation between FSTL3 expression and clinicopathological characters of 130 CRC patients.

Clinicopathological characters			FSTL3 expression		
		n	Low(*n* = 65)	High(*n* = 65)	*p*-value
Age(years)	<60	80	42	38	0.471
	≥60	50	23	27	
Gender	Female	75	26	29	0.594
	Male	55	39	36	
Tumor location	LCC	28	17	11	0.369
	RCC	29	15	14	
	REC	73	33	40	
Tumor differentiation	G1	91	48	43	0.265
	G2	23	8	15	
	G3	16	9	7	
Depth of invasion	T1–T2	16	11	5	0.109
	T3–T4	114	54	60	
Lymph node metastasis	N1	80	50	30	0.000*
	N2	50	15	35	
Stage of III	IIIA	14	10	4	0.008*
	IIIB	72	41	31	
	IIIC	44	14	30	
CEA (ng/ml)	<5.0	98	48	50	0.684
	≥5.0	32	17	15	
Diameter(cm)	<5.0	76	45	31	0.013*
	≥5.0	54	20	34	
Intravascular emboli	No	83	47	36	0.045*
	Yes	47	18	29	
Intestinal obstruction	No	119	59	60	0.753
	Yes	11	6	5	
CA19-9(kU/L)	<35.0	109	54	55	0.812
	≥35.0	21	11	10	

**$p < 0.05$ was considered statistically significant. The P-values of chi-square test.*

gene expression, we established YAP1-knockdown as well as YAP1-overexpression cell clones. According to baseline FSTL3 expression levels (**Figure 2B**), we decided to knockout YAP1 expression in HCT116 cells and to overexpress YAP1 in DLD-1 cells. Effective YAP1 knockout and overexpression was confirmed by qRT-PCR, WB, and immunofluorescence, respectively (**Figures 3B–D**). We found substantially decreased FSTL3 mRNA and protein expression in YAP1 knockout HCT116 cells, whereas YAP1-overexpression in DLD-1 cells displayed increased FSTL3 mRNA and protein levels (**Figures 3B–D**). *In silico* analyses of the human *FSTL3* (*hFSTL3*) gene promoter sequence revealed three potential YAP1 binding sites, upstream to the transcriptional start site of the *hFSTL3* (**Supplementary Figure 1**). Next, we investigated whether YAP1 directly interacts with the *hFSTL3* gene promoter using luciferase reporter-gene assays. We therefore cloned the promoter region of *hFSTL3* into GV238 vector and measured luciferase expression in YAP1-knockout HCT-116 and YAP1-overexpressed DLD-1 cells. We detected decreased luciferase expression in YAP1-knockout HCT-116 cells and increased luciferase expression in YAP1-overexpressed DLD-1 cells (**Figure 3E**). For proof-of-principle, we decided to inhibit YAP1 activity by treating FSTL3-overexpressing DLD-1 and DLD-1-vector control cells with 0.5 μM Verteporfin (VP) for 48 h. The treatment with VP showed substantially reduced FSTL3 expression levels in DLD-1-OE-FSTL3 and DLD-1-vector control cells (**Figure 3F**). Collectively, these data suggest that YAP1 is indeed necessary for transactivation of FSTL3 in CRC cells.

FSTL3 Modulates β-Catenin-Mediated EMT Processes in CRC Cells

The nuclear translocation of β-Catenin is a hallmark of activated Wnt signaling and cytoplasmic β-Catenin protein levels are tightly controlled by a "destruction complex" and the 26S proteasome. Because nuclear translocation of YAP1 is modulated by the Wnt/β-Catenin pathway in melanoma-associated fibroblasts (Liu et al., 2019) and YAP1 is necessary to transactivate FSTL3 gene expression (**Figure 3F**), we hypothesized that elevated FSTL3 expression modulates β-Catenin signaling in CRC. The latter was supported by the fact, that abundant FSTL3 expression is obviously related to the expression of EMT-related genes, including *E*-cadherin (CDH1), *N*-cadherin (CDH2), Fibronectin-1 (FN-1), and Vimentin (VIM) in CRC tissues, illustrated by the GEPIA database (see footnote 2) (**Supplementary Figure 3**). To investigate any possible influence of FSTL3 on β-Catenin, we initially analyzed β-Catenin expression levels in FSTL3 overexpressed DLD-1 cells and found, surprisingly, increased β-Catenin mRNA and protein levels, compared to control cells (**Figures 4A,C**).

Moreover, overexpressed FSTL3 substantially increased nuclear translocation of β-Catenin, suggesting that the β-Catenin signaling pathway was activated (**Figure 4B**). Elevated FSTL3 expression was also linked to increased levels of F-actin polymerization which is well known to play a crucial role in EMT processes of CRC cells. The RNAi-mediated targeting of β-Catenin in FSTL3 overexpressed DLD-1 cells reduced F-actin polymerization (**Figure 4D**). In particular, FSTL3-overexpressed DLD-1 cells extend their antennae-like pseudopodia, which was reversible by targeting β-Catenin using RNAi. Furthermore, the qRT-PCR results demonstrated that FSTL3 overexpression was also significantly linked with diminished expression of *E*-cadherin and increased expression levels of N-Cadherin, FN-1 and Vimentin, compared to those in the control groups, which was counteracted by the β-Catenin knockdown (**Figure 4A**). The WB assays displayed consistent results except for FN1, which was diminished in sh-β-Catenin cells but not upregulated in cells with FSTL3 overexpression (**Figure 4C**). Therefore, HCT-116 sh-FSTL3 cells were utilized to further confirm the relation between FSTL3 and EMT. The qRT-PCR and WB results illustrated enhanced expression of *E*-cadherin and diminished expression levels of β-Catenin, *N*-Cadherin, and Vimentin in the HCT-116 sh-FSTL3 cells compared to the control groups (**Figures 4E,G**). In particular, knock-down of FSTL3, as a more reliable evidence compared to overexpression system, reduced the mRNA and protein level of FN1 (**Figures 4E,G**). Additionally, knock-down of FSTL3 substantially decreased the nuclear translocation of β-Catenin (**Figure 4F**) and reduced F-actin polymerization

TABLE 2 | Univariate and multivariate analysis of 130 CRC patients for DFS and OS.

Variables	DFS				OS			
	Univariate analysis		Multivariate analysis		Univariate analysis		Multivariate analysis	
	HR(95%CI)	*p*-value	HR(95%CI)	*p*-value	HR(95%CI)	*p*-value	HR(95%CI)	*p*-value
Age, years (≥60 vs. <60)	1.080(0.664–1.811)	0.771	NA	NA	1.025(0.599-1.753)	0.930	NA	NA
Gender (male vs. female)	1.076(0.642-1.804)	0.780	NA	NA	1.134(0.663-1.938)	0.646	NA	NA
Tumor location		0.740	NA	NA		0.836	NA	NA
(LCC vs. RCC)	0.757(0.354-1.617)	0.472	NA	NA	0.782(0.350–1.747)	0.550	NA	NA
(LCC vs. REC)	0.819(0.469–1.508)	0.521	NA	NA	0.893(0.469–1.702)	0.731	NA	NA
(RCC vs. REC)	0.924(0.477–1.790)	0.815	NA	NA	0.876(0.442–1.738)	0.705		
Type		0.072		0.899		0.028		0.846
G1 vs. G3	0.600(0.289–1.246)	0.171	0.836(0.382–1.830)	0.654	0.528(0.252–1.105)	0.090	0.794(0.356–1.771)	0.572
G2 vs. G3	1.165(0.504–2.694)	0.720	0.901(0.357–2.274)	0.825	1.151(0.498–2.660)	0.742	0.797(0.313–2.030)	0.634
G1 vs. G2	1.941(1.047–3.597)	0.035	1.077(0.533–2.177)	0.835	2.181(1.165–4.083)	0.015	1.004(0.496–2.033)	0.991
Depth of invasion(T3/T4	0.901(0.428–1.898)	0.784	NA	NA	0.987(0.447-2.180)	0.975	NA	NA
vs. T1/T2)	0.908(0.376–2.195)	0.083	NA	0.681	0.981(0.375-2.563)	0.016	1.345(0.497-3.640)	0.714
Substage	1.650(0.679–4.011)	0.831	1.298(0.517-3.255)	0.579	2.135(0.819-5.565)	0.969	1.952(0.386-9.883)	0.560
IIIA vs. IIIB	0.550(0.322–0.940)	0.269	0.487(0.096-2.464)	0.384	0.459(0.265-0.796)	0.121	0.689(0.182-2.604)	0.419
IIIA vs. IIIC	1.822(1.097–3.024)	0.029	0.632(0.161-2.480)	0.511	1.740(1.029-2.940)	0.006	1.729(0,989-3.020)	0.583
IIIC vs. IIIB		0.020	1.822(1.064-3.119)	0.029		0.039		0.055
Diameter(≥5 cm vs. <5 cm)								
LN metastasis(N1 vs.	1.658(0.997–2.756)	0.051	0.645(0.169–2.465)	0.522	2.113(1.250–3.574)	0.005	0.892(0.242–3.286)	0.864
N2)	3.876(2.302–6.527)	0.000	3.163(1.721–5.815)	0.000	4.608(2.660–7.982)	0.000	3.455(1.852–6.445)	0.000
Intravascular emboli	1.025(0.410–2.562)	0.958	NA	NA	1.014(0.405–2.543)	0.976	NA	NA
Intestinal obstruction								
CEA(≥ 5 ng/ml vs. < 5ng/ml)	0.964(0.530–1.753)	0.903	NA	NA	1.122(0.612–2.055)	0.709	NA	NA
CA199(≥35 kU/L vs.	1.800(0.973–3.331)	0.061	NA	NA	1.617(0.854–3.063)	0.140	NA	NA
<35 kU/L)	2.866(1.659–4.953)	0.000	1.948(1.059–3.586)	0.032	3.674(2.027–6.660)	0.000	2.424(1.279–4.593)	0.007
FSTL3 expression level (High vs. Low)								

HR, hazard ratio; CI, confidence interval; NA, not available.

(**Figure 4H**). Altogether, FSTL3 can activate the β-Catenin pathway to promote EMT-processes in CRC cells.

FSTL3 Regulates Glycolysis via Wnt/β-Catenin Pathway

The GEPIA database (see footnote 2) confirmed that the β-Catenin expression was positively associated with genes related to aerobic glycolysis, including glucose transporter 1 (GLUT1/SLC2A1), lactate dehydrogenase A (LDHA), hexokinase 2 (HK2), and pyruvate kinase isoform 2 (PKM2) (**Supplementary Figure 4**). Meanwhile, the expression of FSTL3 was positively related to GLUT1, LDHA and PKM, but negatively related to HK2 expression (**Supplementary Figure 5**). Therefore, we wondered whether aerobic glycolysis is also involved in the phenotypic changes regulated by FSTL3 expression in CRC cells. The qRT-PCR and WB assays demonstrated that FSTL3 overexpression significantly elevated the levels of GLUT1, LDHA, HK2, and PKM2, compared to the control, while the β-Catenin knockdown was sufficient to decrease the expression levels of GLUT1, LDHA, HK2 and PKM2 in DLD-1 cells (**Figures 5A,B**). HCT-116 cells depleted for FSTL3 obviously decreased mRNA and protein expression of GLUT1, LDHA, HK2, and PKM2 (**Figures 5C,D**). In order to analyze any possible changes related to aerobic glycolysis, we investigated intracellular ATP production, lactate levels as well as glucose uptake in FSTL3 overexpressed and knockdown cells. The abundant FSTL3 expression levels significantly elevated glucose uptake and lactate levels, and promoted ATP production in CRC cells (**Figures 5E–G**). Targeting β-Catenin expression significantly reduced aerobic glycolysis in FSTL3 overexpressed cells, compared to the control. Altogether, FSTL3 is able to regulate aerobic glycolysis via Wnt/β-Catenin pathway in CRC cells.

FSTL3 Promotes CRC Metastasis *in vivo*

In order to investigate the effect of FSTL3 on liver metastasis *in vivo*, CRC cells (HCT-116 Con and HCT-116 shFSTL3, DLD-1 Con and DLD-1 OE-FSTL3) were injected into the distal tip of the spleen using a Hamilton syringe ($n = 5$ per group). To analyze and compare any differences between FSTL3 overexpressed and knockdown CRC cells, we quantify the visible metastatic liver nodules and measured the volume of the largest liver metastasis.

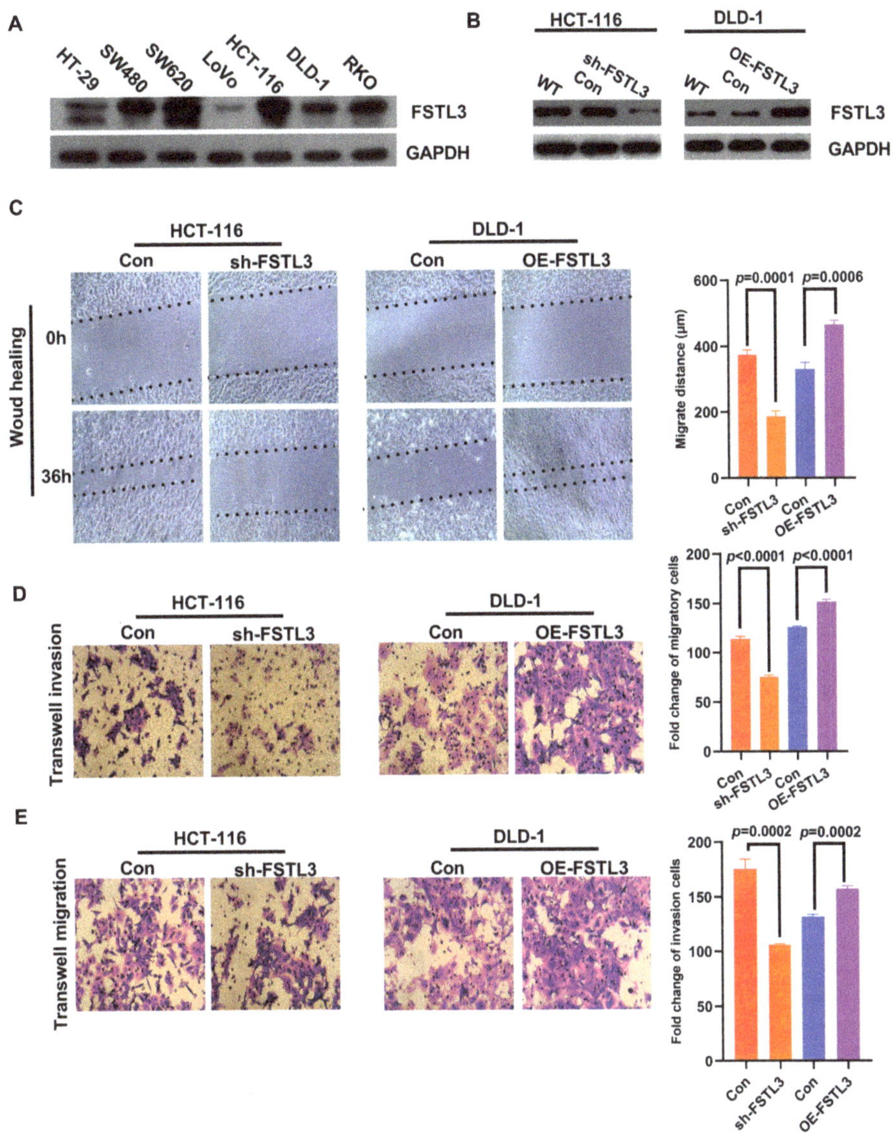

FIGURE 2 | FSTL3 promotes migration and invasion of CRC cells *in vitro*. **(A)** Protein expression levels of FSTL3 in CRC cell lines. **(B)** WB analysis of FSTL3 knockdown and overexpression. **(C)** The wound-healing assays were applied to detect migration capacity (timepoints 0 and 36 h) affected by FSTL3 in HCT-116 and DLD-1 cells. **(D,E)** Transwell assays were utilized to quantify migration and invasion capacity affected by FSTL3 in HCT-116 and DLD-1 cells. Data are presented as the mean ± SD from three independent experiments.

All of the mice successfully formed tumors in the spleen and all of the mice injected with HCT-116 control cells formed liver metastases (**Figure 6A**). The latter was linked to increased visible nodules and larger metastatic volumes (**Figures 6C,D**). In contrast, the injection of FSTL3 knockdown HCT-116 cells not only decreased the rate of liver metastasis but was also linked with significantly reduced volume of the metastatic nodules (**Figures 6C,D**). Additionally, liver metastases appeared in all of the mice injected with DLD-1 OE-FSTL3 cells and in 4 of 5 mice injected with DLD-1 control cells (**Figure 6B**). The total number of liver metastasis were obviously increased in mice injected with FSTL3 high-expression cell lines (HCT-116 Con and DLD-1 OE-FSTL3) compared to those with FSTL3 low-expression (HCT-116 shFSTL3 and DLD-1 Con) (**Figure 6C**). Similarly, the volume of the largest liver metastasis in mice injected with FSTL3 low-expression cells was significantly smaller than that with FSTL3 high-expression (**Figure 6D**). Collectively, these results suggest that FSTL3 is able to enforce the metastatic ability of CRC *in vivo*.

DISCUSSION

Although many advanced CRC patients can have a benefit from regional treatment approaches (e.g., surgery) for isolated liver metastases, the recurrence rate for CRC is still high, unfortunately

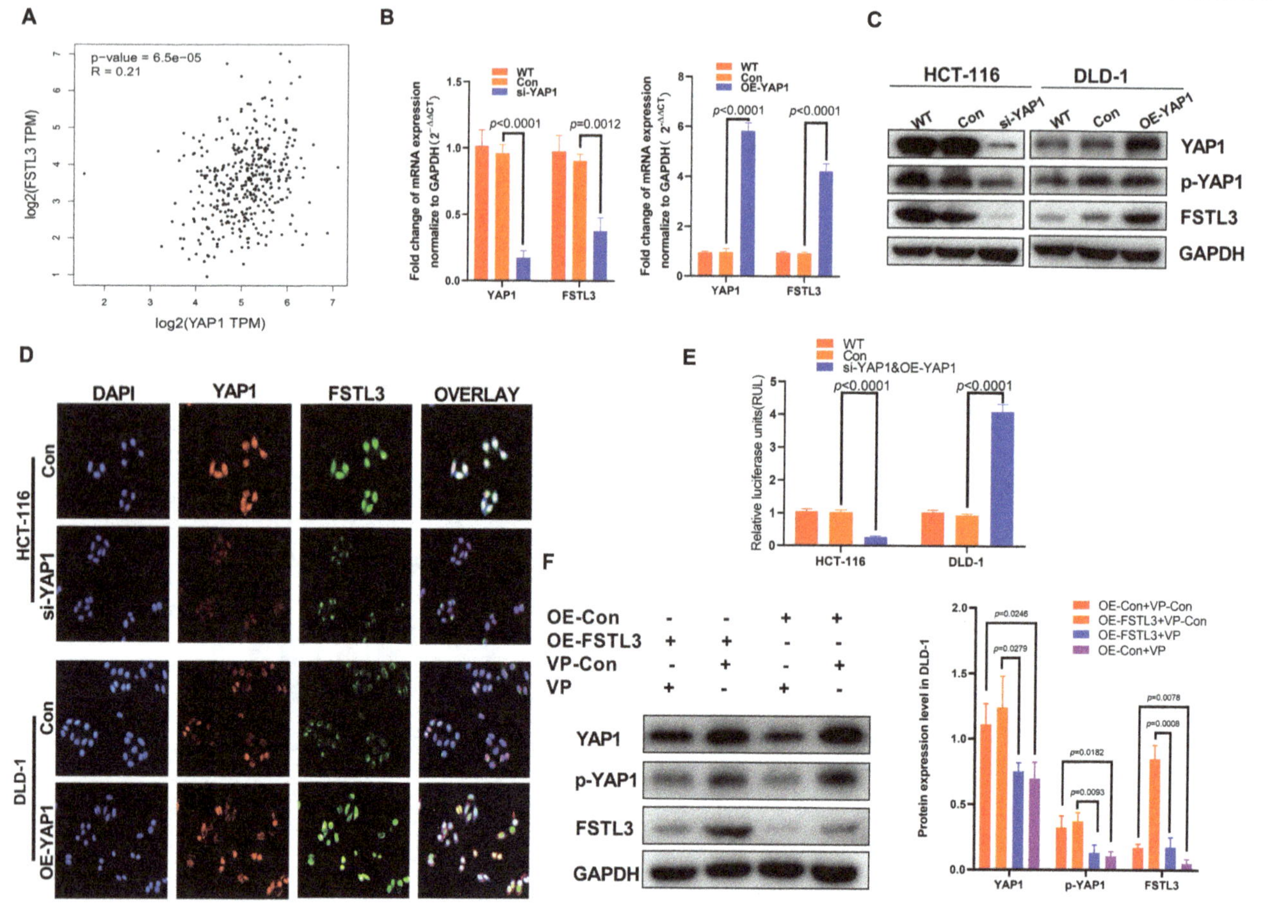

FIGURE 3 | YAP1 modulates the expression of FSTL3 in CRC. **(A)** Data derived from the GEPIA database showed positive correlation between FSTL3 and YAP1 in CRC tissues. **(B)** (left) YAP1 knockdown (siRNA) decreased FSTL3 mRNA expression in HCT116 cells, quantified with qRT-PCR; (right) YAP1 mRNA overexpression in DLD-1 cells promotes FSTL3 expression, quantified with qRT-PCR. **(C)** WB analysis of si-YAP1 and OE-YAP1 in HCT-116 and DLD-1 cells. **(D)** Immunofluorescence displayed elevated FSTL3 expression following YAP1 overexpression in DLD-1 cells. **(E)** Luciferase assays for the *hFSTL3* gene promoter construct. Reporter activation was analyzed in si-YAP1 and OE-YAP1 CRC cells. **(F)** WB analysis determined reduced YAP1 phosphorylation and FSTL3 expression levels in Verteporfin (VP)-treated DLD-1 cells.

(Choti et al., 2002; Abdalla et al., 2004; Fernandez et al., 2004; D'Angelica et al., 2011; Kawaguchi et al., 2020). In recent years it becomes increasingly apparent that the "biological footprint" of a tumor is recognized as an important and useful prognostic factor; hence the molecular profiling has undoubtedly a huge impact on risk stratification and therapy planning in CRC.

Within this study, we investigated the expression and molecular function of FSTL3 in CRC cells. Our data illustrated that abundant FSTL3 expression is a negative prognosticator in CRC patients (n = 130), and is significantly correlated with lymph node metastasis, staging, tumor size and IVE. The ability of cancer cells to migrate *in vivo* has a central role in cancer metastasis and it is believed that a set of specialized cells at the cancer invasive front (CIF) initiates the metastatic cascade through employing a collective mode of migration, rather than single cell migration (Yang et al., 2019). Interestingly, FSTL3 was already shown to localize to CIF, further underlying the here presented significant correlation of FSTL3 expression and lymph node metastasis in CRC. Additionally, the significant correlation of FSTL3 and IVE also reflects the intense invasive ability of cancer cells and is therefore considered as a potential predictor of metastasis.

Different molecular mechanisms have already been attributed to the development and progress of CRC and the most well-studied and dysregulated pathways belong to EGFR, Notch, PI3K/AKT as well as Wnt/β-Catenin signaling (Koveitypour et al., 2019). Wnt/β-Catenin signaling is already recognized for its ability to orchestrate various biological processes such as differentiation, organogenesis, cell proliferation and tissue regeneration. In cancer cells, Wnt is frequently found abnormally activated and accumulating evidences shows that the hyperactivation of Wnt plays an important oncogenic role, especially in CRC, and therefore representing an attractive therapeutic target for CRC treatment (Novellasdemunt et al., 2015). In fact, we found that elevated FSTL3 expression strongly promotes migration and invasion of CRC cells and that FSTL3 exerts these effects by interfering with the Wnt/β-Catenin pathway. Factors that may induce transcriptional activation of

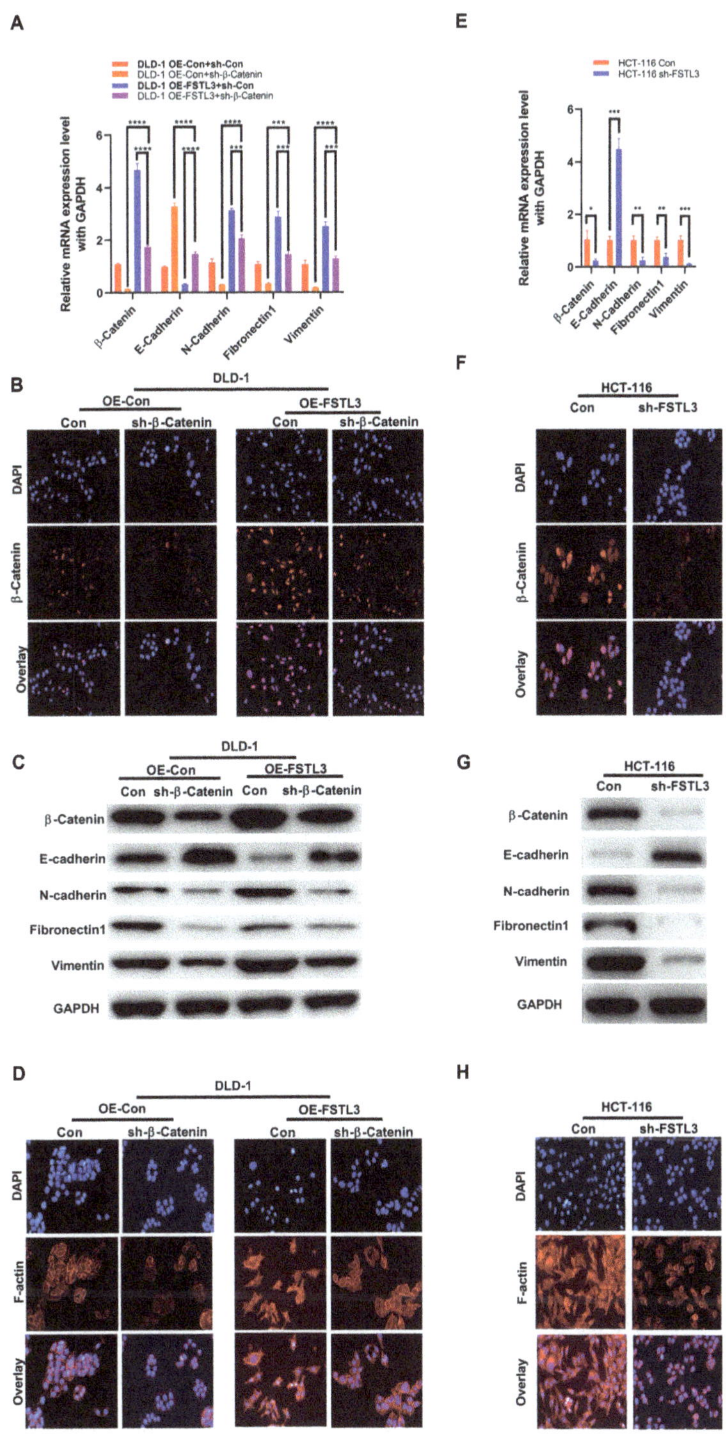

FIGURE 4 | FSTL3 induces β-Catenin-mediated EMT. **(A)** qRT-PCR displayed elevated β-Catenin mRNA expression in DLD-1 cells co-expressed with FSTL3. Impact of FSTL3 and β-Catenin expression on EMT in DLD-1 cells. ****$p < 0.0001$; ***$p < 0.001$. **(B)** Immunofluorescence of ectopically overexpressed FSTL3 promoted expression and nuclear translocation of β-Catenin, compared to control DLD-1 cells. **(C)** WB displayed increased β-Catenin protein expression in cells co-expressed with FSTL3. FSTL3 and β-Catenin expression is linked to the expression of EMT-related proteins in DLD-1cells. **(D)** Immunofluorescence showing that enforced FSTL3 expression increased F-actin levels. β-Catenin depletion decreased F-actin expression in DLD-1 cells, compared to control. **(E)** qRT-PCR displayed the impact of knock-down FSTL3 on β-Catenin and EMT-related genes in HCT-116 cells. ***$p < 0.001$; **$p < 0.01$; *$p < 0.05$. **(F)** Immunofluorescence of ectopically knock-down FSTL3 inhibited expression and nuclear translocation of β-Catenin, compared to control HCT-116 cells. **(G)** WB displayed FSTL3 expression is linked to the expression of β-Catenin and EMT-related proteins in HCT-116 cells. **(H)** Immunofluorescence showing that FSTL3 depletion decreased F-actin expression in HCT-116 cells, compared to control.

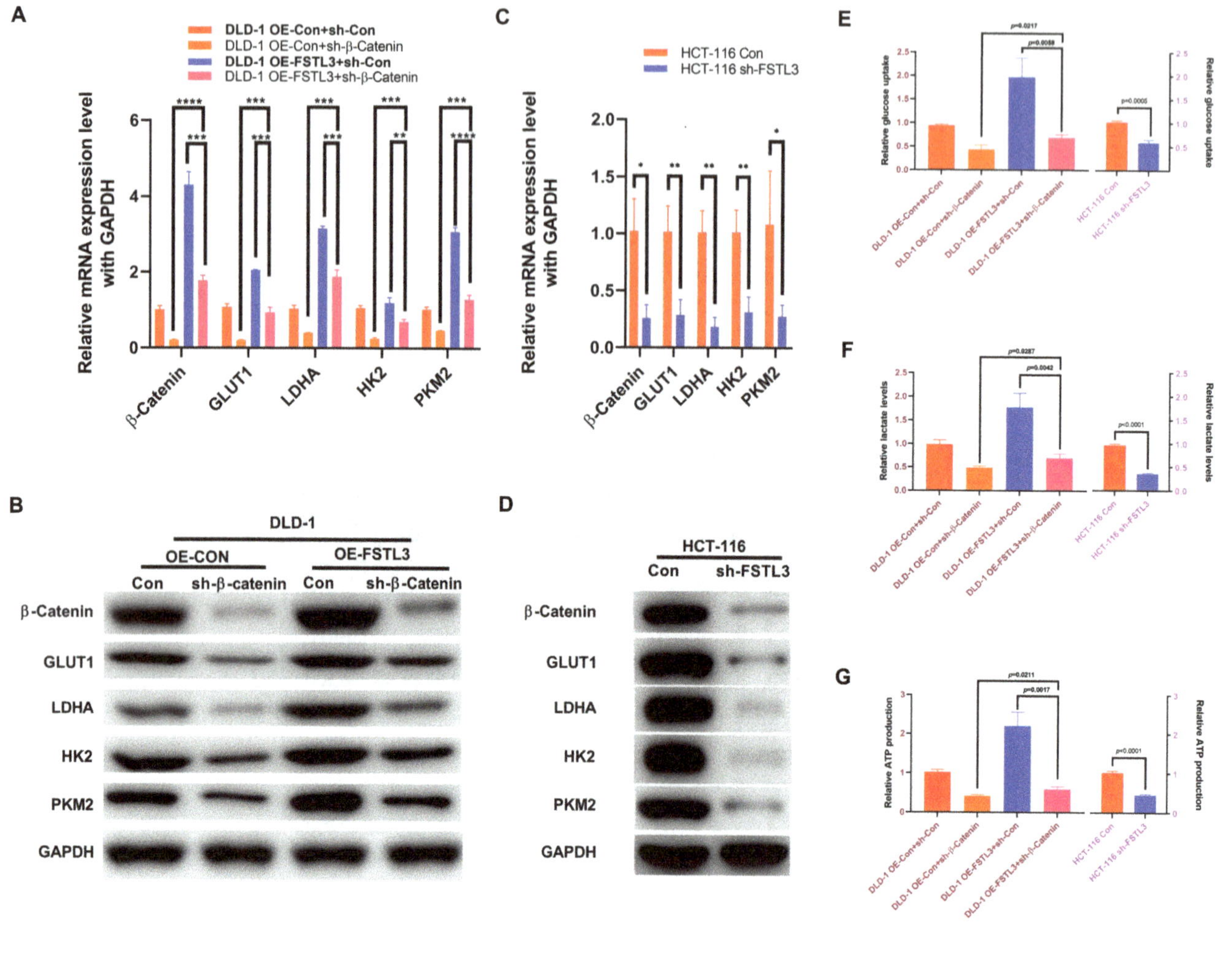

FIGURE 5 | FSTL3 induces β-Catenin-mediated glycolysis. **(A,B)** qRT-PCR and WB assays displayed increased mRNA and protein expression of GLUT1, LDHA, HK2 and PKM2 in FSTL3 overexpressed and/or sh-β-Catenin DLD-1 cells, compared to control. ****$p < 0.0001$; ***$p < 0.001$; **$p < 0.01$. **(C,D)** qRT-PCR and WB assays displayed decreased mRNA and protein expression of GLUT1, LDHA, HK2 and PKM2 in HCT-116 sh-FSTL3 cells, compared to control. **$p < 0.01$; *$p < 0.05$. **(E–G)** Expression of FSTL3 and β-Catenin were significantly connected with glucose uptake, lactate levels and ATP production in DLD-1 cells, compared to control; knock-down FSTL3 significantly reduced glucose uptake, lactate levels and ATP production in HCT-116 cells, compared to control.

FSTL3 in CRC are unknown so far. We therefore performed FSTL3 gene promoter analysis as well as YAP1 knockout studies and found that YAP1, as a transcriptional cofactor, is required for FSTL3 transactivation. Pharmacological inhibition of YAP1 nuclear translocation drastically reduced FSTL3 expression and a positive correlation between YAP1 and FSTL3 mRNA expression was very recently shown in prostate cancer (Lee et al., 2017). Interestingly, in global gene expression analyses, YAP1 was found to transactivate genes that specifically promote cancer cell motility and consequently metastatic formation (Yang et al., 2015; Zhang et al., 2015; Lee et al., 2017; Warren et al., 2018). A possible crosstalk between the HIPPO/YAP1 and Wnt/β-Catenin signaling was already shown to play a key role in the progression course of CRC (Konsavage et al., 2012; Jiao et al., 2017). The similar biological processes mediated by the HIPPO/YAP1 and Wnt/β-Catenin signaling pathways suggest that those may cooperate in concert to regulate each other's activity for precise regulation and fine-tuning of transcriptional target gene activation (Li N. et al., 2019). Another study reported that HIPPO/YAP1 signaling can restrict the Wnt/β-Catenin signaling by increasing Dvl phosphorylation (Varelas et al., 2010). Strikingly, YAP1 gene expression is regulated by Wnt/β-Catenin signaling in CRC cells (Konsavage et al., 2012). The cellular crosstalk between Hippo/YAP1 and Wnt/β-Catenin pathways is not fully understood, but increasing evidence have shown that both are able to coordinately regulate gene expression and signaling with relevance to cancer cell migration and metastatic formation (Azzolin et al., 2014). The importance of this crosstalk is further substantiated by the fact that overexpression of YAP1 or β-Catenin alone cannot lead to tumor development in mice, whereas co-expression of the two resulted in rapid carcinogenesis (Tao et al., 2014). Concurrent nuclear localization of YAP1 and β-Catenin appeared in most liver cancer tissues, suggesting simultaneous activation of these two pathways (Tao et al., 2014).

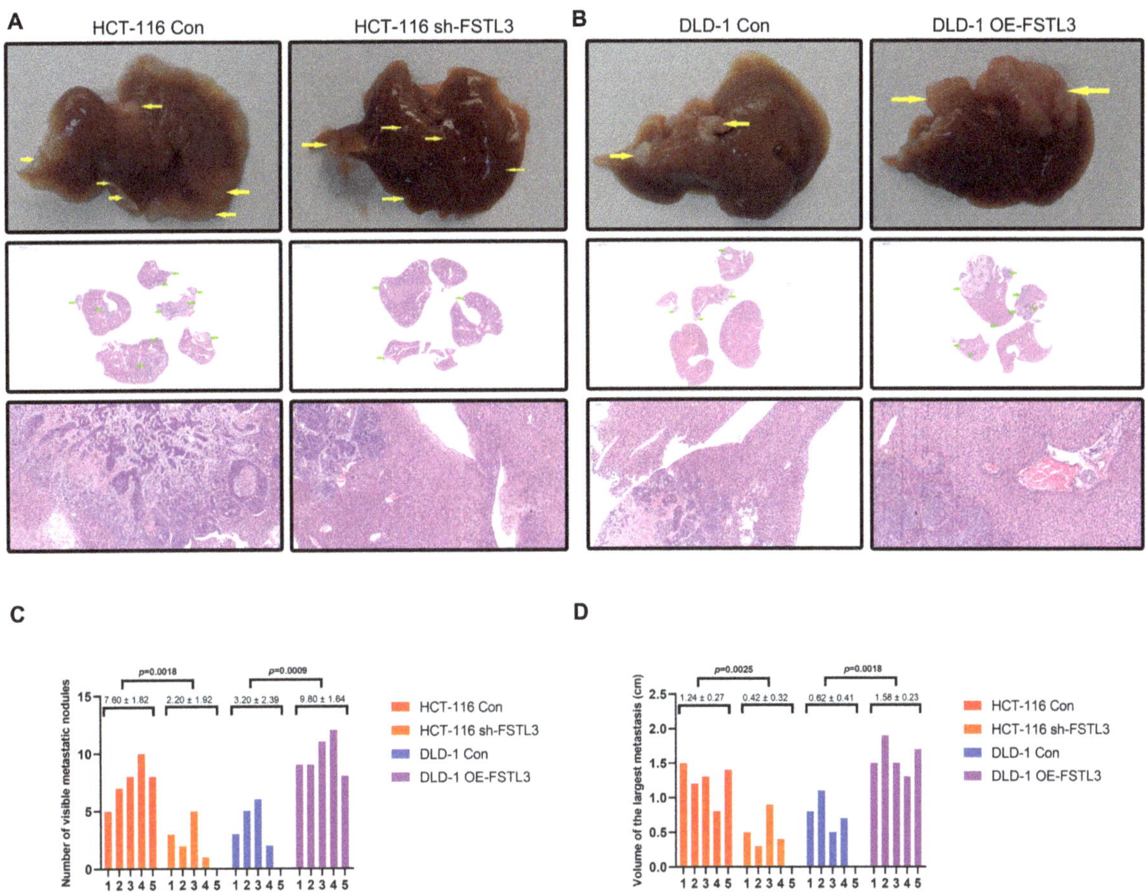

FIGURE 6 | FSTL3 enhances CRC cell metastasis *in vivo*. **(A)** Liver metastases became visible in all of the mice injected with HCT-116 control cells, and in 4 of 5 mice injected with FSTL3-depleted HCT-116 cells (scale bar, top: liver specimen; middle: 5000 μm; bottom: 100 μm). **(B)** Liver metastases were visible in all of the mice injected with DLD-1 overexpressed FSTL3 (OE-FSTL3) cells, and in 4 out of 5 mice injected with DLD-1 control cells (DLD-1 Con) (scale bar, top: liver specimen; middle: 5000 μm; bottom: 100 μm). **(C)** The numbers of hepatic metastatic nodules were notably reduced in mice injected with HCT-116 sh-FSTL3 cells and DLD-1 control cells, compared with the numbers in those injected with HCT-116 control cells and DLD-1 OE-FSTL3 cells ($p = 0.0018$; $p = 0.0009$). **(D)** Volumes of the largest liver metastasis in mice injected with FSTL3-depleted HCT116 cells were significantly smaller than that with FSTL3 overexpressed cells ($p = 0.0025$; $p = 0.0018$).

Because of the fact that β-Catenin can induce YAP1, and YAP1 is able to transactivate FSTL3, we curiously investigated a possible impact of abundant FSTL3 on β-Catenin signaling in CRC and found not only elevated β-Catenin expression levels, but also increased β-Catenin nuclear translocation in FSTL3 overexpressed cells, suggesting a positive feedback loop. Active β-Catenin signaling depends on its nuclear translocation and is strongly linked with EMT processes and aerobic glycolysis in different cancers (Cai et al., 2018; Fang et al., 2019; Zuo et al., 2020). In CRC, dysregulated β-Catenin signaling participates in the regulation of tumor invasion, metastasis formation and aerobic metabolism, and various mutations in crucial regulatory factors of the Wnt/β-Catenin pathway have already been widely noted in CRC (Jiao et al., 2020; Wang et al., 2020; Xue et al., 2020; Zhang et al., 2020).

Our here presented data revealed that FSTL3 promotes EMT processes and enhances aerobic glycolysis by activating β-Catenin to positively affect the migrative/invasive capacity of CRC cells. In fact, EMT is able to drive a series of hybrid states, endowing cancer cells an increased metastatic and aggressive potential and is also associated with significant metabolic rewiring (Ramesh et al., 2020). Cancer cell metabolism is principally characterized by an enhanced uptake/utilization of glucose as well as lactate production. As an important intermediary in numerous metabolic processes, lactate is closely associated with tumor growth, immune escape, angiogenesis and EMT processes (Ippolito et al., 2019; Pennington et al., 2019). Especially the increased lactate production in cancer cells is thought to reduce extracellular pH, thereby promoting the acidification of the tumor microenvironment. An acidic microenvironment with less glucose available is thought to suppress immune cell infiltration and contribute to immune evasion (San-Millán and Brooks, 2017; Harmon et al., 2019). In cancer cells, the persistent activation of aerobic glycolysis can be linked to oncogene activation or loss of tumor suppressors and thereby substantially advancing cancer occurrence and

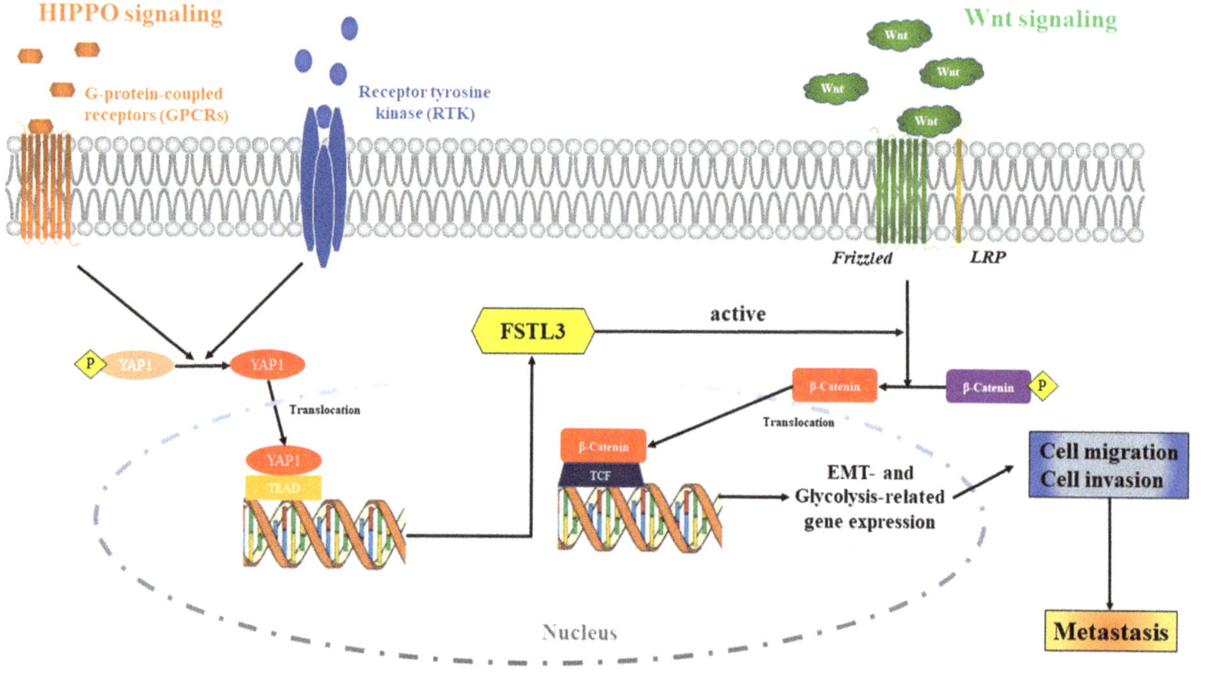

FIGURE 7 | The *Cartoon*: The activation of HIPPO/YAP1 can induce FSTL3 expression, which then promotes EMT and enhanced aerobic glycolysis to affect invasion, migration and metastasis formation of CRC cells by activating the Wnt/β-Catenin pathway. FSTL3 serves as a bridging molecule in the crosstalk between HIPPO/YAP1 and Wnt/β-Catenin pathways and is a crucial regulatory factor of the molecular mechanisms governed by Wnt/β-Catenin in CRC.

progression (Jang et al., 2013). Blocking aerobic glycolysis have therefore been recently considered as a therapeutic strategy to circumvent tumorigenesis (Peng et al., 2019; Zhang et al., 2019). In line with this, we found that FSTL3 significantly elevated the levels of key metabolic enzymes like HK2, PKM2, GLUT1 and LDHA. On the other hand, FSTL3 overexpression in CRC cells that are depleted for β-Catenin, were not able to show up an increase expression of these rate-limiting metabolic enzymes, suggesting that the here presented effects largely depend on active β-Catenin. To gain more insight into any possible changes related to aerobic glycolysis and energy production, we also investigated the intracellular ATP pool, lactate levels as well as glucose uptake in FSTL3 overexpressed CRC cells. We observed that abundant FSTL3 expression was only able to increase ATP pools, lactate and glucose levels in cells positive for β-Catenin expression, whereas β-Catenin depletion circumvented any increase in the presence of FSTL3.

Finally, we analyzed the effects of FSTL3 on metastatic ability in a xenograft mouse model of CRC. We therefore injected CRC cells with showing either elevated FSTL3 (DLD-1) or depleted FSTL3 expression (HCT116) to compare any differences in visible metastatic liver nodules and to measure the largest liver metastases between both mice groups. In mice, injected with DLD-1 OE-FSTL3 cells, we observed an increase in the number of visible metastatic nodules and larger metastatic volumes, whereas injection of HCT-116 shFSTL3 cells displayed reduced nodules and a reduced metastatic volume. A very recent study came to the same conclusion, that FSTL3 is strongly linked with increased metastatic formation in a mice model of lung cancer (Gao et al., 2020). We therefore believe that abundant FSTL3 is able to enforce the metastatic ability of CRC cells *in vivo*.

However, some questions still need to be resolved in future studies. For example, dissecting the specific binding site of YAP1 on the FSTL3 gene promoter needs to be explored in more detail (e.g., ChIP). The conduction of various oncogenic signal pathways is interdependent rather than independent. This interdependence crosstalk among various signal pathways is still not fully understood and should provide new insights to uncover the relevant molecular mechanism. A dual-targeting therapy option in patients suffering from advanced disease become an attractive new strategy in recent years. Finally, the identification and better understanding of new interdependent pathways may pave the way to substantially increase a survival benefit in these difficult-to-treat late therapy stages.

CONCLUSION

The high expression of FSTL3 is a poor prognostic factor for patients with CRC. The activation of YAP1 can induce FSTL3 expression, which then promotes EMT and enhances aerobic glycolysis to affect invasion and metastasis formation of CRC cells by activating the β-Catenin pathway. FSTL3 can serve as a bridging molecule between HIPPO/YAP and Wnt/β-Catenin signaling in CRC (*cartoon*, **Figure 7**). Our findings illustrate that FSTL3 could serve as a crucial regulatory factor of the β-Catenin molecular mechanisms, and reflects therefore a promising therapeutic target for anti-metastatic strategies in

CRC. Pharmacological targeting of YAP1 can counteract FSTL3 expression in CRC.

ETHICS STATEMENT

The studies involving human participants were reviewed and approved by the Medical Ethics Committee of Xiangya Hospital, Central South University. Written informed consent for participation was not required for this study in accordance with the national legislation and the institutional requirements. The animal study was reviewed and approved by the Medical Ethics Committee of Xiangya Hospital, Central South University.

AUTHOR CONTRIBUTIONS

YL and FT contributed to the conception and design of the study. FT, MT, and YL performed the statistical analysis, the experimental operation, and organized the experimental data. DW, ZZ, and QP contributed to data collection and some of the experiments. YL and YH performed the statistical analysis. YL wrote the first draft of the manuscript. YL, WL, FT, and CG wrote sections of the manuscript. All the authors contributed to manuscript revision, read, and approved the submitted version.

Center for Geriatric Disorders (Grant No. 2019SK2335), the Strategy-Oriented Special Project of Central South University of China (Grant No. ZLXD2017003), and the Colorectal Cancer Medical Seed Research Fund of Beijing Bethune Public Welfare Foundation Named "Effect and mechanism of YAP1 on EGFR resistance in K-ras wild-type metastatic colorectal cancer."

ACKNOWLEDGMENTS

YL gratefully acknowledges financial support from China Scholarship Council.

SUPPLEMENTARY MATERIAL

Supplementary Figure 1 | Vector information and partial promoter sequence of human *FSTL3* gene (NM_005860), showing three potential YAP1 binding sites *boxes*).

Supplementary Figure 2 | The data from various databases identified increased FSTL3 expression as a poor prognostic factor in CRC.

Supplementary Figure 3 | Analysis in GEPIA database http://gepia.cancer-pku.cn/) illustrated that expression of FSTL3 is obviously related to EMT-connected proteins, including CDH1, CDH2, FN1, and VIM in CRC tissues.

Supplementary Figure 4 | Analysis in GEPIA database http://gepia.cancer-pku.cn/) illustrated that β-Catenin expression is significantly associated with proteins related to aerobic glycolysis, including SLC2A1, LDHA, HK2, and PKM.

Supplementary Figure 5 | Analysis in GEPIA database http://gepia.cancer-pku.cn/) illustrated that FSTL3 expression is positively associated with expression of SLC2A1, LDHA and PKM, but negatively related to HK2.

Supplementary Table 1 | The primary antibodies used in this study.

Supplementary Table 2 | Primer sequences.

REFERENCES

Abdalla, E. K., Vauthey, J. N., Ellis, L. M., Ellis, V., Pollock, R., Broglio, K. R., et al. (2004). Recurrence and outcomes following hepatic resection, radiofrequency ablation, and combined resection/ablation for colorectal liver metastases. *Ann. Surg.* 239, 818–825; discussion 825–817. doi: 10.1097/01.sla.0000128305.90650.71

Azzolin, L., Panciera, T., Soligo, S., Enzo, E., Bicciato, S., Dupont, S., et al. (2014). YAP/TAZ incorporation in the β-catenin destruction complex orchestrates the Wnt response. *Cell* 158, 157–170. doi: 10.1016/j.cell.2014.06.013

Binnewies, M., Roberts, E. W., Kersten, K., Chan, V., Fearon, D. F., Merad, M., et al. (2018). Understanding the tumor immune microenvironment (TIME) for effective therapy. *Nat. Med.* 24, 541–550. doi: 10.1038/s41591-018-0014-x

Cai, C. F., Ye, G. D., Shen, D. Y., Zhang, W., Chen, M. L., Chen, X. X., et al. (2018). Chibby suppresses aerobic glycolysis and proliferation of nasopharyngeal carcinoma via the Wnt/β-catenin-Lin28/let7-PDK1 cascade. *J. Exp. Clin. Cancer Res.* 37:104. doi: 10.1186/s13046-018-0769-4

Choti, M. A., Sitzmann, J. V., Tiburi, M. F., Sumetchotimetha, W., Rangsin, R., Schulick, R. D., et al. (2002). Trends in long-term survival following liver resection for hepatic colorectal metastases. *Ann. Surg.* 235, 759–766. doi: 10.1097/00000658-200206000-00002

Couto, H. L., Buzelin, M. A., Toppa, N. H., Bloise, E., Wainstein, A. J., and Reis, F. M. (2017). Prognostic value of follistatin-like 3 in human invasive breast cancer. *Oncotarget* 8, 42189–42197. doi: 10.18632/oncotarget.15026

D'Angelica, M., Kornprat, P., Gonen, M., DeMatteo, R. P., Fong, Y., Blumgart, L. H., et al. (2011). Effect on outcome of recurrence patterns after hepatectomy for colorectal metastases. *Ann. Surg. Oncol.* 18, 1096–1103. doi: 10.1245/s10434-010-1409-1

Davidson, B., Abeler, V. M., Hellesylt, E., Holth, A., Shih Ie, M., Skeie-Jensen, T., et al. (2013). Gene expression signatures differentiate uterine endometrial stromal sarcoma from leiomyosarcoma. *Gynecol. Oncol.* 128, 349–355. doi: 10.1016/j.ygyno.2012.11.021

Dongre, A., and Weinberg, R. A. (2019). New insights into the mechanisms of epithelial-mesenchymal transition and implications for cancer. *Nat. Rev. Mol. Cell Biol.* 20, 69–84. doi: 10.1038/s41580-018-0080-4

Fang, Y., Shen, Z. Y., Zhan, Y. Z., Feng, X. C., Chen, K. L., Li, Y. S., et al. (2019). CD36 inhibits β-catenin/c-myc-mediated glycolysis through ubiquitination of GPC4 to repress colorectal tumorigenesis. *Nat. Commun.* 10:3981. doi: 10.1038/s41467-019-11662-3

Fernandez, F. G., Drebin, J. A., Linehan, D. C., Dehdashti, F., Siegel, B. A., and Strasberg, S. M. (2004). Five-year survival after resection of hepatic metastases from colorectal cancer in patients screened by positron emission tomography with F-18 fluorodeoxyglucose (FDG-PET. *Ann. Surg.* 240, 438–447; discussion 447–450. doi: 10.1097/01.sla.0000138076.72547.b1

Ganapathy-Kanniappan, S., and Geschwind, J. F. (2013). Tumor glycolysis as a target for cancer therapy: progress and prospects. *Mol. Cancer* 12:152. doi: 10.1186/1476-4598-12-152

Gao, L., Chen, X., Wang, Y., and Zhang, J. (2020). Up-Regulation of FSTL3, regulated by lncRNA DSCAM-AS1/miR-122-5p Axis, promotes proliferation and migration of non-small cell lung cancer cells. *Onco Targets Ther.* 13, 2725–2738. doi: 10.2147/OTT.S236359

Gavert, N., Sheffer, M., Raveh, S., Spaderna, S., Shtutman, M., Brabletz, T., et al. (2007). Expression of L1-CAM and ADAM10 in human colon cancer cells induces metastasis. *Cancer Res.* 67, 7703–7712. doi: 10.1158/0008-5472.can-07-0991

Harmon, C., Robinson, M. W., Hand, F., Almuaili, D., Mentor, K., Houlihan, D. D., et al. (2019). Lactate-Mediated acidification of tumor microenvironment induces apoptosis of liver-resident NK cells in colorectal liver metastasis. *Cancer Immunol. Res.* 7, 335–346. doi: 10.1158/2326-6066.cir-18-0481

Ippolito, L., Morandi, A., Giannoni, E., and Chiarugi, P. (2019). Lactate: a metabolic driver in the tumour landscape. *Trends Biochem. Sci.* 44, 153–166. doi: 10.1016/j.tibs.2018.10.011

Jang, M., Kim, S. S., and Lee, J. (2013). Cancer cell metabolism: implications for therapeutic targets. *Exp. Mol. Med.* 45:e45. doi: 10.1038/emm.2013.85

Jiao, S., Li, C., Hao, Q., Miao, H., Zhang, L., Li, L., et al. (2017). VGLL4 targets a TCF4-TEAD4 complex to coregulate Wnt and Hippo signalling in colorectal cancer. *Nat. Commun.* 8:14058. doi: 10.1038/ncomms14058

Jiao, Y., Zhou, J., Jin, Y., Yang, Y., Song, M., Zhang, L., et al. (2020). Long non-coding RNA TDRKH-AS1 promotes colorectal cancer cell proliferation and invasion through the β-catenin activated Wnt signaling pathway. *Front. Oncol.* 10:639. doi: 10.3389/fonc.2020.00639

Kalluri, R., and Weinberg, R. A. (2009). The basics of epithelial-mesenchymal transition. *J. Clin. Invest.* 119, 1420–1428. doi: 10.1172/jci39104

Kawaguchi, Y., Kopetz, S., Lillemoe, H. A., Hwang, H., Wang, X., Tzeng, C. D., et al. (2020). A new surveillance algorithm after resection of colorectal liver metastases based on changes in recurrence risk and RAS mutation status. *J. Natl. Compr. Canc. Netw.* 18, 1500–1508. doi: 10.6004/jnccn.2020.7596

Konsavage, W. M. Jr., Kyler, S. L., Rennoll, S. A., Jin, G., and Yochum, G. S. (2012). Wnt/β-catenin signaling regulates Yes-associated protein (YAP) gene expression in colorectal carcinoma cells. *J. Biol. Chem.* 287, 11730–11739. doi: 10.1074/jbc.M111.327767

Koveitypour, Z., Panahi, F., Vakilian, M., Peymani, M., Seyed Forootan, F., Nasr Esfahani, M. H., et al. (2019). Signaling pathways involved in colorectal cancer progression. *Cell Biosci.* 9:97. doi: 10.1186/s13578-019-0361-4

Lee, H. J., Diaz, M. F., Price, K. M., Ozuna, J. A., Zhang, S., Sevick-Muraca, E. M., et al. (2017). Fluid shear stress activates YAP1 to promote cancer cell motility. *Nat. Commun.* 8:14122. doi: 10.1038/ncomms14122

Li, C., Tan, F., Pei, Q., Zhou, Z., Zhou, Y., Zhang, L., et al. (2019). Non-coding RNA MFI2-AS1 promotes colorectal cancer cell proliferation, migration and invasion through miR-574-5p/MYCBP axis. *Cell Prolif.* 52:e12632. doi: 10.1111/cpr.12632

Li, N., Lu, N., and Xie, C. (2019). The Hippo and Wnt signalling pathways: crosstalk during neoplastic progression in gastrointestinal tissue. *FEBS J.* 286, 3745–3756. doi: 10.1111/febs.15017

Li, Y., Zhao, L., Güngör, C., Tan, F., Zhou, Z., Li, C., et al. (2019). The main contributor to the upswing of survival in locally advanced colorectal cancer: an analysis of the SEER database. *Therap. Adv. Gastroenterol.* 12:1756284819862154. doi: 10.1177/1756284819862154

Liu, T., Zhou, L., Yang, K., Iwasawa, K., Kadekaro, A. L., Takebe, T., et al. (2019). The β-catenin/YAP signaling axis is a key regulator of melanoma-associated fibroblasts. *Signal Transduct. Target. Ther.* 4:63. doi: 10.1038/s41392-019-0100-7

Lunt, S. Y., and Vander Heiden, M. G. (2011). Aerobic glycolysis: meeting the metabolic requirements of cell proliferation. *Annu. Rev. Cell Dev. Biol.* 27, 441–464. doi: 10.1146/annurev-cellbio-092910-154237

Mukherjee, A., Sidis, Y., Mahan, A., Raher, M. J., Xia, Y., Rosen, E. D., et al. (2007). FSTL3 deletion reveals roles for TGF-beta family ligands in glucose and fat homeostasis in adults. *Proc. Natl. Acad. Sci. U.S.A.* 104, 1348–1353. doi: 10.1073/pnas.0607966104

Novellasdemunt, L., Antas, P., and Li, V. S. (2015). Targeting Wnt signaling in colorectal cancer. A review in the theme: cell signaling: proteins, pathways and mechanisms. *Am. J. Physiol. Cell. Physiol.* 309, C511–C521. doi: 10.1152/ajpcell.00117.2015

Peng, W., Huang, W., Ge, X., Xue, L., Zhao, W., and Xue, J. (2019). Type Iγ phosphatidylinositol phosphate kinase promotes tumor growth by facilitating Warburg effect in colorectal cancer. *EBioMedicine* 44, 375–386. doi: 10.1016/j.ebiom.2019.05.015

Pennington, Z., Goodwin, M. L., Westbroek, E. M., Cottrill, E., Ahmed, A. K., and Sciubba, D. M. (2019). Lactate and cancer: spinal metastases and potential therapeutic targets (part 2). *Ann. Transl. Med.* 7:221. doi: 10.21037/atm.2019.01.85

Ramesh, V., Brabletz, T., and Ceppi, P. (2020). Targeting EMT in cancer with repurposed metabolic inhibitors. *Trends Cancer* 6, 942–950. doi: 10.1016/j.trecan.2020.06.005

Sánchez-Tilló, E., de Barrios, O., Siles, L., Cuatrecasas, M., Castells, A., and Postigo, A. (2011). β-catenin/TCF4 complex induces the epithelial-to-mesenchymal transition (EMT)-activator ZEB1 to regulate tumor invasiveness. *Proc. Natl. Acad. Sci. U.S.A.* 108, 19204–19209. doi: 10.1073/pnas.1108977108

San-Millán, I., and Brooks, G. A. (2017). Reexamining cancer metabolism: lactate production for carcinogenesis could be the purpose and explanation of the Warburg Effect. *Carcinogenesis* 38, 119–133. doi: 10.1093/carcin/bgw127

Siegel, R. L., Miller, K. D., Goding Sauer, A., Fedewa, S. A., Butterly, L. F., Anderson, J. C., et al. (2020). Colorectal cancer statistics, 2020. *CA Cancer J. Clin.* 70, 145–164. doi: 10.3322/caac.21601

Sleeman, J. P., and Thiery, J. P. (2011). SnapShot: the epithelial-mesenchymal transition. *Cell* 145:162.e1. doi: 10.1016/j.cell.2011.03.029

Sullivan, L. B. (2018). Metabolic frugality marks cancer cells for immune targeting. *Cell* 174, 1344–1346. doi: 10.1016/j.cell.2018.08.023

Tan, F., Huang, Y., Pei, Q., Liu, H., Pei, H., and Zhu, H. (2018). Matrix stiffness mediates stemness characteristics via activating the Yes-associated protein in colorectal cancer cells. *J. Cell. Biochem.* 120, 2213–2225. doi: 10.1002/jcb.27532

Tan, F., Zhu, H., Tao, Y., Yu, N., Pei, Q., Liu, H., et al. (2015). Neuron navigator 2 overexpression indicates poor prognosis of colorectal cancer and promotes invasion through the SSH1L/cofilin-1 pathway. *J. Exp. Clin. Cancer Res.* 34:117. doi: 10.1186/s13046-015-0237-3

Tao, J., Calvisi, D. F., Ranganathan, S., Cigliano, A., Zhou, L., Singh, S., et al. (2014). Activation of β-catenin and Yap1 in human hepatoblastoma and induction of hepatocarcinogenesis in mice. *Gastroenterology* 147, 690–701. doi: 10.1053/j.gastro.2014.05.004

Thiery, J. P., Acloque, H., Huang, R. Y., and Nieto, M. A. (2009). Epithelial-mesenchymal transitions in development and disease. *Cell* 139, 871–890. doi: 10.1016/j.cell.2009.11.007

Tsuchida, K., Arai, K. Y., Kuramoto, Y., Yamakawa, N., Hasegawa, Y., and Sugino, H. (2000). Identification and characterization of a novel follistatin-like protein as a binding protein for the TGF-beta family. *J. Biol. Chem.* 275, 40788–40796. doi: 10.1074/jbc.M006114200

Vander Heiden, M. G., Cantley, L. C., and Thompson, C. B. (2009). Understanding the Warburg effect: the metabolic requirements of cell proliferation. *Science* 324, 1029–1033. doi: 10.1126/science.1160809

Varelas, X., Miller, B. W., Sopko, R., Song, S., Gregorieff, A., Fellouse, F. A., et al. (2010). The Hippo pathway regulates Wnt/beta-catenin signaling. *Dev. Cell* 18, 579–591. doi: 10.1016/j.devcel.2010.03.007

Wang, Z., Yang, Y., Hu, S., He, J., Wu, Z., Qi, Z., et al. (2020). Short-form RON (sf-RON) enhances glucose metabolism to promote cell proliferation via activating β-catenin/SIX1 signaling pathway in gastric cancer. *Cell Biol. Toxicol.* 37, 35–49. doi: 10.1007/s10565-020-09525-5

Warren, J. S. A., Xiao, Y., and Lamar, J. M. (2018). YAP/TAZ activation as a target for treating metastatic cancer. *Cancers (Basel)* 10:115. doi: 10.3390/cancers10040115

Xue, S., Wu, W., Wang, Z., Lu, G., Sun, J., Jin, X., et al. (2020). USP5 promotes metastasis in non-small cell lung cancer by inducing epithelial-mesenchymal transition via Wnt/β-Catenin pathway. *Front. Pharmacol.* 11:668. doi: 10.3389/fphar.2020.00668

Yang, S., Zhang, L., Purohit, V., Shukla, S. K., Chen, X., Yu, F., et al. (2015). Active YAP promotes pancreatic cancer cell motility, invasion and tumorigenesis in a mitotic phosphorylation-dependent manner through LPAR3. *Oncotarget* 6, 36019–36031. doi: 10.18632/oncotarget.5935

Yang, Y., Zheng, H., Zhan, Y., and Fan, S. (2019). An emerging tumor invasion mechanism about the collective cell migration. *Am. J. Transl. Res.* 11, 5301–5312.

Zhang, L., Dong, X., Yan, B., Yu, W., and Shan, L. (2020). CircAGFG1 drives metastasis and stemness in colorectal cancer by modulating YY1/CTNNB1. *Cell Death Dis.* 11:542. doi: 10.1038/s41419-020-2707-6

Zhang, L., Yang, S., Chen, X., Stauffer, S., Yu, F., Lele, S. M., et al. (2015). The hippo pathway effector YAP regulates motility, invasion, and castration-resistant growth of prostate cancer cells. *Mol. Cell. Biol.* 35, 1350–1362. doi: 10.1128/mcb.00102-15

Zhang, S., Cao, L., Li, Z., and Qu, D. (2019). Metabolic reprogramming links chronic intestinal inflammation and the oncogenic transformation in colorectal tumorigenesis. *Cancer Lett.* 450, 123–131. doi: 10.1016/j.canlet.2019.02.045

Zuo, Q., He, J., Zhang, S., Wang, H., Jin, G., Jin, H., et al. (2020). PGC1α suppresses metastasis of HCC by inhibiting Warburg effect via PPARγ-dependent WNT/β-catenin/PDK1 axis. *Hepatology* 73, 644–660. doi: 10.1002/hep.31280

8

Integrated Analysis of the Functions and Prognostic Values of RNA-Binding Proteins in Colorectal Cancer

Ya Wang[1,2], Yuqiao Chen[1,2], Shuai Xiao[3] and Kai Fu[1,2,4,5]**

[1] Institute of Molecular Precision Medicine and Hunan Key Laboratory of Molecular Precision Medicine, Xiangya Hospital, Central South University, Changsha, China, [2] Department of General Surgery, Xiangya Hospital, Central South University, Changsha, China, [3] Department of Gastrointestinal Surgery and Institute of Clinical Medicine, The First Affiliated Hospital, University of South China, Hengyang, China, [4] Center for Medical Genetics & Hunan Key Laboratory of Medical Genetics, School of Life Sciences, Central South University, Changsha, China, [5] Hunan Key Laboratory of Animal Models for Human Diseases, Central South University, Changsha, China

***Correspondence:**
Shuai Xiao
xiaoshuai1982@hotmail.com
Kai Fu
fu_kai@csu.edu.cn

Colorectal cancer (CRC) is one of the most common malignant tumors. Selecting effective treatment for CRC patients, especially in the early stages, remains a challenge because of the lack of adequate biomarkers. Recent evidence suggests that RNA-binding proteins (RBPs) play a vital role in development and progression of carcinogenesis. However, their mechanisms in cancer progression are still limited. The role of RBPs in CRC has been poorly understood. There were 1,542 reported RBPs analyzed between CRC tissues and normal tissues using the Wilcoxon test to identify differentially expressed RBPs (DE RBPs). Then, the potential functions and the prognostic value of these DE RBPs were explored through systematic bioinformatics analysis. There were 177 DE RBPs identified between CRC tissues and normal tissues. A protein–protein interaction network was constructed based on DE RBPs, and critical modules were screened. A regulatory network between prognostic DE RBPs and differentially expressed transcription factors was constructed. Besides, a risk signature was built based on prognostic DE RBPs, which is able to predict overall survival of CRC patients with high accuracy. In conclusion, the results provided a comprehensive understanding of the functions of RBPs in CRC, as well as an RBP-related prognostic signature.

Keywords: colorectal cancer, RNA-binding protein, prognostic signature, overall survival, regulatory network

INTRODUCTION

Colorectal cancer (CRC) is one of the most common malignant tumors and the second cause of tumor-related mortality worldwide (Arnold et al., 2017; Bray et al., 2018). By 2030, the global burden of CRC is expected to increase by 60%, with 2.2 million new cases and 1.1 million deaths (Douaiher et al., 2017). The 5-year survival for CRC patients with local tumor is 90.3% and is 70.4%

Abbreviations: AUC, area under the ROC curve; BP, biological processes; CCs, cellular compartments; CRC, colorectal cancer; DE RBPs, differentially expressed RBPs; FC, fold change; GO, Gene Ontology; HR, hazard ratio; KEGG, Kyoto Encyclopedia of Genes and Genomes; MFs, molecular functions; NSCLC, non-small cell lung cancer; OS, overall survival; PPI, protein–protein interaction; RBPs, RNA-binding proteins; ROC, receiver operating characteristic; TCGA, The Cancer Genome Atlas; TFs, transcription factors.

for patients with locally advanced disease, which declines to 12.5% for patients with metastatic disease (DeSantis et al., 2014). Surgery is the most common treatment for early CRC and locally advanced CRC (Hudson et al., 2013; Angenete, 2019). However, half of the patients will suffer a recurrence within 3 years after surgery (Aghili et al., 2010). Despite some advances in the diagnosis and treatment of CRC over the past few decades, the 5-year overall survival (OS) is only 50–65% (DeSantis et al., 2014). Selecting effective treatment for CRC patients, especially in the early stages, remains a challenge because of the lack of adequate biomarkers. Therefore, further understanding of the pathogenesis of CRC will help us to develop effective means for diagnostic and treatment.

It is widely believed that the development of cancer is partly determined by abnormal transcription events and signaling pathways. Emerging evidence shows that RNA-binding proteins (RBPs) could regulate cell proliferation, differentiation, invasion, metastasis, apoptosis, and angiogenesis and thus play a vital role in the initiation and progression of cancer (Wurth, 2012). RBPs regulate a variety of RNA biogenesis, including RNA splicing, polyadenylation, nucleocytoplasmic transport, mRNA translation, and RNA degradation (Lu et al., 2006; Saunus et al., 2008; Shen and Pili, 2008). So far, several RBPs have been found to be involved in cancer progression. RBPs regulate posttranscriptional genes at different levels of mRNA metabolism, including alternative splicing, localization, stability of mRNA, and so on. For example, Sam68, belonging to STAR (signal transduction and activation of RNA) family of RBPs (Bielli et al., 2011; Fu et al., 2019), regulates alternative splicing of cancer-related mRNA, such as CD44 (Matter et al., 2002), cyclin D1 (Paronetto et al., 2010), and Bcl-x (Paronetto et al., 2007). Cap-binding protein eIF4E (eukaryotic initiation factor 4E) is a crucial regulator of translation initiation (Topisirovic et al., 2011). eIF4E has been reported to be overexpressed in different cancers (Hsieh and Ruggero, 2010). However, overexpression of eIF4E does not lead to an overall increase of protein synthesis but enhances the translation of several mRNAs encoding mainly pro-oncogenic proteins (Silvera et al., 2010). mRNAs regulated by eIF4E overexpression include those involving in cell cycle (cyclin D1, CDK2, c-myc, Bcl-2, survivin) or angiogenesis (vascular endothelial growth factor, fibroblast growth factor 2, platelet-derived growth factor) or invasion (matrix metalloproteinase 9) (Mamane et al., 2004; Hsieh and Ruggero, 2010; Silvera et al., 2010). HuR is a member of the ELAV-like family of RBPs. It contains three RNA-recognition motifs by which it binds specific mRNAs to affect their stability and translation. HuR can stabilize the mRNAs coding for cyclins involved in cell cycle progression to promote the proliferation of cancer cells (Wang et al., 2000; Lal et al., 2004; Guo and Hartley, 2006). HuR also stabilizes the mRNAs coding antiapoptotic proteins such as Bcl-2, SIRT1, and p21 (Abdelmohsen et al., 2007; Ishimaru et al., 2009; Cho et al., 2010). Overexpression of HuR has been observed in multiple cancers, including CRC (Lopez, de Silanes et al., 2003; Denkert et al., 2006). HuR has been reported to augment the stability and translation of COX-2 mRNA in CRC (Dixon et al., 2001; Subbaramaiah et al., 2003). Besides, several other RBPs have been found to be abnormally expressed in CRC, such as RBM3 (Sureban et al., 2008), CUGBP2 (Ramalingam et al., 2008), Musashi-1 (Kudinov et al., 2017), and tristetraprolin (Young et al., 2009). However, the RBPs and their mechanisms in cancer progression remain to be explored. Benefiting from high-throughput screening technology, more than 1,500 RBPs have been identified (Gerstberger et al., 2014). A systematic functional study of RBPs in CRC will not only contribute to our deeper understanding of RBPs, but also provide new ideas for the pathogenesis of CRC. Therefore, an integrated bioinformatics analysis of RBPs in CRC was performed. Abnormally expressed RBPs between CRC tissues and normal tissues from The Cancer Genome Atlas (TCGA) dataset were identified, and then a systematic functional analysis was performed on these RBPs. In addition, a prognostic signature related to RBPs was constructed to predict the survival of CRC patients.

MATERIALS AND METHODS

Data Collection and Identification of Differentially Expressed RBPs

Colorectal cancer samples containing genetic information and clinical information from TCGA-COAD were downloaded. RBP lists were obtained as described (Gerstberger et al., 2014). After data normalization, differentially expressed RBPs (DE RBPs) between normal tissues and tumor tissues were identified through the Wilcoxon test. RBPs with $|\log_2FC$ (fold change) $| \geq 1$ and adjusted $p < 0.05$ were deemed DE RBPs.

Gene Ontology and Kyoto Encyclopedia of Genes and Genomes Functional Enrichment Analyses

Gene Ontology (GO) and Kyoto Encyclopedia of Genes and Genomes (KEGG) enrichment analyses for DE RBPs were performed using an R package "clusterProfiler." GO annotation based on three categories, including biological processes (BPs), cellular compartments (CCs), and molecular functions (MFs). Terms in GO and KEGG with a false discovery rate <0.05 were considered significantly enriched and were visualized by R package "ggplot2."

Protein–Protein Interaction Network Construction and Module Screening

Protein–protein interaction (PPI) network of DE RBPs was constructed using STRING database,[1] and an interaction with a combined score >0.4 was considered as statistically significant. Cytoscape, an open-source bioinformatics software platform, was used to visualize molecular interaction networks. The plug-in Molecular Complex Detection (MCODE) in Cytoscape software was used to cluster a given network based on the topology to find densely connected regions. The PPI networks were drawn with Cytoscape, and the most significant modules in the PPI networks were identified through MCODE with the default criteria, including MCODE score >5, degree cutoff value = 2,

[1]https://string-db.org

node score cutoff value = 0.2, maximum depth = 100, and k-score = 2.

Construction and Validation of a Prognostic Signature Based on DE RBPs

The CRC patients were randomly divided into a training set and a testing set. The training set was used to construct an RBP-related prognostic signature, and the testing set was used to validate its prognostic capability. To explore the putative DE RBPs related to the prognosis of CRC patients, a univariate Cox proportional hazards regression analysis was performed to explore the putative DE RBPs related to OS of CRC patients. The DE RBP with $p < 0.05$ was considered as a prognostic RBP. Then prognostic RBPs were used to construct the risk model for predicting the prognosis for CRC patients based on a multivariate Cox proportional hazards regression analysis. In this risk model, the risk score of each sample was calculated according to the following formula: risk score = expression of RBP 1 × coefficient 1 + expression of RBP 2 × coefficient 2 + expression of RBP n × coefficient n. The median risk score was used as the cutoff value. Patients were then divided into high- and low-risk groups according to the cutoff value. The Kaplan–Meier survival curves were carried out using "survival" R package based on high- and low-risk groups according to the risk model. To validate the prognostic capability of the risk model, the time-dependent receiver operating characteristic (ROC) analyses were performed with "survivalROC" R package.

Association Between the Risk Signature Related to RBPs and Clinicopathological Factors

To assess whether the prognosis signature we constructed is independent of other clinical factors, a univariate Cox proportional hazards regression and a multivariate Cox regression analysis were performed on the RBP-related signature together with gender, age, and stage.

The Regulatory Network Between Prognostic DE RBPs and DE Transcription Factors

To explore the potential molecular mechanisms of prognostic DE RBPs, the regulatory network between prognostic DE RBPs and differentially expressed transcription factor (DE TFs) was constructed. TFs are important molecules that directly regulate gene expression. Hence, exploring DE TFs, which have the potential ability in regulating the prognostic DE RBPs, would help to understand the MFs of the prognostic DE RBPs. The Cristrome Cancer database[2] is a valuable resource for experimental and computational cancer biology research and contains a total of 318 TFs related to cancer (Mei et al., 2017). DE TFs between CRC tissues and normal tissues were identified through the Wilcoxon test. TFs with | $\log_2$FC | ≥1 and adjusted $p < 0.05$ were deemed DE TFs.

[2]http://cistrome.org/

RESULTS

Identification of DE RBPs in CRC Patients

The workflow of the study is illustrated in **Supplementary Figure 1**. RNA sequencing data for CRC and corresponding clinical information were downloaded from TCGA database. There were 1,542 reported RBPs analyzed (Gerstberger et al., 2014). After data normalization, DE RBPs were detected between 47 normal tissues and 473 tumor tissues with an adjusted $p < 0.05$ and $|\log_2 FC| \geq 1$ as the thresholds. A total of 177 DE RBPs were obtained (**Figure 1A** and **Supplementary Table 1**), including 123 upregulated RBPs and 54 downregulated RBPs in tumor tissues (**Figure 1B**).

Functional Enrichment Analysis of the Differentially Expressed RBPs

To explore the potential functions of the DE RBPs, GO, and KEGG enrichment analyses were performed. For BP enrichment, DE RBPs were mostly enriched in ncRNA (non-coding RNAs) metabolic process, RNA phosphodiester bond hydrolysis, and ncRNA processing (**Figure 2A**). For CC enrichment, DE RBPs were mainly involved in cytoplasmic ribonucleoprotein granule, nucleolar part, and ribonucleoprotein granule (**Figure 2A**). For MF enrichment, RBPs are mainly enriched in catalytic activity, acting on RNA, ribonuclease activity, and nuclease activity (**Figure 2A**). The top five most significant GO enrichment terms are shown in **Figure 2B**. KEGG enrichment analysis showed DE RBPs were mainly involved in mRNA surveillance pathway, ribosome biogenesis in eukaryotes, and RNA transport (**Figures 2C,D**).

PPI Network Construction and Critical Module Screening

To further explore the potential functions of DE RBPs, a PPI network was constructed using STRING database and Cytoscape software. The PPI network of DE RBPs was downloaded from STRING database (**Supplementary Figure 2A**) and visualized with Cytoscape (**Supplementary Figure 2B**). Then, the network was further analyzed for critical modules by the plug-in MCODE in Cytoscape (**Figure 3A**), and the top three significant modules were obtained. Module 1 included 21 RBPs, all of which were upregulated RBPs except for DQX1 (**Figure 3B**). Module 2 included 13 RBPs, all of which were upregulated RBPs except for TDRD7 (**Figure 3C**). Module 3 included five downregulated RBPs (**Figure 3D**).

Identification of Prognosis-Related DE RBPs

To explore the putative DE RBPs related to prognosis for CRC patients, a univariate Cox proportional hazards regression analysis was performed to identify survival-related DE RBPs. There were 13 DE RBPs significantly correlated with OS ($p < 0.05$) (**Table 1**).

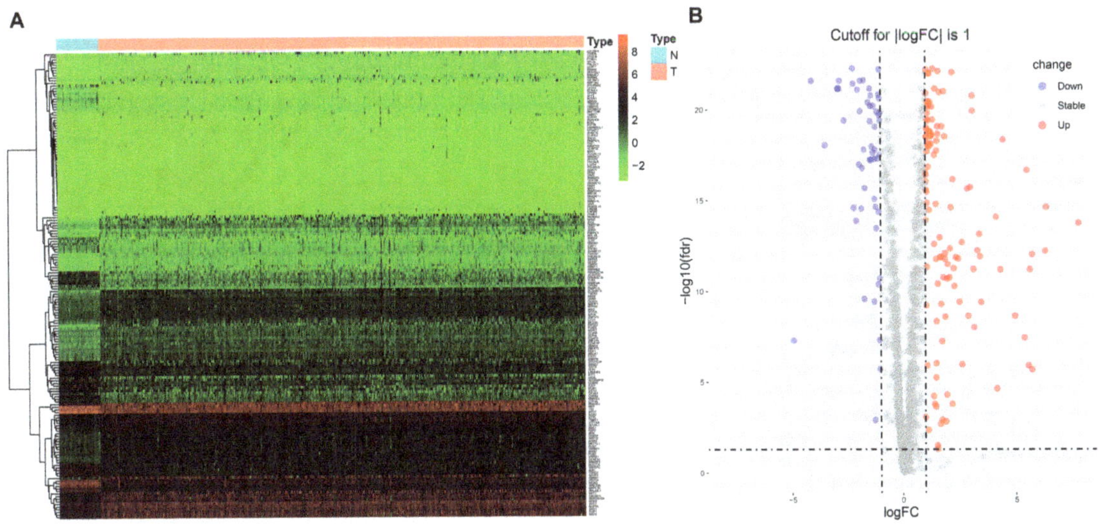

FIGURE 1 | The expression of DE RBPs in CRC based on data from TCGA. **(A)** Heatmap analysis of the differentially expressed RBPs between normal tissues and tumor tissues. Each column represents a tissue sample, and each row represents a differentially expressed RBP. Red indicates high expression, and green indicates low expression. N, normal; T, tumor. **(B)** Volcano plot of differentially expressed RBPs. The horizontal line is for adj $p = 0.05$, and the vertical lines are for $|\log_2 FC| = 1$.

The Regulatory Network Between Prognostic DE RBPs and DE TFs

Three hundred eighteen TFs related to cancer were obtained from The Cristrome Cancer database (see text footnote 2). Then, differentially expressed TFs between CRC tumor tissues and normal tissues were analyzed. A total of 77 differentially expressed TFs were obtained with a threshold that adjusted $p < 0.05$ and $|\log_2 FC| \geq 1$ (**Supplementary Table 2**). Then, a regulatory network based on these 77 DE TFs and 13 prognostic DE RBPs was constructed (**Figure 3E**). The coexpressed genes were identified by calculating the Pearson correlation between DE TFs and prognostic DE RBPs. The screening criteria were set as | Pearson coefficient| > 0.4 and $p < 0.001$.

Construction of a Prognosis Signature Based on RBPs

The 13 prognostic DE RBPs were applied to construct a prognostic model based on multiple Cox regression analysis. Cross-validation was performed to minimize overfitting. A risk-score formula consisting of seven RBPs was obtained as follows: risk score = (−2.01089 × TDRD6) + (−1.06396 × TDRD7) + (−0.83990 × PPARGC1A) + (−0.99781 × PABPC3) + (−1.30029 × LRRFIP2) + (−0.58829 × ZC3H12C) + (0.34108 × PNLDC1). The forest plot for the seven-RBP signature was shown in **Supplementary Figure 3**. The risk scores of patients in the training set and the testing set were calculated with the above formula. The median risk score of the training set was used for the cutoff value, by which the training set and the testing set were divided into high- and low-risk group. The heatmap showed the expression profiles of the seven RBPs in the training group (**Figure 4A**). The ranked risk scores of patients in the training set are shown in **Figure 4B**. The survival status for each patient was plotted, respectively (**Figure 4C**). The expression profiles of the seven RBPs in the testing set are presented in **Figure 4D**. The ranked risk scores of patients and the survival status for each patient in the testing set were plotted, respectively (**Figures 4E,F**). The results suggested that patients in the high-risk group showed a higher mortality rate than those in low-risk group both in the training set and the testing set.

Validation of the RBPs-Related Risk Signature

To investigate the prognostic value of the RBP-related risk signature, Kaplan–Meier survival analysis was performed between high- and low-risk groups in the training set and the testing set. The high-risk group had a significantly poorer OS than that of the low-risk group both in the training set (**Figure 5A**) and the testing set (**Figure 5E**). In addition, the ROC analysis was performed to evaluate the predictive efficiency of the RBP-related prognostic signature. The areas under the ROC curve (AUCs) for the risk signature on OS at 1, 3, and 5 years were 0.712, 0.743, and 0.708 in the training set (**Figures 5B–D**). The AUCs for the risk signature on OS at 1, 3, and 5 years were 0.703, 0.700, and 0.735 in the testing set (**Figures 5F–H**). The Kaplan–Meier analysis and the ROC analysis showed that the risk signature could predict the survival status of patients with high accuracy.

The RBP-Related Prognosis Signature Is an Independent Prognostic Index

To assess whether the prognosis signature we constructed is independent of other clinical factors, a univariate Cox proportional hazards regression and a multivariate Cox regression analysis were performed on the seven-gene signature together with gender, age, stage. Univariate Cox analysis result showed that RBP-related prognosis signature [hazard ratio (HR) = 1.332, 95% confidence interval (CI) = 1.211–1.465,

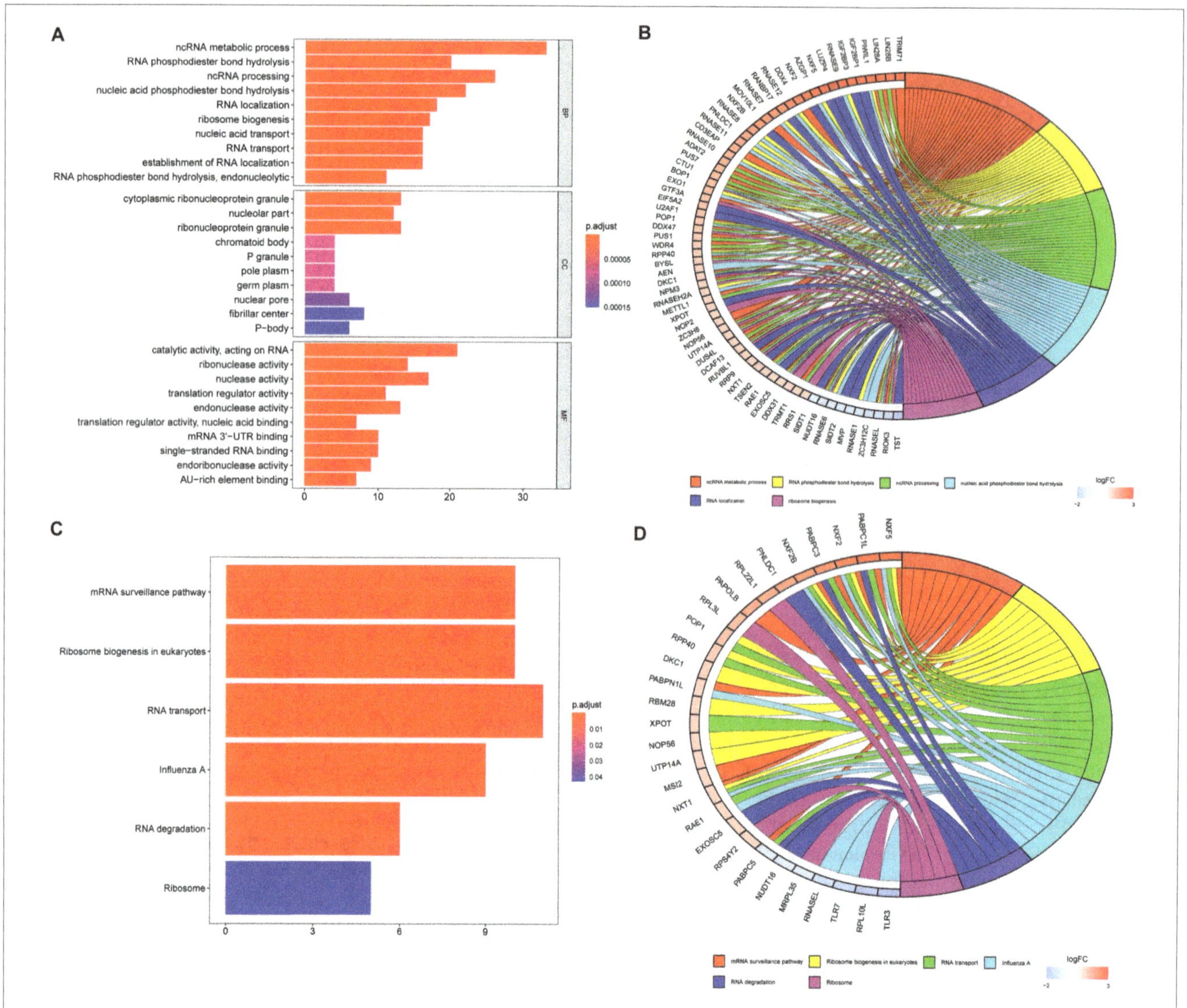

FIGURE 2 | GO and KEGG enrichment analyses of differentially expressed RBPs. **(A)** GO enrichment analysis including biological processes (BP), cellular compartments (CCs), and molecular functions (MFs). **(B)** The top six most significant GO enrichment terms. **(C)** KEGG enrichment analysis. **(D)** The top six most significant KEGG enrichment terms.

$p < 0.001$] was significantly correlated with the survival of patients in the training set (**Table 2**). After multivariable adjustment by other clinical factors, the prognosis signature (HR = 1.252, 95% CI = 1.136–1.380, $p < 0.001$) was still significantly associated with survival of patients (**Table 2**), which suggested that the RBP-related prognosis signature is an independent prognostic factor associated with survival of patients with CRC.

Construction of a Nomogram Based on the Prognostic Signature in the Training Set

To provide a quantitative method to predict the survival probability of CRC patients, a prognostic nomogram was established based on the seven RBPs of the prognostic signature using Cox proportional hazards regression analysis to predict 1-, 3-, and 5-year OS of CRC patients (**Figure 6**). To calculate the probability of survival at a certain point in time, the patient's total score can be obtained by adding the scores corresponding to the values of each predictive variable and then reading the corresponding risk or probability of survival from the total score.

DISCUSSION

RNA-binding proteins play a vital role in the development and progression of carcinogenesis with various mechanisms. However, only a small number of RBPs have been studied in depth to confirm their role in tumor progression. Until now, there is no systematic study on RBPs in CRC. In the present study,

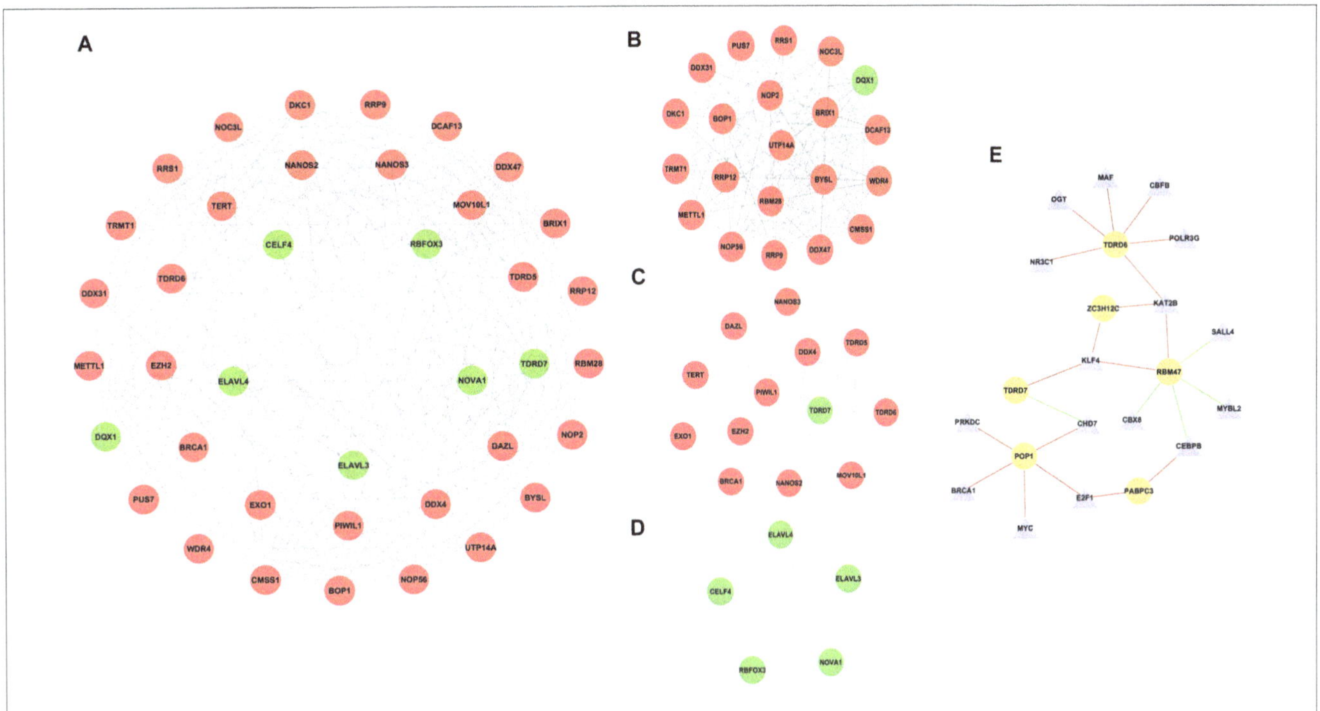

FIGURE 3 | PPI network of differentially expressed RBPs (DE RBPs) and regulatory network based on DE transcription factors and prognostic DE RBPs. **(A)** PPI network including three modules. The three circles from the inside out represent three modules. **(B)** Module 1 in PPI network. **(C)** Module 2 in PPI network. **(D)** Module 3 in PPI network. **(E)** Regulatory network between DE TFs and prognostic DE RBPs. The triangle represents TF, and the cycle represents prognostic DE RBP. The red line represents positive regulation, whereas the green line represents negative regulation.

we identified 177 DE RBPs between CRC tissues and normal tissues from TCGA dataset. To explore the potential functions of the DE RBPs, an integrated analysis was performed. We analyzed signaling pathways these DE RBPs involved in, constructed PPI network, and regulatory network between prognostic DE RBPs and TFs, which would provide a comprehensive understanding of the functions of RBPs in CRC. To further explore the clinical significance, we constructed an RBP-related prognostic model to predict the OS of CRC patients. These results provide novel biomarkers for prognosis of CRC patients.

TABLE 1 | Univariate Cox proportional hazards regression analysis of DE RBPs.

DE RBP	HR	HR.95L	HR.95H	*p*-Value
TDRD6	0.146237	0.031935	0.669646	**0.013267**
POP1	0.547387	0.32844	0.912291	**0.020767**
TDRD7	0.369575	0.198223	0.689049	**0.001738**
LUZP4	9.613842	3.401484	27.17225	**1.96E-05**
PPARGC1B	0.369954	0.164463	0.832203	**0.016215**
PPARGC1A	0.465469	0.28667	0.755786	**0.001987**
PABPC3	0.465077	0.247277	0.874714	**0.017535**
LRRFIP2	0.327354	0.128233	0.83567	**0.019523**
ZC3H12C	0.578625	0.367349	0.911415	**0.01827**
RBM47	0.549608	0.307602	0.982011	**0.043253**
CELF4	27.334	6.51501	114.6809	**6.14E-06**
PNLDC1	1.566855	1.103357	2.225058	**0.012086**
AFF3	4.557023	1.086579	19.11179	**0.038127**

Bold values significantly changed ($p < 0.05$).

For GO enrichment analysis, the BP of DE RBPs is mainly enriched in ncRNA metabolic process, RNA phosphodiester bond hydrolysis, ncRNA processing, nucleic acid phosphodiester bond hydrolysis, RNA localization, ribosome biogenesis, and so on. MicroRNAs, long non-coding RNAs, and small interfering RNA all belong to ncRNA. In recent years, it has become increasingly apparent that ncRNAs play a vital role in human cancer (Esquela-Kerscher and Slack, 2006; Hammond, 2007; Croce, 2009; Gibb et al., 2011). The hyperactivation of ribosome biogenesis, which can be caused by oncogenes or the loss of tumor suppressor genes, plays a vital role in cancer initiation and progression (Orsolic et al., 2016; Truitt and Ruggero, 2017). The upregulation of ribosome biogenesis during G1/S arrest can promote epithelial-to-mesenchymal transition, which is associated with tumor development and metastasis (Prakash et al., 2019). Drugs inhibiting ribosome biogenesis may offer an effective treatment for cancer (Bruno et al., 2017). For KEGG pathway enrichment, DE RBPs are mainly involved in mRNA surveillance pathway, ribosome biogenesis in eukaryotes, RNA transport, and RNA degradation. The mRNA surveillance pathway is a quality control mechanism that detects and degrades abnormal mRNAs (Moore, 2005). Non–sense-mediated mRNA decay (NMD) is one of the most common mRNA surveillance, which is involved in the detection and decay of mRNAs containing premature termination codons (Hentze and Kulozik, 1999). Inhibition of the oncogenic activity of NMD,

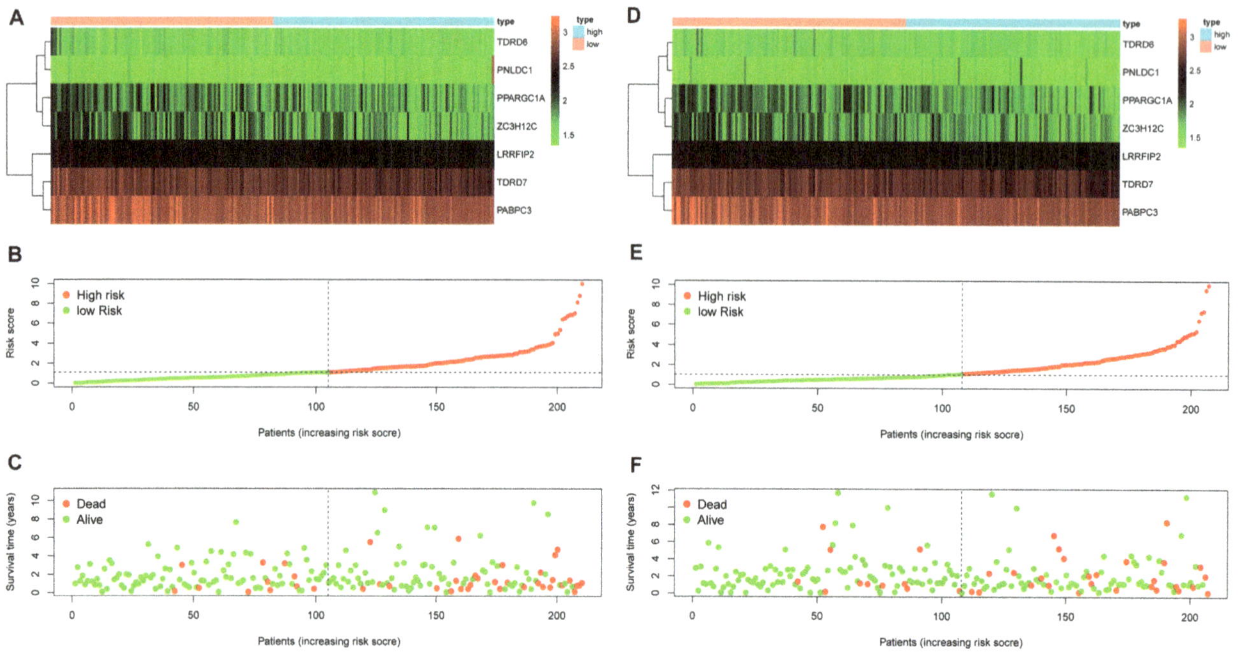

FIGURE 4 | Construction of an RBP-related risk signature and validation of the prognostic value in the testing set. **(A)** Heatmap of the seven-RBP expression profiles in the high- and low-risk groups for the training set. **(B)** The seven RBPs-based risk score distribution in the training set. **(C)** Distribution of the risk score based on the seven-RBP signature for patient survival status in the training set. **(D)** Heatmap of the seven-RBP expression profiles in the high- and low-risk groups for the testing set. **(E)** The seven RBPs-based risk score distribution in the testing set. **(F)** Distribution of the risk score based on the seven-RBP signature for patient survival status in the testing set.

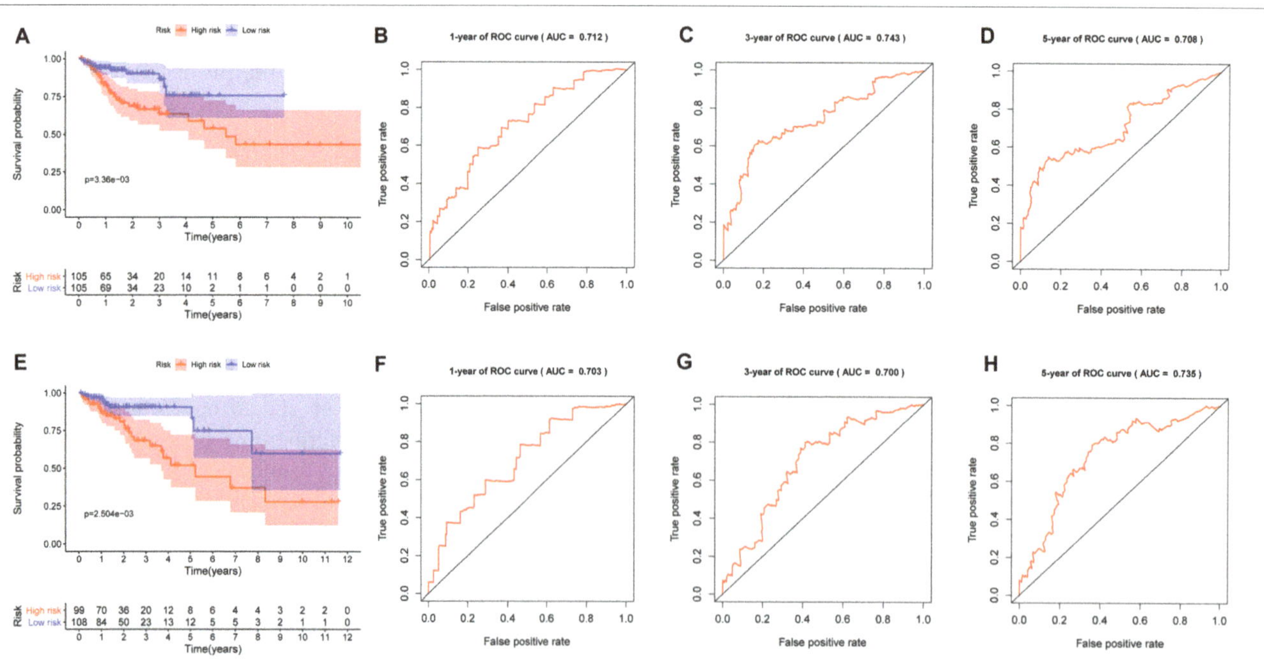

FIGURE 5 | Kaplan–Meier analysis and receiver operating characteristic (ROC) curve analysis in the training set and the testing set. **(A)** Kaplan–Meier analysis of the overall survival of patients in the high- and low-risk groups in the training set based on the RBP-related risk signature. **(B)** ROC curve for 1 year in the training set. **(C)** ROC curve for 3 years in the training set. **(D)** ROC curve for 5 years in the training set. **(E)** Kaplan–Meier analysis of the overall survival of patients in the high- and low-risk groups in the testing set based on the RBP-related risk signature. **(F)** ROC curve for 1 year in the testing set. **(G)** ROC curve for 3 years in the testing set. **(H)** ROC curve for 5 years in the testing set.

TABLE 2 | Univariate and multivariate Cox proportional hazards regression analysis of the RBP-related signature and clinical factors with overall survival in the training set.

Variables	Univariate analysis			Multivariate analysis		
	HR	95% CI	*p*-Value	HR	95% CI	*p*-Value
Gender	1.315	0.701–2.466	0.394	1.050	0.537–2.053	0.887
Age	1.034	1.006–1.063	**0.016**	1.038	1.010–1.067	**0.007**
Stage	2.422	1.656–3.541	**<0.001**	2.486	1.659–3.723	**<0.001**
Risk score	1.332	1.211–1.465	**<0.001**	1.252	1.136–1.380	**<0.001**

Bold values significantly changed ($p < 0.05$).

producing several encoded mutant proteins with deleterious activity, may be an effective strategy for the personalized treatment of microsatellite instability CRC (Bokhari et al., 2018). Tumor suppressor genes are prone to NMD-induced nonsense mutations, which were reported in a series of tumors, including stomach cancer, ovarian cancer, ovarian cancer, breast cancer, and kidney cancer (Popp and Maquat, 2018). RBPs are crucial components in RNA metabolism, resulting in highly organized subcellular localization, mRNA translation, and RNA degradation and then exert regulatory effects on cancer progression (Saunus et al., 2008; Shen and Pili, 2008). These results suggest that DE RBPs may be involved in CRC progression by regulating multiple BPs, such as NRA metabolism, RNA processing, ribosome biogenesis, and mRNA surveillance.

To further explore the potential functions of DE RBP in CRC, PPI network was constructed, and the critical module was screened. Some RBPs among the critical module have been reported to be involved in cancer progression. RRS1, a nuclear protein involved in ribosome biogenesis, has been reported to regulate cancer progression in hepatocellular carcinomas (HCCs) and breast cancer. RRS1 plays a critical role in cell proliferation, colony formation, cell apoptosis, and cell cycle distribution in human HCC cells (Wang et al., 2017). In breast cancer, both the copy number and the mRNA expression of RRS1 increased in cancer tissues compared with normal tissues, and RRS1 overexpression was significantly correlated with lymph node metastasis and poor survival (Song et al., 2018). RRP12 was crucial for the survival of osteosarcoma cell line U2OS during cytotoxic stress via the repression of p53 stability, suggesting that target RRP12 may enhance the chemotherapeutic effect in cancers (Choi et al., 2016). Although some of the RBPs among the crucial modules have been linked to cancer development or resistance to cytotoxic stress, their mRNA targets and mechanism of action are still unclear. In-depth functional research on the RBPs among the critical modules will provide a new way to explore the pathogenesis of CRC, as well as the drug-sensitive targets for CRC treatment. Genes associated with prognosis usually get more attention. In the present study, 13 prognostic DE RBPs were identified by univariate Cox proportional hazards regression analysis (**Table 1**). Some of the identified prognostic DE RBPs have been reported associated with tumor progression, such as RBM47, LUZP4, AFF3, PPARGC1A, PPARGC1B, PABPC3, and PNLDC1. RBM47 has been identified as a suppressor of breast cancer progression and metastasis, and patients with a low level of RBM47 tended to have a poor clinical outcome (Vanharanta et al., 2014), which suppresses the metastasis

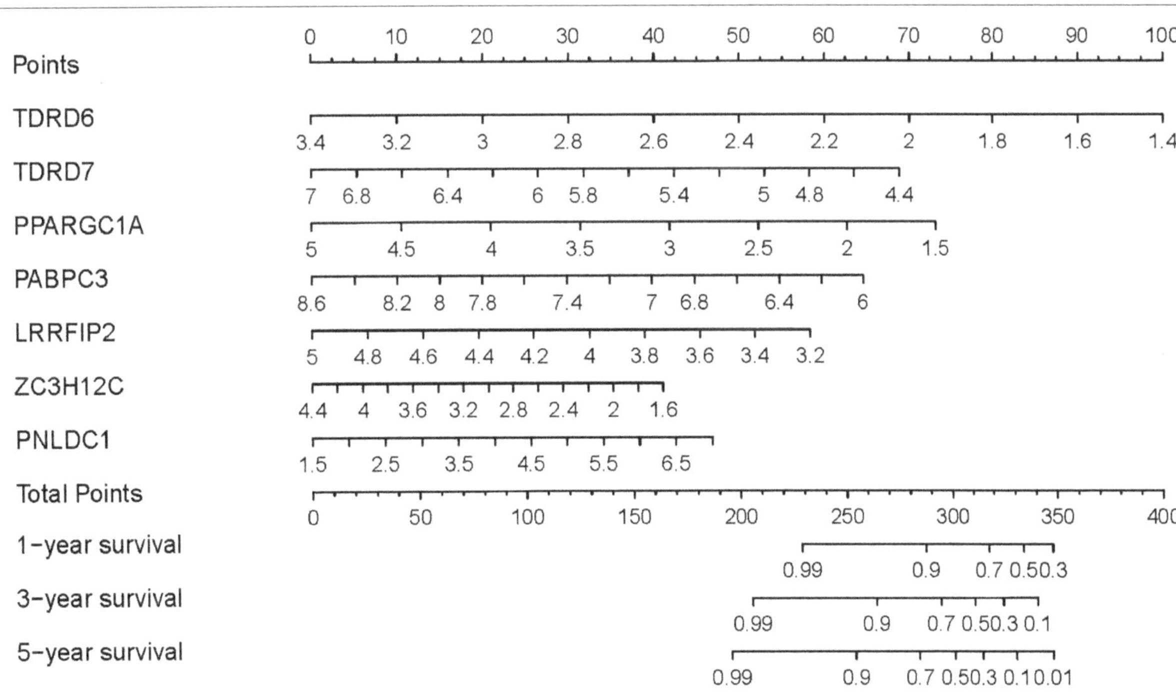

FIGURE 6 | Prognostic nomogram based on the RBP-related signature for prediction of 1-, 3-, and 5-year survival rates.

of breast cancer by stabilizing transcripts of Dickkopf Wnt signaling pathway inhibitor (Vanharanta et al., 2014). Reduced levels of RBM47 have also been observed in non–small cell lung cancer (NSCLC) patients, which correspond to a poorer prognosis and more advanced disease (Shen et al., 2020). RBM47 disrupted NSCLC progression through stabilizing AXIN1 mRNA and consequently suppressing Wnt/β-catenin signaling (Shen et al., 2020). Other mechanisms of RBM47-mediated tumor inhibition in lung cancer have also been reported, RBM47 plays a tumor-suppressive role in lung cancer through inhibiting Nrf2 activity (Sakurai et al., 2016). Downregulation of RBM47 in CRC may promote epithelial–mesenchymal transition and metastasis (Rokavec et al., 2017). RBM47 positively regulates the expression of p53 at the transcriptional level and controls the expression of p21 indirectly through regulation of the p53 promoter activity (Radine et al., 2020). Our analysis also showed RBM47 was downregulated in CRC tissues ($\log_2$FC = -1.59, adjusted p = 3.92 × 10^{-21}; **Supplementary Table 1**), and low level of RBM47 corresponding to a worse prognosis (HR = 0.549608, p = 0.043253; **Table 1**). LUZP4, also called CT-8 or HOM-TES-85, is an mRNA export adaptor required for melanoma proliferation (Viphakone et al., 2015). LUZP4 is upregulated in a range of cancers, including lung cancer, ovarian cancer, and glioma (Türeci et al., 2002). Consistent with these results, the expression of LUZP4 in CRC was also significantly higher than that in normal tissues ($\log_2$FC = 3.28, adjusted p = 5.60 × 10^{-13}; **Supplementary Table 1**). Univariate Cox proportional hazards regression analysis suggested an increased risk for CRC patients while the LUZP4 level was high (HR = 9.613842, p = 0.001738; **Table 1**). AFF3 is a new target of Wnt/β-catenin pathway involved in adrenocortical cancer, acting on transcription and RNA splicing (Lefèvre et al., 2015). Overexpression of AFF3 in breast cancer was associated with tamoxifen resistance and worse OS (Shi et al., 2018). However, downregulation of AFF3 was observed in CRC tissues ($\log_2$FC = −2.92, adjusted p = 2.54 × 10^{-22}; **Supplementary Table 1**). AFF3 may have different roles in cancers. PPARGC1A is upregulated and facilitates lung cancer metastasis (Li et al., 2017). Genetic variants in PPARGC1A and PPARGC1B have been reported in breast tumors and were associated with familial breast cancer susceptibility (Wirtenberger et al., 2006). PABPC3 has been reported to be a breast cancer candidate gene that may be associated with breast cancer (Kim et al., 2017). PNLDC1 mRNA was altered in several tumor types by analyzing more than 6,000 adult and pediatric tumors (Saghafinia et al., 2018). Although these prognostic DE RBPs were documented to be involved in tumor development, the functions and mechanisms of the remaining DE RBPs other than RBM47 have not been fully elucidated. Some identified prognostic DE RBPs have not been associated with cancers, such as CELF4, POP1, TDRD6, TDRD7, LRRFIP2, and ZC3H12C. Even so, LRRFIP2 was identified as a component of the Wnt signaling pathway that mediates or modulates Wnt signaling through interactions with Dvl (Liu et al., 2005). LRRFIP2 may be involved in cancer progression through regulating Wnt signaling pathway.

The functions of some identified prognostic DE RBPs have not been reported. We constructed a regulatory network based on differentially expressed TFs and prognostic DE RBPs by calculating the Pearson correlation, which would contribute to a systematic understanding of prognostic DE RBPs in CRC. As shown in **Figure 3E**, three RBPs (TDRD7, ZC3H12C, and RBM47) may be regulated by KLF4. KLF4 is an evolutionally conserved zinc finger–containing transcription factor that regulates diverse cellular processes such as cell growth, proliferation, and differentiation (Bieker, 2001; Ghaleb et al., 2005). KLF4 displays a tumor-suppressive function, which is downregulated in CRC (Shie et al., 2000b). KLF4 overexpression in CRC cell line reduced transformation, migration, invasion, and tumorigenicity (Dang et al., 2003). Constitutive expression of KLF4 led to the inhibition of DNA synthesis and regulates the cell cycle by blocking G1/S progression (Chen et al., 2001). KLF4 suppresses CRC proliferation through upregulating $p21^{WAF1/Cip1}$ and downregulating cyclin D1 (Shie et al., 2000a). In the present study, KLF4 expression is downregulated in CRC tissues ($\log_2$FC = −2.52, adjusted p = 2.13 × 10^{-22}; **Supplementary Table 2**), which is consistent with previous report. The results suggest that KLF4 may exert a suppression effect through other mechanisms, such as regulating TDRD7, ZC3H12C, and RBM47. We also demonstrated that KAT2B, a histone acetyltransferase to promote transcriptional activation (Ogryzko et al., 1996), may regulate three RBPs (TDRD6, ZC3H12C, and RBM47). Moreover, KAT2B acetylates non-histone proteins (Choudhary et al., 2009; Downey and Baetz, 2016), which has been reported to be a critical regulator of p53-dependent p21 expression in response to multiple p53-activating stresses (Love et al., 2012). KAT2B also plays a role in the development and progression of cancer (Bondy-Chorney et al., 2019). Thus, KAT2B may be involved in CRC progression through regulating TDRD6, ZC3H12C, and RBM47. Although the functions of TDRD6, TDRD7, and POP1 are not clear, the regulatory network will guide further study of the functions of these RBPs. TDRD6 may be regulated by NR3C1, OGT, MAF, CBFB, POLR3G, and KATZB (**Figure 3E**). TDRD7 may be regulated by KLF4 and CHD7 (**Figure 3E**). POP1 may be regulated by CHD7, E2F1, MYC, BRCA1, and PRKDC (**Figure 3E**). Besides, multiple Cox regression analysis was performed to construct a risk signature for predicting survival of CRC patients, including TDRD6, TDRD7, PPARGC1A, PABPC6, LRRFIP2, ZC3H12C, and PNLDC1. Kaplan–Meier survival analysis and ROC analysis were performed in the training set and testing set to evaluate the predictive efficiency of the RBP-related prognostic signature. Results showed that the signature can predict the survival status of patients in TCGA dataset with high accuracy. Subsequently, a nomogram was built based on the RBP-related prognostic signature to predict 1-, 3-, and 5-year OS more intuitively. In summary, we investigated the expression, prognostic values, and potential functions of DE RBPs through comprehensive bioinformatics analysis. Thirteen prognostic RBPs were identified. An RBP-related prognostic model was developed that could act as an independent prognostic signature for CRC. These findings would provide new therapeutic targets and prognostic markers for CRC.

ETHICS STATEMENT

This study was approved by the Ethical Committee of Central South University (China).

AUTHOR CONTRIBUTIONS

SX and KF conceived the concept, instructed data analysis, and revised the manuscript. YW conducted most of the data analysis prepared figures and table, and wrote manuscript draft. YC helped with some analysis and interpretation of data. KF reviewed the manuscript with input from all authors. All authors contributed to the article and approved the submitted version.

ACKNOWLEDGMENTS

The authors thank all patients, investigators, and institutions involved in these studies, especially the Cancer Genome Atlas Program.

REFERENCES

Abdelmohsen, K., Pullmann, R. Jr., Lal, A., Kim, H. H., Galban, S., et al. (2007). Phosphorylation of HuR by Chk2 regulates SIRT1 expression. *Mol. Cell* 25, 543–557. doi: 10.1016/j.molcel.2007.01.011

Aghili, M., Izadi, S., Madani, H., and Mortazavi, H. (2010). Clinical and pathological evaluation of patients with early and late recurrence of colorectal cancer. *Asia Pac. J. Clin. Oncol.* 6, 35–41. doi: 10.1111/j.1743-7563.2010.01275.x

Angenete, E. (2019). The importance of surgery in colorectal cancer treatment. *Lancet Oncol.* 20, 6–7. doi: 10.1016/S1470-2045(18)30679-X

Arnold, M., Sierra, M. S., Laversanne, M., Soerjomataram, I., Jemal, A., and Bray, F. (2017). Global patterns and trends in colorectal cancer incidence and mortality. 66, 683–691. doi: 10.1136/gutjnl-2015-310912

Bieker, J. J. (2001). Krüppel-like factors: three fingers in many pies. *J. Biol. Chem.* 276, 34355–34358. doi: 10.1074/jbc.R100043200

Bielli, P., Busa, R., Paronetto, M. P., and Sette, C. (2011). The RNA-binding protein Sam68 is a multifunctional player in human cancer. *Endocr. Relat. Cancer* 18, R91–R102. doi: 10.1530/ERC-11-0041

Bokhari, A., Jonchere, V., Lagrange, A., Bertrand, R., Svrcek, M., and Marisa, L. (2018). Targeting nonsense-mediated mRNA decay in colorectal cancers with microsatellite instability. *Oncogenesis* 7:70. doi: 10.1038/s41389-018-0079-x

Bondy-Chorney, E., Denoncourt, A., Sai, Y., and Downey, M. (2019). Nonhistone targets of KAT2A and KAT2B implicated in cancer biology (1). *Biochem. Cell Biol.* 97, 30–45. doi: 10.1139/bcb-2017-0297

Bray, F., Ferlay, J., Soerjomataram, I., Siegel, R. L., Torre, L. A., and Jemal, A. (2018). Global cancer statistics 2018: GLOBOCAN estimates of incidence and mortality worldwide for 36 cancers in 185 countries. *CA Cancer J. Clin.* 68, 394–424. doi: 10.3322/caac.21492

Bruno, P. M., Liu, Y., Park, G. Y., Murai, J., Koch, C. E., Eisen, T. J., et al. (2017). A subset of platinum-containing chemotherapeutic agents kills cells by inducing ribosome biogenesis stress. *Nat. Med.* 23, 461–471. doi: 10.1038/nm.4291

Chen, X., Johns, D. C., Geiman, D. E., Marban, E., Dang, D. T., Hamlin, G., et al. (2001). Krüppel-like factor 4 (gut-enriched Krüppel-like factor) inhibits cell proliferation by blocking G1/S progression of the cell cycle. *J. Biol. Chem.* 276, 30423–30428. doi: 10.1074/jbc.M101194200

Cho, S. J., Zhang, J., and Chen, X. (2010). RNPC1 modulates the RNA-binding activity of, and cooperates with, HuR to regulate p21 mRNA stability. *Nucleic Acids Res.* 38, 2256–2267. doi: 10.1093/nar/gkp1229

Choi, Y. J., Lee, H. W., Lee, Y. S., Shim, da, M., and Seo, S. W. (2016). RRP12 is a crucial nucleolar protein that regulates p53 activity in osteosarcoma cells. *Tumour Biol.* 37, 4351–4358. doi: 10.1007/s13277-015-4062-2

Choudhary, C., Kumar, C., Gnad, F., Nielsen, M. L., Rehman, M., Walther, T. C., et al. (2009). Lysine acetylation targets protein complexes and co-regulates major cellular functions. *Science* 325, 834–840. doi: 10.1126/science.1175371

Croce, C. M. (2009). Causes and consequences of microRNA dysregulation in cancer. *Nat. Rev. Genet.* 10, 704–714. doi: 10.1038/nrg2634

Dang, D. T., Chen, X., Feng, J., Torbenson, M., Dang, L. H., and Yang, V. W. (2003). Overexpression of Krüppel-like factor 4 in the human colon cancer cell line RKO leads to reduced tumorigenecity. *Oncogene* 22, 3424–3430. doi: 10.1038/sj.onc.1206413

Denkert, C., Koch, I., von Keyserlingk, N., Noske, A., Niesporek, S., Dietel, M., et al. (2006). Expression of the ELAV-like protein HuR in human colon cancer: association with tumor stage and cyclooxygenase-2. *Mod. Pathol.* 19, 1261–1269. doi: 10.1038/modpathol.3800645

DeSantis, C. E., Lin, C. C., Mariotto, A. B., Siegel, R. L., Stein, K. D., Kramer, J. L., et al. (2014). Cancer treatment and survivorship statistics, 2014. *CA Cancer J. Clin.* 64, 252–271. doi: 10.3322/caac.21235

Dixon, D. A., Tolley, N. D., King, P. H., Nabors, L. B., McIntyre, T. M., Zimmerman, G. A., et al. (2001). Altered expression of the mRNA stability factor HuR promotes cyclooxygenase-2 expression in colon cancer cells. *J. Clin. Invest.* 108, 1657–1665. doi: 10.1172/JCI12973

Douaiher, J., Ravipati, A., Grams, B., Chowdhury, S., Alatise, O., and Are, C. (2017). Colorectal cancer-global burden, trends, and geographical variations. *J. Surg. Oncol.* 115, 619–630. doi: 10.1002/jso.24578

Downey, M., and Baetz, K. (2016). Building a KATalogue of acetyllysine targeting and function. *Brief. Funct. Genomics* 15, 109–118. doi: 10.1093/bfgp/elv045

Esquela-Kerscher, A., and Slack, F. J. (2006). Oncomirs - microRNAs with a role in cancer. *Nat. Rev. Cancer* 6, 259–269. doi: 10.1038/nrc1840

Fu, K., Sun, X., Xia, X., Hobbs, R. P., Guo, Y., Coulombe, P. A., et al. (2019). Sam68 is required for the growth and survival of nonmelanoma skin cancer. *Cancer Med.* 8, 6106–6113. doi: 10.1002/cam4.2513

Gerstberger, S., Hafner, M., and Tuschl, T. (2014). A census of human RNA-binding proteins. *Nat. Rev. Genet.* 15, 829–845. doi: 10.1038/nrg3813

Ghaleb, A. M., Nandan, M. O., Chanchevalap, S., Dalton, W. B., Hisamuddin, I. M., and Yang, V. W. (2005). Krüppel-like factors 4 and 5: the yin and yang regulators of cellular proliferation. *Cell Res.* 15, 92–96. doi: 10.1038/sj.cr.7290271

Gibb, E. A., Brown, C. J., and Lam, W. L. (2011). The functional role of long non-coding RNA in human carcinomas. *Mol. Cancer* 10:38. doi: 10.1186/1476-4598-10-38

Guo, X., and Hartley, R. S. (2006). HuR contributes to cyclin E1 deregulation in MCF-7 breast cancer cells. *Cancer Res.* 66, 7948–7956. doi: 10.1158/0008-5472.CAN-05-4362

Hammond, S. M. (2007). MicroRNAs as tumor suppressors. *Nat. Genet.* 39, 582–583. doi: 10.1038/ng0507-582

Hentze, M. W., and Kulozik, A. E. (1999). A perfect message: RNA surveillance and nonsense-mediated decay. *Cell* 96, 307–310. doi: 10.1016/s0092-8674(00)80542-5

Hsieh, A. C., and Ruggero, D. (2010). Targeting eukaryotic translation initiation factor 4E (eIF4E) in cancer. *Clin. Cancer Res.* 16, 4914–4920. doi: 10.1158/1078-0432.CCR-10-0433

Hudson, M. M., Ness, K. K., Gurney, J. G., Mulrooney, D. A., Chemaitilly, W., Krull, K. R., et al. (2013). Clinical ascertainment of health outcomes among adults treated for childhood cancer. *JAMA* 309, 2371–2381. doi: 10.1001/jama.2013.6296

Ishimaru, D., Ramalingam, S., Sengupta, T. K., Bandyopadhyay, S., Dellis, S., Tholanikunnel, B. G., et al. (2009). Regulation of Bcl-2 expression by HuR in HL60 leukemia cells and A431 carcinoma cells. *Mol. Cancer Res.* 7, 1354–1366. doi: 10.1158/1541-7786.MCR-08-0476

Kim, Y. C., Soliman, A. S., Cui, J., Ramadan, M., Hablas, A., Abouelhoda, M., et al. (2017). Unique features of germline variation in five egyptian familial breast cancer families revealed by exome sequencing. *PLoS One* 12:e0167581. doi: 10.1371/journal.pone.0167581

Kudinov, A. E., Karanicolas, J., Golemis, E. A., and Boumber, Y. (2017). Musashi RNA-binding proteins as cancer drivers and novel therapeutic targets. *Clin. Cancer Res.* 23, 2143–2153. doi: 10.1158/1078-0432.ccr-16-2728

Lal, A., Mazan-Mamczarz, K., Kawai, T., Yang, X., Martindale, J. L., and Gorospe, M. (2004). Concurrent versus individual binding of HuR and AUF1 to common labile target mRNAs. *Embo J.* 23, 3092–3102. doi: 10.1038/sj.emboj.7600305

Lefèvre, L., Omeiri, H., Drougat, L., Hantel, C., Giraud, M., Val, P., et al. (2015). Combined transcriptome studies identify AFF3 as a mediator of the oncogenic effects of β-catenin in adrenocortical carcinoma. *Oncogenesis* 4:e161. doi: 10.1038/oncsis.2015.20

Li, J. D., Feng, Q. C., Qi, Y., Cui, G., and Zhao, S. (2017). PPARGC1A is upregulated and facilitates lung cancer metastasis. *Exp. Cell Res.* 359, 356–360. doi: 10.1016/j.yexcr.2017.08.017

Liu, J., Bang, A. G., Kintner, C., Orth, A. P., Chanda, S. K., Ding, S., et al. (2005). Identification of the Wnt signaling activator leucine-rich repeat in Flightless interaction protein 2 by a genome-wide functional analysis. *Proc. Natl. Acad. Sci. U.S.A.* 102, 1927–1932. doi: 10.1073/pnas.0409472102

Lopez, de Silanes, I., Fan, J., Yang, X., Zonderman, A. B., Potapova, O., et al. (2003). Role of the RNA-binding protein HuR in colon carcinogenesis. *Oncogene* 22, 7146–7154. doi: 10.1038/sj.onc.1206862

Love, I. M., Sekaric, P., Shi, D., Grossman, S. R., and Androphy, E. J. (2012). The histone acetyltransferase PCAF regulates p21 transcription through stress-induced acetylation of histone H3. *Cell Cycle* 11, 2458–2466. doi: 10.4161/cc.20864

Lu, Z., Luo, R. Z., Peng, H., Rosen, D. G., Atkinson, E. N., Warneke, C., et al. (2006). Transcriptional and posttranscriptional down-regulation of the imprinted tumor suppressor gene ARHI (DRAS3) in ovarian cancer. *Clin. Cancer Res.* 12, 2404–2413. doi: 10.1158/1078-0432.CCR-05-1036

Mamane, Y., Petroulakis, E., Rong, L., Yoshida, K., Ler, L. W., and Sonenberg, N. (2004). eIF4E–from translation to transformation. *Oncogene* 23, 3172–3179. doi: 10.1038/sj.onc.1207549

Matter, N., Herrlich, P., and Konig, H. (2002). Signal-dependent regulation of splicing via phosphorylation of Sam68. *Nature* 420, 691–695. doi: 10.1038/nature01153

Mei, S., Meyer, C. A., Zheng, R., Qin, Q., Wu, Q., Jiang, P., et al. (2017). Cistrome cancer: a web resource for integrative gene regulation modeling in cancer. *Cancer Res.* 77, e19–e22. doi: 10.1158/0008-5472.CAN-17-0327

Moore, M. J. (2005). From birth to death: the complex lives of eukaryotic mRNAs. *Science* 309, 1514–1518. doi: 10.1126/science.1111443

Ogryzko, V. V., Schiltz, R. L., Russanova, V., Howard, B. H., and Nakatani, Y. (1996). The transcriptional coactivators p300 and CBP are histone acetyltransferases. *Cell* 87, 953–959. doi: 10.1016/s0092-8674(00)82001-2

Orsolic, I., Jurada, D., Pullen, N., Oren, M., Eliopoulos, A. G., and Volarevic, S. (2016). The relationship between the nucleolus and cancer: current evidence and emerging paradigms. *Semin. Cancer Biol.* 3, 36–50. doi: 10.1016/j.semcancer.2015.12.004

Paronetto, M. P., Achsel, T., Massiello, A., Chalfant, C. E., and Sette, C. (2007). The RNA-binding protein Sam68 modulates the alternative splicing of Bcl-x. *J. Cell Biol.* 176, 929–939. doi: 10.1083/jcb.200701005

Paronetto, M. P., Cappellari, M., Busa, R., Pedrotti, S., Vitali, R., Comstock, C., et al. (2010). Alternative splicing of the cyclin D1 proto-oncogene is regulated by the RNA-binding protein Sam68. *Cancer Res.* 70, 229–239. doi: 10.1158/0008-5472.CAN-09-2788

Popp, M. W., and Maquat, L. E. (2018). Nonsense-mediated mRNA Decay and Cancer. *Curr. Opin. Genet. Dev.* 48, 44–50. doi: 10.1016/j.gde.2017.10.007

Prakash, V., Carson, B. B., Feenstra, J. M., Dass, R. A., Sekyrova, P., Hoshino, A., et al. (2019). Ribosome biogenesis during cell cycle arrest fuels EMT in development and disease. *Nat. Commun.* 10:2110. doi: 10.1038/s41467-019-10100-8

Radine, C., Peters, D., Reese, A., Neuwahl, J., Budach, W., Jänicke, R. U., et al. (2020). The RNA-binding protein RBM47 is a novel regulator of cell fate decisions by transcriptionally controlling the p53-p21-axis. *Cell Death Differ.* 27, 1274–1285. doi: 10.1038/s41418-019-0414-6

Ramalingam, S., Natarajan, G., Schafer, C., Subramaniam, D., May, R., Ramachandran, I., et al. (2008). Novel intestinal splice variants of RNA-binding protein CUGBP2: isoform-specific effects on mitotic catastrophe. *Am. J. Physiol. Gastrointest. Liver Physiol.* 294, G971–G981. doi: 10.1152/ajpgi.00540.2007

Rokavec, M., Kaller, M., Horst, D., and Hermeking, H. (2017). Pan-cancer EMT-signature identifies RBM47 down-regulation during colorectal cancer progression. *Sci. Rep.* 7:4687. doi: 10.1038/s41598-017-04234-2

Saghafinia, S., Mina, M., Riggi, N., Hanahan, D., and Ciriello, G. (2018). Pan-cancer landscape of aberrant DNA methylation across human tumors. *Cell Rep.* 25, 1066.e8–1080.e8. doi: 10.1016/j.celrep.2018.09.082

Sakurai, T., Isogaya, K., Sakai, S., Morikawa, M., Morishita, Y., Ehata, S., et al. (2016). RNA-binding motif protein 47 inhibits Nrf2 activity to suppress tumor growth in lung adenocarcinoma. *Oncogene* 35, 5000–5009. doi: 10.1038/onc.2016.35

Saunus, J. M., French, J. D., Edwards, S. L., Beveridge, D. J., Hatchell, E. C., Wagner, S. A., et al. (2008). Posttranscriptional regulation of the breast cancer susceptibility gene BRCA1 by the RNA binding protein HuR. *Cancer Res.* 68, 9469–9478. doi: 10.1158/0008-5472.CAN-08-1159

Shen, D. J., Jiang, Y. H., Li, J. Q., Xu, L. W., and Tao, K. Y. (2020). The RNA-binding protein RBM47 inhibits non-small cell lung carcinoma metastasis through modulation of AXIN1 mRNA stability and Wnt/β-catentin signaling. *Surg. Oncol.* 34, 31–39. doi: 10.1016/j.suronc.2020.02.011

Shen, L., and Pili, R. (2008). Posttranscription regulation of prostate cancer growth. *Cancer J.* 14, 46–53. doi: 10.1097/PPO.0b013e318162108a

Shi, Y., Zhao, Y., Zhang, Y., AiErken, N., Shao, N., Ye, R., et al. (2018). AFF3 upregulation mediates tamoxifen resistance in breast cancers. *J. Exp. Clin. Cancer Res.* 37:254. doi: 10.1186/s13046-018-0928-7

Shie, J. L., Chen, Z. Y., Fu, M., Pestell, R. G., and Tseng, C. C. (2000a). Gut-enriched Krüppel-like factor represses cyclin D1 promoter activity through Sp1 motif. *Nucleic Acids Res.* 28, 2969–2976. doi: 10.1093/nar/28.15.2969

Shie, J. L., Chen, Z. Y., O'Brien, M. J., Pestell, R. G., Lee, M. E., and Tseng, C. C. (2000b). Role of gut-enriched Krüppel-like factor in colonic cell growth and differentiation. *Am. J. Physiol. Gastrointest. Liver Physiol.* 279, G806–G814. doi: 10.1152/ajpgi.2000.279.4.G806

Silvera, D., Formenti, S. C., and Schneider, R. J. (2010). Translational control in cancer. *Nat. Rev. Cancer* 10, 254–266. doi: 10.1038/nrc2824

Song, J., Ma, Z., Hua, Y., Xu, J., Li, N., Ju, C., et al. (2018). Functional role of RRS1 in breast cancer cell proliferation. *J. Cell. Mol. Med.* 22, 6304–6313. doi: 10.1111/jcmm.13922

Subbaramaiah, K., Marmo, T. P., Dixon, D. A., and Dannenberg, A. J. (2003). Regulation of cyclooxgenase-2 mRNA stability by taxanes: evidence for involvement of p38, MAPKAPK-2, and HuR. *J. Biol. Chem.* 278, 37637–37647. doi: 10.1074/jbc.M301481200

Sureban, S. M., Ramalingam, S., Natarajan, G., May, R., Subramaniam, D., Bishnupuri, K. S., et al. (2008). Translation regulatory factor RBM3 is a proto-oncogene that prevents mitotic catastrophe. *Oncogene* 27, 4544–4556. doi: 10.1038/onc.2008.97

Topisirovic, I., Svitkin, Y. V., Sonenberg, N., and Shatkin, A. J. (2011). Cap and cap-binding proteins in the control of gene expression. *Wiley Interdiscip. Rev. RNA* 2, 277–298. doi: 10.1002/wrna.52

Truitt, M. L., and Ruggero, D. (2017). New frontiers in translational control of the cancer genome. *Nat. Rev. Cancer* 17:332. doi: 10.1038/nrc.2017.30

Türeci, O., Sahin, U., Koslowski, M., Buss, B., Bell, C., Ballweber, P., et al. (2002). A novel tumour associated leucine zipper protein targeting to sites of gene transcription and splicing. *Oncogene* 21, 3879–3888. doi: 10.1038/sj.onc.1205481

Vanharanta, S., Marney, C. B., Shu, W., Valiente, M., Zou, Y., Mele, A., et al. (2014). Loss of the multifunctional RNA-binding protein RBM47 as a source of selectable metastatic traits in breast cancer. *eLife* 3:e02734. doi: 10.7554/eLife.02734

Viphakone, N., Cumberbatch, M. G., Livingstone, M. J., Heath, P. R., Dickman, M. J., Catto, J. W., et al. (2015). Luzp4 defines a new mRNA export pathway in cancer cells. *Nucleic Acids Res.* 43, 2353–2366. doi: 10.1093/nar/gkv070

Wang, J., Li, Z., Zuo, C., Xie, Q., Li, H., Jia, J., et al. (2017). Knockdown of RRS1 by lentiviral-mediated RNAi promotes apoptosis and suppresses proliferation of human hepatocellular carcinoma cells. *Oncol. Rep.* 38, 2166–2172. doi: 10.3892/or.2017.5906

Wang, W., Caldwell, M. C., Lin, S., Furneaux, H., and Gorospe, M. (2000). HuR regulates cyclin A and cyclin B1 mRNA stability during cell proliferation. *Embo J.* 19, 2340–2350. doi: 10.1093/emboj/19.10.2340

Wirtenberger, M., Tchatchou, S., Hemminki, K., Schmutzhard, J., Sutter, C., Schmutzler, R. K., et al. (2006). Associations of genetic variants in the estrogen receptor coactivators PPARGC1A, PPARGC1B and EP300 with familial breast cancer. *Carcinogenesis* 27, 2201–2208. doi: 10.1093/carcin/bgl067

Wurth, L. (2012). Versatility of RNA-binding proteins in cancer. *Comp. Funct. Genomics* 2012:178525. doi: 10.1155/2012/178525

Young, L. E., Sanduja, S., Bemis-Standoli, K., Pena, E. A., Price, R. L., and Dixon, D. A. (2009). The mRNA binding proteins HuR and tristetraprolin regulate cyclooxygenase 2 expression during colon carcinogenesis. *Gastroenterology* 136, 1669–1679. doi: 10.1053/j.gastro.2009.01.010

9

Down Regulation of SIRT2 Reduced ASS Induced NSCLC Apoptosis Through the Release of Autophagy Components *via* Exosomes

Lei Wang[1†], Pei Xu[1†], Xiao Xie[1], Fengqing Hu[1], Lianyong Jiang[1], Rui Hu[1], Fangbao Ding[1], Haibo Xiao[1] and Huijun Zhang[2*]*

[1] Department of Cardiothoracic Surgery, Xinhua Hospital Affiliated to Shanghai Jiao Tong University School of Medicine, Shanghai, China, [2] Department of Cardiothoracic Surgery, Huashan Hospital of Fudan University, Shanghai, China

***Correspondence:**
Haibo Xiao
xiaohaibo@xinhuamed.com.cn
Huijun Zhang
zhanghuijunhp@163.com

† These authors have contributed equally to this work

Metastasis of cancer is the main cause of death in many types of cancer. Acute shear stress (ASS) is an important part of tumor micro-environment, it plays a crucial role in tumor invasion and spread. However, less is known about the role of ASS in tumorigenesis and metastasis of NSCLC. In this study, NSCLC cells were exposed to ASS (10 dyn/cm^2) to explore the effect of ASS in regulation of autophagy and exosome mediated cell survival. Finally, the influence of SIRT2 on NSCLC cell metastasis was verified *in vivo*. Our data demonstrates that ASS promotes exosome and autophagy components releasing in a time dependent manner, inhibition of exosome release exacerbates ASS induced NSCLC cell apoptosis. Furthermore, we identified that this function was regulated by sirtuin 2 (SIRT2). And, RNA immunoprecipitation (RIP) assay suggested SIRT2 directly bound to the 3′UTR of transcription factor EB (TFEB) and facilitated its mRNA stability. TFEB is a key transcription factor involved in the regulation of many lysosome related genes and plays a critical role in the fusion of autophagosome and lysosome. Altogether, this data revealed that SIRT2 is a mechanical sensitive protein, and it regulates ASS induced cell apoptosis by modulating the release of exosomes and autophagy components, which provides a promising strategy for the treatment of NSCLCs.

Keywords: acute shear stress, autophagy, exosome, SIRT2, TFEB, NSCLC, metastasis

INTRODUCTION

Lung cancer stands as the leading cause of cancer-related deaths world-wide (Siegel et al., 2019). Non-small lung cancer (NSCLC) accounts for 87% of all lung cancers, with about 75% of cases diagnosed at a later stage leading to poor prognosis (Cancer Genome Atlas Research Network, 2014). Radiation and chemotherapy are valid available treatment strategies, but these approaches cannot improve the poor 5 years survival

Abbreviations: ASS, acute shear stress; Exo, exosome; NSCLC, non-small lung cancer; SIRT2, sirtuin 2; TFEB, transcription factor EB.

rate of these patients, which ranges from 5 to 31% (Herbst et al., 2018). Metastasis is the key contributor to tumorigenesis in many cancers, including NSCLC (Gassmann et al., 2004; Gupta and Massague, 2006). Metastasis is defined as the migration of cancer cells from its primary site of origin to progressively invade and colonize the neighboring tissues (Steeg, 2016). Cancerous cells migrate either by entering the blood stream directly or through the lymphatic system (Chaffer and Weinberg, 2011). Several proangiogenic factors secreted by the tumor cells aid in the formation and connection with the capillary system which allows intravasation and circulation of these cells in the blood stream (Folkman, 1986; Sitohy et al., 2012). Once in the blood stream, cells encounter multiple stresses due to flow of blood, lymph or other tissue fluids (Tarbell et al., 2014). Shear stress (SS) is a key factor that has previously been associated with organogenesis and maintenance (Rutkowski and Swartz, 2007). In spite of the negative effects of SS, studies have indicated low-shear stress enhances migration, proliferation, and differentiation of circulating tumor cells (CTCs) (Sebastian et al., 2020). Studies have attempted to elucidate how CTCs can survive in such harsh conditions, and it has been suggested that they undergo multiple morphological and molecular changes to adapt and survive under mechanically stressful conditions (Cognart et al., 2020). Interestingly, it has been reported that SS can induce autophagy in different cancer cell types (Fleury et al., 2006; Das et al., 2018). Autophagy has varying roles in multiple cell types, critically cancer cells depend on autophagy to maintain a minimal metabolic requirement and survive under harsh conditions through self-degradation of organelles and protein aggregates (Mowers et al., 2018). In an *in vitro* study by Lien et al. (2013) found that SS (0.5, 6, and 12 dyn/cm^2) increased autophagy which was evident from the acidic vesicular organelle formation, microtubule-associated protein light chain 3 (LC3B) transformation and p62/SQSTM1 degradation in HCC cells. In addition, to protect cells against these autophagic components, cancer cells under acute SS have an alternative protection mechanism through the release of autophagic components through extracellular vesicle (EV) release (Reck et al., 2014). Recently, a study has indicated such release of exosomes are regulated by a member of the sirtuin family, SIRT1. A study by Latifkar et al. (2019), indicated that SIRT1 down-regulation altered the secretome and increased the exosome release in breast cancer cell lines. This study further indicated that SIRT1 reduced the tumorigenesis of breast cancer by altering the lysosomal activity. However, sirtuin's role in NSCLC is still not clear.

The aim of this study is to assess the effect of ASS in NSCLC and to elucidate the role of sirtuins in stress response and survival of cancer cells. Initially, we identified that NSCLCs exposed to ASS (10 dyn/cm^2) clearly shed increased level of exosomes and autophagic components. Interestingly, ASS exposed NSCLCs expressed less SIRT2 and the expression of SIRT1 remained unaffected. Further, it was evident that SIRT2 regulated autophagosome formation, apoptosis, and metastasis by binding and regulating the expression of a key player in the lysosomal biogenesis and autophagy, transcription factor EB (TFEB). Thus, this study aims to elucidate the role SIRT2 and TFEB in NSCLC tumorigenesis and shed light into ASS associated mechanisms, thus aiding in identification of potential target for treatment strategies against NSCLC.

MATERIALS AND METHODS

Clinical Samples

We collected forty pairs of NSCLC tissue samples and healthy lung tissues from the Xin Hua Hospital Affiliated to Shanghai Jiao Tong University School of Medicine. Based on the TNM criteria for NSCLC, we grouped and selected samples for this study. Patients who previously received chemotherapy or radiotherapy were eliminated from the study. All subjects provided written informed consents. This study was approved by the Institutional Review Board of Xin Hua Hospital Affiliated to Shanghai Jiao Tong University School of Medicine and is in compliance with the principles laid down in the Declaration of Helsinki.

Cell Culture

NSCLC cells A549 and H1299 were purchased from American Type Culture Collection (ATCC, Manassas, VI, United States). The cells were cultured in Dulbecco's Eagle Medium (DMEM) with 10% fetal bovine serum (FBS) and 1% penicillin/streptomycin (Invitrogen, Carlsbad, CA) in 37°C and 5% CO_2.

Plasmids and Lentivirus

The pcDNA3.1 vector (Invitrogen, United States) with a full-length cDNA sequence of either SIRT2 or TFEB were used to overexpress SIRT2 or TFEB, respectively. Empty pcDNA3.1 vector and scrambled shRNA or siRNA were used as negative controls. Further, Lipofectamine^{TM} 2000 (Invitrogen, United States) was used to transfect H1299 or A549 cells with the above-mentioned plasmids. Post 48 h of transfection, cells were collected for further use.

Ad-mCherry-GFP-LC3B Transfection

A549 and H1299 cells were seeded onto 24 well plate and cultured in DMEM complete medium till 50% confluence. Further, the complete medium was replaced with viral solution with MOI of 10. Post 24 h, the medium was removed and the cells were washed with PBS and DMEM medium. Further, the cells were continued to be cultured in DMEM medium till use.

Quantitative Real-Time PCR (RT-qPCR)

Total RNA was isolated using the Trizol reagent (Gibco, Carlsbad, CA, United States). Using primescript RT reagent kit, the RNA was reverse transcribed to cDNA, and SYBR-Green qPCR (Invitrogen) was performed using an Applied Biosystems system (Foster City, CA, United States). The primers used for these experiments were SIRT2 Forward: 5′-TGCGGAACT TATTCTCCCAGA-3′; Reverse: 5′-CCAGCCGATACTCGT TCAGC-3′, TFEB Forward: 5′-ACCTGTCCGAGACCTATGGG-3′; Reverse: 5′-CGTCCAGACGCATAATGTTGTC-3′, GAPDH Forward: 5′-GGAGCGAGATCCCTCCAAAAT-3′; Reverse: 5′-GGCTGTTGTCATACTTCTCATGG-3′.The relative abundance of mRNA was normalized to GAPDH and the $2^{-\Delta\Delta CT}$ method was used to analyze expression levels.

Western Blotting Analysis

Total protein was isolated from tissue samples using RIPA buffer (Sigma-Aldrich). After quantification using Bradford assay(Thermo Fisher Scientific, Waltham, United States), 20 μg of total protein were pretreated with loading buffer and loaded in 5–20% SDS-polyacrylamide gel (Bio-Rad Laboratories, Hercules, United States). After migration, the samples were transferred into a nitrocellulose membrane (GE Healthcare Life Science). Subsequently, the membranes were blocked using 5% skim milk in PBS buffer for 1 h. Further, the membranes were incubated overnight at 4°C in the primary antibody diluted in 1% skim milk in PBS buffer. The primary antibodies used were anti-SIRT2 antibody (Cell Signaling Technology, Beverly, CA), anti-TFEB antibody (Abcam, Cambridge, United Kingdom), anti-TSG101 antibody (Abcam, Cambridge, United Kingdom), anti-CD63 antibody (Abcam, Cambridge, United Kingdom), anti-HSP70 antibody (Abcam, Cambridge, United Kingdom), and anti-LC3 antibody (Cell Signaling Technology, Beverly, CA). For housekeeping, anti-β-actin antibody (Sigma, St. Louis, MO) was used. After washes with PBS, the membranes were incubated with HRP-conjugated secondary antibodies (Cell Signaling Technology, Danvers, MA) and were visualized using Odyssey Imaging Systems (LI-COR Biotechnology, Lincoln, United Kingdom).

TUNEL

Using TUNEL detection kit (Beyotime, Hangzhou, China), apoptosis in A549 and H1299 cells were monitored following the manufacturer's protocol. Cells cultured in a 24 well dish were initially incubated with proteinase K followed by TUNEL reaction mixture for 1 h at 37°C. Further, the cells were monitored using a confocal microscope (Leica, Germany). Controls were incubated with DNase I (positive control) or labeling solution (negative control) for 1 h. Percentage of TUNEL positive cells were assessed using MetaMorph image 7.1.2.0 software.

Isolation of Exosomes

Initially, 10% FBS was centrifuged overnight at 100,000 g to remove any existing exosomes. Further, the cells were cultured in medium with the above mentioned FBS for 24 h and the medium was centrifuged at 320 g for 10 min followed by centrifugation at 2,000 g for 15 min which allows removal of any cellular debris. Further, the supernatant was again centrifuged 10,000 *g* for 30 min at 4°C. The supernatant collected from the previous step was again centrifuged at 100,000 *g* for 70 min and the pellet was washed with PBS and recentrifuged at 100,000 *g* for 70 min. The pellet contained exosomes which was further processed for other experiments.

Transmission Electron Microscopy (TEM)

When NSCLC cells (H1299 and A549 cells) reached 90% confluence, cells were collected and centrifuged at 1,500 rpm for 15 min. To the pellet, 0.5% glutaraldehyde fixative was added and incubated for 10 min at 4°C. Further, the samples were centrifuged at 12,000 rpm for 12 min. After discarding the supernatant, 3% glutaraldehyde was added. Finally, 1% osmium tetroxide was used to fix again, dehydration was performed using acetone, and embedding was done using Epson812. Ultra-thin sections were obtained and double staining with uranyl acetate and lead citrate was performed. Finally, exosomes and autophagosomes were observed using TEM.

Nanoparticle Tracking Analysis (NTA)

The isolated exosomes were assessed with NanoSight NS300 (Malvern, Cornell NanoScale Science and Technology Facility) to determine the sizes and concentrations of exosomes in a given sample. Further, the data was assessed using NTA 3.2 Dev Build 3.2.16.

Flow Cytometry of Apoptosis

Annexin V-FITC Apoptosis Detection Kit (Sigma-Aldrich) was used to assess apoptosis rate after exposure to ASS. Cells were suspended in binding buffer and incubated at 37°C. Further, the cells were incubated with 10 μL Annexin V-FITC and 5 μL PI in the dark. Finally, cell apoptosis rate was measured by Flow Cytometer using FlowJo software (Beckman Coulter, Fullerton, CA, United States).

In vitro Invasion Assay

4×10^4 cells were suspended in 200 μL of serum-free medium, and seeded into an upper chamber of the Transwell chamber (8 μm pore size; Millipore, Burlington, MA, United States) which was pre-coated with 20 μg Matrigel (BD Biosciences) while medium supplemented with 10% FBS was added into the lower chamber after 24 h incubation at 37°C. The non-invaded cells in the upper chamber were removed, and the cells that invaded the matrix were fixed with 4% paraformaldehyde for 20 min and stained with 0.5% crystal violet. Finally, the invaded cells are counted under the microscope.

Immunofluorescence Staining (IFC)

Cells were initially washed with PBS and fixed with 4% paraformaldehyde for 10 min. Further, after thorough washing with PBS, the cells were blocked with 1% BSA in PBST (PBS + 0.1% Tween 20) for 30 min. Then, the cells were incubated in primary antibody in 1% BSA in PBST overnight (4°C). The primary antibodies used were anti-LC3B antibody (Cell Signaling Technology, Beverly, CA), anti-LAMP1 antibody (Cell Signaling Technology, Beverly, CA), and anti-TFEB antibody (Abcam, Cambridge, United Kingdom). Further after washes with PBST, the cells were incubated with FITC-conjugated or CY3-conjugated secondary antibodies (Abcam, Cambridge, United Kingdom) for 1 h. The cells were finally incubated with DAPI and imaged using an Olympus microscope at 40× magnification. Images were captured using an Olympus FSX100 microscope and analyzed using Image J software.

RNA Immunoprecipitation (RIP) Assay

After preparing whole-cell lysates from confluent A549 and H1299 cells, equal amounts of lysates and antibodies against SIRT2 or control IgG were loaded onto magnetic beads followed by extensive washing. We performed individual pulldowns at 4°C. Then, we amplified recovered RNA for immunoprecipitation and generated cDNA. The obtained cDNA were used to perform PCR with primers TFEB Forward: 5′-ACC TGTCCGAGACCTATGGG-3′; Reverse: 5′-CGTCCAGACGC ATAATGTTGTC-3′, GAPDH Forward: 5′-GGAGCGAGATC CCTCCAAAAT-3′; Reverse: 5′-GGCTGTTGTCATACTTCTC ATGG-3′.The PCR product was migrated in an agarose gel (1.5%, Biowest, Nuaille, France) and the product was observed using a FluorChem^{TM} Q system (Alpha Innotech, San Jose, CA, United States) and visualized.

Model of Metastases of NSCLC in Nude Mice

BALB/c nude mice were purchased from Shanghai SLAC Laboratory Animal, aged at 4–6 weeks. All animal experiments included in this study were approved by the Ethical Committee for Animal Research of Xin Hua Hospital Affiliated to Shanghai Jiao Tong University School of Medicine. Further, All animal care procedures accorded with institutional and international guidelines. The mice were housed in a controlled temperature of 22 ± 1°C with a 12 h light/12 h dark cycle with lights on from 0600 to 1,800 h. A549 and H1299 cells were cultured as previously mentioned and a suspension of 1×10^6 cells were injected intraperitoneally into the nude mice ($n = 6$ for each cell type). The mice were weighed once every 3 days for 33 days. After 33 days, the mice were sacrificed and lungs and liver were isolated to assess the levels of metastasis.

Histological Analysis

Histological analysis was performed using a previously described protocol. Initially tissues were collected and fixed in 10% formalin followed by paraffin embedding and sectioning into 10 μm slices. The sections were stained using hematoxylin-eosin (H&E) and observed and imaged under a light microscope.

Statistical Analysis

All the data were analyzed using SPSS software. All *in vitro* experiments were repeated at least three times independently. Data are presented as the mean ± standard deviation (SD) unless otherwise stated. $P < 0.05$ was considered significant.

RESULTS

ASS Induced NSCLC Cell Autophagy

To understand the effects of ASS on NSCLC, two epithelial carcinoma cell lines A549 and H1299 were exposed to ASS (10 dyn/cm^2) for 60 min. Further, we performed western blotting analysis from the ASS exposed cell lysates and observed that LC3II/GAPDH ratio was significantly increased in the ASS exposed cells compared to the unexposed (maintained in resting state) control cells (**Figures 1A–C**). Interestingly, there was no significant decrease in the p62 levels in both A549 and H1299 cells. Further, A549 cells expressing EGFP-LC3 (a mammalian ortholog of atg8) were examined. These A549-EGFP-LC3 cells were exposed to ASS (10 dyn/cm^2) for varied periods of time (0, 15, 30, and 60 min). Evidently, with prolonged exposures to ASS, we could clearly observe a exposure time-dependent increase in the number of EGFP-LC3 green puncta in the cells. By 60 min, a significantly high number of green LC3 puncta could be observed in the ASS exposed cells compared to the cells not exposed to ASS (0 min) (**Figures 1D,E**). In order to further characterize ASS induced autophagy, A549 cells were exposed to ASS (10 dyn/cm^2) for varying lengths of time (0, 15, 30, and 60 min), which were further characterized by TEM. TEM has been previously used to trace the process of autophagy, as the autophagosomes can be observed as bi- or multi-layer vacuole like structures encompassing components such as organelles. From the TEM images obtained at different times, it was evident that exposure to ASS increased the formation of autophagosomes in a time-dependent manner. After 60 min of exposure to ASS, it was clear that the cells had increased number of autophagosomes compared to the control (0 min ASS) (**Figure 1F**). These results indicate that ASS could induce autophagy in A549 cells. Next, to further understand the effect of ASS on apoptosis, we performed TUNEL assay on A549 cells. As shown in **Figure 1G**, we could observe an increasing number of TUNEL positive cells after 60 min of exposure to ASS. This further indicated a potential role of ASS in apoptosis.

ASS Promoted Exosomes and Autophagy Related Components Release

As recent studies have revealed that mechanical stress affects exosome release of autophagic components, we were interested to observe the effects of ASS on exosomes (Reck et al., 2014). Initially, using TEM, we clearly observed and characterized the A549 cells derived exosomes (**Figure 2A**). Further, with the aid of a previously published protocol, we isolated the exosomes which were secreted by NSCLC cells; and then confirmed their presence through TEM and NANOSIGHT (**Figures 2B,C**). Exosomes were also isolated from A549 and H1299 cells exposed to ASS (10 dyn/cm^2) and the further exosomes characterized with nanoparticle tracking analysis (NTA). It was evident that shared a similar size between control and ASS exposed group (**Figure 2D**), but the concentration of exosomes were significantly higher in the ASS exposed A549 and H1299 cells (**Figure 2E**). Expression of exosomes maker (TSG101, CD63, and HSP70) and autophagy component maker (LC3I/II) were assessed by western blot analysis. From the western blot analysis, it was clear that exosomes obtained after exposure to ASS, had high expression levels of TSG101, CD63, and HSP70 (**Figures 2F,G,I,J**). Interestingly, we also observed high levels of LC3II in the exosomes obtained from both A549 and H1299 after exposure to ASS (**Figures 2H,K**) compared to the control (static) cell exosomes. These data clearly indicate that ASS promotes exosomes secretion along with release of autophagic components in NSCLC.

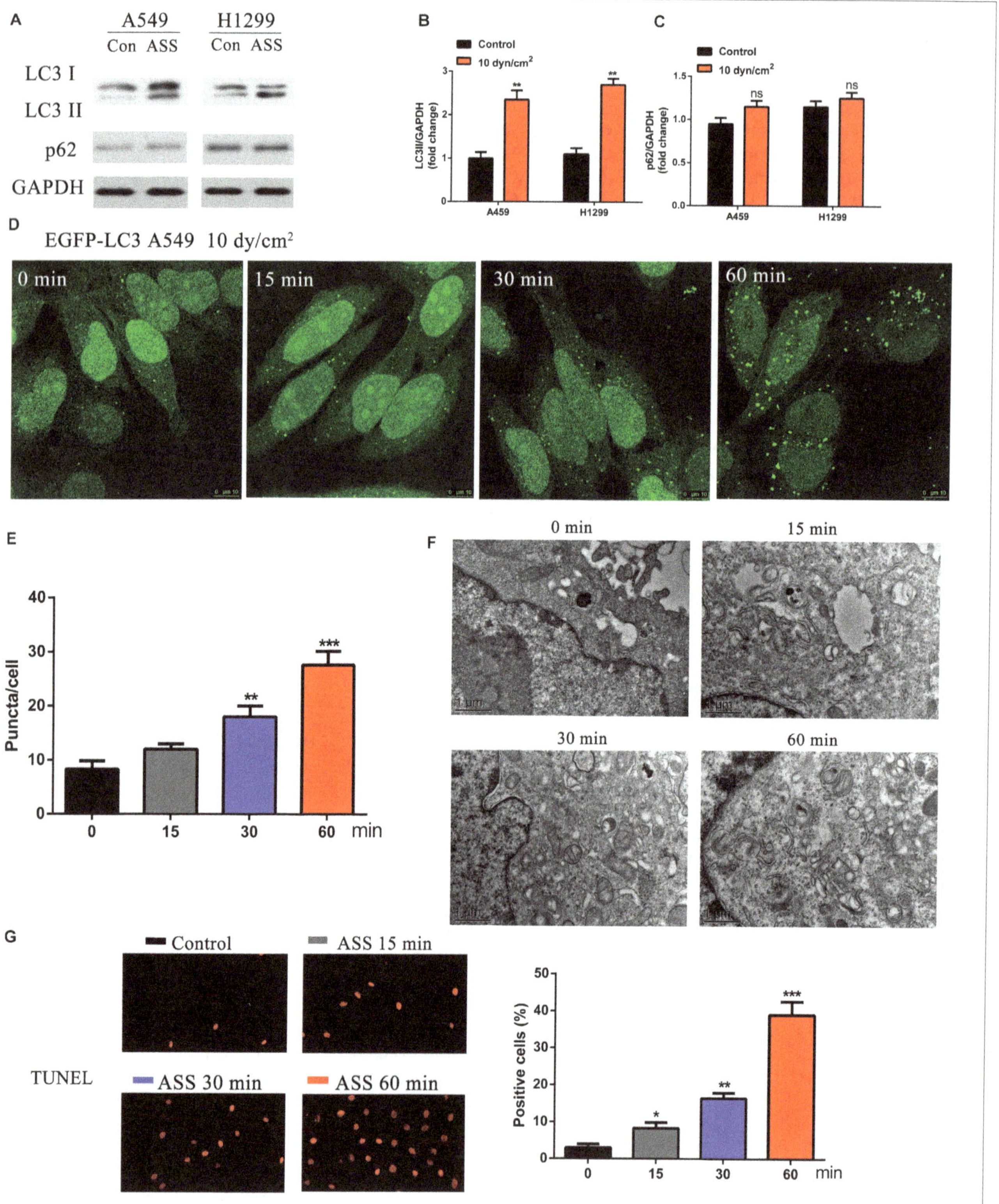

FIGURE 1 | ASS activated NSCLC cell autophagy and promoted cell apoptosis. **(A)** The expression of LC3I/II and p62 were detected by western blot in A549 and H1299 cells treated with ASS (10 dyn/cm^2) for 60 min or incubated at quiet state. All experiments were repeated three times, $^{**}P < 0.01$. **(B)** Quantification of LC3II/LC3I ratio in relation to GAPDH, **(C)** Quantification of p62 levels in relation to GAPDH, **(D,E)** A549 cells expressing EGFP-LC3 were exposed to ASS (10 dyn/cm^2) for indicated times (0, 15, 30, and 60 min); Scale bar, 10 μm. The percentage of cells with EGFP-LC3 puncta were quantified, $^{**}P < 0.01$, $^{***}P < 0.001$. **(F)** TEM images of A549 cells exposed to ASS for 0, 15, 30, and 60 min; Scale bar, 1 μm. **(G)** TUNEL assay was performed after A549 cells were exposed to ASS for indicated times, the percentage of cell apoptosis were quantified by Image Pro Plus software, $^{*}P < 0.05$, $^{**}P < 0.01$, $^{***}P < 0.001$.

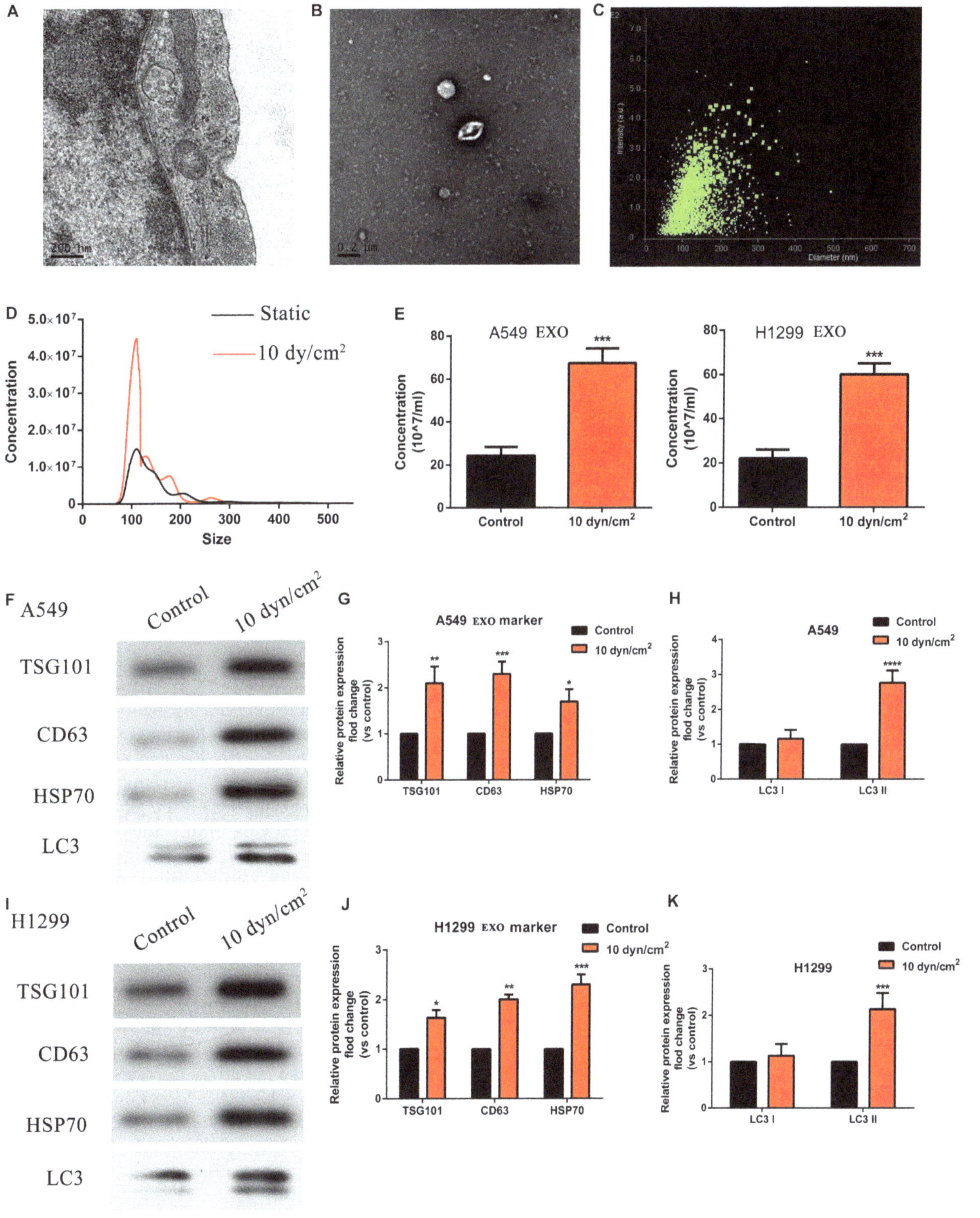

FIGURE 2 | ASS promoted exosomes and autophagy related components release. **(A,B)** A549 cells derived exosomes observed by TEM, Scale bar, 200 nm. **(C)** The intensity and size of exosomes as evaluated by NANOSIGHT. **(D,E)** The concentration of exosomes isolated from A549 and H1299 cells after exposure to ASS for 60 min as acquired by Nanoparticle Tracking Analysis (NTA), $^{***}P < 0.001$. **(F–K)** Expression of exosomes maker (TSG101, CD63, and HSP70) and autophagy component maker (LC3I/II) were measured by western blot analysis, every experiment was repeated in triplicate, $^{*}P < 0.05$, $^{**}P < 0.01$, $^{***}P < 0.001$, $^{****}P < 0.0001$.

Suppression of Exosomes Release by ASS Will Induce NSCLC Cell Apoptosis

To understand the relationship between ASS and exosomes, we further treated the NSCLC cell lines with a known exosome inhibitor GW4689 (Essandoh et al., 2015) for 60 min and then exposed these cells to ASS (10 dyn/cm^2) for 60 min. Exosomes were isolated and assessed by NTA. Interestingly, it was clear that even when cells were exposed to ASS, pretreatment with GW4689 decreased the concentration of exosomes (**Figure 3A**). Further, western blotting analysis confirmed that exosomes from GW4689 pretreatment group showed significantly decreased exosomes markers (TSG101, CD63, and HSP70) and autophagic marker (LC3II) in both A549 and H1299 cells (**Figure 3B**). This indicated that GW4689 was successful in inhibiting exosome secretion in ASS exposed NSCLCs. Further to understand the effect of suppression of exosome release on apoptosis of NSCLC, we performed TUNEL assay. Initially A549 cells were pretreated with GW4689 for 60 min and then the cells were exposed to ASS (10 dyn/cm^2) for 0, 15, 30, and 60 min. By 60 min, in ASS exposed cells, a high number of TUNEL positive cells could be observed (**Figure 3C**). However, in the GW4689 pretreated cells, by 60 min the number of TUNEL positive cells increased even higher than the ASS exposed group (**Figure 3D**). This data was further confirmed by flow cytometry using Annexin V-fluorescein isothiocyanate (FITC) Apoptosis Staining/Detection Kit (**Figures 3E,F**) which indicated that GW4689 pretreatment significantly caused a 30% increase in apoptosis in the ASS exposed cells. Hence, it was clear that ASS increases apoptosis in NSCLC which could be exacerbated by the suppression of exosome secretion.

Role of SIRT2 on ASS Induced Cell Apoptosis

Previously, studies indicated the role of SIRT1 in exosome biogenesis. We were therefore interested to understand the roles of SIRT1 and SIRT2 in ASS associated autophagy and apoptosis. Initially, we performed western blotting analysis of ASS exposed A549 and H1299 cell lysates. It was clear that the increase in ASS exposure did not significantly affect the expression of SIRT1, while the expression of SIRT2 decreased significantly (**Figures 4A,B**). As stated earlier, exposure to ASS increased exosome release, apoptosis and decreased SIRT2 expression levels. Hence, we conducted experiments to assess the function of SIRT2 in exosome release and apoptosis. We overexpressed SIRT2 in A549 cells and observed a decrease in expression of exosome and autophagic markers after exposure to ASS for 60 min, indicating a decrease in the secretion of exosomes and autophagic components (**Figures 4C,D**). These data provided evidence to link our findings that SIRT2 is a negative regulator of the secretion of exosomes and autophagic components. In addition, to assess the impact of ASS and SIRT2 overexpression on apoptosis, we produced A549 cells that were stably overexpressing SIRT2 and performed TUNEL assay and flow cytometric analysis after exposure to ASS. Interestingly, both the TUNEL (**Figure 4E**) and flow cytometric assays (**Figure 4F**) showed that the overexpression of SIRT2 and ASS exposure increased apoptosis, higher than that in the ASS exposure only group. Another key observation was that after exposure to ASS, SIRT2 overexpressed cells mimicked the group of cells which were treated with GW (exosome inhibitor). At the same time, the Transwell assay (**Figure 4G**) revealed that SIRT2 overexpression and ASS exposure can significantly inhibit A549 cell invasion. This indicated that SIRT2 overexpression inhibited cell invasion and decreased secretion of exosome and autophagy factors thus increasing apoptosis in ASS exposed cells.

TFEB Overexpression Regulated Cell Apoptosis, Autophagy, and Invasion

Further, to understand how SIRT2 regulates autophagy, we assessed a downstream target of SIRT2, TFEB (transcription factor EB). A549 cells were exposed to ASS (10 dyn/cm^2) for 0, 15, 30, and 60 min, and assessed for TFEB expression using qRT-PCR and western blotting. It was clear that ASS exposure decreased TFEB expression after 15 min, and both mRNA and protein TFEB levels decreased tremendously after 60 min (**Figures 5A,B**). Similarly, we also performed IFC staining and observed clear TFEB cytoplasmic staining in the control cells, whereas ASS exposed cells displayed decreased TFEB staining (**Figure 5C**). Previously, studies have indicated TFEB's role in lysosomal biogenesis and autophagy (Sardiello et al., 2009; Napolitano and Ballabio, 2016). Hence, with the aid of A549 cells overexpressing TFEB, we performed IFC of key autophagic markers such as LAMP1 and LC3B after exposure to ASS (10 dyn/cm^2). Evidently, ASS exposure clearly decreased LAMP1 expression, whereas TFEB overexpression rescued this inhibition of LAMP1 expression by ASS. Alternatively, ASS exposure increased LC3B expression but TFEB overexpression decreased its expression. Further, we could observe a strong co-localization of LC3B and LAMP1 specifically near the nuclear region in the TFEB overexpressed cell line, after exposure to ASS, indicating a potential increase in the fusion of autophagosome and lysosome (**Figure 5D**). Additionally, using western blotting, we observed that TFEB overexpression decreased exosome and autophagic components secretion after ASS exposure (**Figures 5E,F**). Using TUNEL assay and flow cytometry, we could confirm that TFEB overexpression increased apoptosis when compared to the control cells and thus mimicked the cells treated with GW (exosome inhibitor), after exposure to ASS (**Figures 5G,H**). In addition, through Tranwell assay (**Figure 5I**), we concluded that compared with the control cells, TFEB overexpression cells and the group of cells which were treated with GW significantly inhibited cell invasion, after exposure to ASS. These data indicated that TFEB overexpression decreased secretion of exosomes along with autophagic factors, accelerated autophagosome, and lysosome fusion, and increased apoptosis in ASS exposed NSCLC cells.

SIRT2 Directly Binds and Regulates TFEB Expression

Initially, using *cat*RAPID we assessed the interaction between SIRT2 and 3′ UTR of TEFB. Evidentially, heatmap analysis indicated that SIRT2 and TFEB 3′ UTR associated with a high

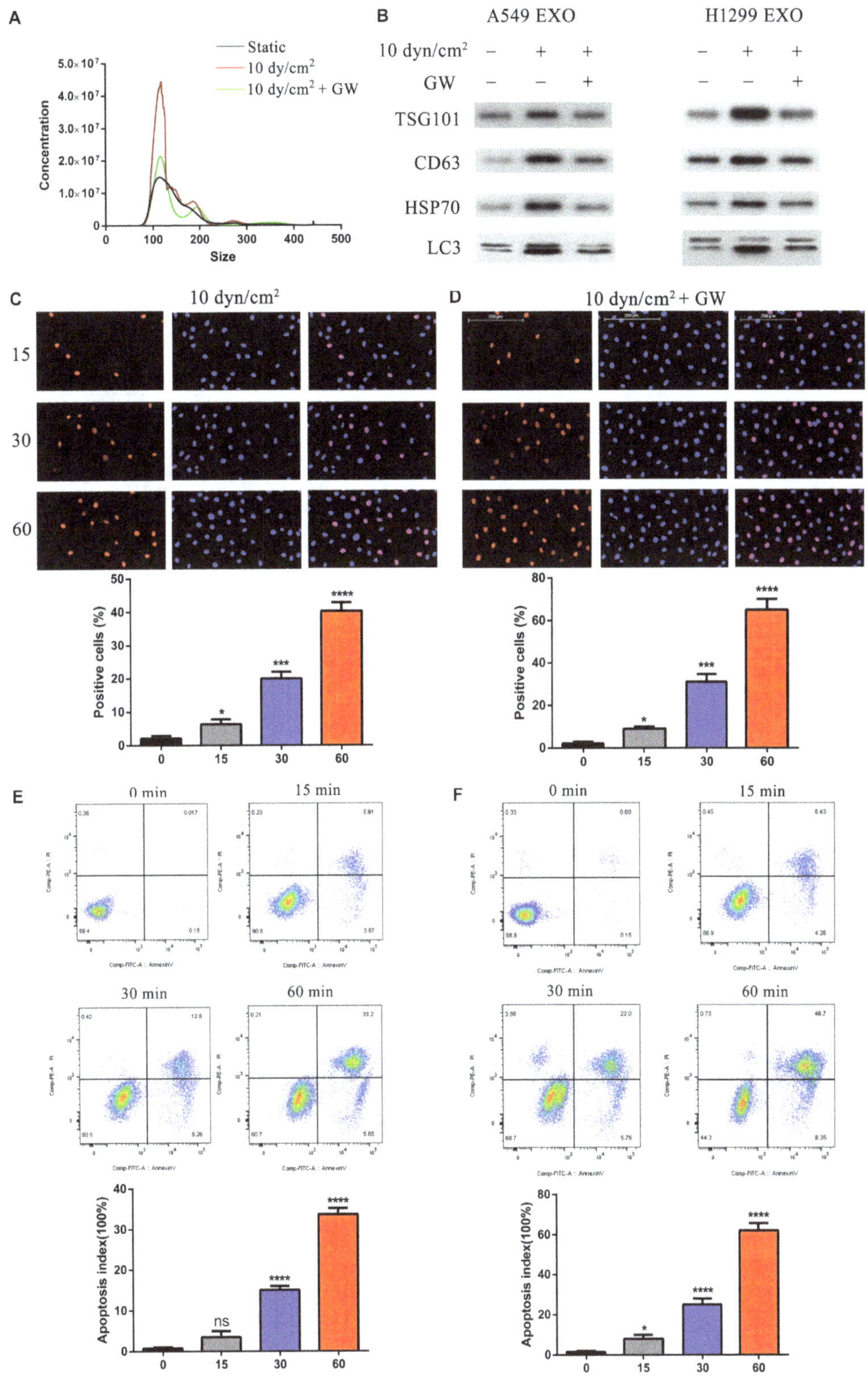

FIGURE 3 | Suppression of exosomes release exacerbated ASS induced NSCLC cell apoptosis. **(A)** A549 and H1299 cells were pretreated with exosome inhibitor GW4689 (GW) for 60 min and then exposed to ASS (10 dyn/cm^2) for 60 min, the concentration of isolated exosomes were detected by NTA. **(B)** The expression of exosomes marker (TSG101, CD63, and HSP70) and secreted autophagy components (LC3 I/II) were analyzed by western blot. **(C–F)** After pretreatment with GW4689 for 60 min, NSCLC cells were exposed to ASS (10 dyn/cm^2) for 0, 15, 30, and 60 min, the percentage of cell apoptosis was evaluated by **(C,D)** TUNEL assay and **(E,F)** flow cytometry using Annexin V-fluorescein isothiocyanate (FITC) Apoptosis Staining/Detection Kit, $^*P < 0.05$, $^{***}P < 0.001$, $^{****}P < 0.0001$.

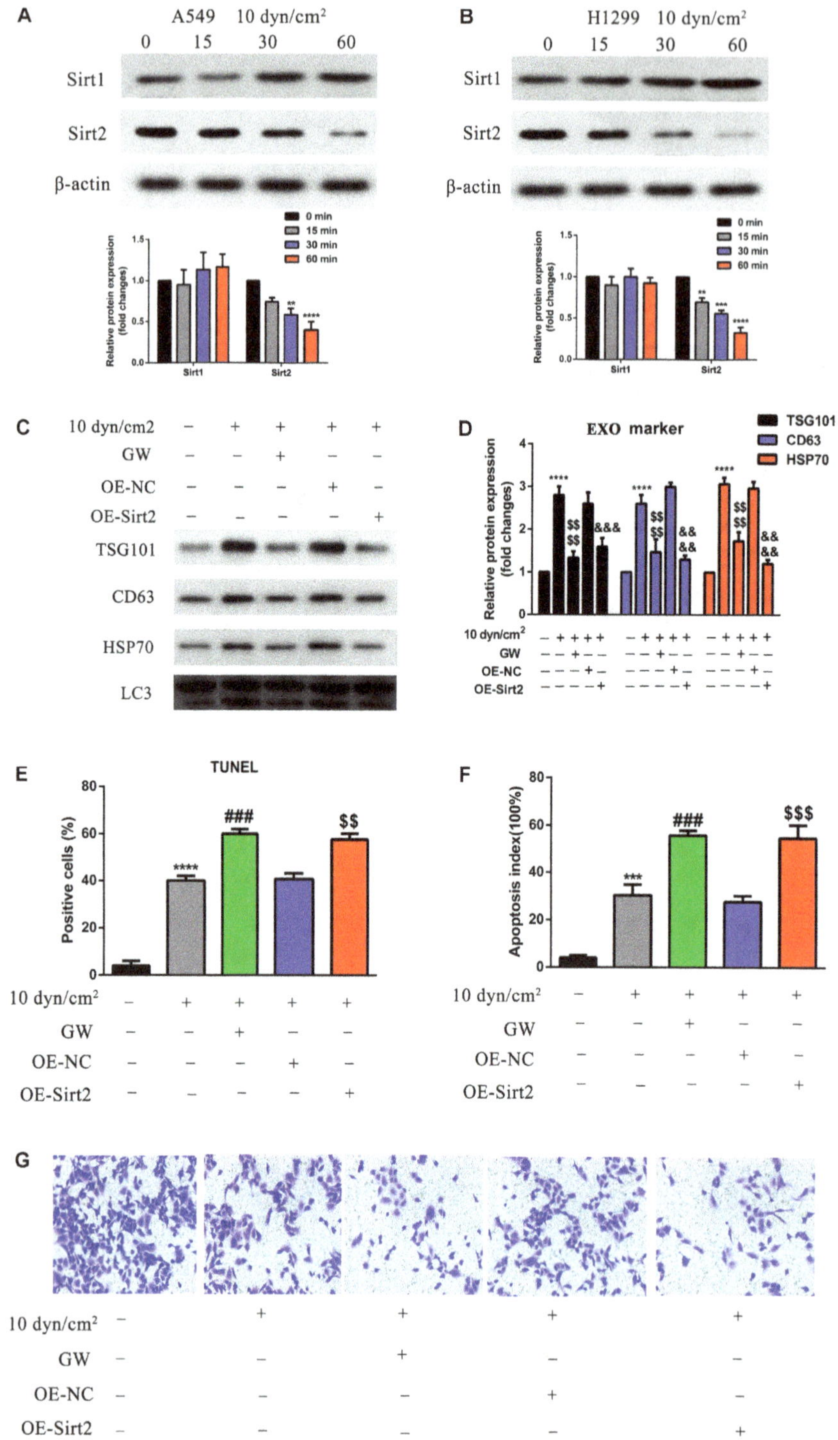

FIGURE 4 | Over expression of SIRT2 reduced exosomes and autophagy component release, promoted ASS induced cell apoptosis, inhibited cell invasion. **(A,B)** A549 and H1299 cells were exposed to ASS (10 dyn/cm^2) for indicated times, and then the expression of SIRT1 and SIRT2 were detected by western blot, each experiment was repeated at least three times, $^{**}P < 0.01$, $^{***}P < 0.001$, $^{****}P < 0.0001$. **(C,D)** After overexpression of SIRT2 or treatment with GW4689, A549 cells were exposed to ASS (10 dyn/cm^2) for 60 min, quantitative analysis of the released exosome (TSG101, CD63, HSP70) and autophagy component (LC3) markers were carried out by western blot, $^{****}P < 0.0001$ compared to control group, $$$$ denote $P < 0.0001$ compared to ASS (10 dyn/cm^2) group, &&&, &&&& denote $P < 0.001$ and $P < 0.0001$ compared to OE-NC group. **(E,F)** Cell apoptosis rate were, respectively, examined by **(E)** TUNEL assay, and **(F)** flow cytometry after the cells were stably overexpressed for SIRT2 or pretreated with GW4689 for 60 min. Further, the cells were exposed to ASS for 60 min, *** and **** denote $P < 0.001$ and $P < 0.0001$ compared to control group,$^{###}$ denote $P < 0.001$ compared to ASS (10 dyn/cm^2) group, $$, $$$ denote $^{**}P < 0.01$ and $P < 0.001$ compared to OE-NC group. **(G)** After overexpression of SIRT2 or treatment with GW4689, A549 cells were exposed to ASS (10 dyn/cm^2) for 60 min, cell invasion was detected by Tranwell assay.

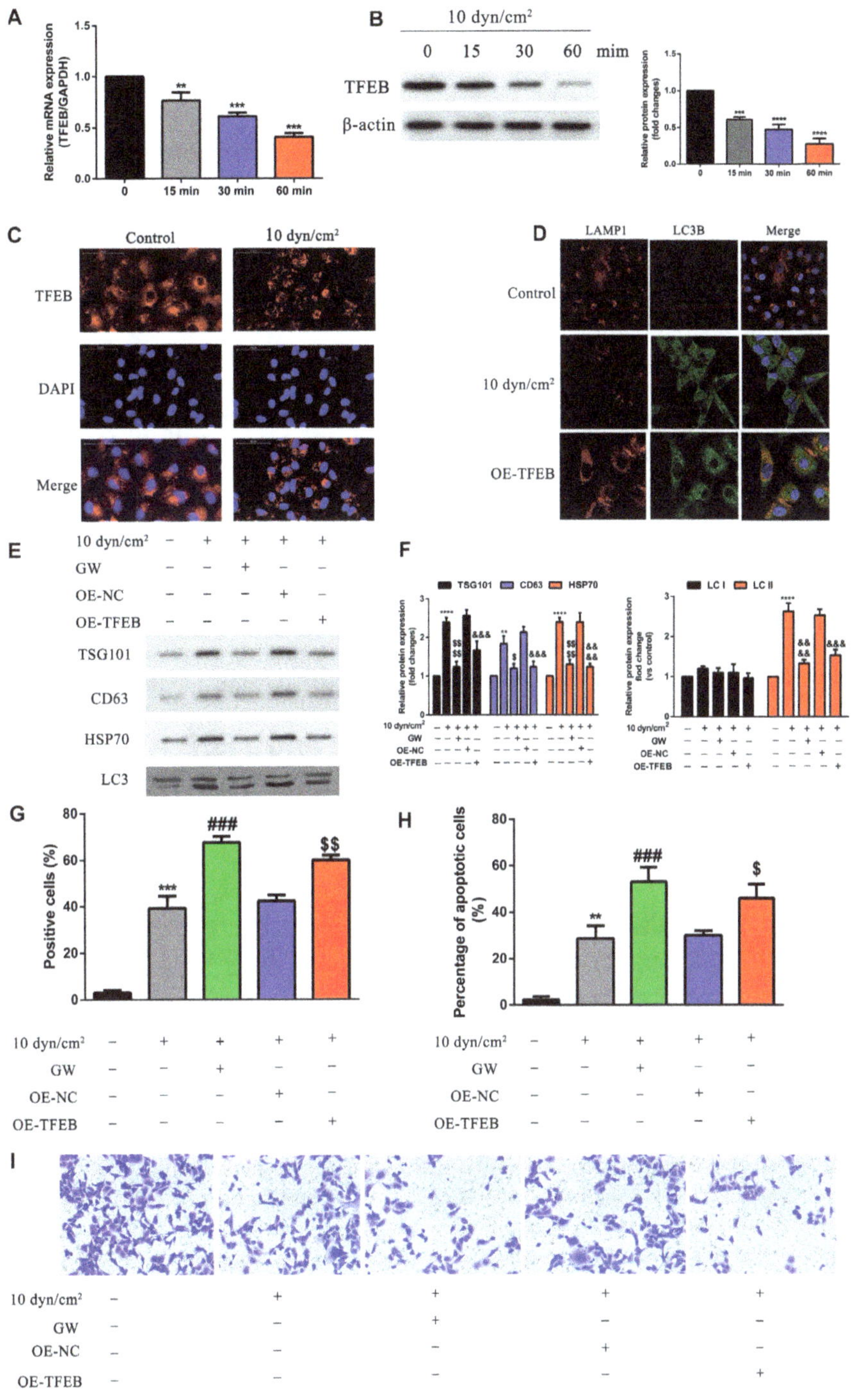

FIGURE 5 | Overexpression of TFEB accelerated fusion of autophagosome and lysosome, inhibited exosomes and autophagy component release, promoted cell apoptosis, regulated cell invasion. **(A,B)** A549 cells exposed to ASS (10 dyn/cm^2) for 0, 15, 30, and 60 min, the expression of TFEB was detected by qRT-PCR and western blot, $^{**}P < 0.01$, $^{***}P < 0.001$, $^{****}P < 0.0001$. **(C)** The expression level of TFEB after exposure to ASS (10 dyn/cm^2) for 60 min were confirmed by cell immunofluorescence. **(D)** Immunofluorescence of LAMP1 and LC3B was performed on A549 cells exposed to ASS (10 dyn/cm^2) for 60 min, the co-localization of LAMP1 puncta and LC3B puncta was observed in the merge image (yellow merge area), magnification, 600×. **(E,F)** A549 cells, after stable overexpression of TFEB or GW4689 treatment, were exposed to ASS (10 dyn/cm^2) for 60 min, then isolated exosomes and autophagic components were identified and quantified by western blot, $^{****}P < 0.0001$ compared to control group, \$, \$\$\$\$ $P < 0.05$ and $P < 0.0001$ compared to ASS (10 dyn/cm^2) group, &&&, &&&& denote $P < 0.001$ and $P < 0.0001$ compared to OE-NC group. **(G,H)** Cell apoptosis was determined by TUNEL assay and flow cytometry, each group was treated the same as panel E, ** and *** denote $P < 0.01$ and $P < 0.001$ compared to control group, $^{###}P < 0.001$ compared to ASS (10 dyn/cm^2) group, \$, \$\$\$ denote $P < 0.05$ and $P < 0.01$ compared to OE-NC group. **(I)** A549 cells, after stable overexpression of TFEB or GW4689 treatment, were exposed to ASS (10 dyn/cm^2) for 60 min, Tranwell assay was used to detect cell invasion.

interaction propensity score of 84. The software also validated that this interaction had a high predictability rate due to the high discriminative power score of 98% (**Figure 6A**). Based on NSCLC tissue samples from TCGA database, we further performed Pearson's correlation analysis to assess the association between SIRT2 and TFEB. Incidentally, SIRT2 and TFEB shared a positive relationship with an *R*-value of 0.41 ($P < 0.0001$) (**Figure 6B**). To further assess the effect of SIRT2 on TFEB, SIRT2 was either overexpressed (OE) or silenced (sh) in A549 cells and exposed to ASS (10 dyn/cm^2) for 60 min. Further, we performed western blotting analysis to assess the levels of TFEB expression. Silencing of SIRT2 in the static cells, significantly decreased TFEB expression levels similar to the expression in cells exposed to ASS (10 dyn/cm^2). However, overexpression of SIRT2, significantly recovered the TFEB expression levels after exposure to ASS (**Figure 6C**). This indicated that TFEB expression levels were SIRT2 dependent. RNA immunoprecipitation studies were also performed to confirm the interaction between SIRT2 and TFEB. Initially, A549 cells were either silenced or overexpressed for SIRT2 expression and after 48 h, we subsequently performed immunoprecipitation experiments on cell lysates using SIRT2 and control igG antibodies. Further, from the immunoprecipitated samples, the levels of target mRNA were assessed through qRT-PCR and semi-quantitative PCR. For the SIRT2 silenced cells, we identified significantly low levels of TFEB mRNA, however, for the cells which were overexpressed for SIRT2, we identified high levels of TFEB mRNA (**Figures 6D,E**). These evidences clearly indicated that SIRT2 promoted TFEB expression through direct binding with TFEB mRNA.

SIRT2 Along With TFEB Regulates Autolysosome Formation, Exosomes, and Autophagy Component Release, Cell Apoptosis, and Invasion

To understand the role of TFEB and its association with autophagy, A549 cells were overexpressed for SIRT2 and silenced for TFEB and exposed to ASS for 60 min. As observed previously, overexpression of SIRT2 or TFEB, significantly decreased secretion of exosomes and autophagy factors, as indicated by western blotting analysis of TSG101, CD63, HSP70, and LC3 (**Figures 7A,B**). However, when SIRT2 was overexpressed but TFEB was silenced, we observed an opposite effect. This indicated that the effect of SIRT2 on secretion of autophagic factors and exosomes were dependent on TFEB expression. Further, using IFC, we could observe that SIRT2 or TFEB overexpression increased LAMP1 expression and co-localization with LC3B. However, when SIRT2 was overexpressed but TFEB was silenced, the expression of LAMP1 significantly decreased along with decrease in co-localization of LAMP1 and LC3B, indicating its effect on autolysosome formation (**Figure 7C**). Subsequently, we checked TFEB's effect on apoptosis using flow cytometry and TUNEL assay. Similar to the previous evidence, overexpression of SIRT2 and silencing of TFEB, significantly decreased the number of apoptotic cells compared to the SIRT2 or TFEB overexpressing cells (**Figures 7D,E**). At the same time, Transwell assay (**Figure 7F**) proved overexpression of SIRT2 and silencing of TFEB, significantly increased cell invasion compared to the SIRT2 or TFEB overexpressing cells. These evidences clearly indicate that TFEB is required for SIRT2's effect on autolysosome formation, exosomes, and autophagy component release, cell apoptosis, and regulated invasion in NSCLCs.

SIRT2 Overexpression Inhibited NSCLC Cell Metastasis *in vivo*

To assess the role of SIRT2 *in vivo* NSCLC cells (A549 and H1299) were transfected with SIRT2 overexpression systems, and were injected into nude mice ($n = 6$ mice per group). Mice were monitored and weighed once every 3 days for 33 days. Compared to the mice injected with NSCLC control cells (A549, H1299; $n = 6$ mice per group), nude mice injected with SIRT2 overexpressing cells had lesser weight loss (**Figures 8A,B**). After 33 days, mice were sacrificed and images were taken of the lung and liver tissues to assess the formation of metastatic nodules (**Figures 8C,D**). Evidentially, SIRT2 over-expression significantly decreased metastatic nodule formation in the mice lung and liver tissues. We subsequently performed hematoxylin and eosin staining of these tissue sections and observed severe metastasis in the NSCLC injected mice models (**Figures 8E,F**). However, mice injected with SIRT2 over-expressing cells showed significantly less metastasis compared to the mice injected with control cells.

SIRT2 and TFEB Are Down-Regulated in Human NSCLC Tissues and Positively Correlated With Overall Survival in TCGA Database

We assessed the expression levels of SIRT2 and TFEB in the TCGA-LUAD database, and observed that both SIRT2 and TFEB were highly expressed in the LUAD patients (**Figures 9A,D**). Further, from the database, two groups were identified based on the SIRT2 and TFEB expression levels. It was evident that increased levels of SIRT2 and TFEB were associated with high survival rate (**Figures 9B,E**). Further, we performed western blotting analysis of the protein samples from patient NSCLC lung tissue and normal lung tissue samples, and observed that NSCLC tissues had significantly lower expression of SIRT2 and TFEB levels (**Figures 9C,F**). Additionally, we also performed IHC staining of the tissue sections and observed significantly low levels of both SIRT2 and TFEB levels in the NSCLC tumor tissues (**Figures 9G,H**). These evidences clearly indicate that SIRT2 and TFEB levels are significantly down-regulated in NSCLC patients and low expression levels of these transcripts are associated with low-survival rates.

DISCUSSION

Exposure to various mechanical stress such as fluid SS (FSS), low SS (LSS), and ASS instigates multiple responses in different cell types. In endothelial cells, SS is necessary for the organization and functional activity of the cells (Girard and Nerem, 1993). However, in cancer cells SS initiates a cascade of protective mechanisms which allows them to migrate, invade, and proliferate in target regions, which is a key process to establish metastasis in cancer. Based on previous studies, LSS

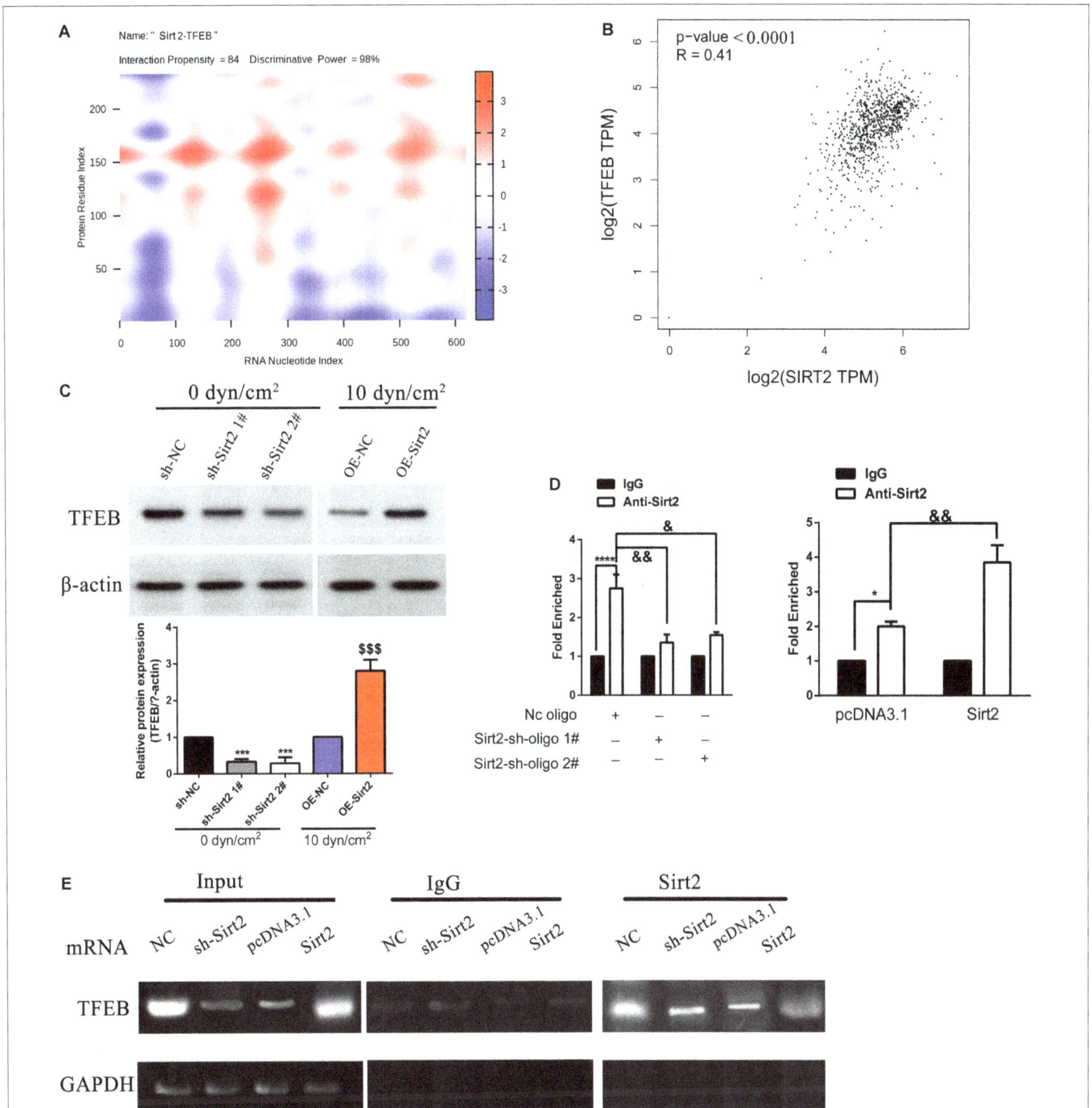

FIGURE 6 | SIRT2 promoted TFEB expression through direct binding with TFEB mRNA. **(A)** Prediction of the interaction between SIRT2 and TFEB 3′ UTR indicated as a heat-map, *cat*RAPID identified the interaction between SIRT2 and TFEB with confidence (Interaction Propensity = 84, Discriminative Power = 98%). **(B)** Based on data from TCGA, Pearson correlation of SIRT2 and TFEB ($P < 0.0001$, $R = 0.41$). **(C)** A549 cells were either stably knocked-down or overexpressed for SIRT2, and then exposed to ASS (0 and 10 dyn/cm^2) for 60 min, the expression of TFEB was determined by western blot, ***$P < 0.001$ compared to sh-NC group, $$$ $P < 0.001$ compared to OE-NC group. **(D,E)** Cellular extracts of NSCLC cells with either stable knockdown or overexpression of SIRT2 were immunoprecipitated with SIRT2 and IgG antibodies, the target TFEB mRNA of the immunoprecipitation was assessed through qRT-PCR and semi-quantitative RT-PCR. *$P < 0.05$, ****$P < 0.0001$.

(5–30 dyn/cm^2) seem to increase migration and invasion of the cancer cells whereas high stress (160 dyn/cm^2) leads to tumor cell death. In our study, use of ASS (10 dyn/cm^2) for 60 min led to a significant increase in migration and invasion of NSCLC cells in our *in vivo* models as indicated by increased metastatic nodules in liver and lung tissues of our nude mice model (**Figure 8B**). Previously, a study by Aung et al. (2014) showed that low level 3D stress on a breast cancer lines increased its migration

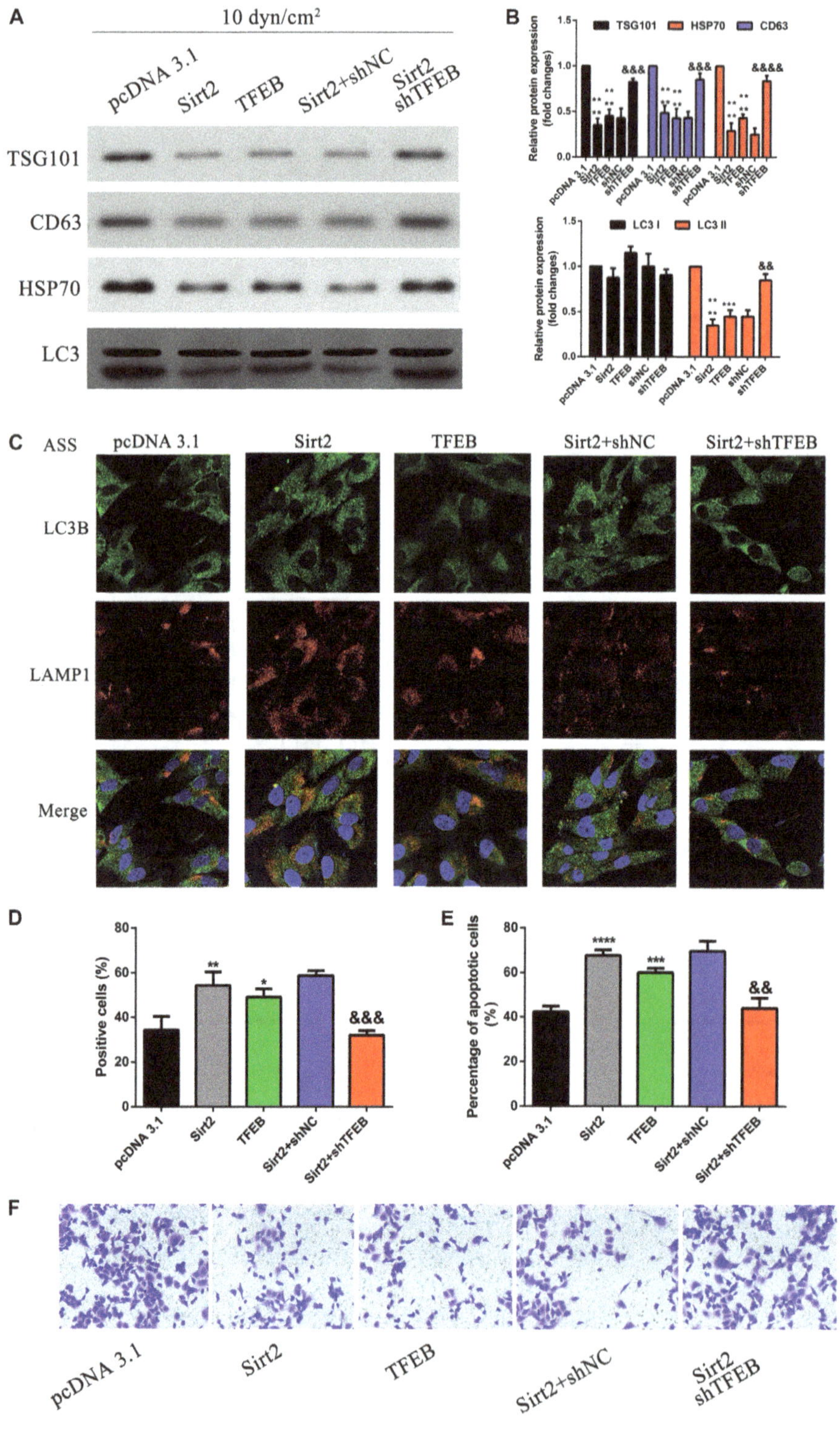

FIGURE 7 | SIRT2 along with TFEB regulates autolysosome formation, exosomes, autophagy component release, cell apoptosis, and invasion. **(A,B)** NSCLC cells transfected with OE-SIRT2, OE-TFEB, or OE-SIRT2/sh-TFEB plasmid were exposed to ASS (10 dyn/cm^2) for 60 min, exosomes which were released were collected and exosome specific markers were detected by western blot, ****$P < 0.0001$ compared to pcDNA3.1 group, &&&, &&&& denote $P < 0.001$ and $P < 0.0001$ compared to shNC group. **(C)** After treatment as previously described, immunofluorescence was performed to detect the fluorescence intensity of LAMP1 and LC3B, the co-localization of LAMP1 and LC3B was observed as yellow region in the merged image, magnification, 600×. **(D,E)** The percentage of cell apoptosis was determined by TUNEL assay and flow cytometry, *, **, *** and **** denotes $P < 0.05$, $P < 0.01$, $P < 0.001$, and $P < 0.0001$ compared to pcDNA3.1 group, &&, &&& denote $P < 0.01$ and $P < 0.001$ compared to SIRT2/shNC group. **(F)** After treatment as previously described, cell invasion was measured by Tranwell assay.

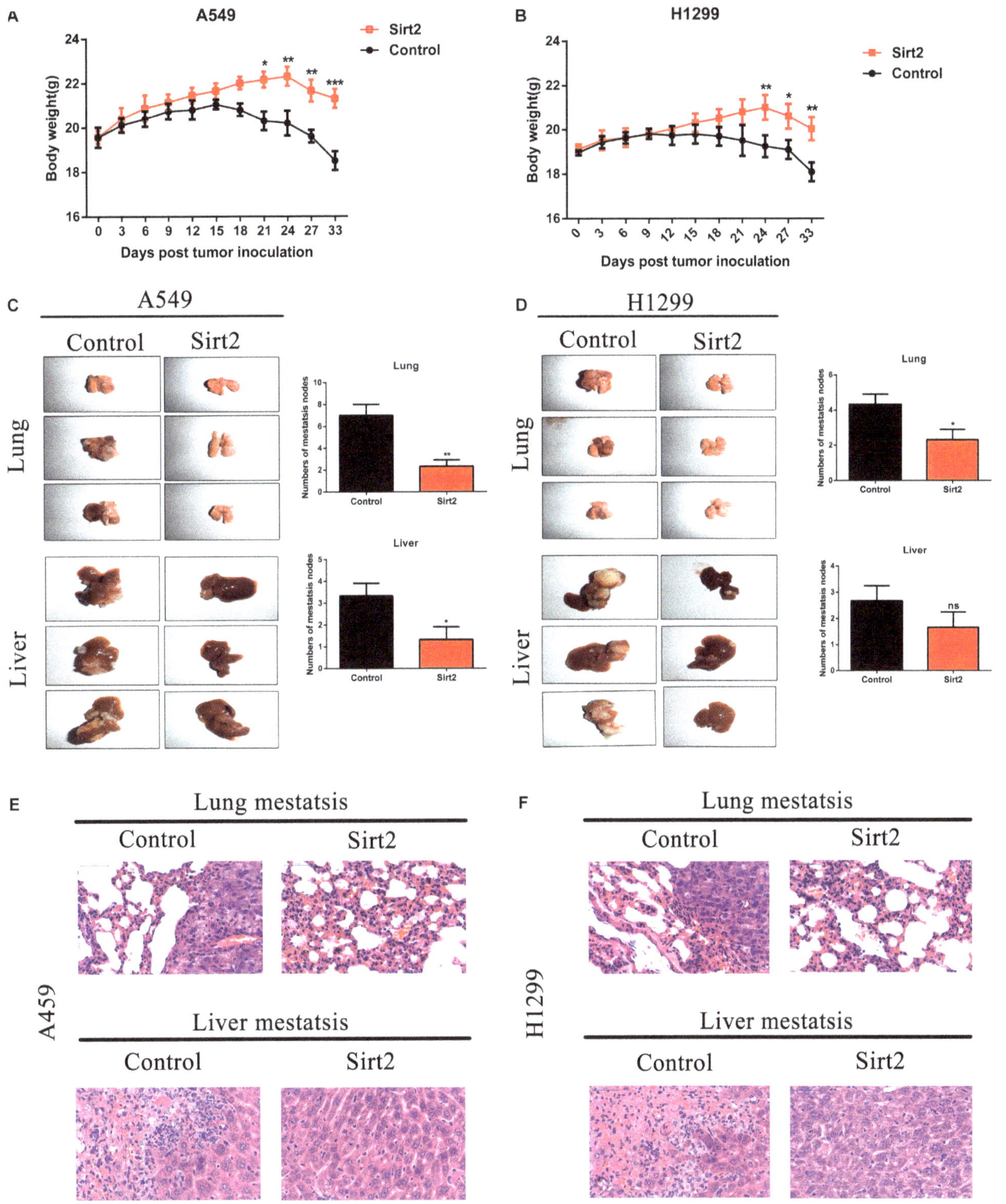

FIGURE 8 | SIRT2 overexpression inhibited NSCLC cell metastasis *in vivo*. **(A,B)** SIRT2 overexpressing A549 cells or H1299 cells were injected into nude mice, the weight of each mouse were detected for every 3 days, after 33 days, the mice were sacrificed and liver and lung metastasis nodules were observed and imaged ($n = 6$ mice per group, $^{*}P < 0.05$, $^{**}P < 0.01$, $^{***}P < 0.001$). **(C,D)** Six weeks after injection with SIRT2 over-expressed A549, H1299, or control cells, representative photos of nude mouse metastatic nodules of lung and liver were imaged. Black arrowheads show metastatic nodules in lungs and livers and the total numbers of metastatic nodules were assessed ($n = 6$ mice per group, $^{*}P < 0.05$, $^{**}P < 0.01$). **(E,F)** Representative images of hematoxylin and eosin staining of lung and liver metastasis nodule, Scale bar, 50 μm.

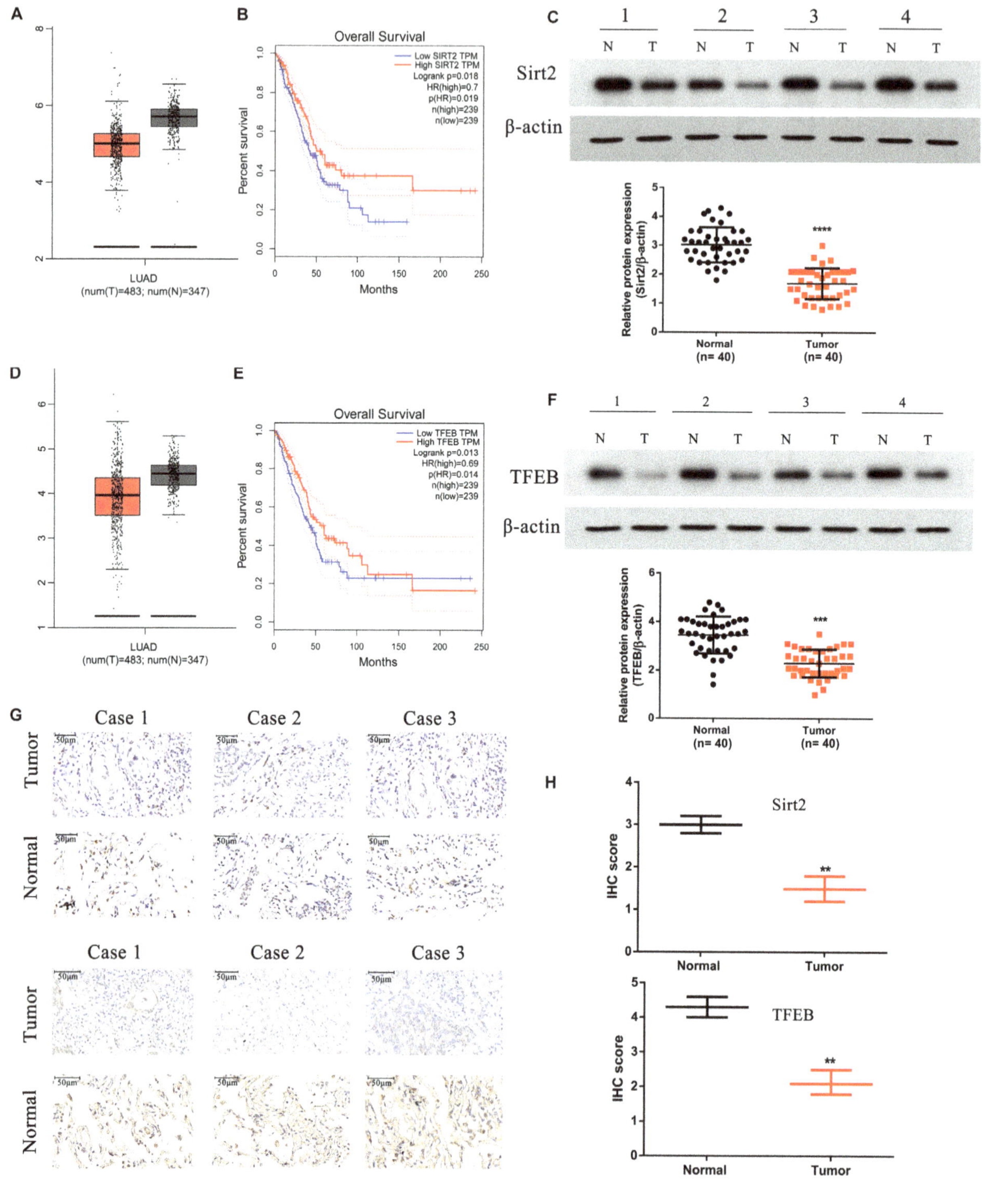

FIGURE 9 | SIRT2 and TFEB are down-regulated in human NSCLC tissues and positively correlated with overall survival in TCGA database. **(A,B)** The expression of SIRT2 in lung adenocarcinoma (LUAD) patients (t = 483, n = 347) and the overall survival (OS) curves of SIRT2^{high} (n = 239) and SIRT2^{low} (n = 239) NSCLC patients. **(C)** Total protein was extracted from human NSCLC tissues (n = 40), SIRT2 was detected by western blot, the upper panel shows SIRT2 expression in four tumor tissues samples with corresponding normal lung tissues samples. And the lower panel indicates the quantification of SIRT2 protein level in NSCLC tissues and corresponding normal lung tissues (n = 40, ****P < 0.0001). **(D,E)** The expression of TFEB in LUAD patients (t = 483, n = 347) and the OS curves of TFEB^{high} (n = 239) and TFEB^{low} (n = 239) NSCLC patients. **(F)** The expression of TFEB was detected in human NSCLC tissues, the upper panel shows the expression of TFEB in four tumor tissues samples with corresponding normal lung tissues samples. And the lower panel indicates the quantification of SIRT2 protein level in NSCLC tissues and corresponding normal lung tissues (n = 40, ***P < 0.001). **(G,H)** IHC staining detected the expression of SIRT2 and TFEB in human NSCLC tissues (n = 40, **P < 0.01).

and invasion in a protease dependent manner. In another study in hepatocellular carcinoma (HCC), it was indicated that this increase in migration and invasion could be through the rearrangement of actin cytoskeleton and integrin signaling which also plays a key role in autophagy (Zeng and Tarbell, 2014). In starved HeLa cells, microfilament and autophagic markers were colocalized and inhibition of microfilaments decreased autophagy as well (Aguilera et al., 2012). Further another study on HepG32 cells, confirmed the role of SS on autophagy and cytoskeletal proteins as FSS seems to induce cytoskeletal remodeling and migration through activation of autophagy (Yan et al., 2019). In our study, we found a significant increase LC3B puncta after increased exposure to ASS (10 dyn/cm^2) for 60 min (**Figures 1A–D**). Further, we observed an increase in secretion of exosomes containing autophagy factors such as LC3B after exposure to ASS (**Figures 2F–K**). Another study indicated that ASS induced formation, accumulation, and fusion of autophagosome with multivesicular body which is then released into the extracellular space through EVs (Wang et al., 2019). We also observed that exposure to ASS increased apoptosis in NSCLCs, however, inhibition of exosome release significantly increased apoptotic rate (**Figures 3C–F**). These results clearly indicated that the cancer cells releases Exosomes with the autophagic components as a protective mechanism against apoptosis.

To understand the mechanism underlying such release in exosomes and autophagic components by NSCLC exposed to ASS, we explored the role of sirtuins, a family of proteins previously identified to be associated with autophagy and lysosomal pathway. A study by Latifkar et al. (2019) (McAndrews et al., 2019), identified sirtuin 1 (SIRT1) levels were significantly decreased in the triple negative breast cancer patients, and from their *in vitro* studies it was evident that the knockdown of SIRT1 significantly increased release of exosomes and autophagic factors. In our study, interestingly we observed no significant decrease in SIRT1 levels, however, we observed a significant decrease in SIRT2 levels in NSCLC cells exposed to ASS (**Figures 4A,B**). Further, overexpression (OE) of SIRT2 significantly decreased exosome and autophagic component release, this effect was similar to the use of autophagic inhibitor (GW4689) (**Figure 4C**). Additionally, it was also evident that OE of SIRT2 increased apoptosis of NSCLCs (**Figure 4E**), thus clearly indicating that SIRT2 is necessary for the anti-tumorigenic effect of ASS.

Next, we were curious as to how SIRT2 regulated autophagy in NSCLCs, and assessed the expression of its down stream target TFEB. In NSCLCs, we observed that TFEB was also highly downregulated, and silencing of SIRT2 decreases TFEB expression (**Figure 6C**). RNA immunoprecipitation assays indicated that SIRT2 binds to the 3′ UTR of TFEB and thus regulates its expression (**Figure 6E**). TFEB has been previously reported to link autophagy and lysosomal biogenesis pathways (Settembre et al., 2011). Specifically, TFEB seems to be phosphorylated by mTOR and the dephosphorylated TFEB migrates to the nucleus where it activates many lysosomal and autophagy related target genes (Napolitano and Ballabio, 2016). Further, TFEB also has been identified to bind to many autophagy associated genes and thus activate autophagosome biogenesis and autophagosome–lysosome fusion (Settembre et al., 2011). In the current study, we observed that TFEB overexpression increased the autophagosome and lysosome fusion as indicated by the increased co-localization of LC3B and LAMP1 near the nucleus. It was also evident that TFEB overexpression decreased exosomes, autophagic component release, and increased apoptosis in ASS exposed NSCLC cells (**Figure 7**).

We also observed that SIRT2 overexpression significantly decreased the levels of metastatic nodules in the lungs and liver of the *in vivo* mice model (**Figures 8C–F**). Further, we observed that SIRT2 and TFEB were downregulated in human NSCLC tissues and their decreased expression correlated with poor prognosis in patients (**Figure 9**).

CONCLUSION

These evidences clearly indicate for the first time, the role of SIRT2 and TFEB in tumorigenesis of NSCLCs. Further, it also sheds light on the protective mechanisms of cancerous cells under exposure to ASS, thus providing potential drug targets for the treatment of NSCLC. Further, studies on LSS in NSCLC could shed more light on the intrinsic mechanisms associated with metastasis and tumorigenesis.

ETHICS STATEMENT

The animal study was reviewed and approved by the Ethical Committee for Animal Research of Xin Hua Hospital Affiliated to Shanghai Jiao Tong University School of Medicine. Written informed consent was obtained from the individual(s), and minor(s)' legal guardian/next of kin, for the publication of any potentially identifiable images or data included in this article.

AUTHOR CONTRIBUTIONS

HX and HZ conceived the project and designed the research. LW, PX, XX, FH, LJ, RH, and FD performed the experiments. LW, PX, HX, and HZ analyzed the data, discussed the research, and wrote the manuscript. All authors contributed to the article and approved the submitted version.

ACKNOWLEDGMENTS

We would like to acknowledge our lab colleagues for their help in cell experiments and animal feeding.

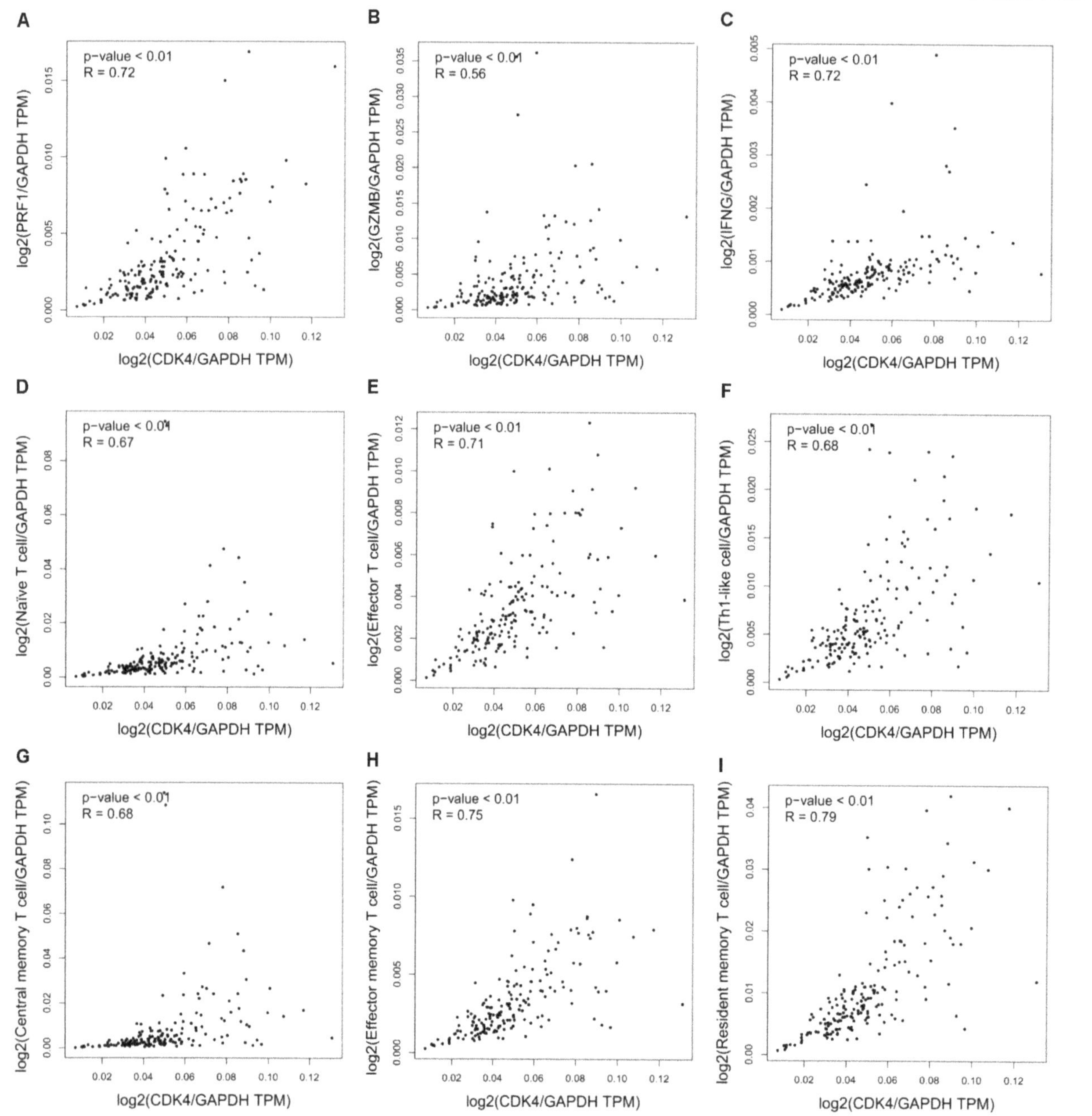

FIGURE 1 | CDK4 correlates with immune regulation in pancreatic cancer. **(A–C)** Correlation analysis of CDK4 and the immune effector molecules PRF1 **(A)**, GZMB **(B)**, and IFNG **(C)** in PAAD. **(D–I)** Correlation analysis of CDK4 and immune cell signatures in PAAD, including naïve T cell signatures **(D)**, effector T cell signatures **(E)**, Th1-like cell signatures **(F)**, central memory T cell signatures **(G)**, effector memory T cell signatures **(H)**, and resident memory T cell signatures **(I)**. *P*-values $\leq$ 0.05 were considered statistically significant.

METHODS

Data on the prognostic potential of CDK4/6 and RB1 in pancreatic cancer were collected from The Cancer Genome Atlas (TCGA)[1] database. The Tumor and Immune System Interaction Database[2] was used to examine the correlation between the abundance of immunomodulators and the expression of investigative genes. Gene Expression Profiling Interactive Analysis 2[3] was used to calculate the prognostic index, including gene expression level and its correlation to patient survival. cBioPortal for Cancer Genomics[4] was used to visualize and compare gene alterations. A one-way ANOVA was used to

[1] http://cancergenome.nih.gov

[2] http://cis.hku.hk/TISIDB

[3] http://gepia2.cancer-pku.cn

[4] http://www.cbioportal.org

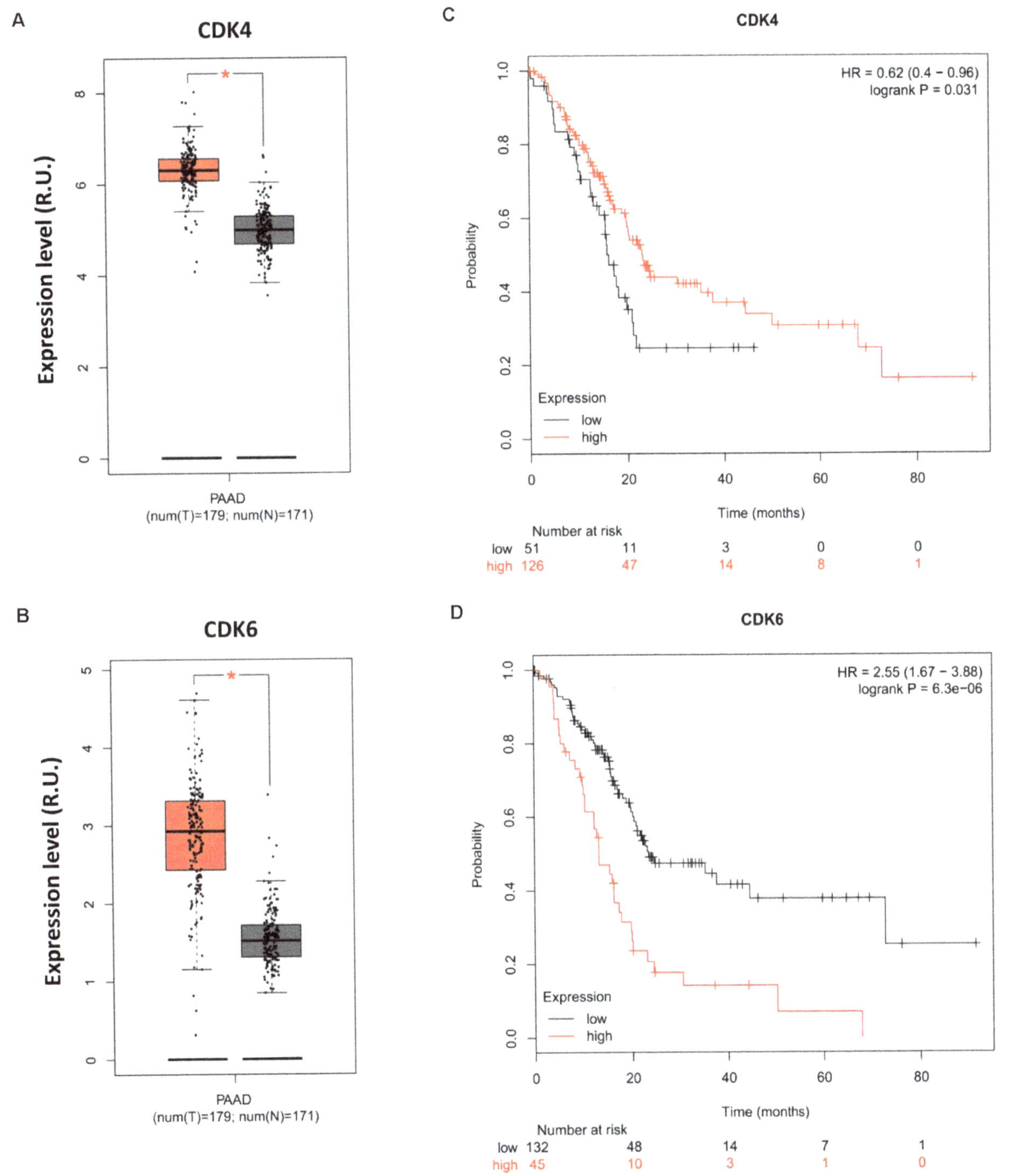

FIGURE 2 | Opposite prognoses of CDK4 and CDK6 in pancreatic cancer. Differential expression analysis of **(A)** CDK4 and **(B)** CDK6 in PAAD. OS analysis of **(C)** CDK4 and **(D)** CDK4 in PDA. *P*-values ≤ 0.05 were considered statistically significant. $*p \leq 0.01$.

analyze the differential expression of CDK4/6 and RB1 and the abundance of immunomodulators. Genes with |log2FC| values > 1 and *q* values < 0.01 were considered statistically significant. Overall survival (OS) analyses of CDK4/6 and RB1 were assessed using the Kaplan–Meier method, with a 50% (median) cutoff for both low and high expression groups. The log-rank test (the Mantel–Cox test) was used for hypothesis testing, and the Cox proportional hazard regression model was used to calculate the hazard ratio. *P*-values ≤ 0.05 were used as a threshold when ranking the data. Spearman correlation analysis was used to analyze the correlation between the pair-wise gene expression of CDK4 and a range

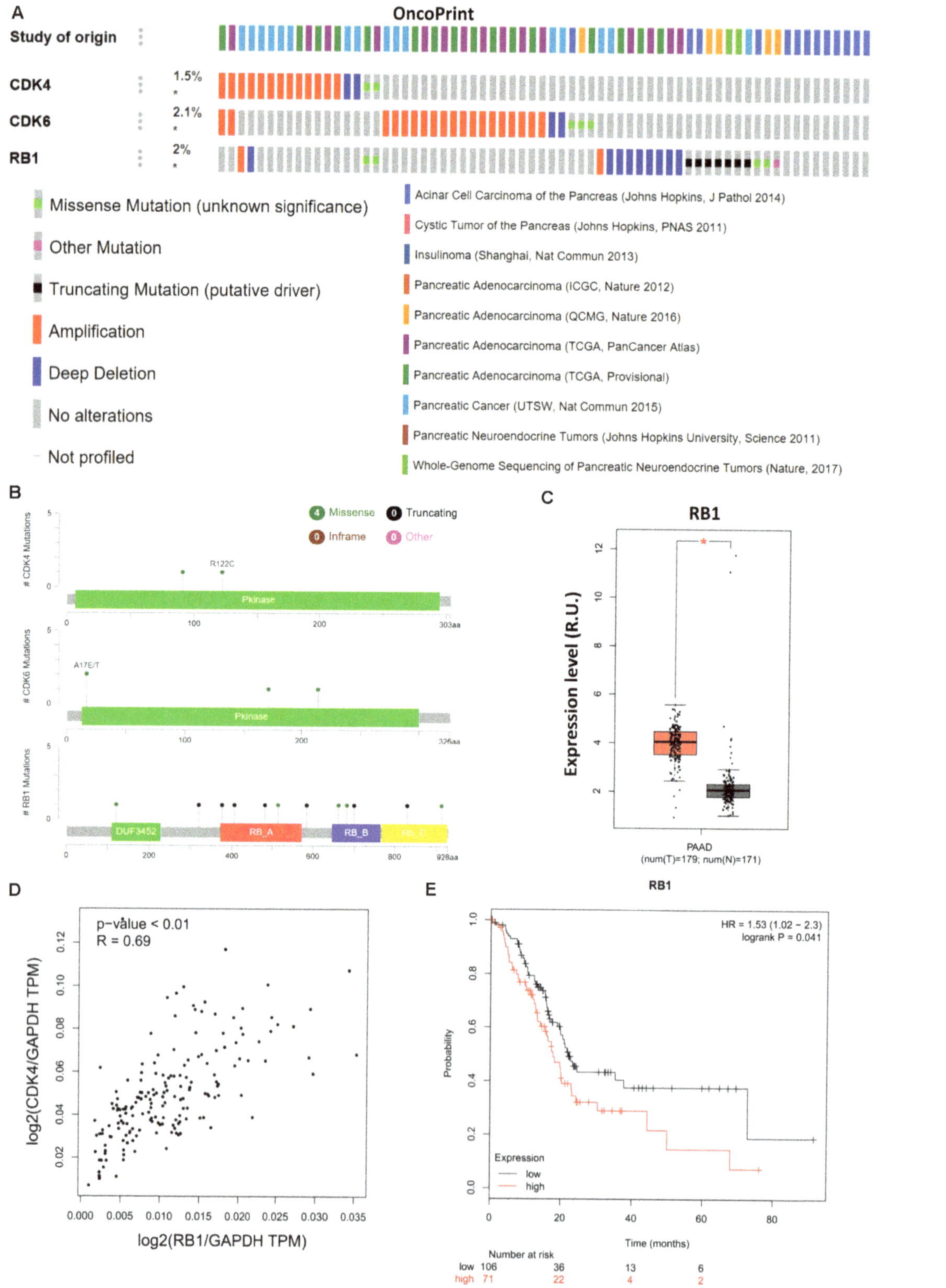

FIGURE 3 | RB1 couples with CDK4 and is related to poor prognosis in pancreatic cancer. **(A)** Landscape of the CDK4/6–RB1 axis in pancreatic cancer. Compact visualization of cases with different genetic alterations, including fusions, amplification, deletions, truncating mutations, and missense mutations. **(B)** Detailed mutational analysis of CDK4, CDK6, and RB1 in pancreatic cancer. **(C)** Differential expression analysis of RB1 in PAAD. **(D)** Correlation analysis of RB1 and CDK4 in PAAD. **(E)** OS analysis of RB1 in PAAD. *P*-values ≤ 0.05 were considered statistically significant. $^{*}p \leq 0.01$.

of immunomodulators. *P*-values < 0.01 were considered as significant. CDK4-related immunomodulators were collected, according to Charoentong et al.

RESULTS

Cyclin-Dependent Kinase 4 Correlates With Immune Regulation in Pancreatic Cancer

Despite the importance of immune activation for cancer therapy (Sanmamed and Chen, 2018), experimental models for PDA therapeutics often fail to recapitulate host defense systems. Chou et al. (2018) used patient-derived tumor xenografts, which must be implanted into immunodeficient mice, to analyze the therapeutic efficacy of CDK4 inhibition on pancreatic cancer. This inevitably bypasses any immune involvement and fails to recapitulate the tumor immune microenvironment. Moreover, previous studies have validated the role of CDK4 in the regulation of cancer immunity and immunotherapy. Goel et al. (2017) reported that CDK4/6 inhibition triggers anticancer immune responses in breast cancer, and Zhang et al. (2018) showed that cyclin D-CDK4 kinase destabilizes programmed death-ligand 1 via the Cul3^{SPOP} complex to control cancer immunosurveillance in melanoma cancer. To determine the immunologic relevance of CDK4 in pancreatic cancer, we integrated all relevant datasets in the TCGA database for bioinformatics analyses. In pancreatic adenocarcinoma (PAAD), the results showed a positive correlation between CDK4 and the immunomodulatory system, including the immune effector molecules PRF1, GZMB, and IFNG (**Figures 1A–C**), as well as immune cells (naïve T cells, effector T cells, Th1-like cells, central memory T cells, effector memory T cells, and resident memory T cells) (**Figures 1D–I**). These data suggest that the outcomes of CDK4-based PDA therapy in immunocompromised models have limited significance to the clinical treatment of PDA.

Opposite Prognoses of Cyclin-Dependent Kinase 4 and 6 in Pancreatic Cancer

Chou et al. (2018) recently highlighted the potential of CDK4 inhibitors as a targeted therapy for pancreatic cancer. However, Palbociclib (PD-0332991, Pfizer), the major CDK4-targeted drug used in the study, is a small molecule inhibitor designed to block the activity of both CDK4 and CDK6 to promote cytostasis (O'Leary et al., 2016). The concomitant effects of this therapy on CDK6 in more relevant physiological models of pancreatic cancer can, therefore, not be discounted. In light of this, we analyzed relevant genomic data and observed the opposite effects of CDK4 and CDK6 on pancreatic cancer prognosis. The expression levels of CDK4 and CDK6 were highly upregulated in PAAD compared with normal tissue (**Figures 2A,B**); however, CDK4 promoted rather than suppressed the OS of PDA patients (**Figure 2C**), whereas high CDK6 expression was associated with poor survival (**Figure 2D**). This phenotype implicates CDK6 as opposed to CDK4 for the poor prognosis of PDA in the clinic and questions the therapeutic benefits of Palbociclib in PDA therapy due to its synergistic effects on CDK4 and CDK6. In light of these data, patient-derived primary cell lines that genetically lack CDK4 and CDK6 should be generated to investigate their significance during Palbociclib treatment and exclude off-target effects. Of note, the combination of palbociclib and gemcitabine was investigated in the study as mentioned earlier, but the therapeutic efficacy of gemcitabine has been reported to be influenced by tumor immune microenvironment during pancreatic cancer therapy (Halbrook et al., 2019), which further highlights the importance of appropriate models in evaluating the CDK4/6-targeted combinational strategy.

Retinoblastoma 1 Is Coupled to Cyclin-Dependent Kinase 4 and Poor Prognosis in Pancreatic Cancer

Cyclin-dependent kinase 4/6 controls the downstream transcriptional signals that regulate cancer cell proliferation through the phosphorylation of their canonical substrate RB1. CDK4/6–phosphorylated RB1 has been shown to promote anticancer immunity by inhibiting nuclear factor-κB activation and programmed death-ligand 1 expression (Jin et al., 2019), further indicating the immunological relevance of palbociclib during cancer treatment. Moreover, aberrant CDK4/6-RB1 signaling has been reported in a range of cancers. Such alterations regulate immune evasion and immunotherapy (Hutcheson et al., 2015). Genomic analyses indicated that a similar phenotype exists in pancreatic cancer in which CDK4 regulates RB1 activation (**Figures 3A,B**). However, Chou et al. (2018) used only 19 whole-genome-sequenced pancreatic cancer patient-derived primary cell lines to exclude the potential impact of RB1 mutations *in vivo*. Although RB1 is highly expressed (**Figure 3C**) and positively related to CDK4 (**Figure 3D**) in PAAD, higher expression of RB1 was related to poor prognosis (**Figure 3E**), contradictory to the previous conclusions. The differential outcomes between genomic analysis and immunohistochemistry staining were caused by the failure to account for immune function and/or alterations in RB1. Hence, the phosphorylation of RB1 as a biomarker when predicting the therapeutic sensitivity of CDK4/6 inhibition requires further clinical and genetic analysis.

CONCLUSION

In summary, we highlight the importance of CDK4 for immune regulation. We further show that elevated CDK4 expression is a favorable prognostic index for cancer patients instead of high CDK6 expression that is close to poor prognosis. RB1 was positively related to CDK4 but linked to a poorer prognosis. These data suggest that the direct anti-tumor effects of CDK4/6 inhibition in xenografts fail to reflect their efficacy in pancreatic cancer patients. The utility of targeting CDK4/6 as a strategy for targeted-immunotherapy in pancreatic cancer now warrants further exploration.

AUTHOR CONTRIBUTIONS

XH conceived this manuscript, conducted the analyses, and interpreted the data. XH and GZ drafted, discussed, and revised the manuscript. Both authors read and approved the final version.

ACKNOWLEDGMENTS

The authors would like to gratefully thank the TCGA http://cancergenome.nih.gov) and other open-access cancer genome databases for data collection, and cBioPortal for Cancer Genomics (http://www.cbioportal.org) and Gene Expression Profiling Interactive Analysis 2 (http://gepia2.cancer-pku.cn) for providing data processing and customizable functions. Especially, XH would like to express deepest thanks to Prof. Guido Kroemer for the cancer immunity-associated technological training in his lab.

REFERENCES

Chou, A., Froio, D., Nagrial, A. M., Parkin, A., Murphy, K. J., Chin, V. T., et al. (2018). Tailored first-line and second-line CDK4-targeting treatment combinations in mouse models of pancreatic cancer. *Gut* 67, 2142–2155. doi: 10.1136/gutjnl-2017-315144

Collisson, E. A., Bailey, P., Chang, D. K., Biankin, A. V., et al. (2019). Molecular subtypes of pancreatic cancer. *Nat. Rev. Gastroenterol. Hepatol.* 16, 207–220.

Goel, S., DeCristo, M. J., Watt, A. C., BrinJones, H., Sceneay, J., Li, B. B., et al. (2017). CDK4/6 inhibition triggers anti-tumour immunity. *Nature* 548, 471–475. doi: 10.1038/nature23465

Halbrook, C. J., Pontious, C., Kovalenko, I., Lapienyte, L., Dreyer, S., Lee, H. J., et al. (2019). Macrophage-released pyrimidines inhibit gemcitabine therapy in pancreatic cancer. *Cell Metab.* 29, 1390.e6–1399.e6.

Hutcheson, J., Witkiewicz, A. K., and Knudsen, E. S. (2015). The RB tumor suppressor at the intersection of proliferation and immunity: relevance to disease immune evasion and immunotherapy. *Cell Cycle* 14, 3812–3819. doi: 10.1080/15384101.2015.1010922

Jin, X., Ding, D., Yan, Y., Li, H., Wang, B., Ma, L., et al. (2019). Phosphorylated RB promotes cancer immunity by inhibiting NF-kappaB activation and PD-L1 expression. *Mol. Cell* 73, 22.e6–35.e6.

Kleeff, J., Korc, M., Apte, M., La Vecchia, C., Johnson, C. D., Biankin, A. V., et al. (2016). Pancreatic cancer. *Nat. Rev. Dis. Primers* 2:16022.

O'Leary, B., Finn, R. S., and Turner, N. C. (2016). Treating cancer with selective CDK4/6 inhibitors. *Nat. Rev. Clin. Oncol.* 13, 417–430. doi: 10.1038/nrclinonc.2016.26

Rubin, S. M. (2013). Deciphering the retinoblastoma protein phosphorylation code. *Trends Biochem. Sci.* 38, 12–19. doi: 10.1016/j.tibs.2012.10.007

Sanmamed, M. F., and Chen, L. (2018). A paradigm shift in cancer immunotherapy: from enhancement to normalization. *Cell* 175, 313–326. doi: 10.1016/j.cell.2018.09.035

van den Heuvel, S., and Dyson, N. J. (2008). Conserved functions of the pRB and E2F families. *Nat. Rev. Mol. Cell. Biol.* 9, 713–724. doi: 10.1038/nrm2469

Zhang, J., Bu, X., Wang, H., Zhu, Y., Geng, Y., Nihira, N. T., et al. (2018). Cyclin D-CDK4 kinase destabilizes PD-L1 via cullin 3-SPOP to control cancer immune surveillance. *Nature* 553, 91–95. doi: 10.1038/nature25015

11

BAP31 Promotes Tumor Cell Proliferation by Stabilizing SERPINE2 in Hepatocellular Carcinoma

Xiyang Zhang[†]*, Dongbo Jiang*[†]*, Shuya Yang*[†]*, Yuanjie Sun, Yang Liu, Jingqi Shi, Chenchen Hu, Jingyu Pan, Tianyue Liu, Boquan Jin and Kun Yang*[*]

Department of Immunology, The Fourth Military Medical University, Xi'an, China

***Correspondence:**
Kun Yang
yangkunkun@fmmu.edu.cn

[†]*These authors share first authorship*

Hepatocellular carcinoma (HCC) patients are mostly diagnosed at an advanced stage, resulting in systemic therapy and poor prognosis. Therefore, the identification of a novel treatment target for HCC is important. B-cell receptor-associated protein 31 (BAP31) has been identified as a cancer/testis antigen; however, BAP31 function and mechanism of action in HCC remain unclear. In this study, BAP31 was demonstrated to be upregulated in HCC and correlated with the clinical stage. BAP31 overexpression promoted HCC cell proliferation and colony formation *in vitro* and tumor growth *in vivo*. RNA-sequence (RNA-seq) analysis demonstrated that serpin family E member 2 (SERPINE2) was downregulated in BAP31-knockdown HCC cells. Coimmunoprecipitation and immunofluorescence assays demonstrated that BAP31 directly binds to SERPINE2. The inhibition of SERPINE2 significantly decreased the BAP31-induced cell proliferation and colony formation of HCC cells and phosphorylation of Erk1/2 and p38. Moreover, multiplex immunohistochemistry staining of the HCC tissue microarray showed positive associations between the expression levels of BAP31, SERPINE2, its downstream gene LRP1, and a tumor proliferation marker, Ki-67. The administration of anti-BAP31 antibody significantly inhibited HCC cell xenograft tumor growth *in vivo*. Thus, these findings suggest that BAP31 promotes tumor cell proliferation by stabilizing SERPINE2 and can serve as a promising candidate therapeutic target for HCC.

Keywords: B-cell receptor-associated protein 31 (BAP31), serpin family E member 2 (SERPINE2), hepatocellular carcinoma (HCC), cell proliferation, molecular target therapy

INTRODUCTION

Liver cancer is ranked the sixth most common diagnosed cancer and the fourth leading cause of cancer death worldwide with 841,000 new cases and 782,000 deaths in 2018 (Bray et al., 2018). Hepatocellular carcinoma (HCC) is the main histological subtype of primary liver cancer accounting for 75–85% of cases (Sia et al., 2017). Several risk factors for HCC have been identified: HBV or HCV infection, aflatoxin exposure, alcohol consumption, smoking, etc. (Budny et al., 2017; Ozakyol, 2017; Fujiwara et al., 2018). However, the specific mechanisms of pathogenesis of HCC remain unclear. Moreover, most of the HCC patients are diagnosed at an advanced stage, which is not the best time for surgery treatment, and thus, the patients have to receive systemic therapy (Villanueva, 2019). Therefore, the identification of a novel treatable target will advance the understanding of the molecular pathogenesis of HCC and provide clues for clinical molecular-targeted therapy.

B-cell receptor-associated protein 31 (BAP31) has been identified as a cancer/testis antigen (Dang et al., 2018) that plays an important role in promoting the development of several types of cancers via diverse molecular mechanisms. The abnormal high expression of BAP31 was initially detected in cervical cancer, and BAP31 expression was positively correlated with the clinical stages of cervical cancer (Dang et al., 2018). Subsequently, Chen et al. (2019) demonstrated that BAP31 can promote the proliferation of gastric cancer cells by interacting with cyclin kinase inhibitor $p27^{kip1}$. Xu et al. (2019) found that miR-451a binds to the 5′-UTR of BAP31, induces the endoplasmic reticulum (ER) stress, and leads to the inhibition of cell proliferation in colorectal cancer. A recent study has shown that BAP31 may promote the migration and invasion of lung cancer cells via the Akt/m-TOR/p70S6K pathway (Wang et al., 2020). However, the function of BAP31 in HCC cells remains unclear.

In this study, the function of BAP31 in HCC was investigated *in vitro* and *in vivo*. BAP31 expression was associated with clinical stages in HCC patients. BAP31 overexpression significantly promoted proliferation and colony formation of HCC cells, and downregulation of BAP31 reversed this process. *In vivo* studies validated the promotion of tumor growth by BAP31 overexpression, and downregulation of BAP31 inhibited tumor growth. The major mechanism of action includes direct BAP31 binding to and upregulation of serpin family E member 2 (SERPINE2), resulting in an increase in the phosphorylation levels of Erk and p38. Inhibition of SERPINE2 attenuated BAP31-induced cell proliferation. Additionally, an anti-BAP31 antibody significantly suppressed HCC cell xenograft tumor formation. Our findings suggest that targeting BAP31 may be an effective strategy for HCC treatment.

MATERIALS AND METHODS

Cell Cultures

The human HCC cell lines Hep3b and MHCC97h were used in this study; Hep3b cell line was purchased from GeneChem Co., Ltd. (Shanghai, China), and MHCC97h cell line was obtained from the Department of Hepatological Surgery, Xijing Hospital (Xi'an, China). Both cell lines had been authenticated by STR profiling and tested for mycoplasma contamination. Cells were cultured in high-glucose Dulbecco's Modified Eagle's Medium (DMEM) (HyClone, USA) supplemented with 10% FBS (Gibco, Gaithersburg, MD, USA) and 1% penicillin/streptomycin (Solarbio, China) under 5% CO_2 at 37°C.

BAP31 Overexpression and Knockdown by Lentivirus Infection

Full-length BAP31 cDNA (NCBI Reference Sequence: NM_005745.7) was cloned into the pCDH-CMV-MCS-EF1-GFP-Puro vector. The GFP-BAP31 lentivirus and vector control were constructed by GeneCreate Co., Ltd. (Wuhan, China). BAP31-specific shRNA (GGTGAACCTCCAGAACAAT) was inserted into the hU6-MCS-Ubiquitin-EGFP-IRES-Puro vector. The BAP31-shRNA lentivirus and vector control were constructed by GeneChem Co., Ltd. (Shanghai, China).

Hep3b and MHCC97h cells were seeded in 96-well plates. After 24 h, 10 μl of virus [diluted in enhanced infection solution (ENi.S.), 1×10^8 TU/ml] and 10 μl of polybrene (E) (diluted polybrene in ENi.S., 50 μg/ml) was added to 80 μl of ENi.S. per well. After 12 h, the infection solution was removed and replaced with fresh medium containing 10% FBS. Puromycin (5 μg/ml) (MP Biomedicals, Shanghai, China) was added into the supernatant to select transfected cells. BAP31 expression was validated by qPCR and western blot.

RNA Isolation, Quantitative Real-Time RT-PCR, and RNA-Sequence Analysis

Total RNA was isolated using TRIzol reagent (Invitrogen, USA). cDNA was generated by PrimeScript RT Master Mix (TaKaRa, Tokyo, Japan), and quantitative real-time PCR was performed using SYBR-green PCR Master Mix (TaKaRa). Human β-actin gene was used as an internal control. PCR assays were performed three times, and the expression of the genes was calculated using the comparative Ct method (ΔΔCt). PCR primers for BCAP31 were 5′-CGGCTGGTGGAGTTGTTAGT-3′ (sense) and 5′-CGGGATTGTTCTGGAGGTT-3′ (antisense) (Sangon Biotech, China).

The differentially expressed genes in BAP31-knockdown cells were identified using RNA-sequence (RNA-Seq) analysis. Total RNA was extracted and sent to LC-Bio Technology Co., Ltd. for sequencing (Hangzhou, China).

The raw sequence data reported in this paper have been deposited in the Genome Sequence Archive (Genomics, Proteomics, and Bioinformatics 2017) in the National Genomics Data Center (Nucleic Acids Res 2020), Beijing Institute of Genomics (China National Center for Bioinformation), Chinese Academy of Sciences, under accession number CRA003471 that is publicly accessible at https://bigd.big.ac.cn/gsa/s/5N91IqLS (Wang et al., 2017; National Genomics Data Center Members and Partners, 2020).

siRNA Interference and Transfection

SERPINE2-siRNA was purchased from GenePharma (Shanghai, China); the siRNA sequences for SERPINE2 were as follows: si-SERPINE2 #1, 5′-GCUAACGCCGUGUUUGUUATT-3′ (sense) and 5′-UAACAAACACGGCGUUA-GCTT-3′ (antisense) and si-SERPINE2 #2, 5′-CCAGGGAUAUGAUUGACAATT-3′ (sense) and 5′-UUGUCAAUCAUAUCCCUGGTT-3′ (antisense). All transient transfections were performed using Attractene Transfection Reagent (QIAGEN, Germany) for 72 h.

Cell Proliferation and Colony Formation Assays

Cells were seeded into a 96-well plate at a density of 5×10^3 cells per well for 1, 2, or 3 days. Cell counting kit-8 (CCK-8) reagent (EnoGene, China) was added at a dilution of 1:10 to each well and incubated for 3 h. The absorbance was then measured at a wavelength of 450 nm using a SpectraMax plate reader (Molecular Devices, USA).

A total of 500 cells were seeded into 60-mm dishes and cultured in DMEM for 2 weeks. The colonies were then fixed with precooled ethanol and stained with a 0.5% crystal violet

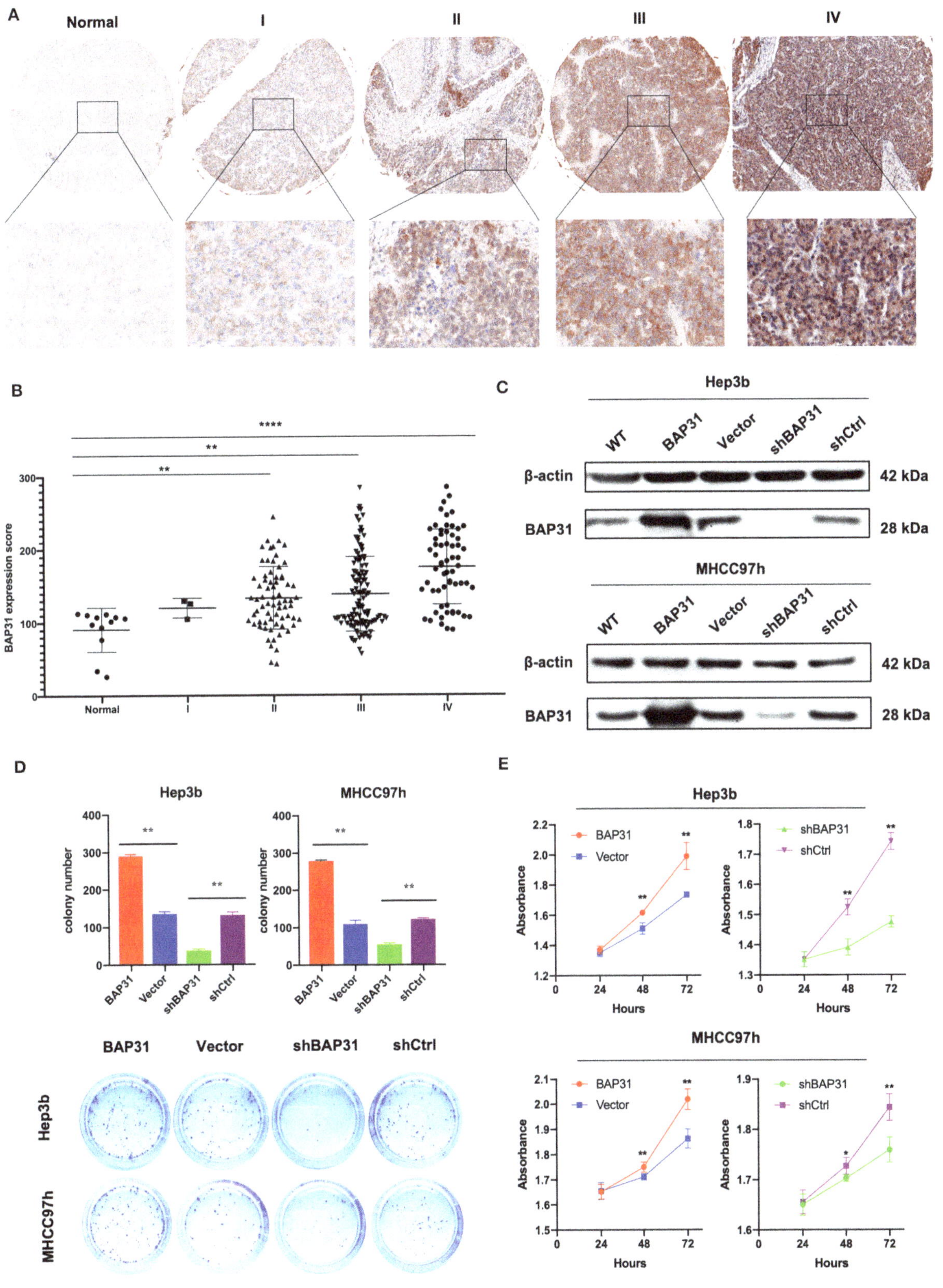

FIGURE 1 | BAP31 expression is increased in HCC patients and involved in HCC cell proliferation *in vitro*. **(A)** Expression of BAP31 in normal liver and HCC tumor tissues at various clinical stages monitored by IHC analysis. **(B)** Expression of BAP31 in 12 normal liver and 248 HCC tumor tissue samples. **(C)** Western blot analysis *(Continued)*

FIGURE 1 | of BAP31expression in Hep3b and MHCC97h cells after stable transfection using lentivirus. **(D)** Colony formation assay using Hep3b and MHCC97h cells. Representative images were acquired, and the colonies were counted. **(E)** Cell viability of Hep3b and MHCC97h cells detected by the cell counting kit-8 assay. *$p < 0.05$; **$p < 0.01$; ****$p < 0.0001$. BAP31, B-cell receptor-associated protein 31; HCC, hepatocellular carcinoma; IHC, immunohistochemistry.

TABLE 1 | Correlation between the expression of BAP31 and clinicopathological parameters in HCC.

Characteristics	BAP31 low expression		BAP31 high expression		P
	N	%	*N*	%	
Gender					0.257
Male	93	76.2	88	69.8	
Female	29	23.8	38	30.2	
Age (years)					0.545
≤50	55	45.1	52	41.3	
>50	67	54.9	74	58.7	
Tumor size					0.002*
T1 or T2	48	39.3	27	21.4	
T3 or T4	74	60.7	99	78.6	
Lymph node					<0.0001*
N0	107	87.7	80	63.5	
N1	15	12.3	46	36.5	
Grade					0.461
–	9	7.4	12	9.5	
1	5	4.1	9	7.2	
2 or 3	108	88.5	105	83.3	
Stage					<0.0001*
I or II	65	53.2	28	22.2	
III or IV	57	46.7	98	77.8	

**Statistically significant.*

solution (Xi'an Hat Biotechnology, China). Each experiment was performed in triplicate and repeated three times.

Western Blot and Immunoprecipitation Assays

For detection of the protein levels of BAP31, SERPINE2, β-actin, Erk1/2, phospho-Erk1/2, p38, and phospho-p38, total protein was extracted using RIPA lysis buffer with protease and phosphatase inhibitors (Beyotime, China) from HCC cell lines. Protein concentrations were determined using a BCA protein assay kit. Proteins with different molecular weight were separated using 10% SDS-PAGE (Epizyme, China) and then transferred to a nitrocellulose membrane. After blocking with 5% non-fat milk (BD Biosciences, USA), the membranes were incubated with antibodies against BAP31 (Proteintech, China; 11200-1-AP; 1:2,000), SERPINE2 (Proteintech; 66203-1-Ig; 1:1,000), β-actin (Proteintech; 60008-1-Ig; 1:5,000), Erk1/2, p38 (Cell Signaling Technology, USA; 9926; 1:1,000), and phospho-Erk1/2, phospho-p38 (Cell Signaling Technology; 9910; 1:1,000).

For immunoprecipitation, a lysis buffer was prepared as follows: 20 mM HEPES, 150 mM NaCl, 2 mM EDTA, 1.5 mM $MgCl_2$, 0.5% NP-40, and protease and phosphatase inhibitor (TargetMol, China). Cells were lysed using lysis buffer, and the supernatant was collected after centrifugation. Anti-BAP31 mouse monoclonal antibody (FMU-BAP31-2, preserved in our laboratory), anti-SERPINE2 antibody (Proteintech; 11303-1-AP), and mouse IgG isotype were added to the lysates with protein A beads and incubated overnight. The beads were collected and subjected to western blot.

Immunofluorescence Assays

Cells were seeded into a 15-mm glass bottom cell culture dish at a cell density of 30%. After three washes with phosphate-buffered saline (PBS), the cells were fixed with 4% formaldehyde and permeabilized with 0.2% Triton X-100 for 10 min. After blocking with 1% BSA, the cells were incubated with an anti-SERPINE2 rabbit polyclonal antibody for 2 h at room temperature. Cells were washed three times in PBS and incubated with mixed Cy5-labeled anti-BAP31 mouse monoclonal antibody and Cy3-labeled donkey anti-rabbit IgG for 1.5 h at room temperature. Cells were rinsed with PBS three times, stained with 4′,6-diamidino-2-phenylindole (DAPI), and analyzed with a confocal laser scanning microscope (Nikon, Japan).

Multiplex Immunohistochemistry Staining

The HCC tissue microarrays LV2089 and LV1221 (Alenabio, China) were deparaffinized in xylene and rehydrated in an ethanol gradient. Microarrays were stained according to Opal 7-plex technology (PerkinElmer) to simultaneously visualize five markers (DAPI was used to stain the nuclei) on the same slide. During each of the six cycles of staining, antigen retrieval (AR) was performed via microwave treatment in AR solution pH 6 or pH 9 (AR6 or AR9) suggested by immunohistochemistry (IHC) validation; blocking was followed by incubation for 15 min at room temperature (RT); primary antibodies [anti-BAP31 mouse monoclonal antibody, anti-SERPINE2 antibody, anti-LRP1 antibody (Abcam; ab92544), and anti-Ki67 antibody (Immunoway; YM6189)] were then incubated for 1 h at RT or overnight at 4°C. Then, HRP-labeled polymer goat anti-mouse and rabbit antibodies were incubated at RT for 10 min followed by 10-min incubation with tyramide signal amplification (TSA) opal fluorophores (Opal 520, Opal 570, Opal 620, or Opal 690). Microwave treatment was performed to remove the antibody–TSA complex at each cycle of staining with AR solution (pH 9 or pH 6). Finally, both microarrays were counterstained with DAPI for 5 min and enclosed in ProLong antifade mounting liquid (Solarbio). The slides were scanned using a PerkinElmer Mantra system (PerkinElmer), and the multispectral images were unmixed using spectral libraries that were previously built from the images stained for each fluorophore (mono-plex) using the inForm advanced image analysis software (inForm 2.4.1, PerkinElmer).

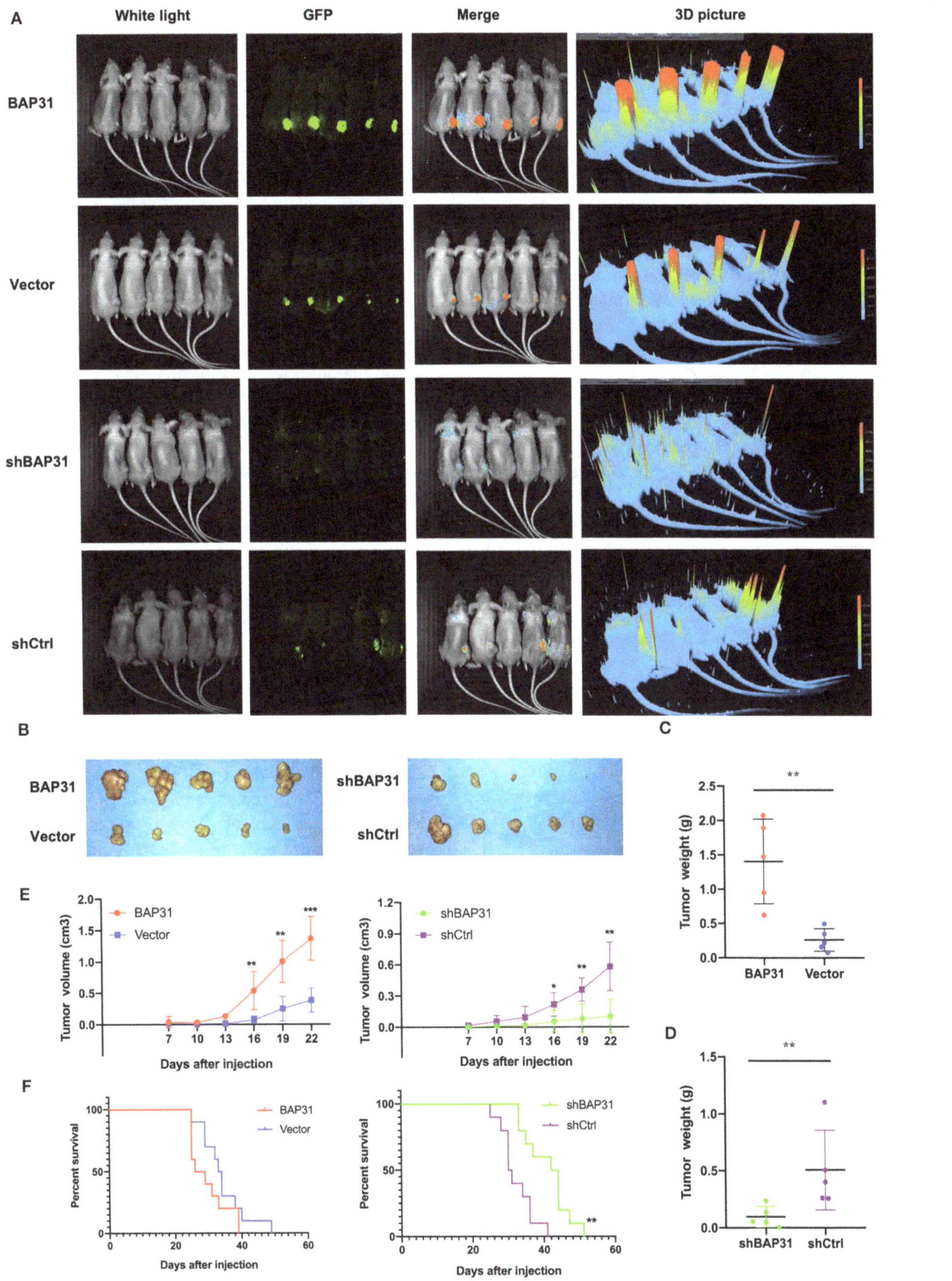

FIGURE 2 | BAP31 promotes HCC cell proliferation *in vivo*. **(A)** BAP31 overexpression, BAP31 knockdown, and the corresponding control Hep3b cells were injected into the right flanks of nude mice. Images of tumors were acquired with FUSION FX Spectra after 20 days. **(B–D)** Images of tumors and tumor weight of nude mice 30

(Continued)

FIGURE 2 | days after subcutaneous injection of Hep3b cells. The results represent the mean ± SD, and $^{**}p < 0.01$ was considered significant; Student's *t*-test was used. **(E)** Growth curve of xenografts of Hep3b cells transfected with BAP31, vector, BAP31shRNA, and scramble shRNA ($n = 5$, mean ± SD). **(F)** Kaplan–Meier survival curve representing the overall survival of the injected mice with BAP31 overexpression or knockdown and control Hep3b cells ($n = 10$, $^{**}p < 0.01$ by log-rank test). BAP31, B-cell receptor-associated protein 31; HCC, hepatocellular carcinoma; IHC, immunohistochemistry. $^{*}p < 0.05$, $^{**}p < 0.01$, and $^{***}p < 0.001$.

Animal Experiments

For tumor xenograft, stable BAP31-overexpressing and -knockdown Hep3b cells were injected subcutaneously (2×10^6 cell per site) into the right flanks of nude mice (8-week-old) (Department of Laboratory Animal Medicine of the Fourth Military Medical University). Hep3b cells transfected with the vector and control shRNAs were used. Five mice were randomly included in each group; mice were examined every 3 days to monitor tumor development. The size of the tumors was estimated with FUSION FX Spectra (Vilber, France), measured using calipers, and calculated as follows: length × width × height; the size was expressed in cubic centimeters. The differences in survival time were observed with 10 mice in each group.

For antibody treatment, anti-BAP31 mouse monoclonal antibody (10 mg/kg), mouse IgG isotype (10 mg/kg), and PBS (same volume as antibody) were intraperitoneally injected two times a week after Hep3b cell injection. This study was approved by the institutional review board of the Fourth Military Medical University.

Statistical Analysis

All experiments were repeated at least three times, and graphs were created by GraphPad Prism software 8.0 (San Diego, CA, USA). Student's *t*-test was used to compare the mean between two groups, and one-way analysis of variance (ANOVA) was used to compare three or more groups. Survival curves were evaluated using the Kaplan–Meier method. Correlations between two genes were analyzed using Pearson's correlation. $P < 0.05$ was considered statistically significant.

RESULTS

BAP31 Expression Is Increased in HCC Patients and Is Involved in HCC Cell Proliferation *in vitro*

To explore BAP31 characteristics in HCC, immunohistochemistry (IHC) staining was performed to determine the expression patterns of BAP31 using two tissue microarrays (LV2089 and LV1221) of 248 available HCC samples and 12 normal controls. The BAP31 expression was significantly increased in HCC tissue compared with that in normal liver tissue and was correlated with the clinical stage (**Figures 1A,B**). To evaluate the clinical significance of BAP31, the relationship between BAP31 expression levels and general characteristics of HCC patients was analyzed, including gender, age, tumor size, lymph node, grade, and tumor stage. The HCC patients were divided into high- and low-expression groups based on the median expression level of BAP31. Statistical analyses indicated that BAP31 expression was associated with the tumor size, lymph node metastasis, and tumor stage (**Table 1**).

To evaluate the function of BAP31 in HCC cells, stable Hep3b and MHCC97h cell lines transfected with BAP31-overexpressing and BAP31-knockdown vectors were established. Western blot assay was performed to test the efficiency of the overexpression and knockdown systems (**Figure 1C**). BAP31 knockdown significantly inhibited the colony formation of Hep3b and MHCC97h cell lines; however, the number of colonies was substantially increased in BAP31-overexpressing cells (**Figure 1D**). Moreover, the effect of BAP31 on HCC cell proliferation was investigated. BAP31 knockdown inhibited proliferation of Hep3b and MHCC97h cells, and ectopic BAP31 expression enhanced proliferation of HCC cells (**Figure 1E**).

BAP31 Promotes HCC Cell Proliferation *in vivo*

To investigate the function of BAP31 *in vivo*, stable BAP31-overexpressing, BAP31-knockdown, and control Hep3b cells were subcutaneously injected in nude mice. Twenty days after the injection, the tumor formation in four groups of mice was estimated with a FUSION FX Spectra imaging system. The tumor size was significantly decreased by BAP31 knockdown in Hep3b cells; the tumor size was substantially increased by BAP31 overexpression (**Figure 2A**). A similar result was observed in the tumors 30 days after the injection (**Figure 2B**). Moreover, the tumor weight of BAP31 knockdown group was significantly lower than that in the control group; conversely, the tumor weight of BAP31 overexpression group was substantially higher than that in the control group (**Figures 2C,D**). Additionally, the tumor growth curve indicated that the depletion of BAP31 expression inhibited tumor formation and development compared with that in the control groups (**Figure 2E**). To evaluate the effect of BAP31 expression on survival of mice, additional four animal groups were included in the study. The Kaplan–Meier survival curve showed that knockdown of BAP31 significantly increased the survival of mice in the xenograft model (**Figure 2F**).

Identification of SERPINE2 as a Novel Downstream Gene Regulated by BAP31 in HCC Cells

To investigate the molecular mechanism of BAP31-mediated regulation of HCC cell proliferation, RNA-Seq was performed in BAP31-knockdown and control Hep3b and MHCC97h cells. The expression heat map profiled that mRNA levels of various genes were changed (**Figure 3A**). An overlap in the Venn diagram showed that 108 genes were upregulated or downregulated after knockdown of BAP31 expression. A total of 13 genes out of 108 were downregulated in both HCC cell lines (**Figure 3B**). These genes included SERPINE2, which is actively involved in tumor cell proliferation and invasion (Buchholz et al., 2003; Fayard et al.,

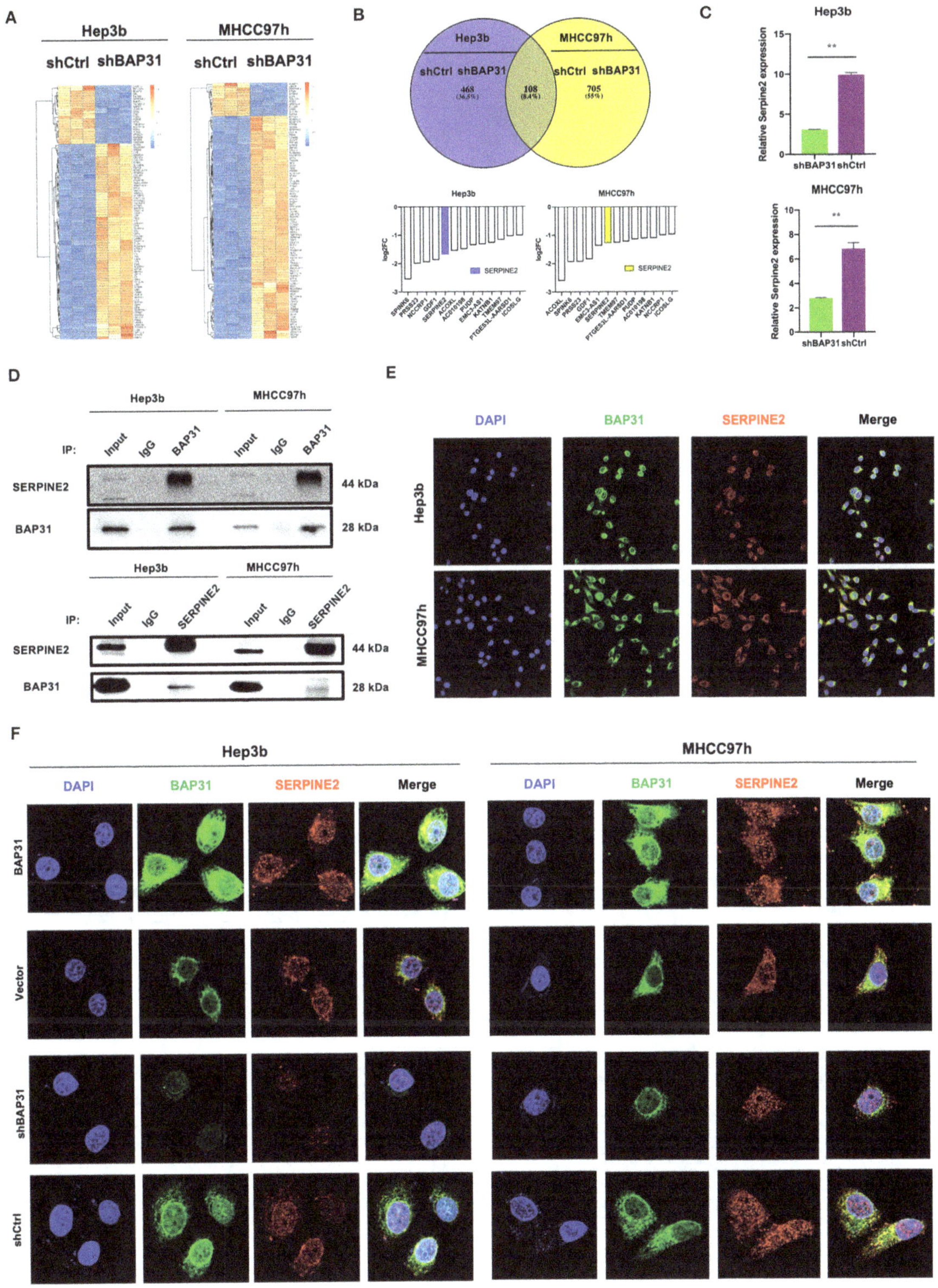

FIGURE 3 | Identification of SERPINE2 as a novel downstream gene regulated by BAP31 in HCC cells. **(A)** Identification of the genes regulated by BAP31 in HCC cells using RNA-Seq analysis. A heat map was constructed based on the genes differentially expressed between the control and BAP31-knockdown cells. **(B)** Comparative intersection analysis of differentially expressed genes in the BAP31-knockdown and control Hep3b and MHCC97h cells. **(C)** qRT-PCR analysis of SERPINE2 expression in the BAP31-knockdown and control HCC cells. **(D)** Lysates of HCC cells expressing the indicated proteins were immunoprecipitated with anti-BAP31, anti-SERPINE2, or mouse IgG isotype antibody, and the immunoprecipitates were probed with the indicated antibodies. **(E,F)** Colocalization of BAP31 (green) with SERPINE2 (red) in wild-type **(E)** and BAP31-overexpression and -knockdown and control **(F)** HCC cells according to confocal microscopy. BAP31, B-cell receptor-associated protein 31; HCC, hepatocellular carcinoma; SERPINE2, serpin family E member 2. ***p* < 0.01.

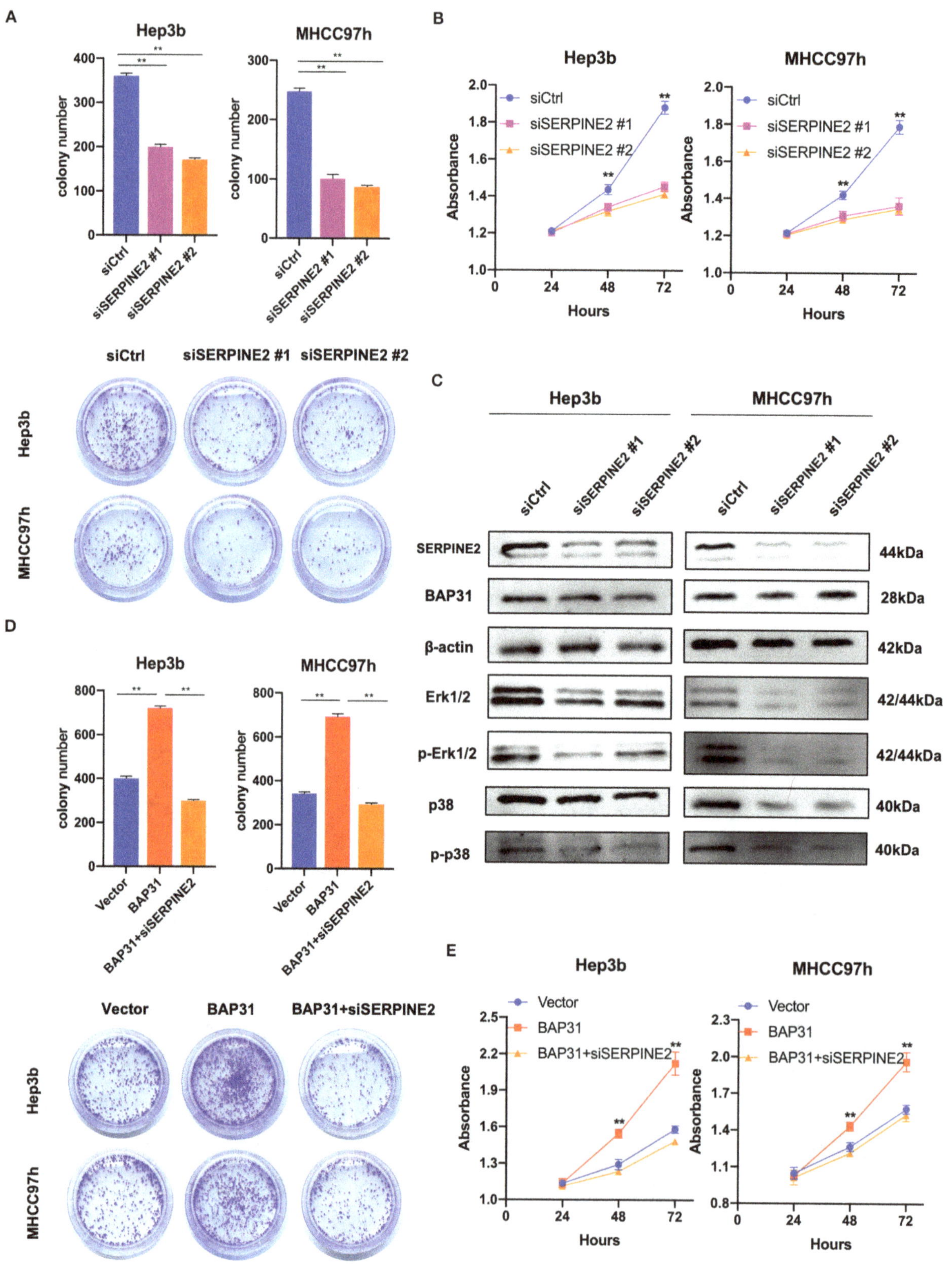

FIGURE 4 | Inhibition of SERPINE2 attenuates BAP31-promoted cell proliferation. **(A)** Colony formation assay using Hep3b and MHCC97h cells that were transiently transfected with SERPINE2 siRNA or control siRNA. Representative images were acquired, and the colony numbers were counted. **(B)** Cell viability of transiently

(Continued)

FIGURE 4 | transfected Hep3b and MHCC97h cells detected by the cell counting kit-8 assay. **(C)** Protein levels of SERPINE2, BAP31, β-actin, Erk1/2, phospho-Erk1/2, p38, and phospho-p38 were monitored by western blot. **(D)** Colony formation assay using BAP31-overexpressing HCC cells that were transiently transfected using SERPINE2 siRNA and control siRNA. **(E)** Cell viability of transiently transfected Hep3b and MHCC97h cells detected by the cell counting kit-8 assay. $^{**}p < 0.01$. BAP31, B-cell receptor-associated protein 31; SERPINE2, serpin family E member 2.

2009; Bergeron et al., 2010; McKee et al., 2012; Wang et al., 2015; Zhang et al., 2020). Therefore, SERPINE2 was selected for further investigation. To confirm these results, qRT-PCR was used to determine that the SERPINE2 mRNA level was significantly decreased after BAP31 knockdown in Hep3b and MHCC97h cells (**Figure 3C**).

To investigate how BAP31 influences SERPINE2, coimmunoprecipitation (co-IP) assay was performed. The results indicated that BAP31 directly interacted with SERPINE2 in Hep3b and MHCC97h cells (**Figure 3D**). Confocal microscopy demonstrated colocalization of BAP31 with SERPINE2 in both HCC cell lines (**Figure 3E**). Moreover, the colocalization area was increased in BAP31-overexpressing HCC cells and decreased in BAP31-knockdown HCC cells compared with that in the corresponding control cells (**Figure 3F**).

Inhibition of SERPINE2 Attenuates BAP31-Promoted Cell Proliferation

SERPINE2 may be a downstream gene regulated by BAP31 in HCC cells; thus, the effect of SERPINE2 on the proliferation of HCC cells was investigated. The SERPINE2-knockdown and control Hep3b and MHCC97h cells were generated using transient transfection with SERPINE2 siRNA or control siRNA. The plate colony formation assay revealed that SERPINE2 contributed to cell proliferation in HCC cells because colony numbers were reduced with SERPINE2 deficiency (**Figure 4A**). Similarly, the CCK8 assay results showed that inhibition of SERPINE2 significantly decreased the HCC cell proliferation (**Figure 4B**). Considering the crucial roles of phosphorylated Erk1/2 and p38 in cell proliferation, the expression levels of these markers were analyzed in SERPINE2-knockdown cells. Western blot showed that the expression levels of Erk1/2, phospho-Erk1/2, and phospho-p38 were significantly decreased when SERPINE2 was knocked down; however, the BAP31 expression was not different in these cells, thus suggesting that SERPINE2 is a downstream gene of BAP31 and may regulate cell proliferation by influencing the phosphorylation of Erk1/2 and p38 (**Figure 4C**).

To investigate the role of SERPINE2 in BAP31-promoted cell proliferation, the function of SERPINE2 in HCC cells was inhibited using SERPINE2 siRNA. The colony formation assay showed that inhibition of SERPINE2 decreased BAP31-induced colony formation (**Figure 4D**). Additionally, CCK8 assay results indicated that inhibition of SERPINE2 attenuated BAP31-promoted cell proliferation (**Figure 4E**).

Multiplex IHC Staining Reveals That BAP31 Is Positively Correlated With SERPINE2, LRP1, and Ki67 in HCC

To determine the relationship between the BAP31 and SERPINE2 expression levels in human HCC, the expression patterns of BAP31, SERPINE2, LRP1 (a downstream gene regulated by SERPINE2), and Ki-67 were analyzed using multiplex IHC staining technology. The HCC tissue microarrays LV2089 and LV1221 were stained using Opal 7-plex technology yielding in the simultaneous visualization of five markers (DAPI was used to stain the nuclei) on the same slide (**Figures 5A,B**). The merged-channel multispectral image and single-channel images of the A5 core of LV2089 are shown in **Figure 5B**. A typical analysis process of a composite image is shown in **Figure 5C**. Briefly, each core was under a supervised successive four-step exploration. First, at the tissue segment stage, the malignant tumor and tumor stroma were distinguished as red and green, respectively; second, at the cell segment stage, all cell nuclei were identified and labeled with green; third, at the phenotype segment stage, the tumor, interstitial, and immune cells were distinguished as red, green, and blue, respectively; finally, at the scoring stage, the expression levels of indicated markers in the tumor cells were calculated. Blue represents no expression, yellow represents 1+ expression, orange represents 2+ expression, and tan represents 3+ expression; each result is presented with a comprehensive *H*-score.

After the analysis of the expression levels of four markers in all available tissue samples, the correlations between the levels of BAP31, SERPINE2, and other markers were calculated. The expression level of BAP31 was positively associated with the expression levels of SERPINE2, its downstream gene LRP1, and tumor cell proliferation marker Ki-67 (**Figures 5D–F**). Moreover, the SERPINE2 expression level was positively associated with LRP1 and Ki-67 (**Figures 5G,H**). Additionally, the LRP1 expression level was correlated with Ki-67 (**Figure 5I**).

Anti-BAP31 Antibody Inhibits HCC Cell-Induced Tumor Formation

To investigate the potential of BAP31 as a molecular target for HCC therapy, the effect of anti-BAP31 antibody on HCC cell-induced tumor formation was assessed. Hep3b cells were subcutaneous injected into mice, and tumor formation was observed on day 22 after the injection. Starting from day 3, mice were intraperitoneally injected twice a week with anti-BAP31 antibody, mouse IgG isotype, or PBS. The anti-BAP31 antibody treatment group developed smaller tumors compared with those in the two control groups (**Figure 6A**). The tumor growth curve indicated that anti-BAP31 antibody significantly inhibited the formation of Hep3b tumor xenograft (**Figure 6B**). Moreover, the tumor weight in the anti-BAP31 antibody treatment group was significantly less than that in the two control groups; the tumor weight in the IgG isotype group was also lower than that in the PBS group (**Figure 6C**). Then, the subcutaneous Hep3b tumors were stained to evaluate the expression levels of BAP31, Ki-67, and SERPINE2. The IHC results showed that anti-BAP31

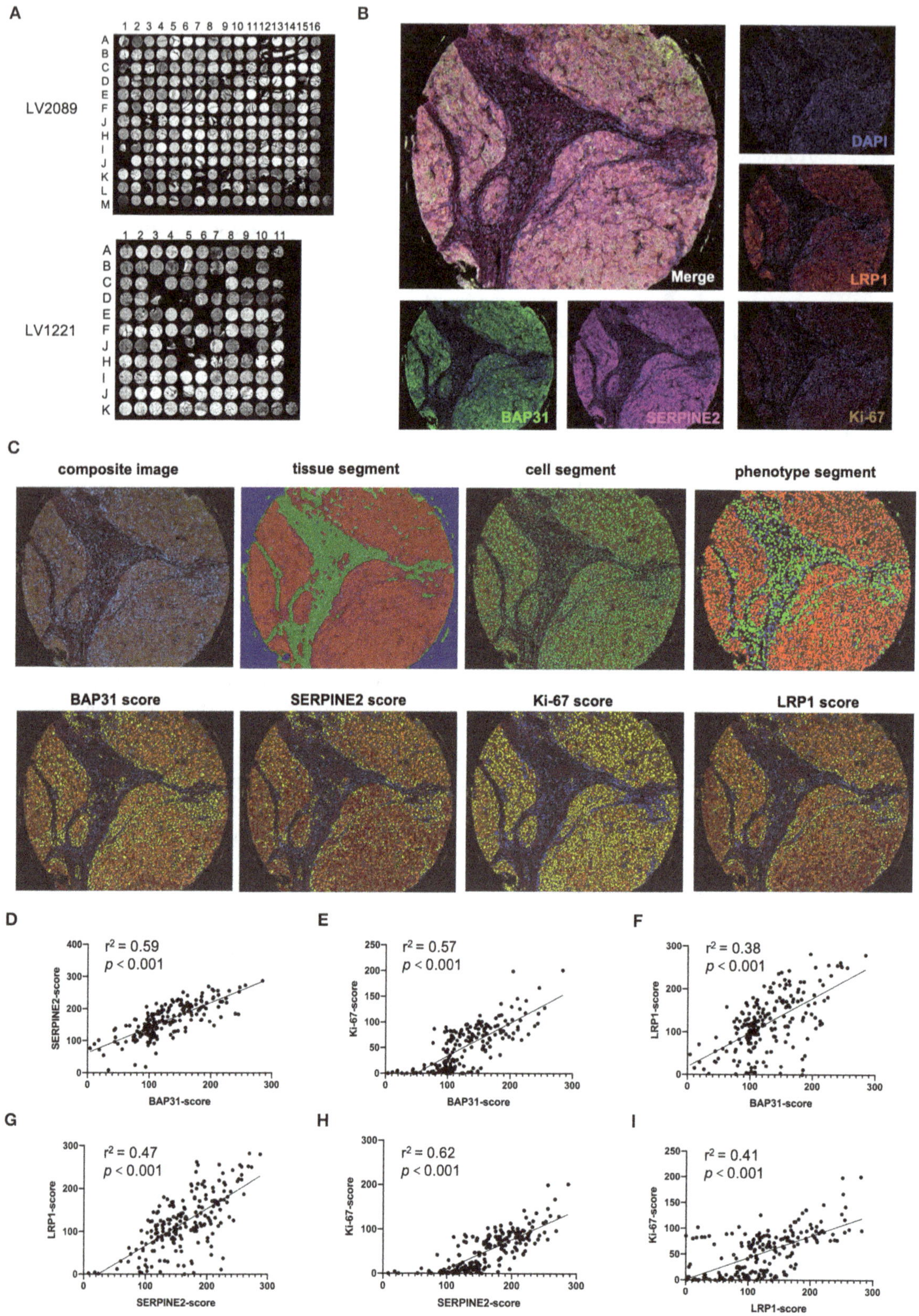

FIGURE 5 | Multiplex IHC staining indicates that BAP31 is positively correlated with SERPINE2, LRP1, and Ki67. **(A)** The HCC tissue microarrays LV2089 and LV1221 were stained using Opal 7-plex technology. **(B)** The merged-channel multispectral image was captured after four-cycle TSA staining and DAPI counterstain and

(Continued)

FIGURE 5 | separated by single channels. Fake colors are assigned as DAPI: blue, BAP31: green, SERPINE2: pink, LRP1: red, and Ki-67: brown (A5 point of LV2089 is shown). **(C)** The typical analysis process of composite image is as follows: first, at the tissue segment stage, the malignant tumor and tumor stroma are distinguished as red and green, respectively; second, at the cell segment stage, the cell nuclei are identified and labeled with green; third, at the phenotype segment stage, the tumor, interstitial, and immune cells are distinguished as red, green, and blue, respectively; finally, at the scoring stage, blue represents no expression, yellow represents 1+, orange represents 2+, and tan represents 3+; each result was assigned a comprehensive *H*-score. **(D–F)** The correlation between the expression levels of BAP31 and SERPINE2, Ki-67, and LRP1 in HCC tumor tissue. **(G,H)** The correlation between the expression levels of SERPINE2 and Ki-67 and LRP1. **(I)** The correlation between the expression levels of LRP1 and Ki-67. BAP31, B-cell receptor-associated protein 31; HCC, hepatocellular carcinoma; IHC, immunohistochemistry; SERPINE2, serpin family E member 2; TSA, tyramide signal amplification; DAPI, 4′,6-diamidino-2-phenylindole.

antibody decreased the number of Ki-67-positive cells and the expression level of SERPINE2 (**Figure 6D**).

To evaluate the effect of anti-BAP31 antibody on the survival of tumor-bearing mice, another three groups of mice were injected with Hep3b and administered with anti-BAP31 antibody, IgG isotype, and PBS. The Kaplan–Meier survival curve showed that the anti-BAP31 antibody treatment group had longer survival time than that in the control groups (**Figures 6E,F**). Finally, to evaluate the safety of anti-BAP31 antibody, hematoxylin and eosin (HE) staining was performed using the heart, liver, lung, and kidney samples of mice. The results showed that there were no significant differences in the histomorphology between the three groups (**Figure 6G**).

DISCUSSION

At present, the common methods of HCC treatment include surgical resection, liver transplantation, vascular intervention, radiofrequency ablation, etc. (Grandhi et al., 2016). However, these treatment methods provide additional benefit for the patients with early stages of HCC (Forner et al., 2018). For the patients diagnosed at an advanced stage, molecular targeting treatment and immunotherapy are more effective treatment options (Sim and Knox, 2018). BAP31 is a cancer/testis antigen that plays important roles in promotion of tumor development and can be a potential treatment target in malignant tumors (Dang et al., 2018). In the present study, the function of BAP31 was investigated in HCC using *in vitro* and *in vivo* experiments; the data demonstrated that targeting BAP31 may be an effective strategy for treatment of advanced HCC.

BAP31 is a membrane protein located on the ER and cell surface that acts as an important molecular chaperone (Kim et al., 2015). Early studies have reported that BAP31 is involved in the vesicular transport of transmembrane proteins: MHC-1, CD81, CD44, cellubrevin, etc. (Annaert et al., 1997; Abe et al., 2009; Eric et al., 2010). Wang et al. (2008) identified the sorting factor role of BAP31: it can recognize newly synthesized CFTRΔF508 and promote its retro-translocation from the ER and degradation by the 26s proteasome system in the cytoplasm. Moreover, Namba et al. (2013) reported that BAP31 could interact with CDIP1 to realize ER stress-mediated mitochondrial apoptosis, and it could also form a complex with mitochondria-localized protein Tom40 to enhance the communication between the ER and mitochondria (Namba, 2019). Of note, Xu J. L. et al. (2018) found deletion of BAP31 in the liver may destroy the ER homeostasis and then induce ER stress. Besides, Xu et al. (2019) demonstrated that silencing BAP31 can induce ER stress in colorectal cancer cells via upregulation of ER stress-related protein GRP78/BIP and activation of its downstream PERK/elF2α/ATF4/CHOP signaling pathway. Our results indicate that BAP31 is expressed at a high level in HCC patients, and its expression is positively correlated with clinical stage of HCC. Moreover, *in vitro* and *in vivo* functional experiments demonstrated that BAP31 can promote cell proliferation and tumor formation of HCC, suggesting that BAP31 may also maintain the ER homeostasis of HCC cells, protect cells from ER stress, and realize the promotion of cell proliferation and tumor formation. However, this hypothesis needed to be validated in further studies.

Moreover, SERPINE2 was identified as a novel downstream gene regulated by BAP31 in HCC, suggesting that BAP31 may influence the development of HCC by directly regulating the transport of SERPINE2. SERPINE2 belongs to the serine protease inhibitor superfamily and is a secreted protein that can inhibit the activity of thrombin, urokinase, plasmin, trypsin, and other serine proteinases (Li et al., 2016).

Previous studies have shown that the abnormal expression of SERPINE2 is involved in the occurrence and development of various cancers: mammary, pancreatic, prostatic, esophagus, gastric, colorectal cancer, etc. Fayard et al. (2009) reported that SERPINE2 can bind to LRP1, stimulate extracellular kinase signal, and regulate the invasion and metastasis of mammary tumor. Buchholz et al. (2003) found that SERPINE2 can enhance the invasion of pancreatic cancer cells by increasing ECM production. McKee et al. (2012) demonstrated that SERPINE2 can decrease the expression of Hh ligand Sonic, regulate Hh signaling, and eventually inhibit cell proliferation in prostate cancer. Moreover, Bergeron et al. (2010) demonstrated that activation of Ras, BRAF, and MEK1 increased the SERPINE2 expression, and SERPINE2 stimulated the ERK signaling to promote the colorectal cancer tumorigenesis. Additionally, Wang et al. (2015) identified SERPINE2 as a prognostic factor and anticancer target for gastric cancer due to its promotion of invasion. Recently, Zhang et al. (2020) reported that SERPINE2 promotes metastasis of esophageal cancer by activating BMP4. In our study, inhibition of SERPINE2 significantly decreased the BAP31-induced cell proliferation and colony formation of HCC cells and the phosphorylation of Erk1/2 and p38, suggesting that SERPINE2 may promote tumor cell proliferation through activation of the MAPK pathway.

In recent years, immunotherapy has gradually become one of the main therapies for various cancers due to beneficial enhancement of the immune function, decrease in the recurrence, and extension of survival (Xu F. et al., 2018; Gavrielatou et al., 2020; Schizas et al., 2020; Topalian et al.,

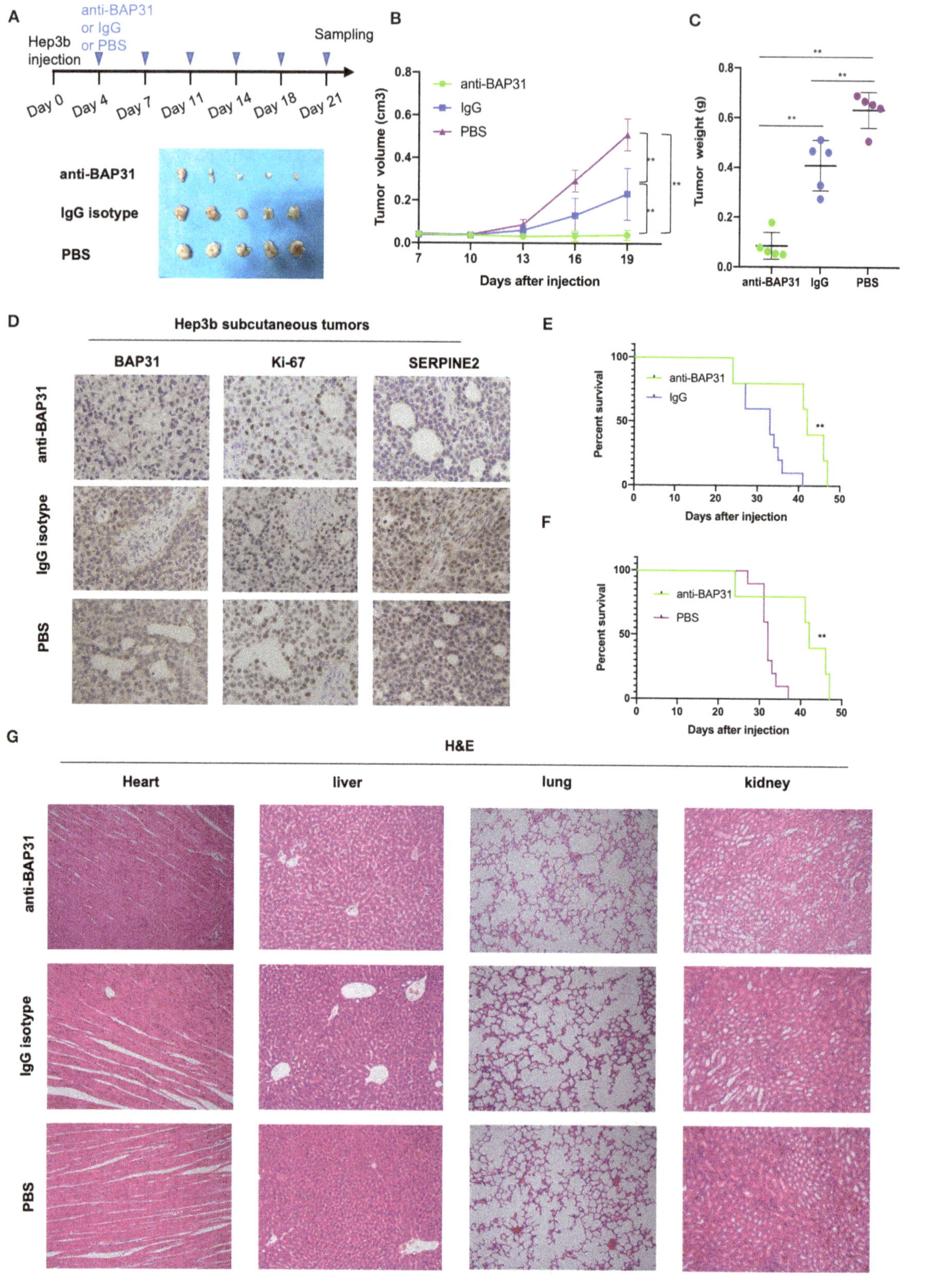

FIGURE 6 | Anti-BAP31 antibody inhibits HCC cell-induced tumor formation. **(A)** Hep3b cells were injected subcutaneously into the right flank of nude mice on day 0. Starting from day 4, anti-BAP31 antibody, mouse IgG isotype, and PBS were administered intraperitoneally twice a week. Images of the xenograft tumors are shown.

(Continued)

FIGURE 6 | (B) Growth curve of xenografts of Hep3b cells treated with anti-BAP31, mouse IgG isotype, and PBS ($n = 5$, mean ± SD). **(C)** Weight of the xenograft tumors was measured. The results represent the mean ± SD, and $^{**}p < 0.01$ was considered to be significant according to Student's *t*-test. **(D)** Expression levels of BAP31, Ki-67, and SERPINE2 in Hep3b subcutaneous tumors were monitored by IHC analysis. **(E,F)** Kaplan–Meier survival curve representing the overall survival of mice injected with Hep3b cells and treated with anti-BAP31 antibody, mouse IgG isotype, and PBS ($n = 10$, $^{**}p < 0.01$ by log-rank test). **(G)** Hematoxylin and eosin staining of the heart, liver, lung, and kidney in various groups of mice. BAP31, B-cell receptor-associated protein 31; HCC, hepatocellular carcinoma; IHC, immunohistochemistry; SERPINE2, serpin family E member 2; PBS, phosphate-buffered saline.

2020; Wculek et al., 2020; Xu et al., 2020). Considering the cancer/testis antigen role of BAP31, the effect of an anti-BAP31 monoclonal antibody developed in-house and produced by a hybridoma on tumor formation in HCC was investigated. The antitumor effect of IgG observed in the study could be caused by the opsonophagocytosis, antibody-dependent cell-mediated cytotoxicity, or complement activation (Shen et al., 1981; Aderem and Underhill, 1999; Hester and Frank, 2019). Anti-BAP31 antibody significantly suppressed the tumor formation of HCC cells *in vivo* compared with that in the IgG isotype and PBS control groups; thus, BAP31 may be a new therapeutic candidate for HCC treatment.

In conclusion, our study demonstrated that BAP31 expression is upregulated in HCC and correlates with the clinical stage. BAP31 promoted cell proliferation by direct regulation of SERPINE2 and activation of the MAPK pathway. Moreover, anti-BAP31 antibody significantly inhibited the tumor formation of HCC cells, suggesting that targeting BAP31 may be a good candidate therapeutic strategy in patients with HCC.

ETHICS STATEMENT

The studies involving human participants were reviewed and approved by Ethics Committee of the Fourth Military Medical University. The patients/participants provided their written informed consent to participate in this study. The animal study was reviewed and approved by Ethics Committee of the Fourth Military Medical University.

AUTHOR CONTRIBUTIONS

KY, XZ, and BJ conceived and designed the project. XZ, DJ, SY, YS, YL, and JS carried out the experimental work. XZ, DJ, SY, CH, JP, and TL analyzed the data. XZ wrote the paper. All authors read and approved the final manuscript.

REFERENCES

Abe, F., Van Prooyen, N., Ladasky, J. J., and Edidin, M. (2009). Interaction of Bap31 and MHC class I molecules and their traffic out of the endoplasmic reticulum. *J. Immunol.* 182, 4776–4783. doi: 10.4049/jimmunol.0800242

Aderem, A., and Underhill, D. M. (1999). Mechanisms of phagocytosis in macrophages. *Annu. Rev. Immunol.* 17, 593–623. doi: 10.1146/annurev.immunol.17.1.593

Annaert, W. G., Becker, B., Kistner, U., Reth, M., and Jahn, R. (1997). Export of cellubrevin from the endoplasmic reticulum is controlled by BAP31. *J. Cell Biol.* 139, 1397–1410. doi: 10.1083/jcb.139.6.1397

Bergeron, S., Lemieux, E., Durand, V., Cagnol, S., Carrier, J. C., Lussier, J. G., et al. (2010). The serine protease inhibitor serpinE2 is a novel target of ERK signaling involved in human colorectal tumorigenesis. *Mol. Cancer* 9:271. doi: 10.1186/1476-4598-9-271

Bray, F., Ferlay, J., Soerjomataram, I., Siegel, R. L., Torre, L. A., and Jemal, A. (2018). Global cancer statistics 2018: GLOBOCAN estimates of incidence and mortality worldwide for 36 cancers in 185 countries. *Cancer J. Clin.* 68, 394–424. doi: 10.3322/caac.21492

Buchholz, M., Biebl, A., Neesse, A., Wagner, M., Iwamura, T., Leder, G., et al. (2003). SERPINE2 (protease nexin I) promotes extracellular matrix production and local invasion of pancreatic tumors *in vivo*. *Cancer Res.* 63, 4945–4951.

Budny, A., Kozłowski, P., Kamińska, M., Jankiewicz, M., Kolak, A., Budny, B., et al. (2017). Epidemiology and risk factors of hepatocellular carcinoma. *Pol. Merkur. Lekarski.* 43, 133–139.

Chen, J., Guo, H., Jiang, H., Namusamba, M., Wang, C., Lan, T., et al. (2019). A BAP31 intrabody induces gastric cancer cell death by inhibiting p27kip1 proteasome degradation. *Int. J. Cancer* 144, 2051–2062. doi: 10.1002/ijc.31930

Dang, E., Yang, S., Song, C., Jiang, D., Li, Z., Fan, W., et al. (2018). BAP31, a newly defined cancer/testis antigen, regulates proliferation, migration, and invasion to promote cervical cancer progression. *Cell Death Dis.* 9:791. doi: 10.1038/s41419-018-0824-2

Eric, B., Eyster, C. A., Kasinath, V., Mandana, M., Donaldson, J. G., Klaus, F., et al. (2010). Membrane-associated RING-CH proteins associate with Bap31 and target CD81 and CD44 to lysosomes. *PLoS ONE* 5:e15132. doi: 10.1371/journal.pone.0015132

Fayard, B., Bianchi, F., Dey, J., Moreno, E., Djaffer, S., Hynes, N. E., et al. (2009). The serine protease inhibitor protease nexin-1 controls mammary cancer metastasis through LRP-1-mediated MMP-9 expression. *Cancer Res.* 69, 5690–5698. doi: 10.1158/0008-5472.CAN-08-4573

Forner, A., Reig, M., and Bruix, J. (2018). Hepatocellular carcinoma. *Lancet* 391, 1301–1314. doi: 10.1016/S0140-6736(18)30010-2

Fujiwara, N., Friedman, S. L., Goossens, N., and Hoshida, Y. (2018). Risk factors and prevention of hepatocellular carcinoma in the era of precision medicine. *J. Hepatol.* 68, 526–549. doi: 10.1016/j.jhep.2017.09.016

Gavrielatou, N., Doumas, S., Economopoulou, P., Foukas, P. G., and Psyrri, A. (2020). Biomarkers for immunotherapy response in head and neck cancer. *Cancer Treat. Rev.* 84:101977. doi: 10.1016/j.ctrv.2020.101977

Grandhi, M. S., Kim, A. K., Ronnekleiv-Kelly, S. M., Kamel, I. R., Ghasebeh, M. A., and Pawlik, T. M. (2016). Hepatocellular carcinoma: from diagnosis to treatment. *Surg. Oncol.* 25, 74–85. doi: 10.1016/j.suronc.2016.03.002

Hester, C. G., and Frank, M. M. (2019). Complement activation by IgG containing immune complexes regulates the interaction of C1q with its ligands. *Mol. Immunol.* 116, 117–130. doi: 10.1016/j.molimm.2019.10.004

Kim, W. T., Hong, S. C., Lee, H. M., Jang, Y. J., and Ryu, C. J. (2015). B-cell receptor-associated protein 31 regulates human embryonic stem cell adhesion, stemness, and survival via control of epithelial cell adhesion molecule. *Stem Cells* 32, 2626–2641. doi: 10.1002/stem.1765

Li, X., Zhao, D., Guo, Z., Li, T., Qili, M., Xu, B., et al. (2016). Overexpression of serpine2/protease nexin-1 contribute to pathological cardiac fibrosis via increasing collagen deposition. *Sci. Rep.* 6:37635. doi: 10.1038/srep37635

McKee, C. M., Xu, D., Cao, Y., Kabraji, S., Allen, D., Kersemans, V., et al. (2012). Protease nexin 1 inhibits hedgehog signaling in prostate adenocarcinoma. *J. Clin. Invest.* 122, 4025–4036. doi: 10.1172/JCI59348

Namba, T. (2019). BAP31 regulates mitochondrial function via interaction with Tom40 within ER-mitochondria contact sites. *Sci. Adv.* 5:eaaw1386. doi: 10.1126/sciadv.aaw1386

Namba, T., Tian, F., Chu, K., Hwang, S. Y., Yoon, K. W., Byun, S., et al. (2013). CDIP1-BAP31 complex transduces apoptotic signals from endoplasmic reticulum to mitochondria under endoplasmic reticulum stress. *Cell. Rep.* 5, 331–339. doi: 10.1016/j.celrep.2013.09.020

National Genomics Data Center Members and Partners (2020). Database resources of the national genomics data center in 2020. *Nucl Acids Res.* (2020) 48:D24–33. doi: 10.1093/nar/gkz913

Ozakyol, A. (2017). Global epidemiology of hepatocellular carcinoma (HCC epidemiology). *J. Gastrointest. Cancer* 48, 238–240. doi: 10.1007/s12029-017-9959-0

Schizas, D., Charalampakis, N., Kole, C., Economopoulou, P., Koustas, E., Gkotsis, E., et al. (2020). Immunotherapy for pancreatic cancer: a 2020 update. *Cancer Treat. Rev.* 86:102016. doi: 10.1016/j.ctrv.2020.102016

Shen, L., Lydyard, P. M., Roitt, I. M., and Fanger, M. W. (1981). Synergy between IgG and monoclonal IgM antibodies in antibody-dependent cell cytotoxicity. *J. Immunol.* 127, 73–78.

Sia, D., Villanueva, A., Friedman, S. L., and Llovet, J. M. (2017). Liver cancer cell of origin, molecular class, and effects on patient prognosis. *Gastroenterology* 152, 745–761. doi: 10.1053/j.gastro.2016.11.048

Sim, H. W., and Knox, J. (2018). Hepatocellular carcinoma in the era of immunotherapy. *Curr. Probl. Cancer* 42, 40–48. doi: 10.1016/j.currproblcancer.2017.10.007

Topalian, S. L., Taube, J. M., and Pardoll, D. M. (2020). Neoadjuvant checkpoint blockade for cancer immunotherapy. *Science* 367:eaax0182. doi: 10.1126/science.aax0182

Villanueva, A. (2019). Hepatocellular carcinoma. *N. Engl. J. Med.* 380, 1450–1462. doi: 10.1056/NEJMra1713263

Wang, B., Heath-Engel, H., Zhang, D., Nguyen, N., Thomas, D. Y., Hanrahan, J. W., et al. (2008). BAP31 interacts with Sec61 translocons and promotes retrotranslocation of CFTRDeltaF508 via the derlin-1 complex. *Cell* 133, 1080–1092. doi: 10.1016/j.cell.2008.04.042

Wang, J., Jiang, D., Li, Z., Yang, S., Zhou, J., Zhang, G., et al. (2020). BCAP31, a cancer/testis antigen-like protein, can act as a probe for non-small-cell lung cancer metastasis. *Sci. Rep.* 10:4025. doi: 10.1038/s41598-020-60905-7

Wang, K., Wang, B., Xing, A. Y., Xu, K. S., Li, G. X., and Yu, Z. H. (2015). Prognostic significance of SERPINE2 in gastric cancer and its biological function in SGC7901 cells. *J. Cancer Res. Clin. Oncol.* 141, 805–812. doi: 10.1007/s00432-014-1858-1

Wang, Y., Song, F., Zhu, J., Zhang, S., Yang, Y., Chen, T., et al. (2017). GSA: genome sequence archive. *Genom. Proteom. Bioinf.* 15, 14–18. doi: 10.1016/j.gpb.2017.01.001

Wculek, S. K., Cueto, F. J., Mujal, A. M., Melero, I., Krummel, M. F., and Sancho, D. (2020). Dendritic cells in cancer immunology and immunotherapy. *Nat. Rev. Immunol.* 20, 7–24. doi: 10.1038/s41577-019-0210-z

Xu, F., Jin, T., Zhu, Y., and Dai, C. (2018). Immune checkpoint therapy in liver cancer. *J. Exp. Clin. Cancer Res.* 37:110. doi: 10.1186/s13046-018-0777-4

Xu, J. L., Li, L. Y., Wang, Y. Q., Li, Y. Q., Shan, M., Sun, S. Z., et al. (2018). Hepatocyte-specific deletion of BAP31 promotes SREBP1C activation, promotes hepatic lipid accumulation, and worsens IR in mice. *J. Lipid. Res.* 59, 35–47. doi: 10.1194/jlr.M077016

Xu, K., Han, B., Bai, Y., Ma, X. Y., Ji, Z. N., Xiong, Y., et al. (2019). MiR-451a suppressing BAP31 can inhibit proliferation and increase apoptosis through inducing ER stress in colorectal cancer. *Cell. Death Dis.* 10:152. doi: 10.1038/s41419-019-1403-x

Xu, Y., Li, Y., Pan, J., Kang, X., Zhang, X., Feng, X., et al. (2020). EM2D9, A monoclonal antibody against integrin α5β1, has potent antitumor activity on endometrial cancer *in vitro* and *in vivo*. *Cancer Lett.* 483, 66–74. doi: 10.1016/j.canlet.2020.02.019

Zhang, J., Luo, A., Huang, F., Gong, T., and Liu, Z. (2020). SERPINE2 promotes esophageal squamous cell carcinoma metastasis by activating BMP4. *Cancer Lett* 469, 390–398. doi: 10.1016/j.canlet.2019.11.011

12

TLRs as a Promise Target Along With Immune Checkpoint Against Gastric Cancer

Lin Cui[1*†], *Xiuqing Wang*[1†] *and Dekai Zhang*[2*]

[1] Department of Gastroenterology and Hepatology, The Second Affiliated Hospital, Harbin Medical University, Harbin, China,
[2] Center for Infectious and Inflammatory Diseases, Texas A&M University, Houston, TX, United States

***Correspondence:**
Lin Cui
949374102@qq.com
Dekai Zhang
dekaiz@hotmail.com

†These authors have contributed equally to this work and share first authorship

Gastric cancer (GC) is one of the most common cancers in the world, and the incidence of gastric cancer in Asia appears to increase in recent years. Although there is a lot of improvement in treatment approaches, the prognosis of GC is poor. So it is urgent to search for a novel and more effective treatment to improve the survival rate of patients. Both innate immunity and adaptive immunity are important in cancer. In the innate immune system, pattern recognition receptors (PRRs) activate immune responses by recognizing pathogen-associated molecular patterns (PAMPs) and damage-associated molecular patterns (DAMPs). Toll-like receptors (TLRs) are a class of pattern recognition receptors (PRRs). Many studies have reported that TLRs are involved in the occurrence, development, and treatment of GC. Therefore, TLRs are potential targets for immunotherapy to gastric cancer. However, gastric cancer is a heterogeneous disorder, and TLRs function in GC is complex. TLRs agonists can be potentially used not only as therapeutic agents to treat gastric cancer but also as adjuvants in conjunction with other immunotherapies. They might provide a promising new target for GC treatment. In the review, we sort out the mechanism of TLRs involved in tumor immunity and summarize the current progress in TLRs-based therapeutic approaches and other immunotherapies in the treatment of GC.

Keywords: gastric cancer, toll-like receptor, agonist, tumor immunity, immunotherapy, immune checkpoint

INTRODUCTION

Gastric cancer (GC), is the second leading cause of cancer death worldwide according to the latest WHO statistics in 2018 (Bray et al., 2018). Early gastric cancer can be removed by EMR (endoscopic mucosal resection) or ESD (endoscopic submucosal dissection), the long-term prognosis is good at present (Ko et al., 2016). What makes GC difficult to treat is due to the patients with GC usually without any early symptoms. GC is usually diagnosed in the late stage when metastasis (Maeda et al., 2015). There are several standard treatments to treat advanced gastric cancer: surgical resection, chemotherapy, radiotherapy, chemoradiation, and targeted therapy. But the 5-year survival rate of patients with GC had no significant improvement. Besides, the patients had some side effects during and after treatment, including nausea, vomiting, reflux, malnutrition, etc. The quality of life of the patients decreased significantly. This makes people with gastric cancer suffer both physically and mentally.

How to improve the survival rate and quality of life of GC patients is an urgent problem to be solved. GC is a heterogeneous disorder and some molecular subsets of it exhibit certain characteristics, suggesting that immunotherapy may be an effective treatment (Jones and Smyth, 2020). According to The Cancer Genome Atlas (TCGA) network, GC is classified into the four following molecular subgroups: Epstein Barr virus (EBV), microsatellite instability (MSI), chromosomal instability (CIN) and genomic stable (GS) gastric cancers. In the MSI and EBV subgroups, programmed death-ligand 1 (PD-Ll) is higher expressed, that demonstrate the potential of immune checkpoint inhibitors to treat these GC subtypes (Cancer Genome Atlas Research Network, 2014).

The diseases treated by immunotherapy are through inducing, enhancing, or suppressing immune responses. Compared with currently used drugs, immunomodulatory therapy has fewer adverse side effects and develop less resistance in the treatment of microbial diseases (Masihi, 2001). Active immunotherapy uses the parts of the immune system to enhance tumor immunity (Jeremy et al., 2016). In tumor immunity, the immune system suppresses tumor growth by recognizing and removing tumor cells (Keir et al., 2008). However, tumors can achieve malignant reproduction by immune escape (Hanahan and Weinberg, 2011). Tumorigenesis usually involves inflammatory responses, both innate and acquired immune systems (Akira et al., 2006). It is shown that activating the innate immune system can offset tumor-induced immunosuppression partly and may improve the prognosis of cancer patients (Marcus et al., 2014).

The highly conserved PRRs are a significant component of the innate immune system. PRRs family includes TLRs, nucleotide oligomerization domain (NOD)-like receptors (NLRs), a retinoic acid-inducible gene I (RIG-I) like receptors (RLRs), and C-type lectin receptors (CLRs) (Castaño-Rodríguez et al., 2014). Potential natural immune targets include TLRs, RLRs, and stimulator of interferon genes (STING) (Li et al., 2017). Furthermore, The activation of TLRs is necessary for inducing the adaptive immunity. Therefore, the induction of the innate immune system may work in identifying and antagonizing tumor cells. Although immunotherapy has not become a standard therapy like surgery or chemoradiotherapy, its role in cancer treatment could be significant. Especially TLRs-based strategy has greatly promoted the immunotherapy of lung cancer, melanoma, and renal cell carcinoma, etc., but the function of TLRs in gastric cancer immunotherapy has just attracted more studies. However, there is no previous review on the immunotherapeutic effect of TLRs in gastric cancer. Thus, we summarized the research status and mechanism of TLRs in immunotherapy of gastric cancer.

TLR STRUCTURE AND SIGNALING PATHWAYS

TLRs are type I transmembrane glycoproteins, whose structure includes a leucine-rich repetitive sequence in the extracellular domain, a transmembrane domain, and a conserved Toll/ IL-1R homologous domain (TIR) in the cytosolic region, as they are homologous with the signaling domain of IL-1R family members. Extracellular domain induces homo-dimerization of intracellular TIR by recognition of ligands (except for TLR1/2 and TLR2/6). Then TLRs recruit TIR domain-containing adaptor proteins including myeloid differentiation primary response protein 88 (MyD88) and TIR-domain containing adaptor-inducing interferon-β (TRIF) that initiate signaling pathways to activate the transcription factors nuclear factor-kappa B (NF-κB), interferon regulatory factor (IRFs), or mitogen-activated protein kinase (MAPK) to regulate the expression of cytokine and chemokine genes including interleukin-2 (IL-2), IL-6, IL-12, monocyte chemoattractant protein-1 (MCP-1), and tumor necrosis factor-α (TNF-α) (Barton and Kagan, 2009), ultimately involved in establishing a regulatory innate and adaptive immune response (Goutagny et al., 2012; Kawasaki and Kawai, 2014).

Ten TLRs have been determined expressed in various human innate immune cells, such as macrophages and dendritic cells. TLRs may be retained or abnormally expressed in cancer cells (Goutagny et al., 2012; Braunstein et al., 2018). Several TLRs have been expressed in human gastric cancer cells. For example, TLR2 expression was up-regulated in human GC cell SGC7901, which was associated with Pam3CSK4 stimulation, indicating that TLR2 might be involved in the proliferation and metastasis of GC, indicating that TLR2 might serve as a novel therapeutic target against GC (Yang et al., 2014). TLR4 was highly expressed in gastric cancer cells related to the aggressiveness of gastric cancer. The activation of TLR4 by lipopolysaccharide (LPS) promoted cancer proliferation but did not influence apoptosis (Yuan et al., 2013). TLR5 activated by flagellin can increase the proliferation of GC cells. The subsequent antagonism of TLR5 appears to counteract this effect, suggesting that TLR5 signaling can significantly enhance the proliferation of GC cells (Song et al., 2011). However, another study found that GC patients with high TLR5 tissue expression can have a better prognosis, particularly who has stage II disease or intestinal-type GC (Kasurinen et al., 2019). Studies have explored that TLR7 expression is low in GC tissues, and stimulating TLR7 could promote the secretion of pro-inflammatory cytokines, and inhibit the proliferation of GC cells (Jiang et al., 2016). Thus, it can be seen that the function of different TLRs in GC is complex and different.

THE MECHANISM UNDERLYING THE ROLE OF TLRs IN TUMOR IMMUNITY

TLRs are the family of transmembrane receptors on innate immune cells such as dendritic cells (DCs) and macrophages. They can recognize PAMPs and DAMPs of necrotic and apoptotic cells from a foreign specific microbe, including antigens from various tumor sources, to initiate an immune response (Barton and Kagan, 2009; Tartey and Takeuchi, 2014). The immune system recognizes tumor cells through tumor antigens. Tumor-specific antigen (TSA) is expressed only in tumor cells. Tumor-associated antigen (TAA) is expressed in both tumor and normal cells. Dendritic cells (DCs) belong to antigen-presenting cells (APCs). TAA/TSA was presented to CTLs by DCs via the MHC class I pathway (Kurts et al., 2010). Antigen presentation triggers CD8+ T cells to differentiate into cytotoxic T lymphocytes (CTLs) and induces CTLs proliferation. Subsequently, CTLs are attracted to the tumor microenvironment. Through T cell receptor (TCR) and MHC class I-bound antigen, CTLs recognize tumor cells then kill them (Hanson et al., 2000). Immune checkpoints including CTLA-4 and PD-1 can suppress the immune attack. CD4+ T cells are activated by DCs via the MHC class II pathway, differentiating into Th1 and Th2 cells. Th1 cells promote antitumor immunity by secreting proinflammatory cytokines (Kalams and Walker, 1998). Regulatory CD4+ T cells (Tregs) are anti-inflammatory cells suppressing the priming, activation, and cytotoxicity of other effector immune cells including Th1 T cells, CTLs and etc. (Ward-Hartstonge and Kemp, 2017). TLR agonists who have anti-tumor effects activate tumor-specific T cell responses by stimulating antigen-presenting cells (APC), including dendritic cells (DCs) (Li et al., 2017). T lymphocyte activity, as the main involved molecules in tumor immune response, can synergistically act on stimulating molecules and inhibiting molecules (Pardoll, 2012). In humans, most TLRs expression is found on DCs and mature macrophages (Hennessy et al., 2010). There is growing evidence that TLRs can be expressed or induced on multiple cells, such as T cells and tumor cells. Along with the anti-tumor effect of TLRs on DCs, new researches have shown that TLR signals from other cell types can play a crucial role in tumor growth, promotion or inhibition (Fukata and Abreu, 2008; So and Ouchi, 2010; Kaczanowska et al., 2013). This also indicates that the role of TLRs in immunotherapy against GC is very important,might represent a new strategy for patients with GC (**Figure 1**).

TLRs IN IMMUNOTHERAPY OF GASTRIC CANCER

TLRs have been detected in both tumor cells and immune cells. They recognize different ligands, respectively, such as lipopolysaccharide (LPS) of bacteria, bacterial flagellin, unmethylated CpG motif of bacterial, etc. So, the activation of TLRs on different cells is complex, which may be anti-tumor, pro-tumor, or dual effects.

TLR2

It has been reported in several literatures that TLR2 is associated with the occurrence of GC. TLR2 is expressed on the plasma membrane and recognizes peptidoglycan, a part of the cell wall of Gram-positive bacteria, thus activating innate immunity. It was shown that TLR2-activated APCs can promote effector cells to attack tumor cells (Akazawa et al., 2010; Prajeeth et al., 2010). The extract of LarixLeptolepis (ELL) may activate TLR2 and fight cancer. It can also activate bone marrow-derived-dendritic cells (BMDCs) to promote a tumor-specific signal and tumor-specific cytotoxic T lymphocytes (CTLs) to fight cancer (Koizumi et al., 2012). Coley's toxin (a mixture of inactivated Streptococcus pyogenes and Serratia marcescens) and BCG (Bacillus Calmette-Guerin), a TLR2 and TLR4 agonist have been used as a drug for long-term cancer treatment (Galluzzi et al., 2012). Also, the BCG cell wall skeleton (BCG-CWS) vaccine has been used as a vaccine and TLR2 ligand for the prevention of tuberculosis and has been demonstrated to enhance immune effect strongly through DCs and is helpful for cancer immunotherapy, including GC (Tsuji et al., 2000).

However, the underlying mechanism remains unclear although some information has been uncovered. After BCG and lymphocyte co-culture, the apoptosis rate, caspase-3 level, LC-3, and Atg-3 protein level were significantly higher than those in BCG and lymphocyte group alone. BCG induces lymphocyte to secrete interferon-γ (IFN-γ). BCG and IFN-γ can also enhance the level of cleavage of caspase-3, LC-3, and Atg-5. Studies have shown that BCG may induce apoptosis and autophagy of gastric cancer cell line MGC-803 by inducing the release of IFN-γ from peripheral blood lymphocytes (Yao et al., 2018).

Glycoprotein 130 (gp130) binds to IL-6 to form a trimer and transmit downstream signals (Tebbutt et al., 2002). In gp130 mutant mice, TLR2 was absent and gastric cancer lesion shrank (Tye et al., 2012). And the study indicated that the expression of TLR2 in gastric epithelial cells and/or GC tissues may be involved.

A cancer vaccine is a new approach to treat a tumor, and a vaccine essentially consists of a tumor-associated antigen (TAA) and adjuvant. TLR2 ligands are potential adjuvants. Gijs et al. demonstrated that conjugation of new TLR2-L Amplivant (TLR2-ligand, a modified Pam3CSK4) to synthetic long peptides (SLPs) induced dendritic cells(DCs) maturation, T cell priming, and anti-tumor immunity strongly (Zom et al., 2018). BPPcysMPEG (TLR2/6 heterodimer agonist) was proved to be a potent stimulus to generate cytotoxic T lymphocytes (CTLs) via cross-priming (Prajeeth et al., 2010). Hu et al. designed and synthesized a conjugated stimulator of interferon genes (STING) and TLR1/2 agonist, Pam3CSK4-CDGSF, which can serve as a adjuvant for vaccine construction to augment antitumor immunotherapy (Hu et al., 2020).

ANXA2m is an O2-regulated protein binding and signaling through TLR2, acting as an adjuvant by inducing DCs maturation, enhancing antigen cross-presentation, and inducing the secretion of proinflammatory cytokines (Andersen et al., 2016). Wu et al. found that lipo-OVA (Ovalbumin fused with the TLR2 agonist, the lipid part of the bacteria) showed a strong anti-tumor effect by activating BMDCs maturation, promoting cross-presentation of tumor antigen, inducing CTL responses, increasing the numbers of CD8+ T cells (Wu et al., 2016). A vaccine comprising bacteria-mimicking tumor cells (BMTC) and P2CSR11/P2CSK11 (TLR2 ligand) promoted anti-tumor immunity by stimulating DCs and enhancing antigen presentation (Akazawa et al., 2018).

Above all, TLR2 and its agonists have been proved in many studies to attack gastric cancer cells. The next step is to apply it to clinical trials and verify the efficacy of TLR2-related immunotherapy.

TLR3

The expression of TLR3 is primarily intracellular. TLR3 was regarded as a potential therapeutic target for multiple cancers. Poly(I:C) which is a classical TLR3 agonist was studied for

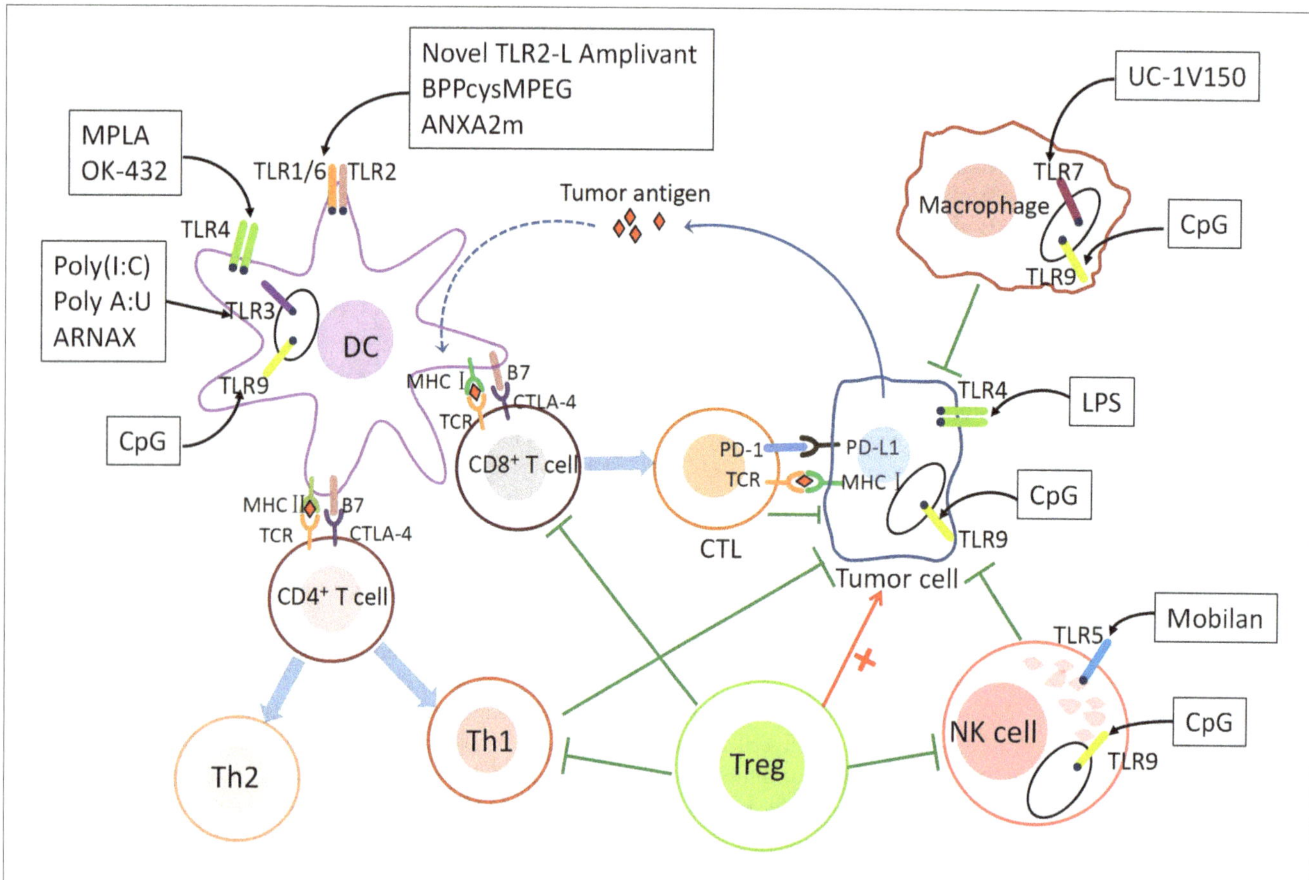

FIGURE 1 | The mechanism underlying the role of TLRs in tumor immunity. TLRs are expressed on different immune cells and cancer cells. The roles of immune cells in tumor immunity. As a class of antigen-presenting cells (APCs), dendritic cells (DCs) recognize tumor antigen and present the antigen to CD8$^+$ T cells through the MHC class I pathway and CD4$^+$ T cells through the MHC class II pathway. After activated by DCs, CD8$^+$ T cells differentiate into cytotoxic T lymphocytes (CTLs) and CD4$^+$ T cells differentiate into Th1 and Th2 cells. CTLs are recruited to the tumor microenvironment (TME) and recognize tumor cells through T cell receptor (TCR) and MHC class I-bound antigen, then kill them. Th1 cells secreting proinflammatory cytokines such as IL-2, TNF-α, and IFN-γ to promote immunity. Immune checkpoints—CTLA-4 and PD-1, can suppress T cell response. NK cells inhibit cancer by directly kill tumor cells and secreting several inflammatory factors. M1 macrophages are pro-inflammatory and M2 Macrophages are anti-inflammatory. Regulatory CD4$^+$ T cells (Tregs) are anti-inflammatory cells suppressing of CTLs, Th1 cells, macrophages, and NK cells. TLRs are expressed both on immune cells and gastric cancer cells. Different TLRs agonists act on different immune and cancer cells to affect tumor immunity—pro-tumor or anti-tumor. Th1 cells, T helper type 1 cells; Th2 cells, T helper type 2 cells; IL-2, interleukin-2; TNF-α, tumor necrosis factor-α; IFN-γ, interferon-γ; CTLA-4, The cytotoxic T-lymphocyte-associated antigen-4; PD-1, Programmed cell death protein 1; PD-L1, Programmed death ligand 1 (PD-L1).The agonists and adjuvants of TLRs are shown in **Tables 1**, **2**.

immunotherapy in recent years. Poly(I:C) was reported that the immune potency of it may be limited by insufficient cellular penetration. Novel immunotherapy was designed based on the cancer vaccine. The Poly(I:C)-DOTAP liposome composite nanoparticles can promote Poly(I:C) into cells and generated corresponding TLR3 signals in BMDCs. In this way, poly(I:C) nanoparticles promoted the tumor properties of TLR3 signals (Wang et al., 2012). The poly(I:C) ligand-receptor complex was internalized into cells by the specific ligand-binding receptors on the surface of tumor cells. TLR3, PKR, RIG-1, and MDA5 was activated by the internalized poly(I:C) simultaneously. The activation of these signaling proteins promotes tumor cells secreting cytokines by the bystander effect and led to the rapid death of tumor cells (Levitzki, 2012). Shime et al. found that TLR3 activated by injection of poly(I:C) to tumor-implant mice converted tumor-supporting macrophages into tumor-killing effectors to shrink the tumor (Shime et al., 2012). Perret et al. demonstrated adding the adjuvant Poly(I:C) to the vaccine increased ratios of tumor antigen-specific effector T cells: regulatory T cells that enhanced the infiltration of CD8+ T-cell, thus promoting anti-tumor immunity. And after treated with OVA+Poly(I:C) vaccine, the tumor growth of EG7 lymphoma was controlled and the survival rate of tumor-bearing mice has enhanced (Perret et al., 2013). Intravaginal (IVAG) instillation of Poly(I:C) after subcutaneous HPV E6/E7 vaccination promoted the proliferation of vaccine-specific CD8+ T cells in the genital mucosa (GM), which may suppress cervical cancer (Domingos-Pereira et al., 2013).

Polyadenylic–polyuridylic acid [poly(A:U)] is also the agonist of TLR3 which can promote immune responses. After surgery for locally advanced gastric cancer, the final results of the 15-year follow-up of phase III clinical trial with 5-fluorouracil

TABLE 1 | The agonists of TLRs in the immunotherapy of gastric cancer.

TLR	TLR agonist/inhibitor	Signal	Effect	Reference
TLR2	ELL	Activate BMDCs and CTLs	Anti-cancer	Koizumi et al., 2012
TLR2/TLR4	Coley toxin BCG	Induce apoptosis and autophagy of gastric cancer cell line MGC-803 (a human gastric cancer cell line)	Anti-cancer	Galluzzi et al., 2012; Yao et al., 2018
TLR3	PolyA:U	Combined with 5-fluorouracil, Adriamycin	Anti-advanced cancer	Jeung et al., 2008
	Poly (I:C)	Overstimulate the immune system	Cause autoimmune and chronic inflammatory diseases	Anders et al., 2005; Lang et al., 2005; Jiang et al., 2008; Zhao et al., 2012; Hafner et al., 2013
TLR4	LPS	promote an suitable environment for the continued proliferation of cancer cells and helping to evade cancer cells from immune surveillance	Pro-cancer	Huang et al., 2005; Tang and Zhu, 2012; Fu et al., 2013; Wang et al., 2013
TLR5	Flagellin	Activate NF-kB	Anti-cancer	Soto et al., 2003; Sfondrini et al., 2006; Rhee et al., 2008; Cai et al., 2011; Burdelya et al., 2012; Garaude et al., 2012
TLR7	Imiquimod	promote the secretion of TNF-α and IL-6, and inhibited cell proliferation in SGC-7901 cells (a human gastric cancer cell line)	Anti-cancer	Jiang et al., 2016
TLR9	Chloroquine(non-specific TLR9 inhibitor)	inhibit the invasion of gastric adenocarcinoma cell line AGS induced by h. pylori DNA.	Anti-cancer	Kauppila et al., 2013

ELL, the extract of larixleptolepis; Coleytoxin, a mixture of inactivated Streptococcus pyogenes and marcescens Serratia; BCG, Bacillus Calmette-Guerrin; poly A:U, Polyadenylic–polyuridylicacid; Chloroquine is a non-specific TLR9 inhibitor, others are all agonists of TLRs.

TABLE 2 | The adjuvants of TLRs in the immunotherapy of gastric cancer.

TLR	Vaccine	Signal	Effect	Reference
TLR2	BCG-CWS	Provide immune enhancement through dendritic cells	Anti-gastric cancer	Tsuji et al., 2000
	TLR2-L Amplivant	Induce DCs maturation,T cell priming	Anti-cancer	Zom et al., 2018
	BPPcysMPEG	Generate CTLs via cross-priming	Anti-cancer	Prajeeth et al., 2010
	ANXA2m	Induce DCs maturation	Anti-cancer	Andersen et al., 2016
	lipo-OVA	Activate BMDCs maturation	Anti-cancer	Wu et al., 2016
TLR3	Poly (I:C) -DOTAP liposome complex nanoparticles	enhance the cellular penetration of poly (I:C) and produce corresponding TLR3 signals in BMDCs.	Anti-cancer	Wang et al., 2012
	ARNAX	Targeting TLR3 in DCs, enhancing DC-priming and CTL proliferation	Anti-cancer	Seya et al., 2019
TLR7	T7-MB	Combined with 5-Fu	Anti-gastric cancer	Wang et al., 2018
TLR9	A nanoscale vaccine	Simulates epitope of gastric cancer specific antigen MG7 and adjuvant CpGODN1645	Anti-cancer	Shi et al., 2005

BCG-CWS, BCG cell wall skeleton; TLR2-L Amplivant, a modified Pam3CSK4, TLR2-ligand; BPPcysMPEG, TLR2/6 heterodimer agonist; ANXA2m, an O2-regulated protein binding and signaling through TLR2; lipo-OVA, ovalbumin fused with a bacterial lipid moiety TLR2 agonist; T7-MB, T7 and MG7-Ag conjugated; T7, TLR7 agonist; MG7-Ag, Monoclonal gastric cancer 7 antigen.

and adriamycin vs. 5-fluorouracil, Adriamycin, and poly(A:U) showed that immunochemotherapy had a survival advantage over chemotherapy alone. But this treatment regimen hasn't become standard therapy for GC patients, which may be due to the lack of platinum drugs in the regimen despite its positive effects (Jeung et al., 2008).

However, poly(I:C) has the opposite effect on cancer. The immune system is overstimulated by poly(I:C), leading to autoimmune and chronic inflammatory diseases. Therefore, we strongly recommend the use of poly(I:C) with alow dose and local injection of particle preparation (Anders et al., 2005; Lang et al., 2005; Jiang et al., 2008; Zhao et al., 2012; Hafner et al., 2013). To overcome the effect, a safe adjuvant, called ARNAX, has been developed which targets for TLR3 in dendritic cells (DCs). Compared to poly(I:C), ARNAX hardly induces the production of proinflammatory cytokines, so it does not result in systemic cytokinemia. The combined use of ARNAX/TAA and anti-PD-L1 Ab can induce the resistance of anti-PD-1 (Takeda et al., 2017). It can enhance anti-tumor immunity by promoting DC-priming and CTL proliferation (Seya et al., 2019).

As an adjuvant, TLR3 agonist is a double-edged sword in gastric cancer. However, it still needs a long time to further perfect the research *in vivo* and *in vitro* before it can be used clinically for gastric cancer.

TLR4

TLR4 is expressed in both tumor and immune cells. The influence of TLR4 on cancer is two-sided, depending on where it is expressed.

Several studies have demonstrated that the expression of TLR4 is increased in various cancer cells and tissues, including gastrointestinal cancers, hepatic cancer, pancreatic cancer, and ovarian cancer (Mai et al., 2013). In gastric cancer, TLR4 is the recognition receptor of helicobacter pylori LPS on gastric epithelial cells (Kawahara et al., 2001; Maeda et al., 2001; Su et al., 2003; Basak et al., 2005). The pro-cancer mechanisms of TLR4 expressing on cancer cells include promoting an environment suitable for the continued proliferation of cancer cells and helping to evade cancer cells from immune surveillance (Huang et al., 2005; Tang and Zhu, 2012; Fu et al., 2013; Wang et al., 2013). For example, LPS-stimulated MC26 (colon cancer) cells supernatants significantly inhibited the function of T cell and NK cell. And in the supernatants, the levels of nitric oxide and IL-6 were higher than controls. So, the production of factors induced by TLR4 signaling is a way to tumor evasion from immune surveillance (Huang et al., 2005). LPS first forms complexes with LPS binding proteins (LBP) and then interacts with monocyte differentiation antigen CD14 and myeloid differentiation protein 2 (MD-2) in turn (Thomas et al., 2002). The complex and TLR4 synergistically induce the MyD88-dependent signaling pathways that lead to transcription factors, which promote inflammation and cancer (Takeda et al., 2003).

Several immune modulators targeting TLR4 have been reported. By binding to and forming a chelate complex with LPS, the TLR4 regulators (antagonists and inhibitors) antagonize the interaction of LPS with CD14 and MD2. TLR4 inhibitors suppress NF-κB signaling, thus reducing inflammation-induced carcinogenesis. For instance, in preclinical models, there is evidence that TLR4 inhibitors can effectively inhibit the development of colon cancer (Kuo et al., 2016) and breast cancer (Yang et al., 2014). It is also suggested as a treatment method for liver cancer (Toffanin et al., 2012). The TLR4 antagonist Ibudilast (AV4II) inhibits the secretion of pro-inflammatory cytokines in neuroinflammation (Ledeboer et al., 2006). This suggests that TLR4 could even be widely used as a primary target for suppressing inflammation-related cancers.

At the same time, activated-TLR4 expressed on immune cells is essential to anti-cancer immunity. Compared with wild-type mice, TLR4-deficient mice grew more tumors after oral tube feeding with carcinogenic polyaromatic aromatic hydrocarbons (PAHs) (Naseemuddin et al., 2012). TLR4 agonists induce maturation of dendritic cells (DCs), promoting the immune response of cancer-antigen specific cytotoxic T cells (Fang et al., 2014), which ultimately kill cancer cells. Mainly based on the mechanism, TLR4 agonists have immunomodulatory effects as adjuvants in vaccines, chronic viral infection therapy, and cancer therapy. Jang et al. identified 60S acidic ribosomal protein P2 (RPLP2) by pull-down assay using human cancer derived proteins that binds to TLR4. Recombinant RPLP2 induced maturation and activation of DCs *in vitro*. This DC-based vaccine has been shown to improve both tumor prevention and tumor treatment *in vivo* (Jang et al., 2020). Monophosphoryllipids A (MPLA) with low toxicity, a modified lipopolysaccharide derivative, retains most of the immune-stimulating activity. It is an immunomodulatory agent that stimulates T cell priming by activating the TRIF-associated TLR4 signaling pathway, not MyD88 (Casella and Mitchell, 2008). MPLA has been approved as part of the hepatitis B and human papillomavirus vaccines (Krieg, 2007), but whether it can have the same effect in gastric cancer remains to be seen. OK-432(Picibanil), an anticancer agent, was reported acting at least partly via TLR4-MD2 signaling pathway and inducing maturation of DCs (Ryoma et al., 2004). In a case report, a squamous cell carcinoma patient was treated with intratumoral injection of OK-432, then the tumor size diminished and no metastasis occurred during a follow-up of 5 years (Akeda et al., 2012). Studies have shown that OK-432 adjuvant immunochemotherapy may have marginal and significant efficacy in stage III or IV patients after radical gastrectomy of gastric cancer (Oba et al., 2016).

As the most classical TLR in gastric cancer caused by helicobacter pylori, TLR4 has great value in immunotherapy of gastric cancer. From the current background, TLR4 stimulation is a double-edged sword, so more researches should be done on gastric cancer patients, and then search for the balance of anti-tumor and pro-tumor in the future.

TLR5

Many studies have suggested that TLR5 is an effective target for antitumor immunotherapy. Bacterial flagellin, a TLR5 agonist, has been demonstrated strong anti-cancer effect in lots of animal models (Soto et al., 2003; Sfondrini et al., 2006; Rhee et al., 2008; Cai et al., 2011; Burdelya et al., 2012; Garaude et al., 2012). The anti-cancer effects of TLR5 agonists stem from the dependence on TLR5 to activate NF-κB. Flagellin is a potent catalyst for NF-κB signaling that mediates natural and acquired anti-tumor immune responses. Nucleoside diphosphate kinase 3(NME3) can enhance flagellin signaling. The expression of NME3 is highly associated with the expression of TLR5 in GC. High NME3 expression reduces the overall survival rate of gastric cancer. In summary, NME3 may strengthen cancer immunotherapy as an unrecognized pro-inflammatory cytokine in TLR5 downstream signaling (Flentie et al., 2018). An adenovirus-based tumor-specific delivery vector, called Mobilan, drives the expression of the TLR5 signaling cassette, which is composed of salmonella flagellin and humanTLR5, which is similar in structure to the clinical-stage TLR5 agonist entolimod. The injection of Mobilan was injected into the primary tumors of transgenic adenocarcinoma mice susceptible to prostate cancer (TRAMP), resulting in a powerful induction of a couple of genes involved in inflammation and mobilization of natural immune cells, to suppress tumor progression (Mett et al., 2018). The high expression of TLR5 in the tissues may determine the better prognosis of patients with GC, especially those with intestinal-type and stage II advanced GC (Kasurinen et al., 2019). Conversely, TLR5 agonist was reported that can induce an inflammatory response and inhibited some tumor progression.

Therefore, the mechanism of TLR5 in immunotherapy of GC deserves further study.

TLR7

TLR7 is expressed on the endosomal membrane (Takeda and Akira, 2015). TLR7 was found low expressed in GC tissues (Jiang et al., 2016). Activating TLR7 can strengthen anti-cancer immunity. Ma et.al developed a bi-functional vector containing a Bcl-2-silencing shRNA and a TLR7-stimulating ssRNA, which promoted apoptosis and inhibited cell growth in MFC cells (a mouse gastric cancer cell line) (Minaga et al., 2017). UC-1V150 which is a TLR7 agonist binds to phospholipids to increase levels of pro-inflammatory cytokines (Wu et al., 2007). A typical TLR7 agonist-imiquimod who has a non-nucleoside imidazolquinoline structure, can be used in immunotherapy of superficial basal cell carcinoma (Papadavid et al., 2007). Imiquimod can induce the expression of TLR7 protein, promote inflammatory cytokines secreting, and inhibited cell proliferation in one of the human gastric cancer cell lines (Jiang et al., 2016). It is also being studied as an adjuvant to anti-tumor vaccines. However, imiquimod lacks the chemical groups that are associated with proteins or peptides. Another TLR7 agonist (T7) has a free carboxyl group that can be attached to amino peptides (Chan et al., 2009). Small molecule T7 was covalently attached to gastric cancer antigen to construct a series of vaccines. After being introduced into animal models, the vaccines could generate immunogenic stimulation and tumor inhibition (Wang et al., 2015). Tumor-associated antigen (TAA) is a target of anti-cancer immunotherapy (Zhang et al., 2006). The monoclonal gastric cancer 7 antigen (MG7-Ag), a TAA in GC, has higher specificity and selectivity compared with existing antigens. T7 and MG7-Ag were conjugated together to construct a new gastric cancer vaccine T7–MB. The inhibition effect of 5-Fu and T7–MB on tumor size and volume by treatment regimen was higher than that of 5-Fu or T7–MB alone (Wang et al., 2018). Overall, either used alone or used as an adjuvant, TLR7 agonist has been shown as an anti-tumor agent in immunotherapy of gastric cancer currently.

TLR9

TLR9 is expressed in many cancer tissues and cell lines, including gastric, hepatocellular, prostate, and colorectal cancers (Damiano et al., 2007; Brignole et al., 2010; So and Ouchi, 2010). TLR9 can play the role of both anti-tumor and pro-tumor. For example, in hepatocellular carcinoma cell lines, the activation of TLR-9 inhibits apoptosis by IL-8, IL-1, IL-6 up-regulation, thereby increasing proliferation and inflammation. In neuroblastoma cells, the activation of TLR-9 results in increased cystatin-dependent apoptotic cell death (Brignole et al., 2010).

TLR-9 can enhance anti-tumor immunity by recognizing Oligodeoxynucleotide(ODN) containing cytosine–guanine dinucleotide (CpG), which is a potential therapeutic agent. Immunosuppressive cells characteristically exist in the immune microenvironment, one of which is Myeloid suppressor cells (MDSC). A large number of MDSCs cluster near the tumor and inhibit the activity of T cells and NK cells. Several reports showed that the agonist CpG ODN of TLR9 can kill tumors by reducing the immunosuppressive activity of monocyte MDSC11-12. At the same time, CpG ODN can be used as a powerful adjuvant to many antigens. CpG ODN promotes the Th1 response (Weiner, 2000; Mccluskie et al., 2002), and when used in combination with the immunogen, enhances immune responses (Yamamoto et al., 2000). It directly activates monocytes/macrophages, DCs, etc., and inducts pro-inflammatory cytokines (Wagner et al., 2000; Gramzinski et al., 2001; Liu et al., 2003). Especially when CpG ODN is tightly bound to the antigen, the activity will be improved. Xu et al. first conducted polyethyleneimine-CpG nanocomplex (CpG@PEI) as an *in situ* vaccine for melanoma *in vivo* therapy (Xu et al., 2020). Shi et al. constructed a nanoscale vaccine that simulates epitope of gastric cancer-specific antigen MG7 and adjuvant CpGODN1645, may have important significance for tumor treatment (Shi et al., 2005).

Kauppila et al. found that Helicobacter pylori DNA can promote the invasion of gastric adenocarcinoma cell line AGS, while chloroquine (non-specific TLR9 inhibitor) can inhibit the invasion induced by Helicobacter pylori DNA (Kauppila et al., 2013). Qin et al. found that in human gastric cancer cells, H. pylori DNA can up-regulate TLR9 expression, promoting cell proliferation, migration, and invasion. In a word, TLR9 is involved in the occurrence and development of gastric cancer (Qin et al., 2019).

A TLR9 agonist can be used as an adjuvant in immunotherapy to make the checkpoint inhibitors more effective. Fumi et al. confirmed that intratumoral administration of 1V270 (TLR7 agonist) or SD-101(TLR9 agonist) and blocking PD-1 can suppress the development of primary tumors and prevent tumor metastasis in the head and neck squamous cell carcinoma (HNSCC) model. This treatment is more effective than any drug alone (Sato-Kaneko et al., 2017). Reilley et al. demonstrated that intratumoral administration of ODN1826 (TLR9 agonist) can synergistically block ctLA-4 and promote the rejection of bilateral implantation of B16 ovalbumin (B16-OVA) melanoma (Reilley et al., 2019).

Above all, we can see that no matter whether the function of TLR9 is pro- or anti-cancer, it is important in the immunotherapy of cancer. How to use its function to treat gastric cancer deserves further study.

CURRENT IMMUNOTHERAPIES FOR GASTRIC CANCER

According to TCGA network classification, gastric cancer is divided into four molecular subtypes: Epstein-Barr virus (EBV), microsatellite instability (MSI), genomically stable (GS), and chromosomal instability (CIN)gastric cancers (Sohn et al., 2017). PD-L1 is more likely expressed on the EBV and MSI subtype (Ma et al., 2016).

At present, trastuzumab targeting HER2 has become the standard therapeutics for advanced gastric cancer as a molecular targeted therapy (Abrahao-Machado and Scapulatempo-Neto, 2016), but the prognosis of patients is still poor. Therefore, immunotherapy for gastric cancer has emerged recently.

Immune Checkpoint Inhibitors

The immune system eliminating cancer cells depends on the cancer-immune cycle, including recognition, stimulation, recruitment, amplification, and final memory to inhibit cell growth. T lymphocytes work together to stimulate and inhibit molecules, which act as immune checkpoints. Through immune checkpoint pathways, T cell suppression signals are released allowing tumors to evade immune surveillance and destruction, thus achieving malignant proliferation (Hanahan and Weinberg, 2011; Pardoll, 2012). Programmed death receptor-1 (PD-1) is mainly expressed on the surface of activated T cells and B cells, and is the receptor involved in cell death. Programmed death receptor-ligand 1 (PD-L1) is binding to PD-1, expressed in antigen-presenting cells(APC), such as macrophages, DCs, and cancer cells. Prolonged TCR stimulation induces the secretion of interferon-γ (IFN-γ) to increased PD-L1 in cancer cells (Buchbinder and Desai, 2016). PD-L1 binding to PD-1 decreases the function and cytotoxicity of effector T cell. The interaction of CD28 on T cells with B7-1/2 on APCs is essential for T cell activation. Cytotoxic T lymphocyte-associated antigen 4 (CTLA-4) has a much higher binding affinity with B7, but not promoting T cell activation (Leach et al., 1996). So the molecule has a non-overlapping inhibitory effect against tumor immunity and participates in the early stage of an immune response of lymphoid organs (Abrahao-Machado and Scapulatempo-Neto, 2016). When immune checkpoint inhibitors are combined with PD-1, PD-L1, and CTLA-4, the function of T lymphocytes can't be suppressed, and the immune response is activated against cancer (Coutzac et al., 2019).

An anti-PD-1 antibody binds to PD-1 to prevent the combination of PD-1 and PD-L1. Blocking the PD-1 pathway inhibits the negative immune regulation of the PD-1 pathway on T cells, then the anti-tumor response is stimulated (Ribas et al., 2015; Nghiem et al., 2016; Bellmunt et al., 2017; Eggermont et al., 2018; Fuchs et al., 2018; Gandhi et al., 2018; Zhu et al., 2018; Chung et al., 2019). Pembrolizumab is a high-affinity anti-PD-1 humanized monoclonal antibody targeting the PD-1 receptor and is already approved for treating GC. A phase 1 study of patients with advanced PD-1 positive GC has shown that pembrolizumab had good antitumor activity and controlled toxicity, which needs further verification in phase 2 and 3 trials (Muro et al., 2016).

Nivolumab, a humanized monoclonal immunoglobulin G4 antibody, is also a PD-1 receptor blocking antibody. It has been approved as a treatment for advanced gastric cancer in Japan. In a phase III randomized study, the ONO-4538-12 (ATTRACTION-2) trial, patients receiving chemotherapy for unresectable late-stage gastric esophageal cancer were divided into the nivolumab 3 mg/kg group and the placebo group (Kang et al., 2017). Nivolumab improved the median overall survival rate. Of patients treated with nivolumab, the recurrence rate was 12% and the tumor reduction rate was 40%. Nivolumab can improve the survival of patients regardless of whether there is PD-L1 expression (Boku et al., 2017). Therefore, regardless of the state of PD-L1, nivolumab is effective for chemotherapeutic gastric cancer.

Anti-PD-L1 antibodies reverse the anti-inflammatory effect of PD-1/PD-L1 pathway and contribute to the anticancer response by binding to PD-L1. Comparative study of Avelumab (anti-PD-L1 antibody) and chemotherapy in the treatment of gastric cancer/gastroesophageal junction cancer showed that the clinical activity of avelumab is not superior to chemotherapy, but avelumab is safer than chemotherapy (Bang et al., 2018).

Durvalumab (the anti–PD-L1 antibody) and tremelimumab (the anti–CTLA-4 antibody) can enhance T cells response to the tumor by blocking the immune checkpoint together, thus generating anti-tumor activity. A Phase Ib/II study in patients with advanced GC showed durvalumab and tremelimumab have a manageable safety profile in the second-line and third-line treatment, with encouraging survival rate compared to durvalumab alone (Kelly et al., 2020).

Ipilimumab is a monoclonal antibody binding to CTLA-4, which can enhance T cells activation and promote tumor immunity. A report compared ipilimumab monotherapy with best supportive care in GC patients who have stabilized during first-line chemotherapy. Compared with the latter, the progression-free survival of the former wasn't improved. In ipilimumab group, the median overall survival rate is ~1 year and ipilimumab has good safety. So, the drugs combined with other therapies for advanced GC is worth for futherstudies (Bang et al., 2017).

It can be seen that not all patients can benefit from immune checkpoint inhibitor therapy alone. As many patients with GC are CIN and GS, the immune signal expresses lowly, and the response to immunotherapy may be weak, but the safety is an advantage compared with traditional radiotherapy and chemotherapy. The combination of immunotherapy inhibitors has been used more and more to improve the response of immunotherapy and has achieved remarkable results.

Checkpoint Blockade Immunotherapy

Checkpoint blocking immunotherapy revolutionizes cancer treatment and improves patient survival and quality of life. However, the effects of this immunotherapy are highly heterogeneous between patients (Chuang et al., 2020). Response rates of patients to checkpoint blockade range from 15 to 30% in most solid tumors (Das and Johnson, 2019). It is urgent to find effective adjuvant treatments to improve the efficacy of immune checkpoint inhibitors. Tumors with low numbers of tumor-infiltrating T cells tend to respond poorly to immune checkpoint blockade therapy (Tsukamoto et al., 2019). As mentioned earlier, TLRs play an important role in immune response. So TLRs agonists may be potential adjuvants for treating overcome checkpoint blockade resistance, to increase efficacy of checkpoint blockade therapy.

It has been shown that the infiltration of CD8+ T cells in tumor site is essential to anti-tumor effect of PD-1 blockade therapy (Tumeh et al., 2014). Many studies have confirmed that TLRs agonists can increase the level of CD8+ T cells or activate CD8+ T cells.

Pam3CSK4, a TLR1/2 ligand, increased Fcγ receptor IV expression on macrophages. The macrophage mediated

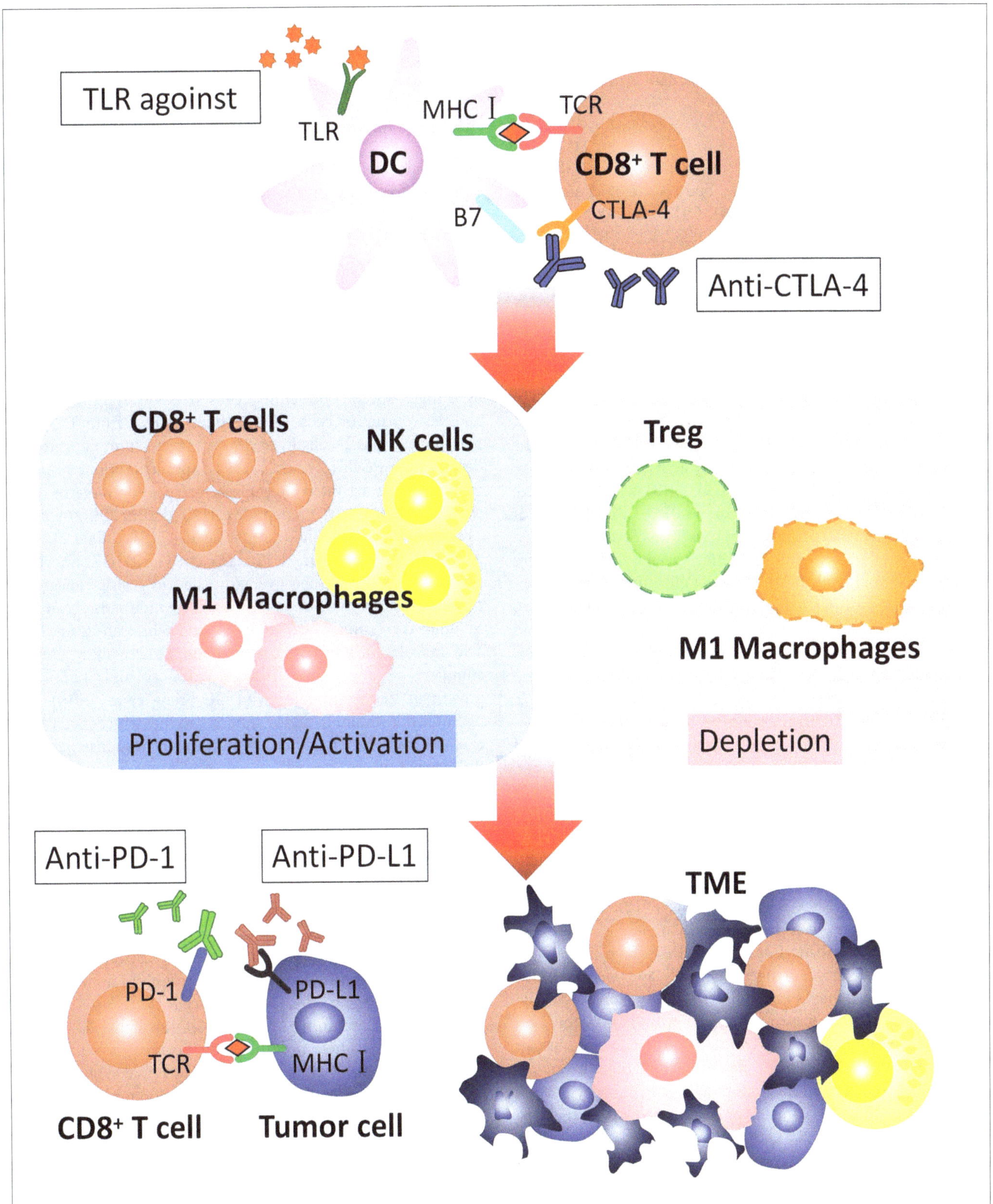

FIGURE 2 | How TLR agonist promotes the efficacy of checkpoint blockade therapy. CTLA-4 is expressed on the surface of $CD8^+$ T cell, combining with B7 on dendritic cells (DCs), to regulate T cell responses. CTLA-4 pathway can be blocked by anti-CTLA-4 antibodies. TLR agonist activates TLR on DC. Activated TLRs pathway can induce proliferation or activation of $CD8^+$ T cells, M1 macrophages and NK-cells, and depletion of M2 macrophages and Tregs. $CD8^+$ T cells, M1

(Continued)

FIGURE 2 | macrophages and NK-cells recognize and kill tumor cells in TME. PD-1 is expressed on CD8+ T cell. PD-L1 is expressed on tumor cell. The combination of PD-1 with PD-L1 inhibits the anti-tumor effect of T cells, that can be blocked by anti-PD-1 or anti-PD-L1 antibodies. TLR agonist and anti-CTLA-4/anti-PD-1/anti-PD-L1 antibodies play a synergistic role in anti-tumor immunotherapy. TLR, toll-like receptor; TCR, T cell receptor; CTLA-4, The cytotoxic T-lymphocyte-associated antigen-4; PD-1, Programmed cell death protein 1; PD-L1, Programmed death ligand 1; TME,Tumor microenvironment.

depletion of Tregs. Through the mechanism, Pam3CSK4 can increase efficacy of anti-CTLA-4 antibody (Chuang et al., 2020). A unique structural domain (UNE-C1) was identified as a novel TLR2/6 ligand that can activate dendritic cells to produce a powerful humoral and cellular immune response *in vivo*. UNE-C1 also showed synergistic effects *in vivo* with tumor antigens and checkpoint inhibitors in different cancer models (Cho et al., 2020). ARNAX, a TLR3 agonist, promoted full priming and proliferation of CTLs and enhanced CD8+ T cell infifiltration into the tumor site through TLR3-TIR domain-containing adaptor molecule-1 (TICAM-1)-IRF3-IFN-β axis in DCs. Therapy using ARNAX/TAA can overcome anti-PD-L1 resistance (Takeda et al., 2017). OVA/TLR4 mAb can enhance the anti-tumor effect of anti-PD-1 mAb by activating OVA-specific CD8+ T-cells (Tsukamoto et al., 2019). CIRP is a TLR4 ligand. SIIN-CIRP up-regulated the expression of PD-L1 on DC, but at the same time enhanced T cell response. It was finally confirmed that the combination of the SIIN-CIRP vaccine with antibodies against PD-1 can inhibit tumor growth (Villanueva et al., 2018).

Combining anti-PD-1 with CMP-001 (a TLR-9 agonist) to treat head and neck squamous cell carcinoma (HNSCC) had a better effect and prolonged the survival time of mouse, compared with anti-PD-1 alone. And CMP-001+anti-PD-1 induced anti-tumor response depends on activation of CD8+ T cells (Cheng et al., 2020). In addition to depending on CD8+ cells, there are other mechanisms that promote the efficacy of checkpoint blockade therapy. CpG is a TLR9 ligand. It can down-regulate PD-1 expresssion on CD8+ T cells by inducing the production of IL-12 from dendritic cells (Yin et al., 2016). Thomas et al. confirmed the combination of CpG with CTLA-4 or PD-1 blockade not only increased the levels of circulating tumor-specific CD8+ T cells, but also reduced the number of Tregs at the tumor site (Mangsbo et al., 2010). Lefitolimod, also a TLR9 agonist, can induce the secretion of IFN-α by qDC. IFN-α increased the number of CD8+ T cells and anti-tumoral M1 macrophages, activated NK-cells and decreased pro-tumoral M2 macrophages inside the TME. In colon carcinoma CT26 model, the combined treatment with lefitolimod and anti-PD-L1 inhibited tumor growth and prolonged survival of the mice (Kapp et al., 2019). Radiation can directly induce upregulation of PD-L1 on tumor cells, and also act as an adaptive resistance mechanism for T cells to release IFNγ in tumor microenvironment. There is a hypothesis that the addition of targeted immunosuppressive PD-1/PD-L1 checkpoint to the radiation /TLR regimen may enhance the antitumor immune response (Walshaw et al., 2020).

In conclusion, TLRs agonists can promote efficacy of checkpoint blockade therapy by inducing or activating CD8+ T cells, M1 macrophages and NK-cells, decreasing M2 macrophages and Tregs, and down-regulating PD-1 expresssion on CD8+ T cells. TLRs agonists are potential adjuvants for checkpoint blockade therapy (**Figure 2**).

Tumor Antigen Vaccine

Tumor-associated antigen (TAAs) can activate the immune response. By generating an immune response, cancer vaccines transform tumor-specific T cells into effector T cells. Therapeutic vaccines can enhance autoimmunity, leading to a stronger anti-tumor immune response. In order to induce tumor-specific T cells, peptides produced by TAAs must be provided to T cells by antigen-specific presenting cells to play an immune role and destroy tumor cells. The peptides derived from TAAs are presented to the T cells by APCs to play an immune role and destroy tumor cells (Steinman, 1991). Specific immune response in GC can be activated by protein and peptide targets. These studies are based on TAA peptide extracted from HER2/neu and MAGE. TAA peptide induces cytotoxic T cells to fight cancers, restricted to MHC class I (Tanaka et al., 1997; Kono et al., 1998). Typical HER2/neu overexpression in gastric cancer and dendritic cells immunizing HER2/neu peptide pulses can lead to tumor regression. The MAGE-3 peptide/chitosan-deoxycholic acid inoculation nanoparticles have been successfully used to stimulate an anti-tumor immune response and inhibit the growth of tumors in mice with GC (Yang et al., 2010). The potential of combining tumor antigen vaccines with conventional chemotherapy to strengthen the anti-cancer response has been the focus of current research.

TLR agonists have been reported that they can contribute to anti-tumor immunity as adjuvants in conjunction with other immunotherapies. It seems that combination therapy is more effective in immunotherapy.

CONCLUSION

The immunotherapy of gastric cancer is a hot topic in recent years. TLRs are expressed not only in natural immune cells but also in non-immune cells, like tumor cells. TLRs play a crucial role in innate immunity. Many studies show that TLRs have complex functions in tumor immunity including pro-tumor and anti-tumor. There is considerable evidence that TLRs play an important role in the occurrence and development of GC, can recognize the composition of Helicobacter pylori, a major cause for GC. TLRs are increasingly being used as immunotherapeutic targets for cancer and infectious diseases. TLR ligands show their anti-tumor activity not only as therapeutic agents directly but also as adjuvants in conjunction with tumor-associated antigen (TAA) or immune checkpoint inhibitors. TLRs agonists are potential adjuvants for checkpoint blockade therapy. Although TLR-based immunotherapy is imperfect and has not been widely used in the clinic yet, elucidating the mechanism of TLR signaling in anti-tumor response and its interaction with other signaling pathways is meaningful. TLRs may provide a promising novel strategy for gastric cancer treatment.

AUTHOR CONTRIBUTIONS

LC performed literature searches, and drafted the manuscript. XW drew figures and supplemented the manuscript. DZ revised the manuscript. LC and DZ developed the idea for this article. All authors have approved the final version of this submission.

REFERENCES

Abrahao-Machado, L. F., and Scapulatempo-Neto, C. (2016). HER2 testing in gastric cancer: an update. *World J. Gastroenterol.* 22, 4619–4625. doi: 10.3748/wjg.v22.i19.4619

Akazawa, T., Inoue, N., Shime, H., Kodama, K., Matsumoto, M., and Seya, T. (2010). Adjuvant engineering for cancer immunotherapy: development of a synthetic TLR2 ligand with increased cell adhesion. *Cancer Sci.* 101, 1596–1603. doi: 10.1111/j.1349-7006.2010.01583.x

Akazawa, T., Ohashi, T., Wijewardana, V., Sugiura, K., and Inoue, N. (2018). Development of a vaccine based on bacteria-mimicking tumor cells coated with novel engineered toll-like receptor. 2 ligands. *Cancer Sci.* 109, 1319–1329. doi: 10.1111/cas.13576

Akeda, T., Yamanaka, K., Kitagawa, H., Kawabata, E., Tsuda, K., Kakeda, M., et al. (2012). Intratumoral injection of OK-432 suppresses metastatic squamous cell carcinoma lesion inducing interferon-γ and tumour necrosis factor-α. *Clin. Exp. Dermatol.* 37, 193–194. doi: 10.1111/j.1365-2230.2011.04151.x

Akira, S., Uematsu, S., and Takeuchi, O. (2006). Pathogen recognition and innate immunity. *Cell* 124, 783–801. doi: 10.1016/j.cell.2006.02.015

Anders, H. J., Zecher, D., Pawar, R. D., and Patole, P. S. (2005). Molecular mechanisms of autoimmunity triggered by microbial infection. *Arthritis Res. Ther.* 7, 215–224. doi: 10.1186/ar1818

Andersen, B. M., Xia, J., Epstein, A. L., Ohlfest, J. R., Chen, W., Blazar, B. R., et al. (2016). Monomeric annexin A2 is an oxygen-regulated toll-like receptor. 2 ligand and adjuvant. *J. Immunother. Cancer* 4:11. doi: 10.1186/s40425-016-0112-6

Bang, Y. J., Cho, J. Y., Kim, Y. H., Kim, J. W., Di Bartolomeo, M., Ajani, J. A., et al. (2017). Efficacy of sequential ipilimumab monotherapy versus best supportive care for unresectable locally advanced/metastatic gastric or gastroesophageal junction cancer. *Clin. Cancer Res.* 23, 5671–5678. doi: 10.1158/1078-0432.Ccr-17-0025

Bang, Y. J., Ruiz, E. Y., Van Cutsem, E., Lee, K. W., Wyrwicz, L., Schenker, M., et al. (2018). Phase III, randomised trial of avelumab versus physician's choice of chemotherapy as third-line treatment of patients with advanced gastric or gastro-oesophageal junction cancer: primary analysis of JAVELIN Gastric 300. *Ann. Oncol.* 29, 2052–2060. doi: 10.1093/annonc/mdy264

Barton, G. M., and Kagan, J. C. (2009). A cell biological view of Toll-like receptor function: regulation through compartmentalization. *Nat. Rev. Immunol.* 9, 535–542. doi: 10.1038/nri2587

Basak, C., Pathak, S. K., Bhattacharyya, A., Mandal, D., Pathak, S., and Kundu, M. (2005). NF-kappaB- and C/EBPbeta-driven interleukin-1beta gene expression and PAK1-mediated caspase-1 activation play essential roles in interleukin-1beta release from *Helicobacter pylori* lipopolysaccharide-stimulated macrophages. *J. Biol. Chem.* 280, 4279–4288. doi: 10.1074/jbc.M412820200

Bellmunt, J., De Wit, R., Vaughn, D. J., Fradet, Y., Lee, J. L., Fong, L., et al. (2017). Pembrolizumab as second-line therapy for advanced urothelial carcinoma. *N. Engl. J. Med.* 376, 1015–1026. doi: 10.1056/NEJMoa1613683

Boku, N., Kang, Y., Satoh, T., Chao, Y., Kato, K., Chung, H., et al. (2017). 617OA Phase. 3 Study of nivolumab (Nivo) in previously treated advanced gastric or gastroesophageal junction (G/GEJ) cancer: Updated results and subset analysis by PD-L1 expression (ATTRACTION-02). *Ann. Oncol.* 28(Suppl. 5), v209–v268. doi: 10.1093/annonc/mdx369

Braunstein, M. J., Kucharczyk, J., and Adams, S. (2018). Targeting toll-like receptors for cancer therapy. *Target. Oncol.* 13, 583–598. doi: 10.1007/s11523-018-0589-7

Bray, F., Ferlay, J., Soerjomataram, I., Siegel, R. L., Torre, L. A., and Jemal, A. (2018). Global cancer statistics. 2018: GLOBOCAN estimates of incidence and mortality worldwide for 36 cancers in 185 countries. *CA Cancer J. Clin.* 68, 394–424. doi: 10.3322/caac.21492

Brignole, C., Marimpietri, D., Di Paolo, D., Perri, P., Morandi, F., Pastorino, F., et al. (2010). Therapeutic targeting of TLR9 inhibits cell growth and induces apoptosis in neuroblastoma. *Cancer Res.* 70, 9816–9826. doi: 10.1158/0008-5472.Can-10-1251

Buchbinder, E. I., and Desai, A. (2016). CTLA-4 and PD-1 pathways: similarities, differences, and implications of their inhibition. *Am. J. Clin. Oncol.* 39, 98–106. doi: 10.1097/coc.0000000000000239

Burdelya, L. G., Gleiberman, A. S., Toshkov, I., Aygun-Sunar, S., Bapardekar, M., Manderscheid-Kern, P., et al. (2012). Toll-like receptor. 5 agonist protects mice from dermatitis and oral mucositis caused by local radiation: implications for head-and-neck cancer radiotherapy. *Int. J. Radiat. Oncol. Biol. Phys.* 83, 228–234. doi: 10.1016/j.ijrobp.2011.05.055

Cai, Z., Sanchez, A., Shi, Z., Zhang, T., Liu, M., and Zhang, D. (2011). Activation of toll-like receptor 5 on breast cancer cells by flagellin suppresses cell proliferation and tumor growth. *Cancer Res.* 71, 2466–2475. doi: 10.1158/0008-5472.Can-10-1993

Cancer Genome Atlas Research Network (2014). Comprehensive molecular characterization of gastric adenocarcinoma. *Nature* 513, 202–209. doi: 10.1038/nature13480

Casella, C. R., and Mitchell, T. C. (2008). Putting endotoxin to work for us: monophosphoryl lipid A as a safe and effective vaccine adjuvant. *Cell. Mol. Life Sci.* 65, 3231–3240. doi: 10.1007/s00018-008-8228-6

Castaño-Rodríguez, N., Kaakoush, N. O., and Mitchell, H. M. (2014). Pattern-recognition receptors and gastric cancer. *Front. Immunol.* 5:336. doi: 10.3389/fimmu.2014.00336

Chan, M., Hayashi, T., Kuy, C. S., Gray, C. S., Wu, C. C., Corr, M., et al. (2009). Synthesis and immunological characterization of toll-like receptor. 7 agonistic conjugates. *Bioconjug. Chem.* 20, 1194–1200. doi: 10.1021/bc900054q

Cheng, Y., Lemke-Miltner, C. D., Wongpattaraworakul, W., Wang, Z., Chan, C. H. F., Salem, A. K., et al. (2020). *In situ* immunization of a TLR9 agonist virus-like particle enhances anti-PD1 therapy. *J. Immunother. Cancer* 8:e000940. doi: 10.1136/jitc-2020-000940

Cho, S., Kim, S. B., Lee, Y., Song, E. C., Kim, U., Kim, H. Y., et al. (2020). Endogenous TLR2 ligand embedded in the catalytic region of human cysteinyl-tRNA synthetase. 1. *J. Immunother. Cancer* 8:e000277. doi: 10.1136/jitc-2019-000277

Chuang, Y. C., Tseng, J. C., Huang, L. R., Huang, C. M., Huang, C. F., and Chuang, T. H. (2020). Adjuvant effect of toll-like receptor 9 activation on cancer immunotherapy using checkpoint blockade. *Front. Immunol.* 11:1075. doi: 10.3389/fimmu.2020.01075

Chung, H. C., Ros, W., Delord, J. P., Perets, R., Italiano, A., Shapira-Frommer, R., et al. (2019). Efficacy and safety of pembrolizumab in previously treated advanced cervical cancer: results from the phase II KEYNOTE-158 study. *J. Clin. Oncol.* 37, 1470–1478. doi: 10.1200/jco.18.01265

Coutzac, C., Pernot, S., Chaput, N., and Zaanan, A. (2019). Immunotherapy in advanced gastric cancer, is it the future? *Crit. Rev. Oncol. Hematol.* 133, 25–32. doi: 10.1016/j.critrevonc.2018.10.007

Damiano, V., Caputo, R., Garofalo, S., Bianco, R., Rosa, R., Merola, G., et al. (2007). TLR9 agonist acts by different mechanisms synergizing with bevacizumab in sensitive and cetuximab-resistant colon cancer xenografts. *Proc. Natl. Acad. Sci. U.S.A.* 104, 12468–12473. doi: 10.1073/pnas.0705226104

Das, S., and Johnson, D. B. (2019). Immune-related adverse events and anti-tumor efficacy of immune checkpoint inhibitors. *J. Immunother. Cancer* 7:306. doi: 10.1186/s40425-019-0805-8

Domingos-Pereira, S., Decrausaz, L., Derr,é, L., Bobst, M., Romero, P., Schiller, J. T., et al. (2013). Intravaginal TLR agonists increase local vaccine-specific CD8 T cells and human papillomavirus-associated genital-tumor regression in mice. *Mucosal Immunol.* 6, 393–404. doi: 10.1038/mi.2012.83

Eggermont, A. M. M., Blank, C. U., Mandala, M., Long, G. V., Atkinson, V., Dalle, S., et al. (2018). Adjuvant pembrolizumab versus placebo in resected stage III melanoma. *N. Engl. J. Med.* 378, 1789–1801. doi: 10.1056/NEJMoa1802357

Fang, H., Ang, B., Xu, X., Huang, X., Wu, Y., Sun, Y., et al. (2014). TLR4 is essential for dendritic cell activation and anti-tumor T-cell response enhancement by DAMPs released from chemically stressed cancer cells. *Cell. Mol. Immunol.* 11, 150–159. doi: 10.1038/cmi.2013.59

Flentie, K., Gonzalez, C., Kocher, B., Wang, Y., Zhu, H., Marasa, J., et al. (2018). Nucleoside diphosphate kinase-3 (NME3) enhances TLR5-induced NFκB activation. *Mol. Cancer Res.* 16, 986–999. doi: 10.1158/1541-7786.Mcr-17-0603

Fu, H. Y., Li, C., Yang, W., Gai, X. D., Jia, T., Lei, Y. M., et al. (2013). FOXP3 and TLR4 protein expression are correlated in non-small cell lung cancer: implications for tumor progression and escape. *Acta Histochem.* 115, 151–157. doi: 10.1016/j.acthis.2012.06.002

Fuchs, C. S., Doi, T., Jang, R. W., Muro, K., Satoh, T., Machado, M., et al. (2018). Safety and efficacy of pembrolizumab monotherapy in patients with previously treated advanced gastric and gastroesophageal junction cancer: phase. 2 clinical KEYNOTE-059 trial. *JAMA Oncol.* 4:e180013. doi: 10.1001/jamaoncol.2018.0013

Fukata, M., and Abreu, M. T. (2008). Role of Toll-like receptors in gastrointestinal malignancies. *Oncogene* 27, 234–243. doi: 10.1038/sj.onc.1210908

Galluzzi, L., Vacchelli, E., Eggermont, A., Fridman, W. H., Galon, J., Sautès-Fridman, C., et al. (2012). Trial watch: experimental toll-like receptor agonists for cancer therapy. *Oncoimmunology* 1, 699–716. doi: 10.4161/onci.20696

Gandhi, L., Rodríguez-Abreu, D., Gadgeel, S., Esteban, E., Felip, E., De Angelis, F., et al. (2018). Pembrolizumab plus chemotherapy in metastatic non-small-cell lung cancer. *N. Engl. J. Med.* 378, 2078–2092. doi: 10.1056/NEJMoa1801005

Garaude, J., Kent, A., Van Rooijen, N., and Blander, J. M. (2012). Simultaneous targeting of toll- and nod-like receptors induces effective tumor-specific immune responses. *Sci. Transl. Med.* 4:120ra116. doi: 10.1126/scitranslmed.3002868

Goutagny, N., Estornes, Y., Hasan, U., Lebecque, S., and Caux, C. (2012). Targeting pattern recognition receptors in cancer immunotherapy. *Target. Oncol.* 7, 29–54. doi: 10.1007/s11523-012-0213-1

Gramzinski, R. A., Doolan, D. L., Sedegah, M., Davis, H. L., Krieg, A. M., and Hoffman, S. L. (2001). Interleukin-12- and gamma interferon-dependent protection against malaria conferred by CpG oligodeoxynucleotide in mice. *Infect. Immun.* 69, 1643–1649. doi: 10.1128/iai.69.3.1643-1649.2001

Hafner, A. M., Corthésy, B., and Merkle, H. P. (2013). Particulate formulations for the delivery of poly(I:C) as vaccine adjuvant. *Adv. Drug Deliv. Rev.* 65, 1386–1399. doi: 10.1158/1535-7163.Mct-12-1019

Hanahan, D., and Weinberg, R. A. (2011). Hallmarks of cancer: the next generation. *Cell* 144, 646–674. doi: 10.1016/j.cell.2011.02.013

Hanson, H. L., Donermeyer, D. L., Ikeda, H., White, J. M., Shankaran, V., Old, L. J., et al. (2000). Eradication of established tumors by CD8+ T cell adoptive immunotherapy. *Immunity* 13, 265–276. doi: 10.1016/s1074-7613(00)00026-1

Hennessy, E. J., Parker, A. E., and O'neill, L. A. (2010). Targeting toll-like receptors: emerging therapeutics? *Nat. Rev. Drug Discov.* 9, 293–307. doi: 10.1038/nrd3203

Hu, H. G., Wu, J. J., Zhang, B. D., Li, W. H., and Li, Y. M. (2020). Pam(3)CSK(4)-CDG(SF) augments antitumor immunotherapy by synergistically activating TLR1/2 and STING. *Bioconjug. Chem.* 31, 2499–2503. doi: 10.1021/acs.bioconjchem.0c00522

Huang, B., Zhao, J., Li, H., He, K. L., Chen, Y., Chen, S. H., et al. (2005). Toll-like receptors on tumor cells facilitate evasion of immune surveillance. *Cancer Res.* 65, 5009–5014. doi: 10.1158/0008-5472.Can-05-0784

Jang, G. Y., Kim, Y. S., Lee, S. E., Lee, J. W., Han, H. D., Kang, T. H., et al. (2020). Improvement of DC-based vaccines using adjuvant TLR4-binding. 60S acidic ribosomal protein P2 and immune checkpoint inhibitors. *Cancer Immunol. Immunother.* doi: 10.1007/s00262-020-02759-6. [Epub ahead of print].

Jeremy, C., Xie, W., Charles, Z., and Jon, B. (2016). Immunotherapy and cell therapy for cancer. *Chin. J. Pharmacol. Toxicol.* 30, 87–94

Jeung, H. C., Moon, Y. W., Rha, S. Y., Yoo, N. C., Roh, J. K., Noh, S. H., et al. (2008). Phase III trial of adjuvant. 5-fluorouracil and adriamycin versus. 5-fluorouracil, adriamycin, and polyadenylic-polyuridylic acid (poly A:U) for locally advanced gastric cancer after curative surgery: final results of. 15-year follow-up. *Ann. Oncol.* 19, 520–526. doi: 10.1093/annonc/mdm536

Jiang, J., Dong, L., Qin, B., Shi, H., Guo, X., and Wang, Y. (2016). Decreased expression of TLR7 in gastric cancer tissues and the effects of TLR7 activation on gastric cancer cells. *Oncol. Lett.* 12, 631–636. doi: 10.3892/ol.2016.4617

Jiang, Q., Wei, H., and Tian, Z. (2008). Poly I:C enhances cycloheximide-induced apoptosis of tumor cells through TLR3 pathway. *BMC Cancer* 8:12. doi: 10.1186/1471-2407-8-12

Jones, J. O., and Smyth, E. C. (2020). Gastroesophageal cancer: navigating the immune and genetic terrain to improve clinical outcomes. *Cancer Treat. Rev.* 84:101950. doi: 10.1016/j.ctrv.2019.101950

Kaczanowska, S., Joseph, A. M., and Davila, E. (2013). TLR agonists: our best frenemy in cancer immunotherapy. *J. Leukoc. Biol.* 93, 847–863. doi: 10.1189/jlb.1012501

Kalams, S. A., and Walker, B. D. (1998). The critical need for CD4 help in maintaining effective cytotoxic T lymphocyte responses. *J. Exp. Med.* 188, 2199–2204. doi: 10.1084/jem.188.12.2199

Kang, Y. K., Boku, N., Satoh, T., Ryu, M. H., Chao, Y., Kato, K., et al. (2017). Nivolumab in patients with advanced gastric or gastro-oesophageal junction cancer refractory to, or intolerant of, at least two previous chemotherapy regimens (ONO-4538-12, ATTRACTION-2): a randomised, double-blind, placebo-controlled, phase 3 trial. *Lancet* 390, 2461–2471. doi: 10.1016/s0140-6736(17)31827-5

Kapp, K., Volz, B., Oswald, D., Wittig, B., Baumann, M., and Schmidt, M. (2019). Beneficial modulation of the tumor microenvironment and generation of anti-tumor responses by TLR9 agonist lefitolimod alone and in combination with checkpoint inhibitors. *Oncoimmunology* 8:e1659096. doi: 10.1080/2162402x.2019.1659096

Kasurinen, A., Hagström, J., Laitinen, A., Kokkola, A., Böckelman, C., and Haglund, C. (2019). Evaluation of toll-like receptors as prognostic biomarkers in gastric cancer: high tissue TLR5 predicts a better outcome. *Sci. Rep.* 9:12553. doi: 10.1038/s41598-019-49111-2

Kauppila, J. H., Karttunen, T. J., Saarnio, J., Nyberg, P., Salo, T., Graves, D. E., et al. (2013). Short DNA sequences and bacterial DNA induce esophageal, gastric, and colorectal cancer cell invasion. *APMIS* 121, 511–522. doi: 10.1111/apm.12016

Kawahara, T., Teshima, S., Oka, A., Sugiyama, T., Kishi, K., and Rokutan, K. (2001). Type I Helicobacter pylori lipopolysaccharide stimulates toll-like receptor. 4 and activates mitogen oxidase. 1 in gastric pit cells. *Infect. Immun.* 69, 4382–4389. doi: 10.1128/iai.69.7.4382-4389.2001

Kawasaki, T., and Kawai, T. (2014). Toll-like receptor signaling pathways. *Front. Immunol.* 5:461. doi: 10.3389/fimmu.2014.00461

Keir, M. E., Butte, M. J., Freeman, G. J., and Sharpe, A. H. (2008). PD-1 and its ligands in tolerance and immunity. *Annu. Rev. Immunol.* 26, 677–704. doi: 10.1146/annurev.immunol.26.021607.090331

Kelly, R. J., Lee, J., Bang, Y. J., Almhanna, K., Blum-Murphy, M., Catenacci, D. V. T., et al. (2020). Safety and efficacy of durvalumab and tremelimumab alone or in combination in patients with advanced gastric and gastroesophageal junction adenocarcinoma. *Clin. Cancer Res.* 26, 846–854. doi: 10.1158/1078-0432.Ccr-19-2443

Ko, W. J., Song, G. W., Kim, W. H., Hong, S. P., and Cho, J. Y. (2016). Endoscopic resection of early gastric cancer: current status and new approaches. *Transl. Gastroenterol. Hepatol.* 1:24. doi: 10.21037/tgh.2016.03.22

Koizumi, S., Masuko, K., Wakita, D., Tanaka, S., Mitamura, R., Kato, Y., et al. (2012). Extracts of larix leptolepis effectively augments the generation of tumor antigen-specific cytotoxic T lymphocytes via activation of dendritic cells in TLR-2 and TLR-4-dependent manner. *Cell Immunol.* 276, 153–161. doi: 10.1016/j.cellimm.2012.05.002

Kono, K., Rongcun, Y., Charo, J., Ichihara, F., Celis, E., Sette, A., et al. (1998). Identification of HER2/neu-derived peptide epitopes recognized by gastric cancer-specific cytotoxic T lymphocytes. *Int. J. Cancer.* 78, 202–208. doi: 10.1002/(sici)1097-0215(19981005)78:2<202::aid-ijc14>3.0.co;2-c

Krieg, A. M. (2007). Toll-free vaccines? *Nat. Biotechnol.* 25, 303–305. doi: 10.1038/nbt0307-303

Kuo, W. T., Lee, T. C., and Yu, L. C. (2016). Eritoran suppresses colon cancer by altering a functional balance in toll-like receptors that bind lipopolysaccharide. *Cancer Res.* 76, 4684–4695. doi: 10.1158/0008-5472.Can-16-0172

Kurts, C., Robinson, B. W., and Knolle, P. A. (2010). Cross-priming in health and disease. *Nat. Rev. Immunol.* 10, 403–414. doi: 10.1038/nri2780

Lang, K. S., Recher, M., Junt, T., Navarini, A. A., Harris, N. L., Freigang, S., et al. (2005). Toll-like receptor engagement converts T-cell autoreactivity into overt autoimmune disease. *Nat. Med.* 11, 138–145. doi: 10.1038/nm1176

Leach, D. R., Krummel, M. F., and Allison, J. P. (1996). Enhancement of antitumor immunity by CTLA-4 blockade. *Science* 271, 1734–1736. doi: 10.1126/science.271.5256.1734

Ledeboer, A., Mahoney, J. H., Milligan, E. D., Martin, D., Maier, S. F., and Watkins, L. R. (2006). Spinal cord glia and interleukin-1 do not appear to mediate persistent allodynia induced by intramuscular acidic saline in rats. *J. Pain.* 7, 757–767. doi: 10.1016/j.jpain.2006.04.001

Levitzki, A. (2012). Targeting the immune system to fight cancer using chemical receptor homing vectors carrying polyinosine/cytosine (PolyIC). *Front. Oncol.* 2:4. doi: 10.3389/fonc.2012.00004

Li, K., Qu, S., Chen, X., Wu, Q., and Shi, M. (2017). Promising targets for cancer immunotherapy: TLRs, RLRs, and STING-mediated innate immune pathways. *Int. J. Mol. Sci.* 18:404. doi: 10.3390/ijms18020404

Liu, N., Ohnishi, N., Ni, L., Akira, S., and Bacon, K. B. (2003). CpG directly induces T-bet expression and inhibits IgG1 and IgE switching in B cells. *Nat. Immunol.* 4, 687–693. doi: 10.1038/ni941

Ma, C., Patel, K., Singhi, A. D., Ren, B., Zhu, B., Shaikh, F., et al. (2016). Programmed death-ligand. 1 expression is common in gastric cancer associated with epstein-barr virus or microsatellite instability. *Am. J. Surg. Pathol.* 40, 1496–1506. doi: 10.1097/pas.0000000000000698

Maeda, H., Kobayashi, M., and Sakamoto, J. (2015). Evaluation and treatment of malignant ascites secondary to gastric cancer. *World J. Gastroenterol.* 21, 10936–10947. doi: 10.3748/wjg.v21.i39.10936

Maeda, S., Akanuma, M., Mitsuno, Y., Hirata, Y., Ogura, K., Yoshida, H., et al. (2001). Distinct mechanism of Helicobacter pylori-mediated NF-kappa B activation between gastric cancer cells and monocytic cells. *J. Biol. Chem.* 276, 44856–44864. doi: 10.1074/jbc.M105381200

Mai, C. W., Kang, Y. B., and Pichika, M. R. (2013). Should a Toll-like receptor. 4 (TLR-4) agonist or antagonist be designed to treat cancer? TLR-4: its expression and effects in the ten most common cancers. *Onco. Targets. Ther.* 6, 1573–1587. doi: 10.2147/ott.S50838

Mangsbo, S. M., Sandin, L. C., Anger, K., Korman, A. J., Loskog, A., and Tötterman, T. H. (2010). Enhanced tumor eradication by combining CTLA-4 or PD-1 blockade with CpG therapy. *J. Immunother.* 33, 225–235. doi: 10.1097/CJI.0b013e3181c01fcb

Marcus, A., Gowen, B. G., Thompson, T. W., Iannello, A., Ardolino, M., Deng, W., et al. (2014). Recognition of tumors by the innate immune system and natural killer cells. *Adv. Immunol.* 122, 91–128. doi: 10.1016/b978-0-12-800267-4.00003-1

Masihi, K. N. (2001). Fighting infection using immunomodulatory agents. *Expert Opin. Biol. Ther.* 1, 641–653. doi: 10.1517/14712598.1.4.641

Mccluskie, M. J., Weeratna, R. D., Payette, P. J., and Davis, H. L. (2002). Parenteral and mucosal prime-boost immunization strategies in mice with hepatitis B surface antigen and CpG DNA. *FEMS Immunol. Med. Microbiol.* 32, 179–185. doi: 10.1111/j.1574-695X.2002.tb00551.x

Mett, V., Komarova, E. A., Greene, K., Bespalov, I., Brackett, C., Gillard, B., et al. (2018). Mobilan: a recombinant adenovirus carrying Toll-like receptor. 5 self-activating cassette for cancer immunotherapy. *Oncogene* 37, 439–449. doi: 10.1038/onc.2017.346

Minaga, K., Takenaka, M., Kitano, M., Chiba, Y., Imai, H., Yamao, K., et al. (2017). Rescue EUS-guided intrahepatic biliary drainage for malignant hilar biliary stricture after failed transpapillary re-intervention. *Surg. Endosc.* 31, 4764–4772. doi: 10.1007/s00464-017-5553-6

Muro, K., Chung, H. C., Shankaran, V., Geva, R., Catenacci, D., Gupta, S., et al. (2016). Pembrolizumab for patients with PD-L1-positive advanced gastric cancer (KEYNOTE-012): a multicentre, open-label, phase. 1b trial. *Lancet Oncol.* 17, 717–726. doi: 10.1016/s1470-2045(16)00175-3

Naseemuddin, M., Iqbal, A., Nasti, T. H., Ghandhi, J. L., Kapadia, A. D., and Yusuf, N. (2012). Cell mediated immune responses through TLR4 prevents DMBA-induced mammary carcinogenesis in mice. *Int. J. Cancer* 130, 765–774. doi: 10.1002/ijc.26100

Nghiem, P. T., Bhatia, S., Lipson, E. J., Kudchadkar, R. R., Miller, N. J., Annamalai, L., et al. (2016). PD-1 blockade with pembrolizumab in advanced merkel-cell carcinoma. *N. Engl. J. Med.* 374, 2542–2552. doi: 10.1056/NEJMoa1603702

Oba, M. S., Teramukai, S., Ohashi, Y., Ogawa, K., Maehara, Y., and Sakamoto, J. (2016). The efficacy of adjuvant immunochemotherapy with OK-432 after curative resection of gastric cancer: an individual patient data meta-analysis of randomized controlled trials. *Gastric Cancer* 19, 616–624. doi: 10.1007/s10120-015-0489-9

Papadavid, E., Stratigos, A. J., and Falagas, M. E. (2007). Imiquimod: an immune response modifier in the treatment of precancerous skin lesions and skin cancer. *Expert Opin. Pharmacother.* 8, 1743–1755. doi: 10.1517/14656566.8.11.1743

Pardoll, D. M. (2012). The blockade of immune checkpoints in cancer immunotherapy. *Nat. Rev. Cancer.* 12, 252–264. doi: 10.1038/nrc3239

Perret, R., Sierro, S. R., Botelho, N. K., Corgnac, S., Donda, A., and Romero, P. (2013). Adjuvants that improve the ratio of antigen-specific effector to regulatory T cells enhance tumor immunity. *Cancer Res.* 73, 6597–6608. doi: 10.1158/0008-5472.Can-13-0875

Prajeeth, C. K., Jirmo, A. C., Krishnaswamy, J. K., Ebensen, T., Guzman, C. A., Weiss, S., et al. (2010). The synthetic TLR2 agonist BPPcysMPEG leads to efficient cross-priming against co-administered and linked antigens. *Eur. J. Immunol.* 40, 1272–1283. doi: 10.1002/eji.200939790

Qin, X. R., Wu, J., Yao, X. Y., Huang, J., and Wang, X. Y. (2019). Helicobacter pylori DNA promotes cellular proliferation, migration, and invasion of gastric cancer by activating toll-like receptor 9. *Saudi J. Gastroenterol.* 25, 181–187. doi: 10.4103/sjg.SJG_309_18

Reilley, M. J., Morrow, B., Ager, C. R., Liu, A., Hong, D. S., and Curran, M. A. (2019). TLR9 activation cooperates with T cell checkpoint blockade to regress poorly immunogenic melanoma. *J. Immunother Cancer.* 7:323. doi: 10.1186/s40425-019-0811-x

Rhee, S. H., Im, E., and Pothoulakis, C. (2008). Toll-like receptor. 5 engagement modulates tumor development and growth in a mouse xenograft model of human colon cancer. *Gastroenterology* 135, 518–528. doi: 10.1053/j.gastro.2008.04.022

Ribas, A., Puzanov, I., Dummer, R., Schadendorf, D., Hamid, O., Robert, C., et al. (2015). Pembrolizumab versus investigator-choice chemotherapy for ipilimumab-refractory melanoma (KEYNOTE-002): a randomised, controlled, phase. 2 trial. *Lancet Oncol.* 16, 908–918. doi: 10.1016/s1470-2045(15)00083-2

Ryoma, Y., Moriya, Y., Okamoto, M., Kanaya, I., Saito, M., and Sato, M. (2004). Biological effect of OK-432 (picibanil) and possible application to dendritic cell therapy. *Anticancer Res.* 24, 3295–3301.

Sato-Kaneko, F., Yao, S., Ahmadi, A., Zhang, S. S., Hosoya, T., Kaneda, M. M., et al. (2017). Combination immunotherapy with TLR agonists and checkpoint inhibitors suppresses head and neck cancer. *JCI Insight.* 2:e93397. doi: 10.1172/jci.insight.93397

Seya, T., Takeda, Y., and Matsumoto, M. (2019). A Toll-like receptor. 3 (TLR3) agonist ARNAX for therapeutic immunotherapy. *Adv. Drug Deliv. Rev.* 147, 37–43. doi: 10.1016/j.addr.2019.07.008

Sfondrini, L., Rossini, A., Besusso, D., Merlo, A., Tagliabue, E., Mènard, S., et al. (2006). Antitumor activity of the TLR-5 ligand flagellin in mouse models of cancer. *J. Immunol.* 176, 6624–6630. doi: 10.4049/jimmunol.176.11.6624

Shi, R., Hong, L., Wu, D., Ning, X., Chen, Y., Lin, T., et al. (2005). Enhanced immune response to gastric cancer specific antigen peptide by coencapsulation with CpG oligodeoxynucleotides in nanoemulsion. *Cancer Biol. Ther.* 4, 218–224. doi: 10.4161/cbt.4.2.1472

Shime, H., Matsumoto, M., Oshiumi, H., Tanaka, S., Nakane, A., Iwakura, Y., et al. (2012). Toll-like receptor. 3 signaling converts tumor-supporting myeloid cells to tumoricidal effectors. *Proc. Natl. Acad. Sci. U.S.A.* 109, 2066–2071. doi: 10.1073/pnas.1113099109

So, E. Y., and Ouchi, T. (2010). The application of toll like receptors for cancer therapy. *Int. J. Biol. Sci.* 6, 675–681. doi: 10.7150/ijbs.6.675

Sohn, B. H., Hwang, J. E., Jang, H. J., Lee, H. S., Oh, S. C., Shim, J. J., et al. (2017). Clinical significance of four molecular subtypes of gastric cancer identified by the cancer genome atlas project. *Clin. Cancer Res.* doi: 10.1158/1078-0432.Ccr-16-2211. [Epub ahead of print].

Song, E. J., Kang, M. J., Kim, Y. S., Kim, S. M., Lee, S. E., Kim, C. H., et al. (2011). Flagellin promotes the proliferation of gastric cancer cells via the Toll-like receptor. 5. *Int. J. Mol. Med.* 28, 115–119. doi: 10.3892/ijmm.2011.656

Soto, L. J. III, Sorenson, B. S., Kim, A. S., Feltis, B. A., Leonard, A. S., and Saltzman, D. A. (2003). Attenuated Salmonella typhimurium prevents the establishment of unresectable hepatic metastases and improves survival in a murine model. *J. Pediatr. Surg.* 38, 1075–1079. doi: 10.1016/s0022-3468(03)00196-9

Steinman, R. M. (1991). The dendritic cell system and its role in immunogenicity. *Annu. Rev. Immunol.* 9, 271–296. doi: 10.1146/annurev.iy.09.040191.001415

Su, B., Ceponis, P. J., Lebel, S., Huynh, H., and Sherman, P. M. (2003). Helicobacter pylori activates Toll-like receptor 4 expression in gastrointestinal epithelial cells. *Infect. Immun.* 71, 3496–3502. doi: 10.1128/iai.71.6.3496-3502.2003

Takeda, K., and Akira, S. (2015). Toll-like receptors. *Curr. Protoc. Immunol.* 109, 14.12.1–14.12.10. doi: 10.1002/0471142735.im1412s109

Takeda, K., Kaisho, T., and Akira, S. (2003). Toll-like receptors. *Annu. Rev. Immunol.* 21, 335–376. doi: 10.1146/annurev.immunol.21.120601.141126

Takeda, Y., Kataoka, K., Yamagishi, J., Ogawa, S., Seya, T., and Matsumoto, M. (2017). A TLR3-specific adjuvant relieves innate resistance to PD-L1 blockade without cytokine toxicity in tumor vaccine immunotherapy. *Cell Rep.* 19, 1874–1887. doi: 10.1016/j.celrep.2017.05.015

Tanaka, F., Fujie, T., Tahara, K., Mori, M., Takesako, K., Sette, A., et al. (1997). Induction of antitumor cytotoxic T lymphocytes with a MAGE-3-encoded synthetic peptide presented by human leukocytes antigen-A24. *Cancer Res.* 57, 4465–4468.

Tang, X., and Zhu, Y. (2012). TLR4 signaling promotes immune escape of human colon cancer cells by inducing immunosuppressive cytokines and apoptosis resistance. *Oncol. Res.* 20, 15–24. doi: 10.3727/096504012x13425470196092

Tartey, S., and Takeuchi, O. (2014). "Toll-like receptors: role in inflammation and cancer," in *Cancer and Inflammation Mechanisms: Chemical, Biological, and Clinical Aspects* (Hoboken, NJ: Wiley Press), 83–102.

Tebbutt, N. C., Giraud, A. S., Inglese, M., Jenkins, B., Waring, P., Clay, F. J., et al. (2002). Reciprocal regulation of gastrointestinal homeostasis by SHP2 and STAT-mediated trefoil gene activation in gp130 mutant mice. *Nat. Med.* 8, 1089–1097. doi: 10.1038/nm763

Thomas, C. J., Kapoor, M., Sharma, S., Bausinger, H., Zyilan, U., Lipsker, D., et al. (2002). Evidence of a trimolecular complex involving LPS, LPS binding protein and soluble CD14 as an effector of LPS response. *FEBS Lett.* 531, 184–188. doi: 10.1016/s0014-5793(02)03499-3

Toffanin, S., Cornella, H., Harrington, A., and Llovet, J. M. (2012). HCC Is promoted by bacterial translocation and TLR-4 signaling: a new paradigm for chemoprevention and management. *Hepatology* 56, 1998–2000. doi: 10.1002/hep.26080

Tsuji, S., Matsumoto, M., Takeuchi, O., Akira, S., Azuma, I., Hayashi, A., et al. (2000). Maturation of human dendritic cells by cell wall skeleton of *Mycobacterium bovis bacillus* Calmette-Guérin: involvement of toll-like receptors. *Infect. Immun.* 68, 6883–6890. doi: 10.1128/iai.68.12.6883-6890.2000

Tsukamoto, H., Kubota, K., Shichiku, A., Maekawa, M., Mano, N., Yagita, H., et al. (2019). An agonistic anti-Toll-like receptor. 4 monoclonal antibody as an effective adjuvant for cancer immunotherapy. *Immunology* 158, 136–149. doi: 10.1111/imm.13095

Tumeh, P. C., Harview, C. L., Yearley, J. H., Shintaku, I. P., Taylor, E. J., Robert, L., et al. (2014). PD-1 blockade induces responses by inhibiting adaptive immune resistance. *Nature* 515, 568–571. doi: 10.1038/nature13954

Tye, H., Kennedy, C. L., Najdovska, M., Mcleod, L., Mccormack, W., Hughes, N., et al. (2012). STAT3-driven upregulation of TLR2 promotes gastric tumorigenesis independent of tumor inflammation. *Cancer Cell.* 22, 466–478. doi: 10.1016/j.ccr.2012.08.010

Villanueva, L., Silva, L., Llopiz, D., Ruiz, M., Iglesias, T., Lozano, T., et al. (2018). The Toll like receptor. 4 ligand cold-inducible RNA-binding protein as vaccination platform against cancer. *Oncoimmunology* 7:e1409321. doi: 10.1080/2162402x.2017.1409321

Wagner, H., Häcker, H., and Lipford, G. B. (2000). Immunostimulatory DNA sequences help to eradicate intracellular pathogens. *Springer Semin. Immunopathol.* 22, 147–152. doi: 10.1007/s002810000025

Walshaw, R. C., Honeychurch, J., Choudhury, A., and Illidge, T. M. (2020). Toll-like receptor agonists and radiation therapy combinations: an untapped opportunity to induce anticancer immunity and improve tumor control. *Int. J. Radiat. Oncol. Biol. Phys.* 108, 27–37. doi: 10.1016/j.ijrobp.2020.04.020

Wang, C., Zhuang, Y., Zhang, Y., Luo, Z., Gao, N., Li, P., et al. (2012). Toll-like receptor. 3 agonist complexed with cationic liposome augments vaccine-elicited antitumor immunity by enhancing TLR3-IRF3 signaling and type I interferons in dendritic cells. *Vaccine* 30, 4790–4799. doi: 10.1016/j.vaccine.2012.05.027

Wang, L., Zhao, Y., Qian, J., Sun, L., Lu, Y., Li, H., et al. (2013). Toll-like receptor-4 signaling in mantle cell lymphoma: effects on tumor growth and immune evasion. *Cancer* 119, 782–791. doi: 10.1002/cncr.27792

Wang, X., Liu, Y., Diao, Y., Gao, N., Wan, Y., Zhong, J., et al. (2018). Gastric cancer vaccines synthesized using a TLR7 agonist and their synergistic antitumor effects with. 5-fluorouracil. *J. Transl. Med.* 16:120. doi: 10.1186/s12967-018-1501-z

Wang, X. D., Gao, N. N., Diao, Y. W., Liu, Y., Gao, D., Li, W., et al. (2015). Conjugation of toll-like receptor-7 agonist to gastric cancer antigen MG7-Ag exerts antitumor effects. *World J. Gastroenterol.* 21, 8052–8060. doi: 10.3748/wjg.v21.i26.8052

Ward-Hartstonge, K. A., and Kemp, R. A. (2017). Regulatory T-cell heterogeneity and the cancer immune response. *Clin. Transl. Immunol.* 6:e154. doi: 10.1038/cti.2017.43

Weiner, G. J. (2000). Immunostimulatory DNA sequences and cancer therapy. *Springer Semin. Immunopathol.* 22, 107–116. doi: 10.1007/s002810000022

Wu, C. C., Hayashi, T., Takabayashi, K., Sabet, M., Smee, D. F., Guiney, D. D., et al. (2007). Immunotherapeutic activity of a conjugate of a Toll-like receptor 7 ligand. *Proc. Natl. Acad. Sci. U.S.A.* 104, 3990–3995. doi: 10.1073/pnas.0611624104

Wu, C. C., Liu, S. J., Chen, H. W., Shen, K. Y., and Leng, C. H. (2016). A Toll-like receptor. 2 agonist-fused antigen enhanced antitumor immunity by increasing antigen presentation and the CD8 memory T cells population. *Oncotarget* 7, 30804–30819. doi: 10.18632/oncotarget.9001

Xu, Y., Ma, S., Si, X., Zhao, J., Yu, H., Ma, L., et al. (2020). Polyethyleneimine-CpG nanocomplex as an *in situ* vaccine for boosting anticancer immunity in melanoma. *Macromol. Biosci.* doi: 10.1002/mabi.202000207. [Epub ahead of print].

Yamamoto, S., Yamamoto, T., Iho, S., and Tokunaga, T. (2000). Activation of NK cell (human and mouse) by immunostimulatory DNA sequence. *Springer Semin. Immunopathol.* 22, 35–43. doi: 10.1007/s002810050013

Yang, H., Wang, B., Wang, T., Xu, L., He, C., Wen, H., et al. (2014). Toll-like receptor. 4 prompts human breast cancer cells invasiveness via lipopolysaccharide stimulation and is overexpressed in patients with lymph node metastasis. *PLoS ONE* 9:e109980. doi: 10.1371/journal.pone.0109980

Yang, J., Li, Z. H., Zhou, J. J., Chen, R. F., Cheng, L. Z., Zhou, Q. B., et al. (2010). Preparation and antitumor effects of nanovaccines with MAGE-3 peptides in transplanted gastric cancer in mice. *Chin. J. Cancer* 29, 359–364. doi: 10.5732/cjc.009.10541

Yao, K., Wang, W., Li, H., Lin, J., Tan, W., Chen, Y., et al. (2018). Bacillus Calmette Guérin (BCG) activates lymphocyte to promote autophagy and apoptosis of gastric cancer MGC-803 cell. *Cell. Mol. Biol.* 64, 11–16.

Yin, P., Liu, X., Mansfield, A. S., Harrington, S. M., Li, Y., Yan, Y., et al. (2016). CpG-induced antitumor immunity requires IL-12 in expansion of effector cells and down-regulation of PD-1. *Oncotarget* 7, 70223–70231. doi: 10.18632/oncotarget.11833

Yuan, X., Zhou, Y., Wang, W., Li, J., Xie, G., Zhao, Y., et al. (2013). Activation of TLR4 signaling promotes gastric cancer progression by inducing mitochondrial ROS production. *Cell Death Dis.* 4:e794. doi: 10.1038/cddis.2013.334

Zhang, D., Chen, Y., and Fan, D. (2006). MG7 mimotope-based DNA vaccination for gastric cancer. *Expert Rev. Vaccines* 5, 223–231. doi: 10.1586/14760584.5.2.223

Zhao, X., Ai, M., Guo, Y., Zhou, X., Wang, L., Li, X., et al. (2012). Poly I:C-induced tumor cell apoptosis mediated by pattern-recognition receptors. *Cancer Biother. Radiopharm.* 27, 530–534. doi: 10.1089/cbr.2012.1226

Zhu, A. X., Finn, R. S., Edeline, J., Cattan, S., Ogasawara, S., Palmer, D., et al. (2018). Pembrolizumab in patients with advanced hepatocellular carcinoma previously treated with sorafenib (KEYNOTE-224): a non-randomised, open-label phase 2 trial. *Lancet Oncol.* 19, 940–952. doi: 10.1016/s1470-2045(18)30351-6

Zom, G. G., Willems, M., Khan, S., Van Der Sluis, T. C., Kleinovink, J. W., Camps, M. G. M., et al. (2018). Novel TLR2-binding adjuvant induces enhanced T cell responses and tumor eradication. *J. Immunother Cancer.* 6:146. doi: 10.1186/s40425-018-0455-2

13

Hypermethylation and Downregulation of UTP6 are Associated with Stemness Properties, Chemoradiotherapy Resistance and Prognosis in Rectal Cancer: A Co-expression Network Analysis

Yiyi Zhang[1†], Qiao Gao[2†], Yong Wu[1†], Yong Peng[1], Jinfu Zhuang[1], Yuanfeng Yang[1], Weizhong Jiang[3], Xing Liu[1] and Guoxian Guan[1*]*

[1] Department of Colorectal Surgery, The First Affiliated Hospital of Fujian Medical University, Fuzhou, China, [2] Fujian Maternity and Child Health Hospital, Affiliated Hospital of Fujian Medical University, Fuzhou, China, [3] Department of Colorectal Surgery, Fujian Medical University Union Hospital, Fuzhou, China

***Correspondence:**
Guoxian Guan
fjxhggx@163.com
Xing Liu
fjmufylx@163.com

† These authors have contributed equally to this work

Background: To identify the hub genes associated with chemoradiotherapy resistance in rectal cancer and explore the potential mechanism.

Methods: Weighted gene co-expression network analysis (WGCNA) was performed to identify the gene modules correlated with the chemoradiotherapy resistance of rectal cancer.

Results: The mRNA expression of 31 rectal cancer patients receiving preoperative chemoradiotherapy was described in our previous study. Through WGCNA, we demonstrated that the chemoradiotherapy resistance modules were enriched for translation, DNA replication, and the androgen receptor signaling pathway. Additionally, we identified and validated UTP6 as a new effective predictor for chemoradiotherapy sensitivity and a prognostic factor for the survival of colorectal cancer patients using our data and the GSE35452 dataset. Low UTP6 expression was correlated with significantly worse disease-free survival (DFS), overall survival (OS), and event- and relapse-free survival both in our data and the R2 Platform. Moreover, we verified the UTP6 expression in 125 locally advanced rectal cancer (LARC) patients samples by immunohistochemical analysis. The results demonstrated that low UTP6 expression was associated with worse DFS and OS by Kaplan-Meier and COX regression model analyses. Gene set enrichment and co-expression analyses showed that the mechanism of the UTP6-mediated chemoradiotherapy resistance may involve the regulation of FOXK2 expression by transcription factor pathways.

Conclusion: Low expression of the UTP6 was found to be associated with chemoradiotherapy resistance and the prognosis of colorectal cancer possibly via regulating FOXK2 expression by transcription factor pathways.

Keywords: rectal cancer, chemoradiotherapy, weighted gene co-expression network analysis, UTP6, prognosis

INTRODUCTION

Preoperative chemoradiotherapy (CRT) and radical surgery have become the standard of care for stage II/III rectal cancer patients (Heald et al., 1982). The benefits of this multimodality therapy have been well documented, including tumor downsizing and downstaging, increased radical resection, and reduced local recurrence (Sauer et al., 2004, 2012; van Gijn et al., 2011). However, the treatment may increase the perioperative mortality rates by 48% (Rahbari et al., 2013). Moreover, 15% to 45% of the rectal cancers would are estimated to develop resistance to CRT, and might be exposed to CRT-related toxicitiestoxicity without oncological benefit (Ha et al., 2017). Therefore, the identification of valid biomarkers for colorectal cancer (CRC) with resistance to CRT has become imperative.

Currently, high-throughput sequencing is commonly used to screen and identify differentially expressed genes (DEGs). Conventional molecular biology methodology evaluates the variations in and functions of genes independently. Weighted gene co-expression network analysis (WGCNA) is an unbiased systematic biological approach, which clarifies the transcriptome function at a system-level, determines gene-gene correlations, and identifies gene modules with a high correlation across microarray data. It also bridges the gap between individual genes and tumorigenesis and progression (Zhang and Horvath, 2005; Langfelder and Horvath, 2008; Tian et al., 2017). WGCNA can facilitate the network-based gene screening approaches that screen key biomarkers associated with clinical traits in various cancers. However, this efficient bioinformatics approach has not yet been adopted to explore network-centric genes associated with CRT resistance in rectal cancer patients.

In this context, this study aimed to screen the relevant hub genes for CRT in our expression profile using WGCNA. Then, the hub genes were verified using testing data sets and patient tissue samples.

MATERIALS AND METHODS

Subjects and Collection

In total, 31 locally advanced rectal cancer (LARC) patients receiving preoperative CRT between March 2016 to December 2016 in Fujian Medical University Union Hospital, China were enrolled as the internal dataset in this study, which was used for the gene-chip analysis. The CRT, treatment, and follow-up protocol were described in a previous study (Zhang et al., 2017). All patients received preoperative CRT and underwent R0 resection of primary colorectal tumors after neoadjuvant CRT. And the samples were collected at diagnosis and without any treatment before biopsy from colonoscopy. The chemoradiotherapy protocol was as follows: preoperative radiotherapy consisted of 45 Gy to the pelvis for 5 weeks (180 cGy/25 fractions) and a tumor boost of 5.4 Gy. Concomitant chemotherapy was administered with oral capecitabine (825 mg/m^2 twice daily from day 1 to day 14 per cycle).

Moreover, to further validate the UTP6 expression in the LARC patients' colonoscopic samples before CRT. Consecutive LARC patients who underwent CRT and radical resection between 2011 and 2014 were identified. A total of 125 patients were enrolled in the present study. This study was approved by the Institutional Review Board of Fujian Medical University Union Hospital (2013051).

RNA Extraction, Quality Control, Labeling, Array Hybridization, and Data Analysis

Total RNA was extracted from the tissue mentioned previously using Trizol reagent (Invitrogen), according to the manufacturer's protocol. RNA quantity and quality were measured by a NanoDrop ND-1000 and RNA integrity was assessed by standard denatured agarose gel electrophoresis. Sample labeling and array hybridization were performed according to the human GeneChip Analysis protocol (Affymetrix, Santa Clara, CA). The scanned data obtained from each microarray were normalized to correct for small differences in the amounts of each of the cRNA probes applied to the microarray and were processed for signal values using Affymetrix software (LIMS 5.0). The differentially expressed mRNAs were identified through fold-change filtering. Hierarchical clustering was performed using Agilent Gene Spring GX software (version 11.5.1). The upregulated and downregulated mRNA groups were defined as the mRNA expression in the CRT-responsive group compared with the CRT-non-responsive group. The Gene Ontology (GO) functional analysis and Kyoto Encyclopedia of Genes and Genomes (KEGG) pathway analysis were performed using standard enrichment computation method.

Data Collection From the Gene Expression Omnibus and the Cancer Genome Atlas Database

Datasets were downloaded from the Gene Expression Omnibus (GEO) database[1] on December 19, 2019. The GSE35452 dataset included mRNA expression gene microarray of 46 rectal cancer patients receiving preoperative CRT and biopsy specimens were collected before preoperative CRT, which was used as the external validation dataset. Cancer stem cells are regarded as having self-renewal and differentiation properties and are one of the integral factors mediating the response to CRT (Baumann et al., 2008; Wahab et al., 2017). GSE14773 and GSE24747 were used to determine the hub gene expression in CRC stem cells. The GSE14773 dataset included one cell line with markers of CRC stem cells, high CD44, and CD166 expression, and the other one was a parental control CRC cell. The GSE24747 dataset included two groups, CD133 + and CD133-, CACO-2 cells. DNA methylation is considered an important component in gene

Abbreviations: WGCNA, weighted gene co-expression network analysis; CRT, chemoradiotherapy; CRC, colorectal cancer; LARC, local advanced rectal cancer; GEO, Gene Expression Omnibus; TCGA, the cancer genome atlas; PPI, protein-protein interaction; GSEA, Gene set enrichment analysis; ROC, receiver operating characteristic curve.

[1] https://www.ncbi.nlm.nih.gov/geo/

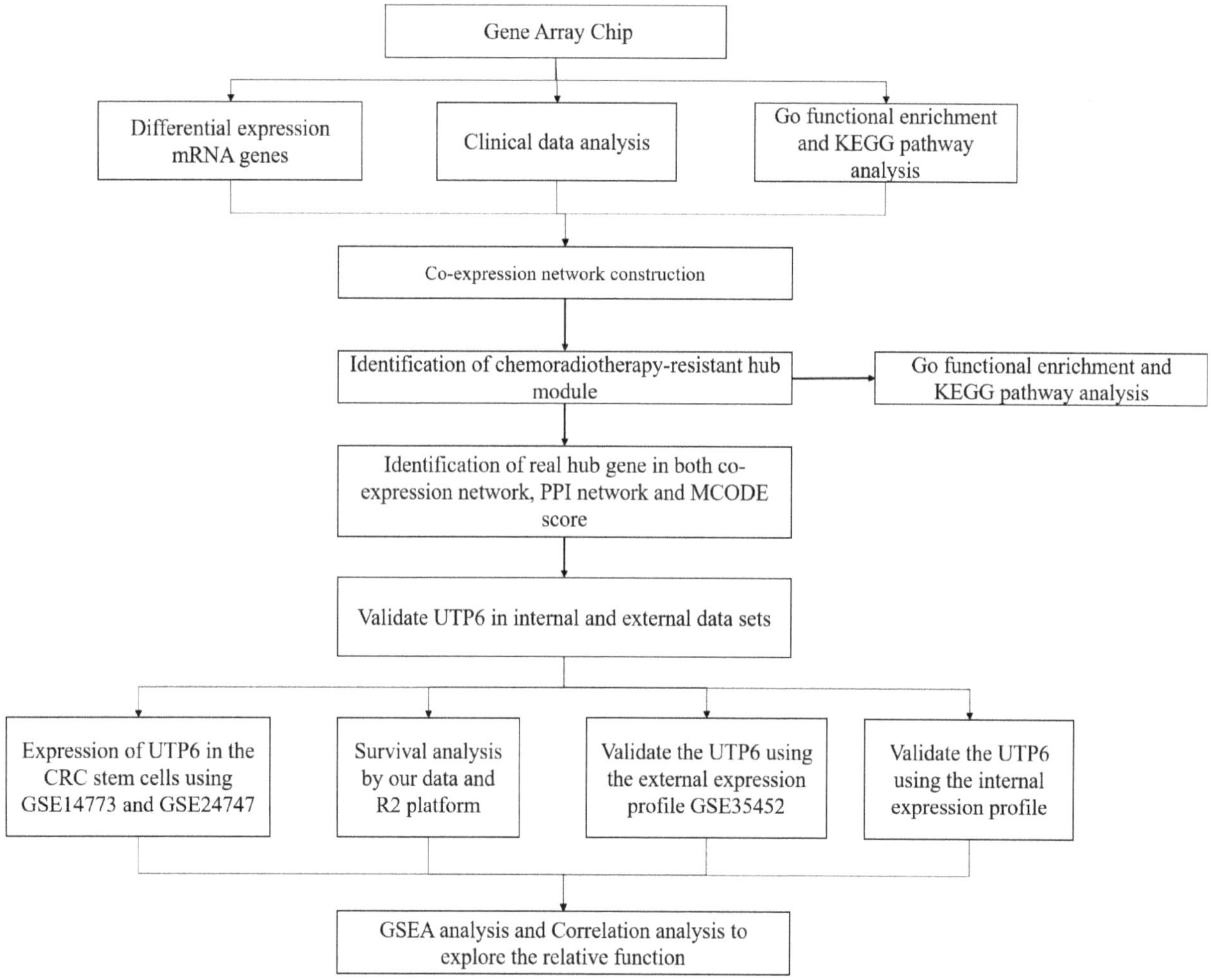

FIGURE 1 | Workflow diagram of data preparation, processing, analysis, and validation in this study.

expression regulation, and high levels of DNA promoter region methylation result in transcriptional silencing. Additionally, promoter regions methylation is reported to be associated with the CRT-resistance and considered as a predictor for CRT (Wilting and Dannenberg, 2012; Ivanova et al., 2013). The GSE104271 dataset was utilized to explore whether the hub genes were regulated by DNA methylation. As described by Huang et al. (2018) previously, FIBP knockdown cell lines were defined as cancer cells compared to cancer stem cells. The methylation data of the CRT-resistant genes CRC and normal colon tissues were obtained from The Cancer Genome Atlas (TCGA) in the UALCAN database[2] (Chandrashekar et al., 2017). A flow diagram of the present study is shown in **Figure 1**.

Definitions

Tumor response to CRT was graded according to the American Joint Committee on Cancer pathological tumor regression grade (AJCC TRG) (Amin et al., 2017; Benson et al., 2018); that is, TRG 0, no residual tumor cells; TRG 1, single cells or small groups of cells; TRG 2, residual cancer with the desmoplastic response; and TRG 3, minimal evidence of tumor response. Pathological complete response (pCR) was defined as the absence of viable tumor cells in the resected specimen, either at the primary site or in the lymph nodes. Venous blood samples were obtained within 1 week before CRT.

Co-expression Network Construction

The WGCNA algorithm was previously described in detail (Zhang and Horvath, 2005). Briefly, first, we identified the qualification of the profile data. The co-expression network was constructed using the "WGCNA" package in R software (Horvath and Dong, 2008; Mason et al., 2009). Next, the correlation matrix was established and the soft threshold power was determined by analysis of the network topology. Then, the topological overlap matrix (TOM) was established (Yip and Horvath, 2007; Ivanova et al., 2013; Botía et al., 2017). Based on the phenotypic data

[2]http://ualcan.path.uab.edu/

of the groups, we calculated each module p-value by the t-test gene significance.

CRT-Resistance Modules and Hub Gene Identification

To explore the relevant modules, we examined the association between module eigengenes (MEs) and CRT-resistance using Pearson's correlation analysis. To identify the hub genes, the CRT-resistance model with the highest correlation coefficient ($P < 0.05$) in the data set was chosen, and the module also had the highest specific weight of all of the modules. The hub genes in the module were defined by module connectivity as measured by thean absolute value of the >0.3 in Pearson's correlation >0.3 analysis. The protein–protein interaction (PPI) network was constructed by all genes in the CRT-resistance module, nd PPI network analysis was performed to screen the hub genes by Cytoscape. And the top 10 values were included for further analysis.

Statistical analysis was performed using SPSS software (version. 23 SPSS Inc., Chicago, IL, United States) and R software (version. 3.4.1). The continuous variables were reported as means and standard deviation from the analysis of variance test. The survival outcomes were assessed using Kaplan-Meier and log-rank analyses. Receiver operating characteristic (ROC) curve analysis was performed. Finally, the prognostic significance of the hub genes in CRC patients was analyzed using the R2: Genomics Analysis and Visualization Platform,[3] on January, 03, 2020. The optimal cutoff points for the expression of UTP6 and FTSJ3 were calculated and determined using Cut-off Finder[4] Visit and download data, 2019.12.26). Budczies et al. (2012), a new bio-informatics tool for biomarker assessment and outcome-based cut-point optimization, which identified the cut-off with the minimum p-values from log-rank $\chi 2$ statistics in terms of disease-free survival (DFS). A P-value of <0.05 was considered statistically significant.

Gene Set Enrichment Analysis and Co-expression Gene Analysis

To explore the potential function of UTP6 in LARC patients, gene set enrichment analysis (GSEA) was performed in the patients in our previous datasets. A P-value of <0.05 and an enrichment score (ES) of >0.3 were set as the cutoff criteria. To further explore the correlation between UTP6 and relevant genes in the GSEA results, we analyzed the co-expressed genes in the TCGA data in the UALCAN dataset (Visit and download data, 2020.02.01).

Immunohistochemical Analysis of UTP6 in the LARC Patients' Sample

The protein expression of UTP6 in specimens obtained before and after CRT in 125 LARC patients was assessed using the immunohistochemical streptavidin-biotin complex method (Zhang et al., 2018). Phosphate-buffered saline (PBS) was used as the negative control and the image of the positive control from GE Healthcare Life Sciences. Immunoreactivity was scored by semi-quantitative analysis, and the fields were randomly selected in five directions (up, center, down, left, and right) under high magnification (*400). The color was determined based on the intensity score as follows: 0 (no staining), 1 (light yellow), 2 (brown), and 3 (deep brown). The percentage of positive cells was scored as 0 (<5%), 1 (5–25%), 2 (25–50%), 3 (50–75%), and 4 (>75%). The mean value was calculated for each case with the aforementioned scoring methods and the final score was obtained by multiplying these two scores. The score between 0 and 4 was defined as the low expression and >4 was defined as high expression. All analyses were performed in a double-blind manner.

RESULTS

Cluster Analysis

A gene chip array was used to examine the gene expression profiles in primary tumor cells. A supervised hierarchical cluster analysis of the gene expression profiling data showed that the two groups had a clustering trend (**Figures 2A,B**). A total of 18419 genes were detected in the gene chip array. The SAM for the DEGs revealed that the two groups significantly differed in genes related to tumor cell biology, including 798 upregulated genes and 450 downregulated genes.

GO Enrichment and KEGG Analysis

GO enrichment analysis was performed to investigate the molecular mechanism of the differently expressed genes involved in the resistance to CRT in LARC patients. We detected the top significant GO-enriched terms and KEGG terms in both the significantly upregulated and downregulated genes in rectal cancer patients (**Figures 2C–F**). The results showed that the top three significant GO terms for the upregulated genes were related to pancreatic A cell differentiation, muscle contraction, and type B pancreatic cell differentiation involved in the immune response. Among the downregulated genes, the top three significant GO terms were related to the ER-associated ubiquitin-dependent protein catabolic process, mRNA processing, and RNA splicing. Moreover, the top three significant KEGG terms in the upregulated genes were related to neuroactive ligand-receptor interaction, lysine degradation, and olfactory transduction involved in the immune response. In the downregulated genes, the top three significant GO terms were related to protein processing in the endoplasmic reticulum, amino sugar and nucleotide sugar metabolism, and the proteasome.

Development of Weighted Co-expression Network and Identification of Key Modules

To identify the hub genes, a weighted co-expression network was utilized to analyze our data (**Figure 3A**). A total of 31 modules were identified, as shown in **Figure 3C**. We further analyzed the relationship between CRT-resistance and the modules

[3] http://r2.amc.nl

[4] http://molpath.charite.de/cutoff/

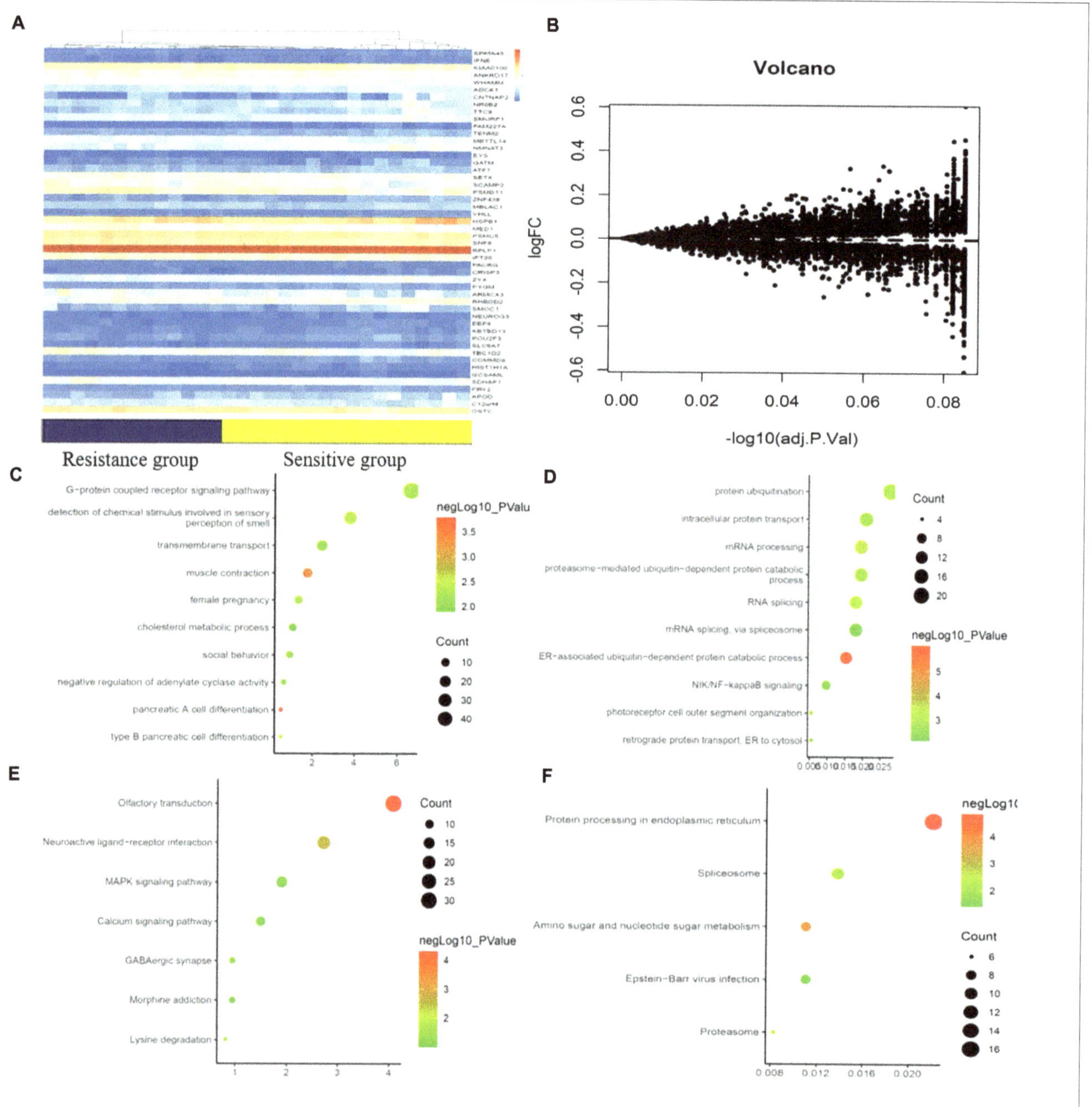

FIGURE 2 | mRNAs expression profile comparison between chemotherapy-resistance and chemotherapy-sensitivity groups. Gene Ontology (GO) functional and Kyoto Encyclopedia of Genes and Genomes (KEGG) pathway analysis of the differentially expressed genes. **(A)** The hierarchical clustering of all targets values of mRNA expression profiling among samples. **(B)** Between the chemotherapy-resistance and chemotherapy-sensitivity group. The purple dots indicated the up-regulated genes of mRNAs and the green dots indicated the down-regulated genes of mRNAs. **(C)** GO functional analysis of the top ten functional classifications of the upregulated genes. **(D)** GO functional analysis of the top ten functional classifications of the downregulated genes. **(E)** KEGG pathway analysis of the top ten significant pathways of upregulated genes. **(F)** KEGG pathway analysis of the top ten pathways of downregulated genes.

(**Figure 3C**). Among these modules, the module shown in dark turquoise (**Figure 3C**) had the strongest negative association with CRT-resistance ($r = -0.45$, $P = 0.01$), while the light cyan module showed the highest positive association with CRT-resistance ($r = 0.25$, $P = 0.18$). Then, we selected the dark turquoise module as the hub module. GO and KEGG enrichment analyses were conducted to explore the functions of the dark turquoise module. The results demonstrated that the dark turquoise module was mainly enriched for translation, DNA replication, and the androgen receptor signaling pathway (**Figure 3B**).

Hub Gene Identification

Through co-expression analysis, 92 genes in the dark turquoise module were considered genes with high module connectivity. Then, the genes were analyzed by the PPI network and 59 genes in the dark turquoise module were identified as hub genes in

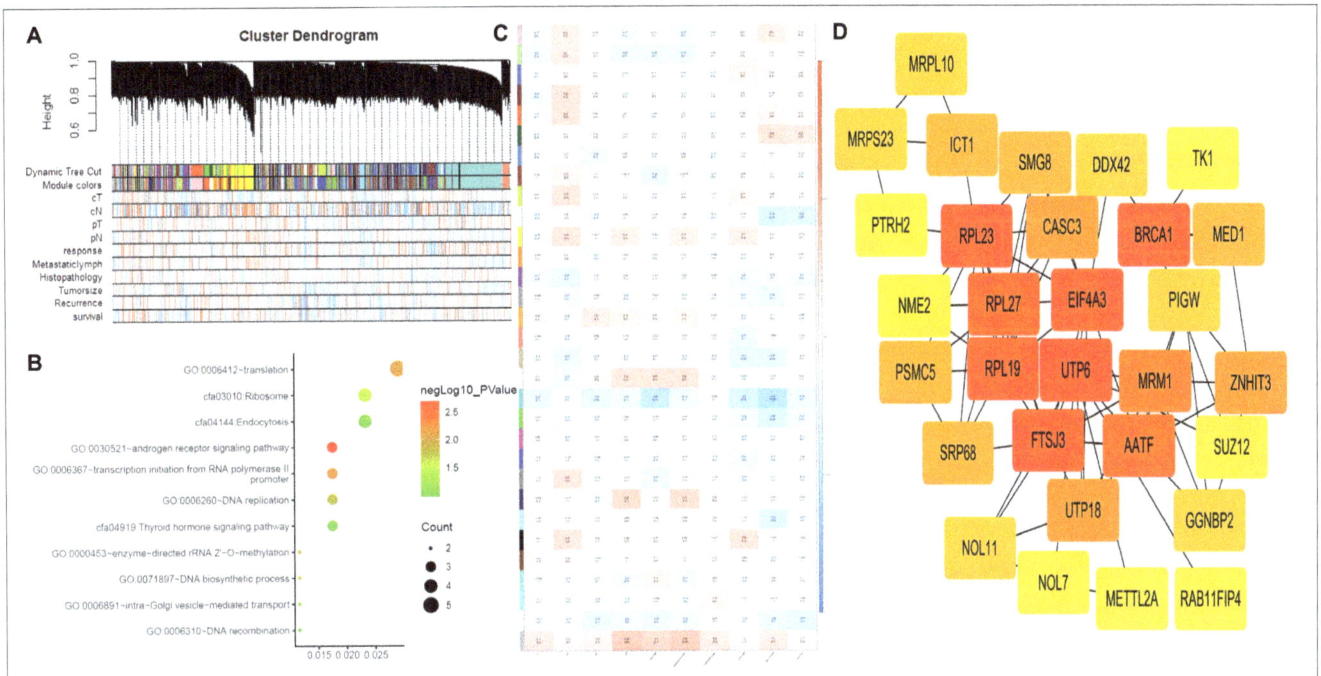

FIGURE 3 | Weighted gene co-expression network analysis and hub gene screened. **(A)** Dendrogram of all expressed genes in the top 25% of variance clustered based on a dissimilarity measure (1-TOM). **(B)** KEGG pathway and GO functional analysis of the pathways of genes in darkturquoise modules. **(C)** Heatmap of the correlation between module eigengenes and CRT-resistance. **(D)** PPI network of genes that had the highest score in the PPI degree in the darkturquoise module. The color intensity in each node was proportional to the degree of connectivity in the weighted gene co-expression network.

the co-expression network. Ten hub genes were analyzed by the degree of PPI and the correlation between clinical traits and module connectivity was analyzed? (**Figure 3D** and **Table 1**). Finally, we chose the most associated genes, *UTP6* and *FTSJ3*, as the actual hub genes.

Hub Gene Validation

To validate the hub genes, we examined the expression of UTP6 and FTSJ3 in rectal cancer tissues of CRT-resistant and CRT-sensitive cases in our datasets. In the internal testing data sets, the relative expression of UTP6 (6.46 ± 0.40 vs. 6.07 ± 0.40, P = 0.02; **Figure 4A**) and FTSJ3 (6.21 ± 0.32 vs. 5.75 ± 0.47, P < 0.01, **Supplementary Figure 1A**) was significantly increased in the CRT-sensitive tissues. The ROC curve demonstrated that both UTP6 (P = 0.02, AUC = 0.76, **Figure 4D**) and FTSJ3 (P < 0.01, AUC = 0.79, **Supplementary Figure 1D**) could efficiently discriminate CRT-resistant from CRT-sensitive rectal cancer cases. Moreover, Pearson's analysis was conducted to determine whether the hub gene expression was associated with the TRG grade. The results demonstrated that UTP6 (r = −0.35, P = 0.02, **Figure 4C**) and FTSJ3 (r = −0.37, P = 0.04, **Supplementary Figure 1C**) had significant associations with the TRG grade.

TABLE 1 | Hub genes.

Genes	Clinical trait relationship (cor. geneTraitSignificance)	Degree in PPI network
UTP6	−0.43	12
RPL23	−0.23	11
RPL19	−0.23	10
EIF4A3	−0.21	10
FTSJ3	−0.50	10
BRCA1	−0.22	10
RPL27	−0.21	9
AATF	−0.19	8
MRM1	−0.33	7
ZNHIT3	−0.28	6

PPI, protein–protein interaction.

We further explored the prognostic impact of UTP6 and FTSJ3 on the survival of LARC patients. Cut-off Finder was used to identify the cutoff values for UTP6 and FTSJ3. Cut-off Finder identified 6.18 and 5.97 as the cutoff values for UTP6 and FTSJ3 expression, respectively (**Supplementary Figure 2**). After a median follow-up period of 42 months (range, 4 – 47 months), low expressions of UTP6 and FTSJ3 were associated with significantly worse disease-free survival (DFS) compared to high expression (UTP6 low expression VS. high expression: 50.0% vs. 100.0%, P < 0.001; FTSJ3 low expression VS. high expression: 54.5% vs. 100.0%, P < 0.001), as shown in **Figure 4F** and **Supplementary Figure 1F**. Similarly, a high expression of UTP6 and FTSJ3 were correlated with better overall survival (OS) compared to low expression (UTP6 high expression VS. low expression: 100.0%, vs. 50.0%, P < 0.001; FTSJ3 high expression VS. low expression: 100.0% vs. 57.7%, P < 0.001), as demonstrated in **Figure 4G** and **Supplementary Figure 1G**.

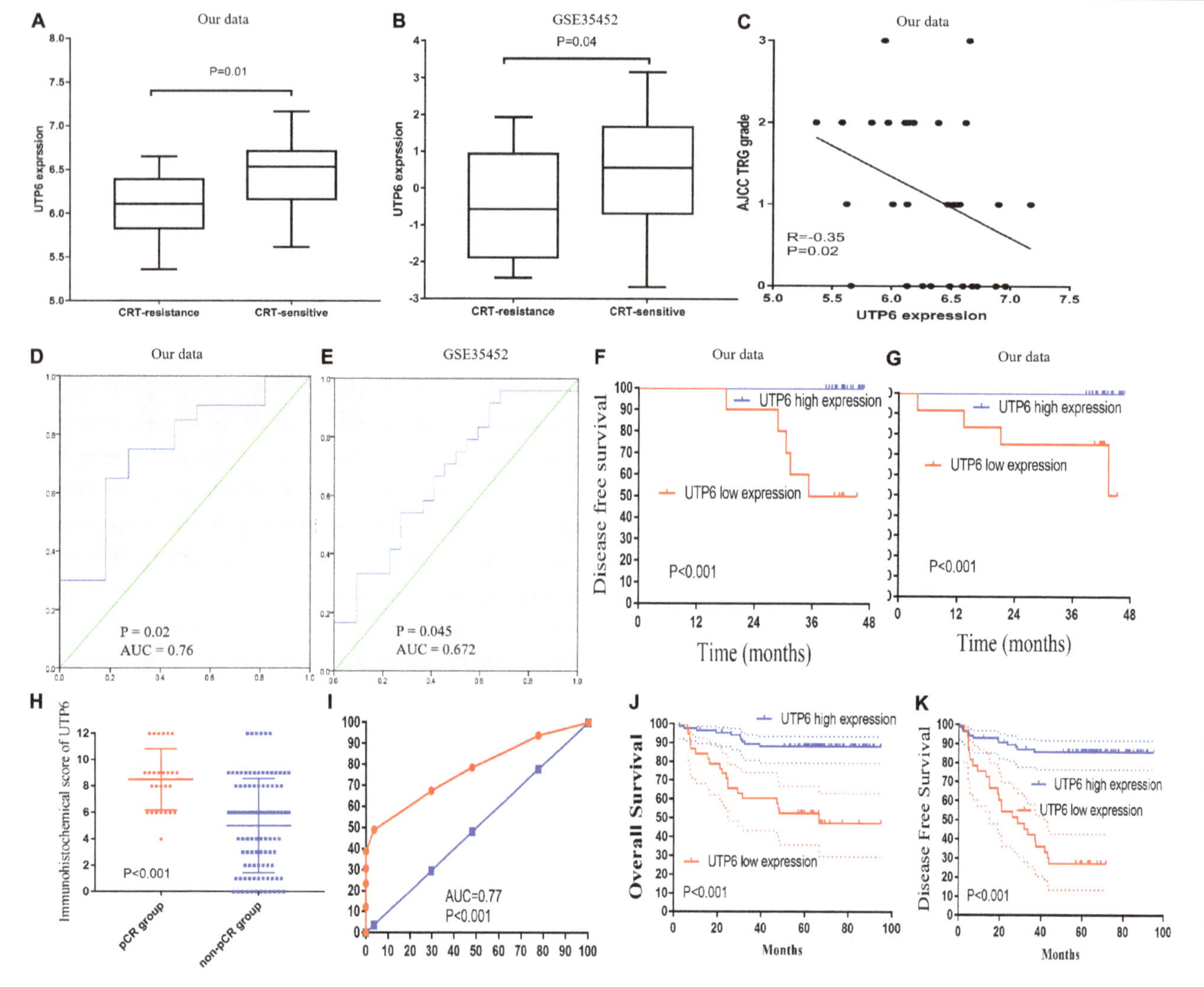

FIGURE 4 | Validation of UTP6. **(A)** In our data (6.46 ± 0.40 vs. 6.07 ± 0.40, $P = 0.02$) and **(B)** GSE35452 (0.45 ± 1.51 vs. −0.47 ± 1.45, $P = 0.042$). **(C)** Pearson's correlation analysis between the AJCC TRG grade and UTP6 expression. ROC curves and AUC statistics to evaluate the predictive efficiency of the UTP6 in our data and external data to distinguish CRT-resistance from CRT-sensitive CRC cases from **(D)** our data and **(E)** GSE35452. The disease-free survival **(F)** and overall survival **(G)** between low and high expression of UTP6. **(H)** UTP6 expression in the pCR and non-pCR group in the LARC patients' sample. **(I)** ROC curves and AUC statistics to evaluate the predictive efficiency of the UTP6 in LARC patients' samples to distinguish pCR from non-pCR LARC cases. The overall survival **(J)** and disease-free survival **(K)** between low and high expression of UTP6 in LARC patients' sample.

Hub Gene Validation in External Data

To validate the hub genes in our data set, we examined the expression level of UTP6 and FTSJ3 by comparing the rectal cancer tissues of CRT-resistant and-sensitive cases using an external dataset. In the external GSE35452 database, UTP6 expression was significantly higher in the CRT-sensitive tissues compared to the CRT-resistant tissues (0.45 ± 1.51 vs. −0.47 ± 1.45, $P = 0.042$; **Figure 4B**), but the expression of FTSJ3 was not statistically different between the two groups (0.11 ± 0.40 vs. −0.05 ± 0.53, $P = 0.246$; **Supplementary Figure 1B**). Thus, we chose UTP6 as the "real" hub gene for further analysis. ROC analysis revealed that UTP6 could efficiently discriminate CRT-resistant from CRT-sensitive cases ($P = 0.045$, AUC = 0.672; **Figure 3E**). However, FTSJ3 could not efficiently distinguish CRT-resistant from CRT-sensitive cases ($P = 0.12$, AUC = 0.63; **Supplementary Figure 1D**).

The R2 were utilized to plot Kaplan-Meier curves by using datasets "Tumor Colon-Sieber-290- MAS5.0-u133p2", "Tumor Colon MVRM -SieberSmith-345- fRMA (bc) - u133p2", "Tumor Colon-Smith-232-MAS5.0-u133p2", "Tumor Colon (KRAS mut)-Hase-59- MAS5.0-u133p2", "Tumor Colon CIT (Combat)-Marisa-566- rma-u133p2", "Tumor Colon MSI-status (Core Exon)-Sveen-95-rma-sketch- huex10p", "Mixed Colon Adenocarcinoma-TCGA-174 custom-agg4502a073", "Tumor Colon (Core-Transcript)-Sveen-333-rma-sketch-huex10p" and "Tumor Colon (Core-Exon)-Sveen-333-rma- sketch-huex10p". Low UTP6 expression was correlated with significantly worse event and relapse-free survival (all $P < 0.05$; **Figures 5A–H**).

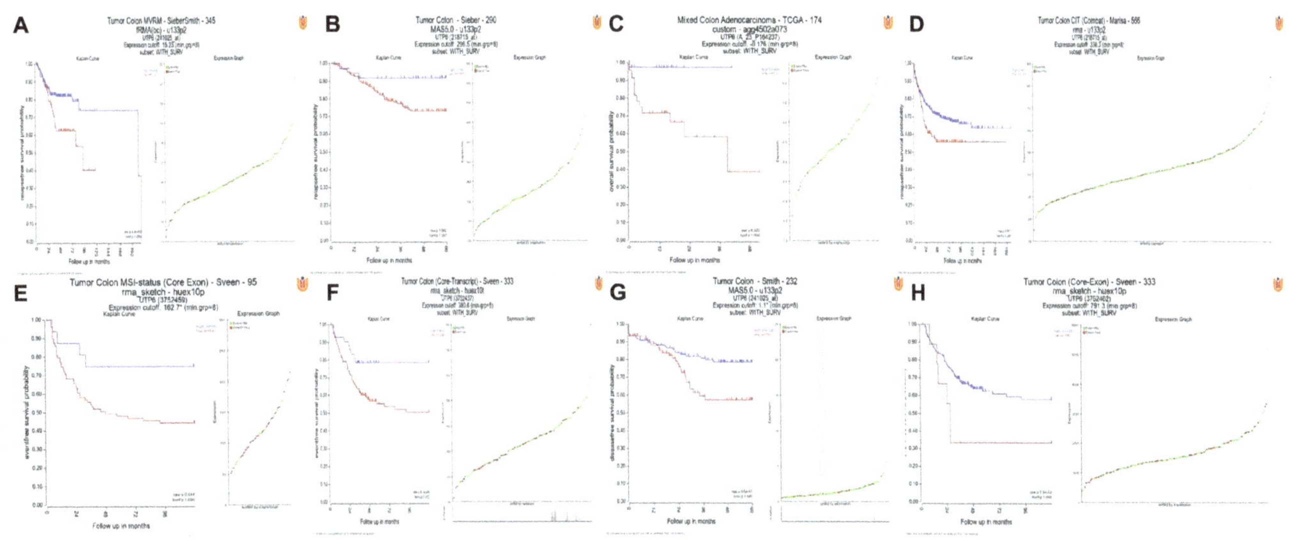

FIGURE 5 | High UTP6 expression was associated with a better event-, disease-, and relapse-free survival. **(A–H)** High UTP6 expression was associated with a significantly better event-, disease- and relapse-free survival (both $P < 0.05$).

UTP6 Validation in LARC Patients' Sample

To further verify UTP6 expression in the tumor samples, colonoscopy samples were collected from LARC patients before CRT. The immunohistochemical analysis demonstrated that higher UTP6 scores were associated with better prognosis in LARC patients following CRT. The 3-year OS rate of the low-UTP6 group was significantly lower than that in the high-UTP6 group (60.5% vs. 89.5%; $P < 0.01$, **Figure 4J**). Lower UTP6 scores were correlated with better DFS (**Figure 4K**). The 3-year DFS rate for the low-UTP6 group was significantly higher than that in the high-UTP6 group (42.4% vs. 87.1%; $P < 0.01$). Moreover, we compared the UTP6 expression in the pCR and non-pCR group. The results revealed that the relative expression of UTP6 was significantly increased in the pCR group ($P < 0.01$; **Figure 4H**). The ROC curve demonstrated that UTP6 could efficiently discriminate pCR from non-pCR LARC cases ($P < 0.001$, AUC = 0.77, **Figure 4I**). In addition, we detected the UTP6 expression in the rectal cancer tissues and adjuvant cancer tissues, the result demonstrated that UTP6 expression value was similar in rectal cancer and adjacent cancer tissues ($P = 0.571$, **Supplementary Figure 3**).

To explore the prognostic impact of UTP6 on the OS and DFS of LARC patients, a Cox regression analysis was performed. Univariate analysis revealed that tumor size ($P = 0.004$), ypTNM stage ($P < 0.001$), AJCC TRG grade ($P = 0.013$), UTP6 expression ($P < 0.001$), CD133 expression ($P < 0.001$), and the pre-CRT-CA19-9 level ($P = 0.012$) were independently associated with DFS in LARC patients following CRT and TME (**Table 2**). Multivariate Cox regression analysis demonstrated that UTP6 expression (HR = 0.398, 95%CI: 0.280 – 0.567, $P < 0.001$) and CD133 expression (HR = 1.205, 95%CI: 1.077 - 1.348, $P = 0.001$) were the independent predictors of DFS in LARC patients following CRT, as shown in **Table 2**.

Upon the univariate analysis of the predictors of OS, tumor size ($P = 0.006$), ypTNM stage ($P < 0.001$), AJCC grade ($P = 0.003$), UTP6 expression ($P < 0.001$), the pre-CRT-CA19-9 level ($P = 0.012$), CD133 expression ($P < 0.001$), and tumor differentiation ($P = 0.013$) were independently associated with OS in LARC patients following CRT and TME (**Table 3**). The results from the multivariate Cox regression model demonstrated that UTP6 expression (HR = 0.398, 95%CI: 0.280 – 0.567, $P < 0.001$) and CD133 expression (HR = 1.185, 95%CI: 1.026 - 1.367, $P = 0.021$) were the independent predictors of OS in LARC patients following CRT, as shown in **Table 3**.

Association of UTP6 Expression With Patient Characteristics and Perioperative Clinicopathological Parameters in the LARC Patients Following CRT

No significant differences were observed between UTP6 low expression group and UTP6 high expression group in terms of gender, age, American Society of Anesthesiologists (ASA) grade, interval time between CRT and surgery, distance from the anal verge, clinical T stage, clinical N stage, pre-CRT CEA level, and pre-CRT CA199 level, as shown in **Table 4**.

No significant differences were observed between UTP6 low expression group and UTP6 high expression group in terms of pathological type, postoperative complication, circumferential resection margin (CRM) involvement, tumor differentiation, perineural invasion, vascular invasion, and organ preservation procedure (**Table 5**). Compared to the UTP6 low expression group, the UTP6 high expression group was associated with an increased metastasis to the lymph nodes (0.45 ± 1.4 vs. 3.1 ± 7.1, $P < 0.001$), pathological T stage, pathological N stage (all $P < 0.01$), and poorer TRG grade ($P < 0.01$). In the training dataset, in the high-risk

TABLE 2 | Cox regression analysis of predictive factors for disease-free survival in the training dataset patients with LARC following CRT (*n* = 125).

Variables	Univariate analysis			Multivariate analysis		
	HR	95% CI	*P*-value	HR	95% CI	*P*-value
Sex, male/female	0.961	0.504–1.833	0.905			
Age	1.002	0.976–1.027	0.904			
ASA	0.972	0.579–1.633	0.915			
Distance from the anal verge	0.976	0.872–1.093	0.677			
Tumor size	1.334	1.094–1.627	0.004	1.073	0.869–1.323	0.513
Pathological TNM stage	1.808	1.333–2.451	<0.001	1.260	0.846–1.878	0.256
AJCC grade	1.537	1.094–2.159	0.013	0.724	0.444–1.181	0.196
Interval time between CRT and surgery	0.982	0.860–1.121	0.785			
DRM involvement	5.137	0.683–38.652	0.112			
CRM involvement	4.226	0.573–31.150	0.157			
Pre-CRT cT stage	1.093	0.636–1.880	0.747			
Pre-CRT cN stage	1.073	0.382–3.011	0.893			
Organ preservation	1.386	0.583–3.297	0.460			
Pre-CRT CEA level	0.955	0.513–1.778	0.885			
Pre-CRT CA19-9 level	2.422	1.210–4.849	0.012	1.625	0.711–3.711	0.250
UTP6 expression	0.385	0.283–0.525	<0.001	0.730	0.650–0.820	<0.001
Postoperative complications	1.152	0.532–2.494	0.720			
Tumor differentiation	1.986	0.878–4.492	0.099			
Histopathology			0.425			
Expanding	Reference	Reference				
Infiltrating	0.678	0.163–2.820	0.593			
Ulcering	1.417	0.236–8.494	0.703			
CD133 expression	1.218	1.093–1.356	<0.001	1.205	1.077–1.348	0.001
FOXK2 expression	1.024	0.895–1.172	0.726			

LARC, locally advanced rectal cancer; CRT, neoadjuvant chemoradiotherapy; HR, hazard ratio; CI, confidential interval; ASA, American Society of Anesthesiologists; AJCC, American Joint Committee on Cancer; CEA, Carcinoembryonic Antigen; CRM, circumferential resection margin; DRM, distal resection margin.

score group a larger tumor size was seen (2.7 ± 1.2 vs. 3.5 ± 1.6, *P* = 0.002), more lymph nodes were retrieved (11.2 ± 8.7 vs. 15.7 ± 13.8, *P* = 0.028), and poorer histopathology was observed (*P* = 0.026) compared with UTP6 low expression group.

Analysis DNA Promoter Region Methylation of UTP6 in CRC Tissues and Expression, Promoter Methylation of UTP6 in CRC Stem Cells

To explore whether UTP6 was modulated by methylation, we evaluated data on the methylation of the *UTP6* promoter region in CRC and normal colon tissues. Based on the ULACAN database, methylation of the *UTP6* promoter was decreased in normal colon tissue compared to CRC tissue (0.0409 ± 0.0013 vs. 0.0441 ± 0.0005, *P* = 0.017, **Figure 6A**). Further, the expression and promoter methylation levels of *UTP6* were analyzed in CRC stem and non-stem cells. The relative UTP6 expression was significantly reduced in CRC stem cells compared to CRC non-stem cells (GSE14773: 10.33 ± 0.13 vs. 10.80 ± 0.14; *P* = 0.04; GSE24747: 3.44 ± 0.09 and 3.81 ± 0.00, *P* = 0.03; **Figures 6C,D**). We analyzed promoter methylation in CRC stem cells in the GSE104271 dataset. The results demonstrated that the UTP6 promoter was hypermethylated at cg10893370 (stem cell vs. non-stem cell: 0.06 ± 0.00 vs. 0.09 ± 0.00, *P* = 0.008, **Figure 6B**) and cg13453082 (0.05 ± 0.01 vs. 0.08 ± 0.00, *P* = 0.03, **Figure 6B**) sites in CRC stem cells.

GSEA and Co-expression Gene Analysis

GSEA was conducted to investigate the potential mechanism of the UTP6-mediated CRT-resistance in CRC. Our data demonstrated that the negatively correlated KEGG pathways were enriched for the ABC transporter signaling pathway (**Figures 7A–C**). The positively correlated pathways included transcription factor pathways and cell cycle signaling pathways. To further explore the mechanism of the UTP6-mediated CRT response, the genes co-expressed with UTP6 in the TCGA colon tumor data from ULACAN were analyzed. The results demonstrated that FOXK2 was significantly correlated with UTP6 (*r* = 0.55, *P* < 0.01; **Figure 7D**).

DISCUSSION

To date, reliable molecular markers for CRT-resistance in LARC patients are still unavailable. In this study, a gene chip array was performed to detect the gene expression in LARC patients who received CRT. Then WGCNA, an advanced methodology for multigene analysis, was conducted to identify the gene co-expression modules associated with CRT resistance. UTP6 was identified and validated as a hub gene correlated with CRT

TABLE 3 | Cox regression analysis of predictive factors for overall survival in the training dataset patients with LARC following CRT (*n* = 125).

Variables	Univariate analysis			Multivariate analysis		
	HR	95% CI	*P*-value	HR	95% CI	*P*-value
Sex, male/female	1.173	0.554–2.484	0.676			
Age	0.987	0.958–1.017	0.388			
ASA	0.915	0.483–1.733	0.785			
Distance from the anal verge	0.997	0.877–1.134	0.962			
Tumor size	1.394	1.102–1.764	0.006	1.071	0.795–1.442	0.653
Pathological TNM stage	1.934	1.379–2.713	<0.001	1.132	0.733–1.748	0.577
AJCC grade	1.869	1.236–2.827	0.003	1.073	0.614–1.874	0.805
Interval time between CRT and surgery	0.927	0.787–1.093	0.367			
DRM involvement	6.957	0.879–55.039	0.066			
CRM involvement	4.390	0.595–32.402	0.147			
Pre-CRT cT stage	0.804	0.431–1.500	0.492			
Pre-CRT cN stage	3.738	0.508–27.480	0.195			
Organ preservation	1.925	0.783–4.731	0.154			
Pre-CRT CEA level	1.109	0.533–2.306	0.782			
Pre-CRT CA19-9 level	2.738	1.245–6.021	0.012	1.578	0.538–4.625	0.406
UTP6 expression	0.507	0.356–0.723	<0.001	0.822	0.722–50.9	0.003
Postoperative complications	0.738	0.257–2.122	0.573			
Tumor differentiation	2.955	1.260–6.931	0.013	1.190	0.363–3.895	0.774
Histopathology			0.209			
Expanding	Reference	Reference				
Infiltrating	0.915	0.124–6.753	0.930			
Ulcering	2.699	0.281–25.961	0.390			
CD133 expression	1.248	1.097–1.421	0.001	1.185	1.026–1.367	0.021
FOXK2 expression	1.117	0.955–1.307	0.167			

LARC, locally advanced rectal cancer; CRT, neoadjuvant chemoradiotherapy; HR, hazard ratio; CI, confidential interval; ASA, American Society of Anesthesiologists; AJCC, American Joint Committee on Cancer; CEA, Carcinoembryonic Antigen; CRM, circumferential resection margin; DRM, distal resection margin.

resistance. High UTP6 expression was correlated with better survival in CRC patients. UTP6 was hypermethylated in CRC tissues, especially in the CRC stem cell subpopulation. The underlying mechanism of UTP6 in maintaining CRC stemness might involve transcription factor pathways, especially FOXK2.

Currently, microarray expression profiling has been utilized to screen biomarkers in patients with CRT-resistant rectal cancer. Conventional molecular biology methodology identifies DEGs, but it is difficult to correlate biological information provided by gene names with biological functions independently. WGCNA has emerged as an effective method to discover the relationship between networks, genes, phenotypes, and biological sample information, thus avoiding the shortcomings of the traditional methods (Bakhtiarizadeh et al., 2018; Gao et al., 2016; Magani et al., 2018).

Herein, we performed WGCNA to identify the actual hub gene in our patient cohort. The results demonstrated that the dark turquoise module was chosen as the hub module and enriched for translation, DNA replication, and androgen receptor signaling pathways. Those pathways are involved in multi-drug resistant CRT tumors, indicating that the dark turquoise module was significantly associated with CRT-resistance. As described previously (Liu et al., 2017; Wang et al., 2018), PPI network analysis and clinical trait correlation were performed to screen for the actual hub gene. The results suggested that the UTP6 gene had the highest correlation coefficient. We further analyzed the expression of UTP6 in our previous data and testing data set (GSE35452), which showed that UTP6 was the relevant gene for CRT-sensitivity. ROC analysis showed that UTP6 could effectively discriminate between CRT-resistant and -sensitive cases. To our knowledge, this was the first study to identify and verify UTP6 as an effective new marker for the prediction of CRT response.

Having shown that UTP6 was associated with CRT-resistance and survival in CRC patients, the underlying mechanism remained unclear. Cancer stem cells are widely known as tumor-initiating cells due to stem cell properties. Increasing evidence has shown that cancer stem cells are involved in the resistance to conventional cytotoxic therapies, radio- and chemotherapy (Baumann et al., 2008; Wahab et al., 2017). Herein, we evaluated the relative UTP6 expression in two independent data sets including CRC stem cells and parental cells (GSE14773 and GSE24747). The results demonstrated that the expression of UTP6 was significantly decreased in CRC stem cells compared to CRC non-stem cells.

DNA methylation, a main epigenetic modification in the mammalian genome (Baylin et al., 2001; Herman and Baylin, 2003), may inactivate genes and affect the CRT response (Wilting and Dannenberg, 2012; Ivanova et al., 2013). Several studies have reported that DNA methylation could promote drug or

TABLE 4 | Baseline characteristics in patients with LARC following CRT stratified by UTP6 expression (*n* = 125).

Characteristics	UTP6 low expression (*n* = 85)	UTP6 low expression (*n* = 40)	*P*-value
Sex (%)			0.421
Male	58 (68.2)	24 (60.0)	
Female	27 (31.8)	16 (40.0)	
Age (years)	58.3 ± 10.9	57.1 ± 14.9	0.620
ASA score (%)			0.980
1	59 (69.4)	28 (70.0)	
2	21 (24.7)	10 (25.0)	
3	5 (5.9)	2 (5.0)	
Distance from the anal verge (cm)	6.4 ± 3.0	6.7 ± 2.0	0.603
Interval time between CRT and surgery (weeks)	8.3 ± 2.5	8.4 ± 1.5	0.797
Pre-CRT cT stage (%)			0.236
T2	5 (5.9)	0 (0.0)	
T3	35 (41.2)	15 (37.5)	
T4	45 (52.9)	25 (62.5)	
Pre-CRT cN stage (%)			0.222
N0	11 (12.9)	2 (5.0)	
N+	74 (87.1)	38 (95.0)	
Pre-CRT CEA (%)			0.702
<5.0 ng/ml	50 (58.8)	22 (55.0)	
≥5.0 ng/ml	35 (41.2)	18 (45.0)	
Pre-CRT CA19-9 (%)			0.306
<37.0 ng/ml	73 (85.9)	31 (77.5)	
≥37.0 ng/ml	12 (14.1)	9 (22.5)	

LARC, locally advanced rectal cancer; CRT, neoadjuvant chemoradiotherapy; ASA, American Society of Anesthesiologists; CEA, Carcino Embryonic Antigen.

TABLE 5 | Operative and postoperative outcomes in patients with LARC following CRT stratified by UTP6 expression (*n* = 125).

Characteristics	UTP6 high expression (*n* = 85)	UTP6 low expression (*n* = 40)	*P*-value
Pathological type (%)			0.445
Ulcering	80 (94.1)	35 (8735)	
Expanding	3 (3.5)	3 (7.5)	
Infiltrating	2 (2.4)	2 (6.0)	
Histopathology (%)			0.026
Adenocarcinoma	80 (94.1)	32 (80.0)	
Mucinous or signet ring cell carcinoma	5 (5.9)	8 (20.0)	
Tumor differentiation (%)			0.077
Well to moderately differentiated	78 (91.8)	32 (80.0)	
Poorly differentiated and others	7 (8.2)	8 (20.0)	
Postoperative complications (%)	16 (18.8)	5 (12.5)	0.450
Organ preservation (%)	76 (89.4)	33 (82.5)	0.389
Lymph nodes retrieved	11.2 ± 8.7	15.7 ± 13.8	0.028
Metastatic lymph nodes	0.45 ± 1.4	3.1 ± 7.1	<0.001
CRM involvement (%)	1 (1.2)	2 (5.0)	0.240
Tumor size (cm)	2.7 ± 1.2	3.5 ± 1.6	0.002
Pathological T stage (%)			<0.001
0	27 (31.8)	0 (0.0)	
1	7 (8.2)	2 (5.0)	
2	15 (17.6)	10 (25.0)	
3	35 (41.2)	23 (57.5)	
4	1 (1.2)	5 (12.5)	
Pathological N stage (%)			0.001
0	72 (84.7)	22 (55.0)	
1	9 (10.6)	11 (27.5)	
2	4 (4.7)	7 (17.5)	
Pathological M stage (%)			0.036
0	84 (98.8)	36 (90.0)	
1	1 (1.2)	4 (10.0)	
TRG (%)			<0.001
0	27 (31.8)	0 (0.0)	
1	27 (31.8)	11 (27.5)	
2	25 (29.4)	23 (57.5)	
3	6 (7.1)	6 (15.0)	
Nerval invasion (%)	0 (0.0)	0 (0.0)	1.000
Vascular invasion (%)	2 (2.4)	0 (0.0)	1.000

LARC, locally advanced rectal cancer; CRT, neoadjuvant chemoradiotherapy; CRM, circumferential resection margin; DRM, distal resection margin; TRG, tumor regression grade; pCR: pathological complete response.

radiation resistance (Su et al., 2011), and thus, could be used to predict treatment response. In the present study, we found hypermethylation in colon cancer tissue and the cg10893370 and cg13453082 sites located in the UTP6 promoter in CRC stem cells. These results indicated that the hypermethylation of UTP6 may result in a decreased expression of UTP6 in CRC stem cells and that the downregulation UTP6 expression in cancer stem cells may be due to hypermethylation of the promoter sites. Several studies have reported that DNA methylation could affect gene expression in the transcriptome, which is involved in CRT-resistance in various cancer stem cells (Kurscheid et al., 2015; Kostopoulou et al., 2018). Importantly, DNA methylation can be reversed by anti-tumor drugs, such as decitabine (Ariazi et al., 2017; Flotho et al., 2018). The findings suggest that the combination of demethylation therapy targeting *UTP6* and cancer stem cells during CRT might be beneficial to rectal cancer patients.

UTP6 (also known as HCA66) is an essential component of the UTPB, a large complex composed of six proteins Utp1/Pwp2, Utp6, Utp12/Dip2, Utp13, Utp18, and Utp21 (Grandi et al., 2002; Krogan et al., 2004). Ferraro et al. (2011) reported that Apafl could bind with UTP6 and participate in the regulation of centrosomal microtubule nucleation, spindle assembly, cell migration, and mitochondrial network organization. Meanwhile, UTP6 has been proposed as a promising prognostic indicator in bladder cancer (Shivakumar et al., 2017). A previous study reported that UTPB was the consist of the UTP6, which is an important complex in regulating ribosome synthesis (Hunziker et al., 2016; Zhang et al., 2016). Herein, we found that UTP6 was not only related to the ABC transporter signal pathway, but also transcription factor pathways, which are associated with CRT resistance (Shinto et al., 2014; McCoy et al., 2015). Pearson's correlation analysis showed that the expression of UTP6 was correlated with that of FOXK2, which is a transcription factor known as an anti-oncogene (Shan et al., 2016; de Moraes et al., 2019). The results indicated that the anti-chemoradiotherapy resistance effect of UTP6 may be related to FOXK2 expression. Unfortunately, the precise mechanism of UTP6 involved in CRT sensitivity in rectal cancer patients is still unclear.

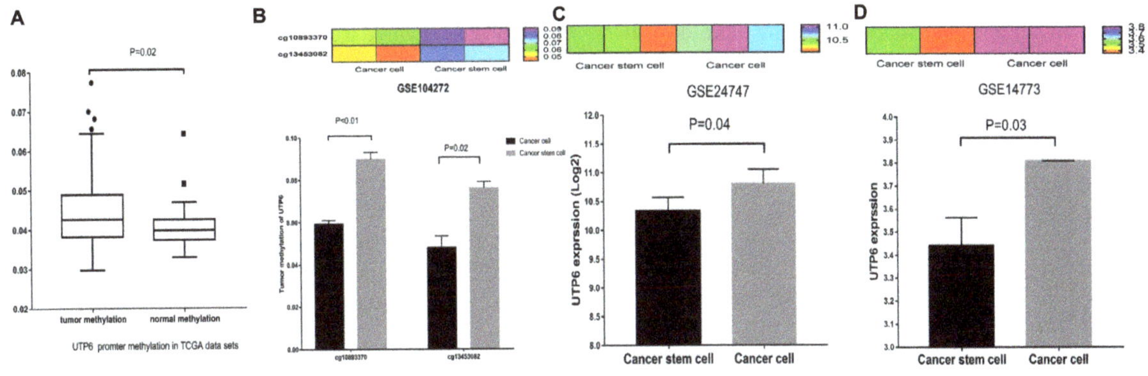

FIGURE 6 | UTP6 had increased promoter hypermethylation in colon tumors, lower expression in CRC stem cells. **(A)** From the TCGA database. UTP6 had increased promoter hypermethylation in colon cancer. **(B)** UTP6 had higher promoter methylation levels in cg10893370 and cg13453082 sites in CRC stem cells. Heat map and bar graph showed that CRC non-stem cells had higher UTP6 expression compared with CRC stem cells in GSE24747 **(C)** and GSE14773 **(D)**.

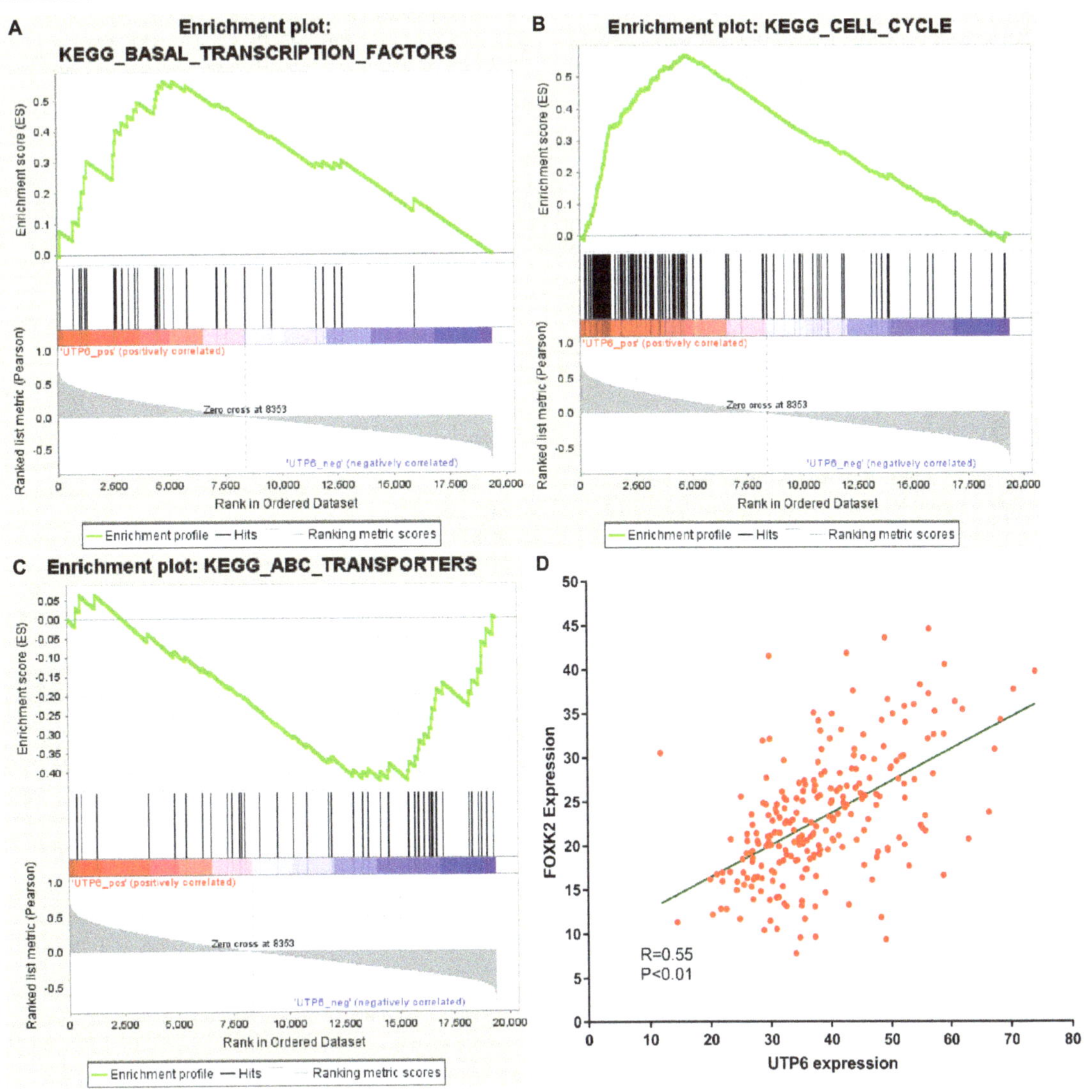

FIGURE 7 | GSEA using our data and co-expression analysis between UTP6 and FOXK2 in the TCGA colon tumor dataset. **(A)** Transcription factors pathway. **(B)** Cell cycle. **(C)** ABC transportanters. **(D)** Co-expression analysis between UTP6 and FOXK2 in the TCGA colon tumor dataset.

There were several limitations to our study. Although the underlying mechanism of UTP6 was explored by bioinformatics analysis, the results warrant further confirmation by *in vitro* or *in vivo* experiments. To our knowledge, this was the first study to explore CRT-resistance-related genes through WGCNA using a patient cohort with complete clinicopathological and follow-up data. The present study provided insight into the role of UTP6 in CRT-sensitive in rectal cancer patients.

CONCLUSION

Through WGCNA, UTP6 was identified and validated as a hub gene and a valid novel predictor for CRT-sensitivity. High expression of UTP6 associated with better survival in LARC patients. UTP6 was hypermethylated in CRC tissues, especially in CRC stem cells subpopulation. GSEA demonstrated that the mechanism underlying UTP6 maintains CRC stemness might be involved in the transcription factors pathway especially FOXK2. Further research is needed to confirm the above findings.

ETHICS STATEMENT

Studies relative to humans in this article were approved by the Ethics Committee of The Fujian Medical University Union Hospital. The patients/participants provided their written informed consent to participate in this study. Written informed consent was obtained from the individual(s) for the publication of any potentially identifiable images or data included in this article.

AUTHOR CONTRIBUTIONS

YZ, QG, YW, GG, and XL designed and performed the experiments, analyzed the data, and wrote the manuscript. YP, JZ, and YY performed the experiments. All authors read and approved the final manuscript.

SUPPLEMENTARY MATERIAL

Supplementary Figure 1 | Validation of FTSJ3. **(A)** In our data (6.21 ± 0.32 vs. 5.75 ± 0.47, $P < 0.01$) and **(B)** GSE35452 (0.11 ± 0.40 vs. −0.05 ± 0.53, $P = 0.246$). **(C)** Person analysis between the AJCC TRG grade and FTSJ3 expression. ROC curves and AUC statistics to evaluate the predictive efficiency of the FTSJ3 in our data and external data to distinguish CRT-resistance from CRT−sensitive CRC cases from **(D)** our data and **(E)** GSE35452. The disease-free survival **(F)** and overall survival **(G)** between low and high expression of FTSJ3.

Supplementary Figure 2 | The result of Cut-off Finder. Plot of the OR of the UTP6 **(A)** and FTSJ3 **(D)** expression and the optimal cutoff value. And the optimal cutoff value is compared to the gene expression. ROC curves and AUC analysis to evaluate the predictive efficiency of the optimal cutoff of the UTP6 **(B)** and FTSJ3 **(E)** expression. The classification using UTP6 **(C)** and FTSJ3 **(F)** expression and patients' DFS status. And the optimal cutoff value is compared to the gene expression. OR, odds ratio; DFS, disease-free survival.

REFERENCES

Amin, M. B., Edge, S., Greene, F., Byrd, D. R., Brookland, R. K., Washington, M. K., et al. (2017). *AJCC Cancer Staging Manual,* 8th Edn. Chicago, IL: Springer.

Ariazi, E. A., Taylor, J. C., Black, M. A., Nicolas, E., Slifker, M. J., Azzam, D. J., et al. (2017). A new role for ERα: silencing via dna methylation of Basal, stem cell, and EMT genes. *Mol. Cancer Res.* 15, 152–164. doi: 10.1158/1541-7786.mcr-16-0283

Bakhtiarizadeh, M. R., Hosseinpour, B., Shahhoseini, M., Korte, A., and Gifani, P. (2018). Weighted gene co-expression network analysis of endometriosis and identification of functional modules associated with its main hallmarks. *Front. Genet.* 9:453. doi: 10.3389/fgene.2018.00453

Baumann, M., Krause, M., and Hill, R. (2008). Exploring the role of cancer stem cells in radioresistance. *Nat. Rev. Cancer* 8, 545–554. doi: 10.1038/nrc2419

Baylin, S. B., Esteller, M., Rountree, M. R., Bachman, K. E., Schuebel, K., and Herman, J. G. (2001). Aberrant patterns of DNA methylation, chromatin formation and gene expression in cancer. *Hum. Mol. Genet.* 10, 687–692. doi: 10.1093/hmg/10.7.687

Benson, A. B., Venook, A. P., Al-Hawary, M. M., Cederquist, L., Chen, Y. J., Ciombor, K. K., et al. (2018). Rectal cancer, version 2.2018, NCCN clinical practice guidelines in oncology. *J. Natl. Compr. Cancer Netw.* 16, 874–901. doi: 10.6004/jnccn.2018.0061

Botía, J. A., Vandrovcova, J., Forabosco, P., Guelfi, S., D'Sa, K., Hardy, J., et al. (2017). An additional k-means clustering step improves the biological features of WGCNA gene co-expression networks. *BMC Syst. Biol.* 11:47. doi: 10.1186/s12918-017-0420-6

Budczies, J., Klauschen, F., Sinn, B. V., Győrffy, B., Schmitt, W. D., Darb-Esfahani, S., et al. (2012). Cutoff Finder: a comprehensive and straightforward Web application enabling rapid biomarker cutoff optimization. *PLoS One* 7:e51862. doi: 10.1371/journal.pone.0051862

Chandrashekar, D. S., Bashel, B., Sah, B., Creighton, C. J., Ponce-Rodriguez, I., Bvsk, C., et al. (2017). UALCAN: a portal for facilitating tumor subgroup gene expression and survival analyses. *Neoplasia* 19, 649–658.

de Moraes, G. N., Ldt, C., Maia, R. C., Lam, E. W., and Sharrocks, A. D. (2019). FOXK2 transcription factor and its emerging roles in cancer. *Cancers (Basel)* 11:393. doi: 10.3390/cancers11030393

Ferraro, E., Pesaresi, M. G., De Zio, D., Cencioni, M. T., Gortat, A., Cozzolino, M., et al. (2011). Apaf1 plays a pro-survival role by regulating centrosome morphology and function. *J. Cell Sci.* 124(Pt 20), 3450–3463.

Flotho, C., Sommer, S., and Lübbert, M. (2018). DNA-hypomethylating agents as epigenetic therapy before and after allogeneic hematopoietic stem cell transplantation in myelodysplastic syndromes and juvenile myelomonocytic leukemia. *Semin. Cancer Biol.* 51, 68–79. doi: 10.1016/j.semcancer.2017.10.011

Gao, B., Shao, Q., Choudhry, H., Marcus, V., Dong, K., Ragoussis, J., et al. (2016). Weighted gene co-expression network analysis of colorectal cancer liver metastasis genome sequencing data and screening of anti-metastasis drugs. *Int. J. Oncol.* 49, 1108–1118. doi: 10.3892/ijo.2016.3591

Grandi, P., Rybin, V., Bassler, J., Petfalski, E., Strauss, D., Marzioch, M., et al. (2002). 90S pre-ribosomes include the 35S pre-rRNA, the U3 snoRNP, and 40S subunit processing factors but predominantly lack 60S synthesis factors. *Mol. Cell* 10, 105–115. doi: 10.1016/s1097-2765(02)00579-8

Ha, Y. J., Tak, K. H., Kim, C. W., Roh, S. A., Choi, E. K., Cho, D. H., et al. (2017). PSMB8 as a candidate marker of responsiveness to preoperative radiation therapy in rectal cancer patients. *Int. J. Radiat. Oncol. Biol. Phys.* 98, 1164–1173. doi: 10.1016/j.ijrobp.2017.03.023

Heald, R. J., Husband, E. M., and Ryall, R. D. (1982). The mesorectum in rectal cancer surgery–the clue to pelvic recurrence. *Br. J. Surg.* 69, 613–616. doi: 10.1002/bjs.1800691019

Herman, J. G., and Baylin, S. B. (2003). Gene silencing in cancer in association with promoter hypermethylation. *N. Engl. J. Med.* 349, 2042–2054. doi: 10.1056/nejmra023075

Horvath, S., and Dong, J. (2008). Geometric interpretation of gene coexpression network analysis. *PLoS Comput. Biol.* 4:e1000117. doi: 10.1371/journal.pcbi.1000117

Huang, Y. F., Niu, W. B., Hu, R., Wang, L. J., Huang, Z. Y., Ni, S. H., et al. (2018). FIBP knockdown attenuates growth and enhances chemotherapy in colorectal cancer via regulating GSK3β-related pathways. *Oncogenesis* 7:77.

Hunziker, M., Barandun, J., Petfalski, E., Tan, D., Delan-Forino, C., Molloy, K. R., et al. (2016). UtpA and UtpB chaperone nascent pre-ribosomal RNA and U3 snoRNA to initiate eukaryotic ribosome assembly. *Nat. Commun.* 7:12090.

Ivanova, T., Zouridis, H., Wu, Y., Cheng, L. L., Tan, I. B., Gopalakrishnan, V., et al. (2013). Integrated epigenomics identifies BMP4 as a modulator of cisplatin sensitivity in gastric cancer. *Gut* 62, 22–33. doi: 10.1136/gutjnl-2011-301113

Kostopoulou, O. N., Mohammad, A. A., Bartek, J., Winter, J., Jung, M., Stragliotto, G., et al. (2018). Glucocorticoids promote a glioma stem cell-like phenotype and resistance to chemotherapy in human glioblastoma primary cells: biological and prognostic significance. *Int. J. Cancer* 142, 1266–1276. doi: 10.1002/ijc.31132

Krogan, N. J., Peng, W. T., Cagney, G., Robinson, M. D., Haw, R., Zhong, G., et al. (2004). High-definition macromolecular composition of yeast RNA-processing complexes. *Mol. Cell* 13, 225–239. doi: 10.1016/s1097-2765(04)00003-6

Kurscheid, S., Bady, P., Sciuscio, D., Samarzija, I., Shay, T., Vassallo, I., et al. (2015). Chromosome 7 gain and DNA hypermethylation at the HOXA10 locus are associated with expression of a stem cell related HOX-signature in glioblastoma. *Genome Biol.* 16:16.

Langfelder, P., and Horvath, S. (2008). WGCNA: an R package for weighted correlation network analysis. *BMC Bioinformatics* 9:559. doi: 10.1186/1471-2105-9-559

Liu, J., Li, H., Sun, L., Wang, Z., Xing, C., and Yuan, Y. (2017). Aberrantly methylated-differentially expressed genes and pathways in colorectal cancer. *Cancer Cell Int.* 17:75. doi: 10.1186/s12935-017-0444-4

Magani, F., Bray, E. R., Martinez, M. J., Zhao, N., Copello, V. A., Heidman, L., et al. (2018). Identification of an oncogenic network with prognostic and therapeutic value in prostate cancer. *Mol. Syst. Biol.* 14:e8202. doi: 10.15252/msb.20188202

Mason, M. J., Fan, G., Plath, K., Zhou, Q., and Horvath, S. (2009). Signed weighted gene co-expression network analysis of transcriptional regulation in murine embryonic stem cells. *BMC Genomics* 10:327. doi: 10.1186/1471-2164-10-327

McCoy, M. J., Hemmings, C., Miller, T. J., Austin, S. J., Bulsara, M. K., Zeps, N., et al. (2015). Low stromal Foxp3+ regulatory T-cell density is associated with complete response to neoadjuvant chemoradiotherapy in rectal cancer. *Br. J. Cancer* 113, 1677–1686. doi: 10.1038/bjc.2015.427

Rahbari, N. N., Elbers, H., Askoxylakis, V., Motschall, E., Bork, U., Büchler, M. W., et al. (2013). Neoadjuvant radiotherapy for rectal cancer: meta-analysis of randomized controlled trials. *Ann. Surg. Oncol.* 20, 4169–4182. doi: 10.1245/s10434-013-3198-9

Sauer, R., Becker, H., Hohenberger, W., Rödel, C., Wittekind, C., Fietkau, R., et al. (2004). Preoperative versus postoperative chemoradiotherapy for rectal cancer. *N. Engl. J. Med.* 351, 1731–1740.

Sauer, R., Liersch, T., Merkel, S., Fietkau, R., Hohenberger, W., Hess, C., et al. (2012). Preoperative versus postoperative chemoradiotherapy for locally advanced rectal cancer: results of the German CAO/ARO/AIO-94 randomized phase III trial after a median follow-up of 11 years. *J. Clin. Oncol.* 30, 1926–1933. doi: 10.1200/jco.2011.40.1836

Shan, L., Zhou, X., Liu, X., Wang, Y., Su, D., Hou, Y., et al. (2016). FOXK2 elicits massive transcription repression and suppresses the hypoxic response and breast cancer carcinogenesis. *Cancer Cell* 30, 708–722.

Shinto, E., Hase, K., Hashiguchi, Y., Sekizawa, A., Ueno, H., Shikina, A., et al. (2014). CD8+ and FOXP3+ tumor-infiltrating T cells before and after chemoradiotherapy for rectal cancer. *Ann. Surg. Oncol.* 21(Suppl. 3), S414–S421.

Shivakumar, M., Lee, Y., Bang, L., Garg, T., Sohn, K. A., and Kim, D. (2017). Identification of epigenetic interactions between miRNA and DNA methylation associated with gene expression as potential prognostic markers in bladder cancer. *BMC Med. Genomics* 10(Suppl. 1):30. doi: 10.1186/s12920-017-0269-y

Su, L. J., Mahabir, S., Ellison, G. L., McGuinn, L. A., and Reid, B. C. (2011). Epigenetic contributions to the relationship between cancer and dietary intake of nutrients, bioactive food components, and environmental toxicants. *Front. Genet.* 2:91. doi: 10.3389/fgene.2011.00091

Tian, F., Zhao, J., Fan, X., and Kang, Z. (2017). Weighted gene co-expression network analysis in identification of metastasis-related genes of lung squamous cell carcinoma based on the Cancer Genome Atlas database. *J. Thorac. Dis.* 9, 42–53. doi: 10.21037/jtd.2017.01.04

van Gijn, W., Marijnen, C. A., Nagtegaal, I. D., Kranenbarg, E. M., Putter, H., Wiggers, T., et al. (2011). Preoperative radiotherapy combined with total mesorectal excision for resectable rectal cancer: 12-year follow-up of the multicentre, randomised controlled TME trial. *Lancet Oncol.* 12, 575–582. doi: 10.1016/s1470-2045(11)70097-3

Wahab, S. M. R., Islam, F., Gopalan, V., and Lam, A. K. (2017). The identifications and clinical implications of cancer stem cells in colorectal cancer. *Clin. Colorectal Cancer* 16, 93–102. doi: 10.1016/j.clcc.2017.01.011

Wang, X., Ghareeb, W. M., Lu, X., Huang, Y., Huang, S., and Chi, P. (2018). Coexpression network analysis linked H2AFJ to chemoradiation resistance in colorectal cancer. *J. Cell. Biochem.* 120, 10351–10362. doi: 10.1002/jcb.28319

Wilting, R. H., and Dannenberg, J. H. (2012). Epigenetic mechanisms in tumorigenesis, tumor cell heterogeneity and drug resistance. *Drug Resist. Updat.* 15, 21–38. doi: 10.1016/j.drup.2012.01.008

Yip, A. M., and Horvath, S. (2007). Gene network interconnectedness and the generalized topological overlap measure. *BMC Bioinformatics* 8:22.

Zhang, B., and Horvath, S. (2005). A general framework for weighted gene co-expression network analysis. *Stat. Appl. Genet. Mol. Biol.* 4:Article17. doi: 10.2202/1544-6115.1128

Zhang, C., Sun, Q., Chen, R., Chen, X., Lin, J., and Ye, K. (2016). Integrative structural analysis of the UTPB complex, an early assembly factor for eukaryotic small ribosomal subunits. *Nucleic Acids Res.* 44, 7475–7486.

Zhang, Y., Sun, Y., Xu, Z., Chi, P., and Lu, X. (2017). Is neoadjuvant chemoradiotherapy always necessary for mid/high local advanced rectal cancer: a comparative analysis after propensity score matching. *Eur. J. Surg. Oncol.* 43, 1440–1446. doi: 10.1016/j.ejso.2017.04.007

Zhang, Y., Xu, Z., Sun, Y., Chi, P., and Lu, X. (2018). Knockdown of KLK11 reverses oxaliplatin resistance by inhibiting proliferation and activating apoptosis via suppressing the PI3K/AKT signal pathway in colorectal cancer cell. *Onco Targets Ther.* 11, 809–821. doi: 10.2147/OTT.S151867 doi: 10.2147/ott.s151867

14

Cisplatin-Resistant Gastric Cancer Cells Promote the Chemoresistance of Cisplatin-Sensitive Cells via the Exosomal RPS3-Mediated PI3K-Akt-Cofilin-1 Signaling Axis

Meng-Yao Sun[1†], *Bo Xu*[1†], *Qiu-Xue Wu*[1†], *Wen-Lian Chen*[2], *Si Cai*[1*], *Hui Zhang*[3*] and *Qing-Feng Tang*[1,4*]

[1] *Department of Clinical Laboratory and Central Laboratory, Putuo Hospital, Shanghai University of Traditional Chinese Medicine, Shanghai, China,* [2] *Cancer Institute, Longhua Hospital, Shanghai University of Traditional Chinese Medicine, Shanghai, China,* [3] *Research Center for Traditional Chinese Medicine Complexity System, Institute of Interdisciplinary Integrative Medicine Research, Shanghai University of Traditional Chinese Medicine, Shanghai, China,* [4] *Department of Clinical Laboratory, Jiading Branch of Shanghai General Hospital, Shanghai, China*

***Correspondence:**
Qing-Feng Tang
tangqingfeng126@126.com
Hui Zhang
zhanghuiman@126.com
Si Cai
13774245929@139.com

† These authors have contributed equally to this work

Cisplatin is an important agent in first-line chemotherapy against gastric cancer (GC). However, consequential drug resistance limits its effectiveness for the treatment of GC. In this study, a cisplatin resistant gastric cancer cell line SGC7901R was determined by LC-MS/MS with increased exosomal levels of RPS3 protein. SGC7901R cell-derived exosomes were readily taken up by cisplatin-sensitive SGC7901S cells, thus triggering off a phenotype of chemoresistance in the receptor cells. Subsequently, it was demonstrated that exosomal RPS3 was essential for inducing chemoresistance of receptor cells as shown by the acquisition of this phenotype in SGC7901S cells with enforced expression of RPS3. Further mechanism study demonstrated that cisplatin-resistant gastric cancer cell-derived exosomal RPS3 enhanced the chemoresistance of cisplatin-sensitive gastric cancer cells through the PI3K-Akt-cofilin-1 signaling pathway. All these findings demonstrated that cisplatin-resistant gastric cancer cells communicate with sensitive cells through the intercellular delivery of exosomal RPS3 and activation of the PI3K-Akt-cofilin-1 signaling pathway. Targeting exosomal RPS3 protein in cisplatin-resistant gastric cancer cells may thus be a promising strategy to overcome cisplatin resistance in gastric cancer.

Keywords: gastric cancer, cisplatin resistance, exosome, RPS3, PI3K-Akt-cofilin-1

INTRODUCTION

Gastric cancer ranks as the second most common malignant disease and the third leading cause of cancer-associated mortality in developing countries (Bray et al., 2018). Chemotherapy is one of the principal therapeutic approaches used for the treatment of gastric cancer. Chemoresistance has been identified as a major problem in the process of cancer treatment. Cisplatin (DDP) is widely used as a front-line chemotherapeutic agent for gastric cancer; however, chemoresistance limits the effectiveness of chemotherapy and results in treatment failure in the majority of cases (Guo et al., 2015; Zhang and Fan, 2017). In the past few years, some reports have partly shown the underlying mechanisms of cisplatin resistance in gastric cancer. However, the molecular mechanisms underlying cisplatin resistance remain to be further investigated.

Exosomes are a subset of extracellular microvesicles secreted from different types of cells (Zhang J. et al., 2015). More and more reports have indicated that exosomes play important roles in tumor growth, metastasis, angiogenesis, and immune regulation by acting as information communicators between different types of cells (Brinton et al., 2015; Meehan and Vella, 2016; Ruivo et al., 2017). Importantly, exosomes have recently been discovered anticipating in the regulation of chemoresistance in cancers (Sousa et al., 2015; Sharma, 2017; Butera et al., 2018). As is known to all, exosomes are nanosized vesicles (about 100 nm) loading a variety of kinds of cargo, including DNA, mRNA, miRNA, circRNA, and proteins (Colombo et al., 2014). Some reports have demonstrated that chemotherapy can change the exosomal composition secreted from tumor cells (Kreger et al., 2016; Ning et al., 2017; Bandari et al., 2018), however, which exosomal cargos play key roles in regulating chemoresistance is not well understood.

In this study, a cisplatin-resistant gastric cancer cell line SGC7901 (SGC7901R) was established, and the exosomal protein expression levels in SGC7901R cells and sensitive (SGC7901S) cells were investigated by LC-MS/MS and compared. RPS3 (ribosomal protein S3) was one of the highly expressed proteins in the exosome of SGC7901R cells in comparison with SGC7901S cells, which sparked our interest to explore the role and mechanism of exosomal RPS3 protein in transmitting a chemoresistance phenotype from cisplatin-resistant to cisplatin-sensitive gastric cancer cells.

It has been proposed that many ribosomal proteins (RPs) may act as cancer genes in human, such as high expression of RPL6 in human gastric cancer cell (Wu et al., 2011). RPL11 expression is a potential biomarker for predicting 5-FU sensitivity (Kawahata et al., 2020). Moreover, RPS15A could promote GC progression via activation of the Akt pathway (Liu et al., 2019). RPS3 has been demonstrated to be involved in DDP resistance of oral squamous cell carcinoma (Huang et al., 2019). However, the effects of RPS3 in DDP resistance of GC were unknown. Our previous study demonstrated that the PI3K/Akt pathway functions as a crucial pathway in the regulation of DDP resistance of GC by modulating PP1- and PP2A-mediated mitochondrial translocation of cofilin-1 (Tang et al., 2016). In addition, it was reported that RP mutations suppress the activity of the AKT pathway (Antunes et al., 2015). Therefore, we speculated that the mechanism of RPS3-related GC resistance to DDP may be associated with the PI3K/Akt signaling pathway, which finally induced PP1- and PP2A-mediated mitochondrial translocation of cofilin-1.

MATERIALS AND METHODS

Establishment of Cisplatin-Resistant Cell Lines

The human gastric cancer cell lines SGC7901 and BGC-823 were obtained from the Cell Bank of Type Culture Collection of the Chinese Academy of Sciences (Shanghai, China). The cells were cultured in RPMI1640 medium (Gibco, Thermo Fisher Scientific, Inc.) supplemented with 10% fetal bovine serum (FBS, Gibco, Thermo Fisher Scientifics, Inc.) and incubated at 37°C in a humidified incubator with 5% CO_2. Cisplatin-resistant SGC7901R and BGC823R cells were established by continuous exposure to stepwise-increasing concentrations of cisplatin (Sigma-Aldrich, Merck KGaA, Darmstadt, Germany). Cells that were viable in the cell culture medium with a high concentration of cisplatin (1,000 μg/L) were designated as cisplatin-resistant cells. Parental cells, denoted as SGC7901S and BGC-823S, were cultured under the same conditions without treatment.

Exosome Isolation and Characterization

Gastric cancer cells were cultured in freshly prepared RPMI1640 medium containing exosome-free FBS for 48 h until cells had reached 90% confluence. Cell culture supernatants were collected and filtered using 0.22-μm pore filters (Merck KGaA), followed by differential centrifugation at 4°C: 300 × *g* for 10 min to remove cells, 2,000 × *g* for 15 min to remove cell debris, and 10,000 × *g* for 30 min to remove large particles. Then, the pellets containing exosomes were collected by spinning at 100,000 × *g* for 70 min. After washing with PBS, the pellets were dealt using ultracentrifugation (Beckman 70Ti rotor). The morphology of exosomes was examined via transmission electron microscopy. The number and size distribution of exosomes were detected by a LM10 nanoparticle characterization system (NanoSight, Malvern Instruments). The exosomal protein concentration was measured by the BCA method, and exosome-associated protein markers of HSP70, CD63, and CD9 expression were analyzed by Western blotting.

Exosome Labeling and Treatment

8×10^4 of SGC7901S cells were seeded in 12-well plates and incubated at 37°C with red fluorescent dye CM-Dil (Invitrogen; Thermo Fisher Scientific, Inc.) at 37°C for 1 h, washed with PBS, and centrifuged at 110,000 × *g* at 4°C for 70 min to remove excess dye. Exosomes from SGC7901R cells were pre-labeled with the green fluorescent dye PKH-67 (Invitrogen; Thermo Fisher Scientific, Inc.) at 37°C for 1 h, washed with PBS, and centrifuged at 110,000 × *g* at 4°C for 70 min to remove excess dye. Unlabeled exosomes were used as a negative control. The CM-Dil-labeled SGC7901S cells were incubated with PKH-67-labeled exosomes or unlabeled control exosomes for 4 h. Then, SGC7901S cells were fixed with 4% paraformaldehyde at room temperature for 1 h. Nuclear staining was performed with DAPI (40, 6-diamidino-2-phenylindole) at room temperature for 10 min. Incorporation of exosomes into targeted SGC7901S cells was visualized by fluorescence microscopy (Zeiss AG, Germany).

Cell Proliferation Analysis

Cells were seeded in 96-well plates (5,000 cells/well) [MULTISCIENCES (LIANKE) BIOTECH, China] and exposed to increasing concentrations of cisplatin for 48 h at 37°C. The concentrations of cisplatin used for the drug dose-response curve analysis of cells were 0, 125, 250, 500, 1,000, 2,000, 4,000, 8,000, and 16,000 μg/L. The proliferative ability of cells was determined with a Cell Counting Kit-8 (CCK-8) (MedChemExpress, Monmouth Junction, United States) according to the manufacturer's protocols. Exosomes were isolated from cells and cancer cells following transfection with oligonucleotides (described below). For exosome treatment analysis, each well in a 96-well plate was seeded with 1,000 cells and loaded with exosomes at 100 μg/mL for 48 h for functional analysis at 37°C, and the untreated cells served as the control. The cell culture medium was then removed, and a fresh medium containing the IC50 concentration of cisplatin was added to each well for 48 h. At the end of treatment, cell proliferation was measured.

LC-MS/MS Analysis

20 μg proteins from each sample was denatured using 8 M urea, reduced with 10 mM dithiothreitol (DTT), and alkylated using 100 mM iodoacetamide. The samples were then proteolytically digested with endoproteinase LysC overnight at room temperature, followed by digestion with trypsin for 15 h at 37°C. The resulting peptide mixtures were extracted using a peptide extract solution (50% ACN, 0.1% TFA) for 30 min at 37°C. Then, the samples were dried and solubilized in the sample loading buffer containing 0.1% formic acid. Each sample of about 3–5 μg was analyzed by reversed-phase nano-liquid chromatography-tandem mass spectrometry (LC-MS/MS) (Thermo Scientific). The source data from three technical replicates of each sample were analyzed by searching the Uniprot human database with MaxQuant and Perseus software. Label-free quantitative (LFQ) values represent protein abundance. The false discovery rate (FDR) values at the protein and peptide levels were set to 1%. Only those proteins quantified in at least two out of three replicates in at least one group remain for further analysis. The multiple-sample ANOVA test was executed and corrected for multiple-hypothesis testing using a cutoff of FDR < 0.05.

RT-qPCR

Total RNA from cells was extracted using TRIzol (Invitrogen; Thermo Fisher Scientific, Inc.). cDNA was produced by reverse transcription using the SuperScript® III RT-PCR kit according to the manufacturer's instructions (Thermo Fisher Scientific, Inc.). The amplification of fluorescence signals was detected by a fluorescence thermal cycler (Bio-Rad Laboratories, Inc., United States). RT-qPCR was performed (Novoprotein, Shanghai, China) using the following primers: RPS3 sense, 5′-GCGAGTTACACCAACCAGGA-3′ and antisense, 5′-ATGAACCGCAGCACACCATA-3′; β-actin sense, 5′-AGCAGCATCGCCCCAAAGTT-3′ and antisense, 5′-GGGCACGAAGGCTCATCATT-3′. B-Actin was set as an internal control for cellular mRNAs. The parameters for PCR quantification were as follows: 2 min at 95°C, followed by 40 cycles of 15 s at 95°C and 30 s at 60°C. The results of qPCR were defined using the quantification cycle (Cq), and $2^{-\Delta\Delta Cq}$ was used to calculate the relative expression levels (Livak and Schmittgen, 2001).

Western Blotting

Cellular proteins were extracted with RIPA lysis buffer (Beyotime Institute of Biotechnology). Protein concentration was determined by the BCA method. A total of 40 μg of protein for each group was separated on 12% SDS-PAGE gels and transferred to 0.45-μm PVDF membranes (EMD Millipore). Membranes were then blocked with 5% BSA and incubated with primary antibodies at 4°C overnight against HPS70 (4876, CST), CD9 (ab92726, CST), CD63 (ab193349, Abcam), RBP4 (ab233138, Abcam), RPSA (ab133645, Abcam), RPS3(9538, CST), RPS20 (ab133776, Abcam), RPS14 (ab246916, Abcam), RPL4 (ab234829, Abcam), RPL13 (ab134961, Abcam), HSPD1 (ab46798, Abcam), HSPA8 (8444, CST), P-gp (13342, CST), p-cofilin-1 (3313, CST), cofilin-1 (5175, CST), PP1 (sc-7482, Santa Cruz), PP2A (9780, CST). Anti-β-actin (ab179467, Abcam) and anti-GAPDH (2118, CST) were used as the internal control. Anti-COX IV (11967, CST) was used as loading control for mitochondrial proteins. The membranes were then incubated at 37°C for 1 h with an HRP-conjugated secondary antibody (ab97051, Abcam). Bands were visualized by chemiluminescence according to the manufacturer's protocols.

Plasmid Construction and Cell Transfection

The recombinant plasmids containing the pcDNA3.1 empty vector, pcDNA3.1-RPS3, pLV4-shRNA/RPS3, and the non-targeting control pLV4-shRNA-negative control (NC) were produced by GeneChem, Inc. (Shanghai Genechem Company Ltd., China). All the transfections were performed using Lipofectamine 3000 reagent (Invitrogen; Thermo Fisher Scientific, Inc.) in accordance with the manufacturer's instructions.

ICP-MS Analysis

SGC-7901R or SGC-7901S cells were digested and collected. 500 μL ddH_2O was added, and the cells were broken by freezing and thawing with liquid nitrogen repeatedly followed by sonication. The samples were centrifuged at 14,000 rpm/min for 10 min, and the supernatant was collected, dried under vacuum for 24 h, and dissolved in PBS. The dissolved samples were digested by 2 mL nitric acid followed by 1 mL perchloric acid, cooled down, set to a constant volume of 10 mL, and ultrafiltrated. The ultrafiltrated samples (10 mL) were diluted using a Gilson ASPEC XLi program to deliver 1.8 mL of iridium internal standard (0.005 mg/mL, in 1% nitric acid) and mixed thoroughly. Intracellular accumulation of DDP in each cell sample was determined by ultrasensitive multi-collector inductively coupled with mass spectrometry (ICP-MS) as previously described (Lavilla et al., 2009).

Flow Cytometry Analysis

Cells were plated in 6-well plates at 2×10^5 cells/well in RPMI 1,640 medium with 10% FBS. The cells were collected and re-suspended gently in 400 μL binding buffer. 5 μL Annexin V FITC was added to the above cell solution, gently vortexed, and incubated for 10 min at 4°C avoiding the light. 10 μL propidium iodide (PI) was added and cultured for another 5 min. Flow cytometry was then conducted using FACSCalibur Flow Cytometry (BD Biosciences, United States), and the results were analyzed with CellQuest software.

Tumor Mouse Model

SGC-7901S cells were harvested in serum-free PBS, and 100 μL single-cell suspensions (2×10^7 cells/mL) were injected into the subcutaneous area of male BALB/c nude mice (4–6 weeks old, SLAC Laboratory Lab, Shanghai, China). When the tumors reached an average size of 100 mm^3, the mice were randomized into 5 groups ($n = 5$). Mice in group 1 were administered with normal saline daily, mice in group 2 were administered with 10 μg/mL DDP, and mice in groups 3, 4, and 5 proceeded administration of control exosomes, shRNA/RPS3 exosomes, and over/RPS3 exosomes, plus 10 μg/mL DDP, respectively. The length and width of tumors were recorded every 7 days. After 35 days, animals were sacrificed by cervical dislocation in deep anesthesia of CO_2, and primary tumors were surgically removed and weighed. Tumor sizes were evaluated using the formula: length $\times$ width^2 $\times$ 0.52. The primary tumors were analyzed by TUNEL assay, and p-PI3K, p-AKT, PP1, and PP2A proteins were detected by immunohistochemistry. All experimental protocols were reviewed and approved by the Animal Experimentation Ethics Committee of Shanghai University of Traditional Chinese Medicine.

TUNEL Assay

TUNEL assay (a DeadEnd^{TM} Colorimetric TUNEL System kit, Promega Corp.) was performed to detect the apoptosis of the subcutaneous tumors in accordance with the manufacturer's instructions.

Immunohistochemistry (IHC)

Paraffin-embedded tumor tissue samples were selected for IHC. IHC for p-PI3K (ab182651, Abcam), p-AKT (4060, CST), PP1 (sc-7482, Santa Cruz), and PP2A (9780, CST) was carried out using a rabbit monoclonal or polyclonal primary antibody overnight at 4°C, an HRP-conjugated goat anti-rabbit IgG secondary antibody (1: 1,000, ab150077, Abcam) for 1 h at 37°C, and DAB staining solution (ab64238, Abcam) for 10 min at room temperature. The staining results were assessed with a Nikon E80i microscope (Nikon Corp.).

Tissue Immunofluorescence

Dissected tissues were fixed in a mixture of 2% PFA and 20% sucrose solution for 24 h at room temperature and then embedded in Tissue-Tek O.C.T. (Electron Microscopy Sciences). Blocks were frozen in a dry ice and ethanol bath. For immunofluorescence, 6-μm O.C.T. tissue cryosections were stained with antibodies against P-cofilin-1 (3313, CST). Secondary antibodies conjugated to Alexa Fluor 594 (A-11032, 1: 1,000) were used (Life Technologies). Nuclear staining was done with DAPI (40, 6-diamidino-2-phenylindole). Immunofluorescence images were taken with fluorescence microscopy (Zeiss AG, Germany) (Qin et al., 2020).

Statistical Analysis

All data are presented as the mean ± standard error of the mean from at least three independent experiments. A Student's t-test, one-way analysis of variance, and a Tukey's *post hoc* test were performed using GraphPad Prism 8.0 software. $P < 0.05$ was considered as statistically significant difference.

RESULTS

SGC7901R Exosomes Induce a Cisplatin-Resistant Phenotype in SGC7901S Cells

Several studies have demonstrated that chemoresistant tumor cells can release exosomes to chemosensitive tumor cells and transmit drug resistance during tumorigenesis (Kreger et al., 2016; Ning et al., 2017; Bandari et al., 2018). To analyze whether SGC7901R cell-derived exosomes may confer a malignant phenotype on cisplatin-sensitive tumor cells, exosomes from the culture medium of SGC7901R and SGC7901S cells were isolated. Purified exosomes from the cultures exhibited typical cup-shaped morphology by transmission electron microscopy analysis (**Figure 1A**). Using the LM10 nanoparticle characterization system, we detected the size and particle number of the purified exosomes. The mean size of SGC7901R exosomes and SGC7901S exosomes were both between 100 and 200 nm (**Figure 1B**), which corresponded with the reported size of exosomes (Kim et al., 2011). Moreover, the particle numbers for two tumor cell-derived exosomes were both more than 2.0×10^7 particles/ml (**Figure 1B**). No significant difference in exosome quantities extracted from SGC7901R and SGC7901S cells was discovered. Next, the exosome markers were detected by Western blotting. Both of the two tumor cell-derived exosomes showed positive expression of exosome markers, including HSP70, CD63, and CD9 (**Figure 1C**).

To demonstrate that exosomes could be taken up by the recipient cells, CMDil-labeled SGC7901S cells (Red) were incubated with PKH67-labeled exosomes (green) derived from SGC7901R cells. In **Figure 1D**, we showed that PKH67 green fluorescence signals were visible around the nuclei and were also in the cytoplasm of SGC7901S cells following exposure to SGC7901R-derived exosomes. However, the negative control did not exhibit any green fluorescence (data not shown). This suggested the effective uptake of PKH67-labeled exosomes by SGC7901S cells. Subsequently, to investigate whether SGC7901R exosomes were responsible for the spread of chemoresistance, SGC7901S cells were incubated with SGC7901R exosomes for 48 h and then treated with DDP for chemosensitivity analysis. CCK-8 assays revealed that SGC7901R-exosome treatment significantly reduced the chemosensitivity of SGC7901S cells (**Figure 1E**). DDP had significantly lower inhibitory effects on SGC7901 + SGC7901/DDP-exos (IC50 = 3.145 μg/mL), relative to SGC7901 (IC50 = 0.8341 μg/mL) ($p < 0.001$). We used another gastric cancer cell line BGC823 to investigate whether BGC823R exosomes were responsible for the spread of chemoresistance. We detected BGC823R exosome treatment

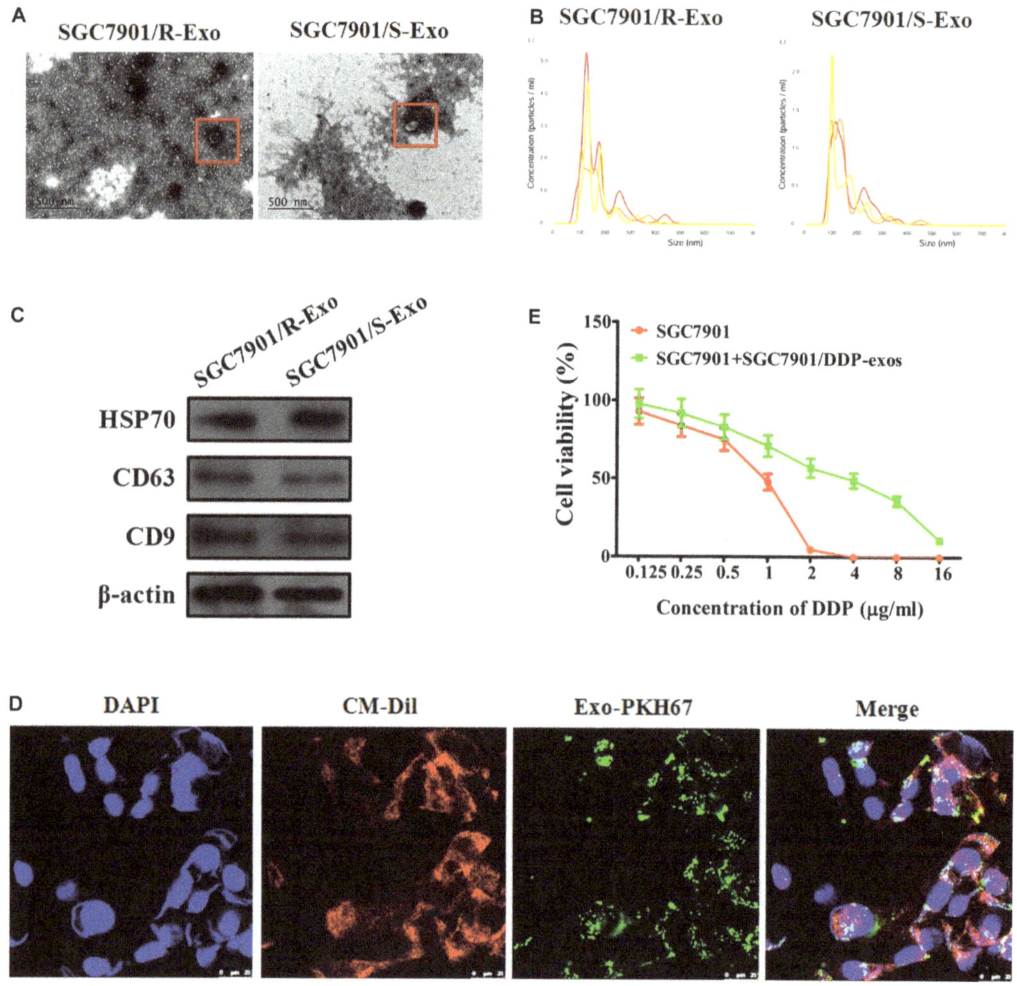

FIGURE 1 | Effect of exosomes derived from SGC7901R cells on the proliferation of SGC7901S cells. **(A)** Exosome isolation from the cell culture medium of SGC7901R and SGC7901S cells was analyzed for the phenotype (purity and shape) by transmission electron microscopy. The red frames indicate the representative exosomes. Scale bar, 500 nm. **(B)** SGC7901R and SGC7901S cells were analyzed for size and particle number by the LM10 nanoparticle characterization system. Representative images were provided. **(C)** Western blotting was performed to detect the exosome markers, including HSP70, CD63, and CD9. β-Actin was used as an internal control. **(D)** Fluorescence imaging showed the delivery of PKH67-labeled exosomes (green) to CM-Dil-labeled SGC7901S cells (red). Cellular nuclei were stained with DAPI. Exosomes were derived from SGC7901R cells. Yellow arrows represented delivered exosomes in the representative images. Scale bar, 25 μm. **(E)** CCK-8 assay was performed to observe the effect of cisplatin (DDP) on the proliferation of indicated cells (SGC7901S cells or SGC7901S cells pretreated with exosomes derived from SGC7901R cells). The concentrations of cisplatin (DDP) used for the drug dose-response curve analysis of indicated cells was 0, 125, 250, 500, 1,000, 2,000, 4,000, 8,000, and 16,000 μg/L. Each experiment was performed in triplicate. All the data are shown as mean ± SD.

significantly reduced the chemosensitivity of BGC823S cells (**Supplementary Figure 4**).

Cisplatin-Resistant Gastric Cancer Cell Line SGC7901R Exhibits Upregulated Levels of RPS3 Protein

Since SGC7901R exosomes can induce the cisplatin-resistant phenotype of SGC7901S cells, it was very necessary to compare the contents in the exosomes of SGC7901R and SGC7901S cells. Although the exosomes contain a variety of kinds of cargo, including DNA, mRNA, miRNA, circRNA, and proteins, here in our study we just consider the protein contents that might play key roles in cisplatin-resistance delivery. By LC-MS/MS analysis methods (**Figure 2A**), we detected the differentially expressed proteins in SGC7901R cell exosomes and SGC7901S cells exosomes. The cluster analysis in **Figure 2B** demonstrated that many differentially expressed proteins were discovered between SGC7901R cell exosomes and SGC7901S cell exosomes. By GO function and KEGG pathway analysis, many important proteins were screened out, including RBP4, RPSA, RPS3, and RPS20 (**Supplementary Figures 1–3**). Next, Western blotting was performed to validate the significant differentially expressed proteins in the exosomes of SGC7901R and SGC7901S cells (**Figures 2C–E**). Considering that the difference was the most significant and acting as an important joint of the PPI network, as well as the preliminary experiments (data not shown), RPS3 was selected as the targets for further research. RPS3 protein level was

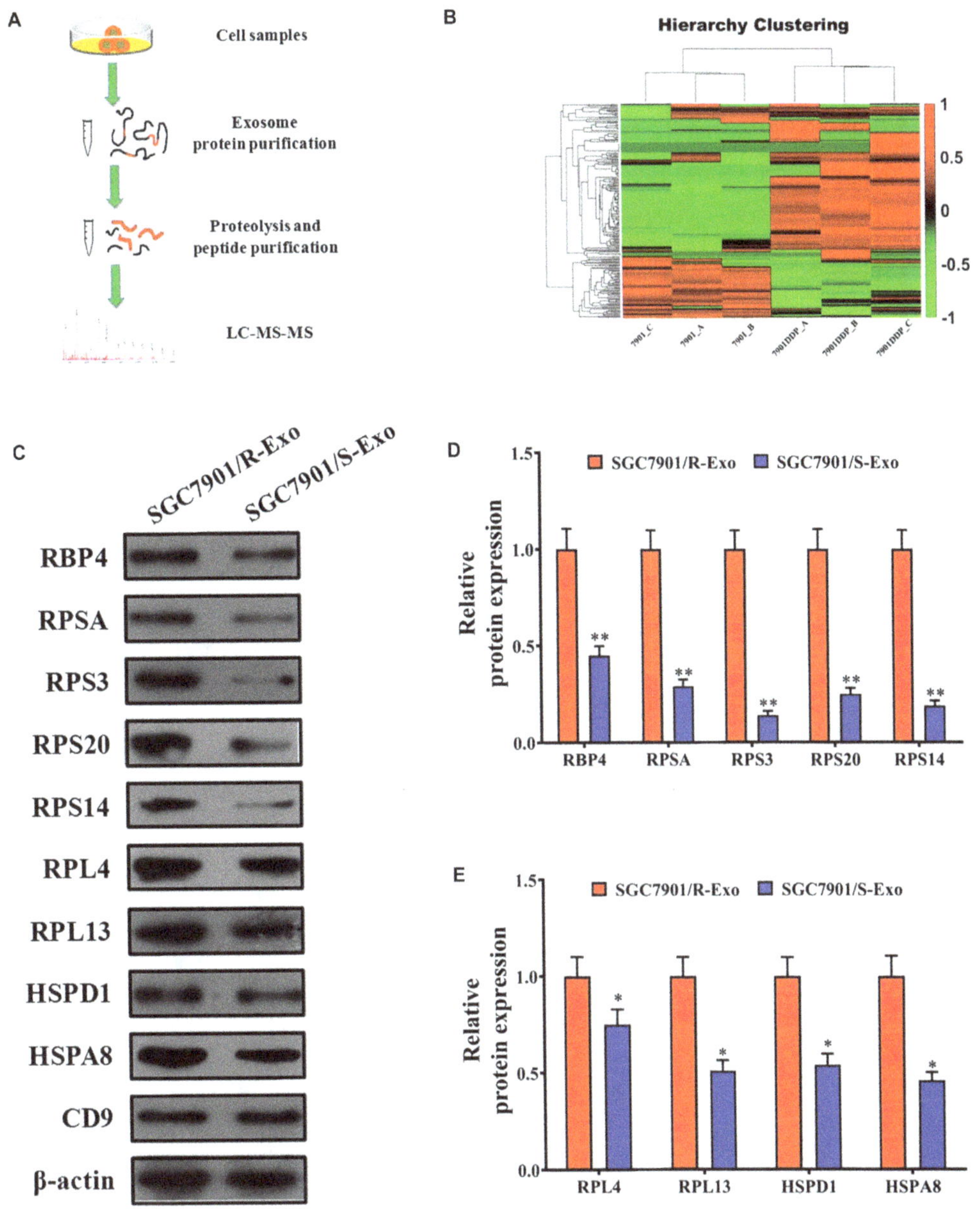

FIGURE 2 | RPS3 was an important differentially expressed protein between SGC7901R cells exosomes and SGC7901S cells exosomes. **(A)** The schematic procedure of searching the differentially expressed proteins between SGC7901R cells exosomes and SGC7901S cell exosomes by LC-MS/MS analysis methods. **(B)** LC-MS/MS and cluster analysis of the differentially expressed proteins between SGC7901R cell exosomes and SGC7901S cell exosomes. Red represents high scores, and green represents low scores. The color brightness of each unit is associated with differences in multiples (log 2[AR/N]). **(C–E)** Western blotting was performed to validate the differentially expressed proteins in the exosomes of SGC7901R and SGC7901S cells. Each experiment was performed in triplicate. All the data are shown as mean ± SD. Student's *t*-test was used to analyze the data. $^{*}P < 0.05$, $^{**}P < 0.01$ vs. SGC7901/R-Exo.

also significantly upregulated in the exosomes of BGC823R cells when compared to BGC823S cells (**Supplementary Figure 5**).

Exosomal Transfer of RPS3 Promotes the Cisplatin Chemoresistance in SGC7901S Cells

To further validate that exosomal RPS3 is involved in the induction of a cisplatin-resistant phenotype, RPS3 was overexpressed or knockdown in SGC7901R cells (**Figures 3A,B**). Then, the exosomes derived from RPS3-overexpressing or -silencing SGC7901R cells were isolated. Western blotting results showed that RPS3 protein was enriched in exosomes derived from RPS3-overexpressing SGC7901R cells but downregulated in exosomes derived from RPS3-silencing SGC7901R cells (**Figures 3C,D**).

To evaluate whether the exosomal transfer of RPS3 promotes the DDP chemoresistance in SGC7901S cells,

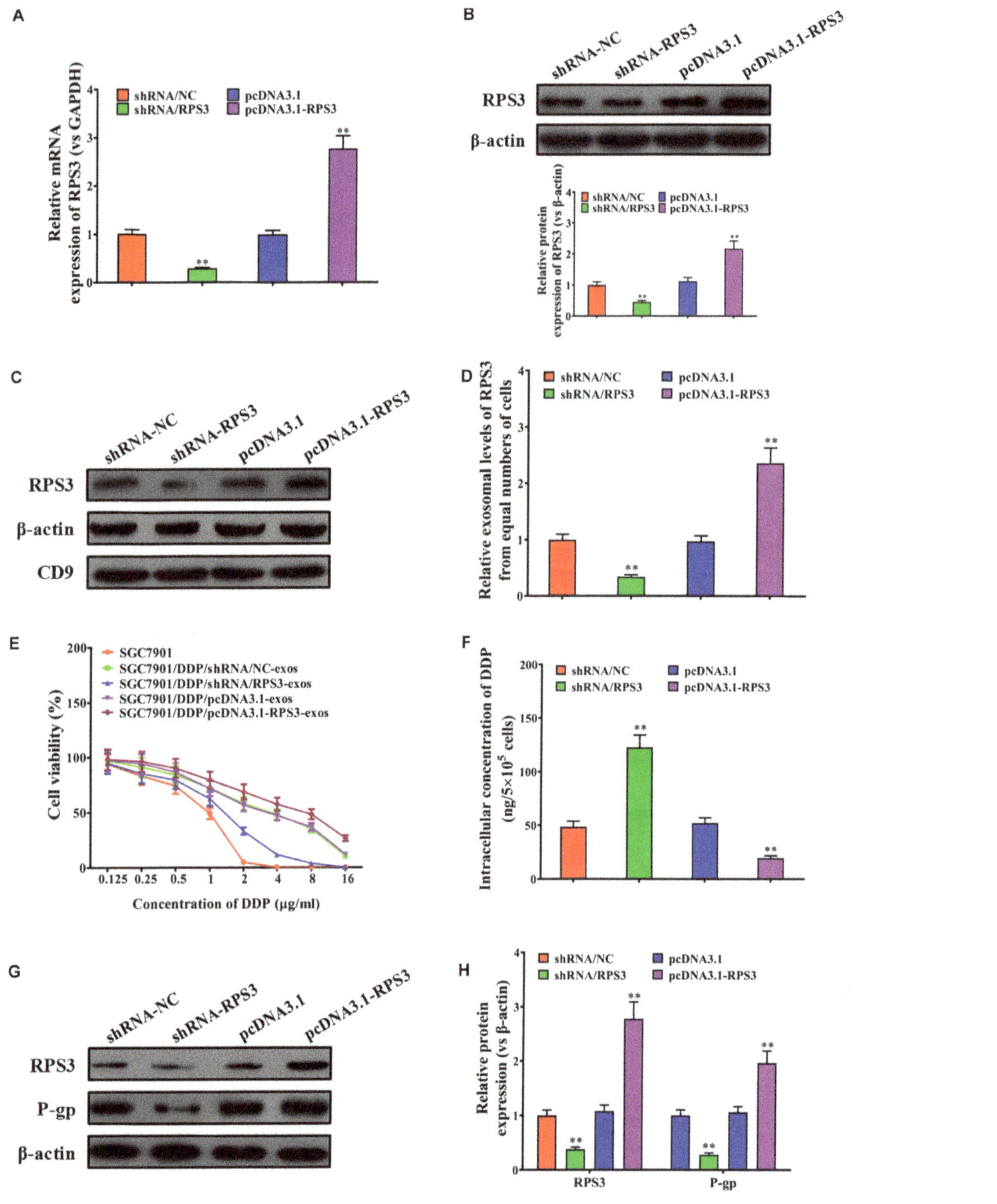

FIGURE 3 | RPS3 overexpression confers DDP-resistant phenotypes from SGC7901R cells to SGC7901S cells. **(A)** RT-qPCR was performed to observe the effect of RPS3 knockdown and overexpression on the mRNA expression of RPS3 in SGC7901R cells. **(B)** Western blotting was performed to observe the effect of RPS3 knockdown and overexpression on the protein expression of RPS3 in SGC7901R cells. **(C,D)** Western blotting and quantitative analysis were performed to observe the effect of RPS3 knockdown and overexpression on the exosomal expression of RPS3 protein in SGC7901R cells. β-Actin was used as cellular control, and CD9 was set as the marker of exosomes. **(E)** CCK-8 assay was performed to observe the effect of cisplatin (DDP) on the proliferation of indicated cells: SGC7901S, SGC7901S + SGC7901R-shRNA/NC-exos, SGC7901S + SGC7901R-shRNA/RPS3-exos, SGC7901S + SGC7901R-pcDNA3.1-exos, SGC7901S + SGC7901R-pcDNA3.1-RPS3-exos. The concentrations of DDP used for the drug dose-response curve analysis of indicated cells were 0, 125, 250, 500, 1,000, 2,000, 4,000, 8,000, and 16,000 μg/L. Each experiment was performed in triplicate. **(F)** ICP-MS analysis was applied to see the effect of exosomes from indicated cells (SGC7901SR-shRNA/NC, SGC7901SR-shRNA/RPS3, SGC7901SR-pcDNA3.1, and SGC7901SR-pcDNA3.1-RPS3) on the DDP concentration in the cellular of SGC7901S cells. **(G,H)** Western blotting and quantitative analysis were performed to observe the effect of exosomes from indicated cells (SGC7901SR-shRNA/NC, SGC7901SR-shRNA/RPS3, SGC7901SR-pcDNA3.1, and SGC7901SR-pcDNA3.1-RPS3) on the P-gp protein expression in SGC7901S cells. β-Actin was used as cellular control. All the data are shown as mean ± SD. Student's *t*-test was used to analyze the data. $^{**}P < 0.01$ vs. SGC7901R-shRNA/NC.

SGC7901S cells were pretreated with exosomes isolated from RPS3-overexpressing or -silencing SGC7901R cells. The results of CCK-8 assay revealed that the proliferation of SGC7901S cells was significantly reduced by RPS3-silencing SGC7901R cell exosome treatment but increased by RPS3-overexpressing SGC7901R cell exosome treatment following incubation with cisplatin (**Figure 3E**). Then, using ICP-MS for determination of the changed intracellular cisplatin concentration in SGC-7901S cells, we found that, when 6.73 μg/mL cisplatin exposed to above cells for 48 h, the intracellular accumulation of cisplatin increased in SGC7901S cells pretreated with RPS3-silencing SGC7901R cell exosomes but reduced in SGC7901S cells pretreated with RPS3-overexpressing SGC7901R cell exosomes compared with the control exosomes (**Figure 3F**). In addition, RPS3 and P-gp were both reduced in SGC7901S cells pretreated with RPS3-silencing SGC7901R cell exosomes but increased in SGC7901S cells pretreated with RPS3-overexpressing SGC7901R cell exosomes (**Figures 3G,H**). These results indicated that exosomal transfer of RPS3 protein may be involved in the induction of a cisplatin-resistant phenotype.

RPS3-Rich Exosomes From SGC7901R Cells Decreased the Apoptosis of SGC7901S Cells Induced by Cisplatin via Affecting the Mitochondrial Translocation of Cofilin-1

Flow cytometry was performed to see the effect of exosomes derived from RPS3-overexpressing or -silencing SGC7901R cells on the cell cycle and apoptosis of SGC-7901S cells following incubation with cisplatin. The results showed that pretreatment of exosomes derived from RPS3-silencing SGC7901R cells led to the reduction of SGC-7901S cells in G2/M phages compared with the control exosomes, while the exosomes derived from RPS3-overexpressing SGC7901R cells did the opposite effect (**Figures 4A,B**). In addition, pretreatment of exosomes derived from RPS3-silencing SGC7901R cells increased cisplatin-induced cell apoptosis of SGC-7901S cells compared with the control exosomes, while the exosomes derived from RPS3-overexpressing SGC7901R cells did the opposite effect (**Figures 4C,D**). Exosomes derived from RPS3-silencing BGC823R cells also induced cisplatin-related cell apoptosis in BGC823S cells compared with the control exosomes (**Supplementary Figure 6**). Furthermore, by Western blotting analysis, we showed that RPS3-rich exosomes from RPS3-overexpressing SGC7901R cells reduced the mitochondrial translocation of cofilin-1 in SGC-7901S cells compared with the control exosomes, while RPS3-reduced exosomes from RPS3-silencing SGC7901R cells did the opposite effect (**Figures 4E–H**). Immunofluorescence analysis also demonstrated that RPS3-rich exosomes from RPS3-overexpressing SGC7901R cells inhibited the translocation of cofilin-1 into the mitochondria (**Supplementary Figure 8**). These data implied that RPS3-rich exosomes from SGC7901R cells decreased the apoptosis of SGC7901S cells induced by cisplatin via affecting the mitochondrial translocation of cofilin-1.

Overexpression of RPS3 Directly in SGC7901S Cells Exhibits Similar Effects to Treatment With SGC7901R Exosomes

Our above data suggested that RPS3 expression levels were significantly elevated in SGC7901R cells, and SGC7901R-exosome treatment was proposed to confer cisplatin-resistant phenotypes to SGC7901S cells. To further investigate the role of RPS3 in the regulation of cisplatin chemoresistance, RPS3 was directly overexpressed or knockdown in SGC7901S cells. RT-qPCR and Western blotting analysis demonstrated that RPS3 was successfully overexpressed or knockdown in RPS3-overexpressing or -silencing SGC7901S cells (**Figures 5A,B**). Next, the CCK-8 assay revealed that the proliferation of SGC7901S cells was significantly reduced by RPS3 silencing but increased by RPS3 overexpressing following incubation with cisplatin compared with the controls (**Figure 5C**). Then, the ICP-MS analysis demonstrated that, when 6.73 μg/mL cisplatin was exposed to the above cells for 48 h, the intracellular accumulation of cisplatin increased in RPS3-silencing SGC7901S cells but reduced in RPS3-overexpressing SGC7901S cells compared with their controls (**Figure 5D**). Subsequently, we detected the protein expression of P-gp in RPS3-overexpressing or -silencing SGC7901R cells; the results showed that P-gp was reduced in RPS3-silencing SGC7901S cells but increased in RPS3-overexpressing SGC7901S cells compared with their controls (**Figures 5E,F**). These results indicated that overexpression of RPS3 directly in SGC7901S cells also exhibits similar effects to treatment with SGC7901R exosomes.

Next, flow cytometry results showed that knockdown of RPS3 directly in SGC7901S cells led to the reduction of SGC-7901S cells in G2/M phages, while the overexpression of RPS3 directly in SGC7901S cells did the opposite effect (**Figure 5G**). In addition, knockdown of RPS3 directly in SGC7901S cells increased cisplatin-induced cell apoptosis of SGC-7901S cells, while the overexpression of RPS3 in SGC7901S cells did the opposite effect (**Figure 5H**). Furthermore, RPS3-overexpressing SGC7901S cells reduced the mitochondrial translocation of cofilin-1, while RPS3-silencing SGC7901S cells did the opposite effect (**Figure 5J**). Additionally, we also found that RPS3-overexpressing SGC7901S cells reduced the expression of PP1 and PP2A and increased the expression of p-PI3K and p-Akt, while RPS3-silencing SGC7901S cells did the opposite effect (**Figures 5I,J**); these results were consistent with that in BGC823S cells (**Supplementary Figure 7**). These data suggested that RPS3 overexpression directly in SGC7901S cells decreased the apoptosis of SGC7901S cells induced by cisplatin via affecting the mitochondrial translocation of cofilin-1 and the expression of PP1 and PP2A, which were closely associated with PI3K-Akt signaling pathway. LY294002 was then used to inhibit the PI3K-Akt signaling pathway of SGC7901S cells. Western blotting analysis indicated that the RPS3 overexpression significantly inhibited cofilin-1(M) expression in SGC7901S. However, the levels of cofilin-1(M) did not noticeably change in LY294002-treated RPS3-overexpressed SGC7901S cells (**Supplementary Figure 9**), suggesting that RPS3

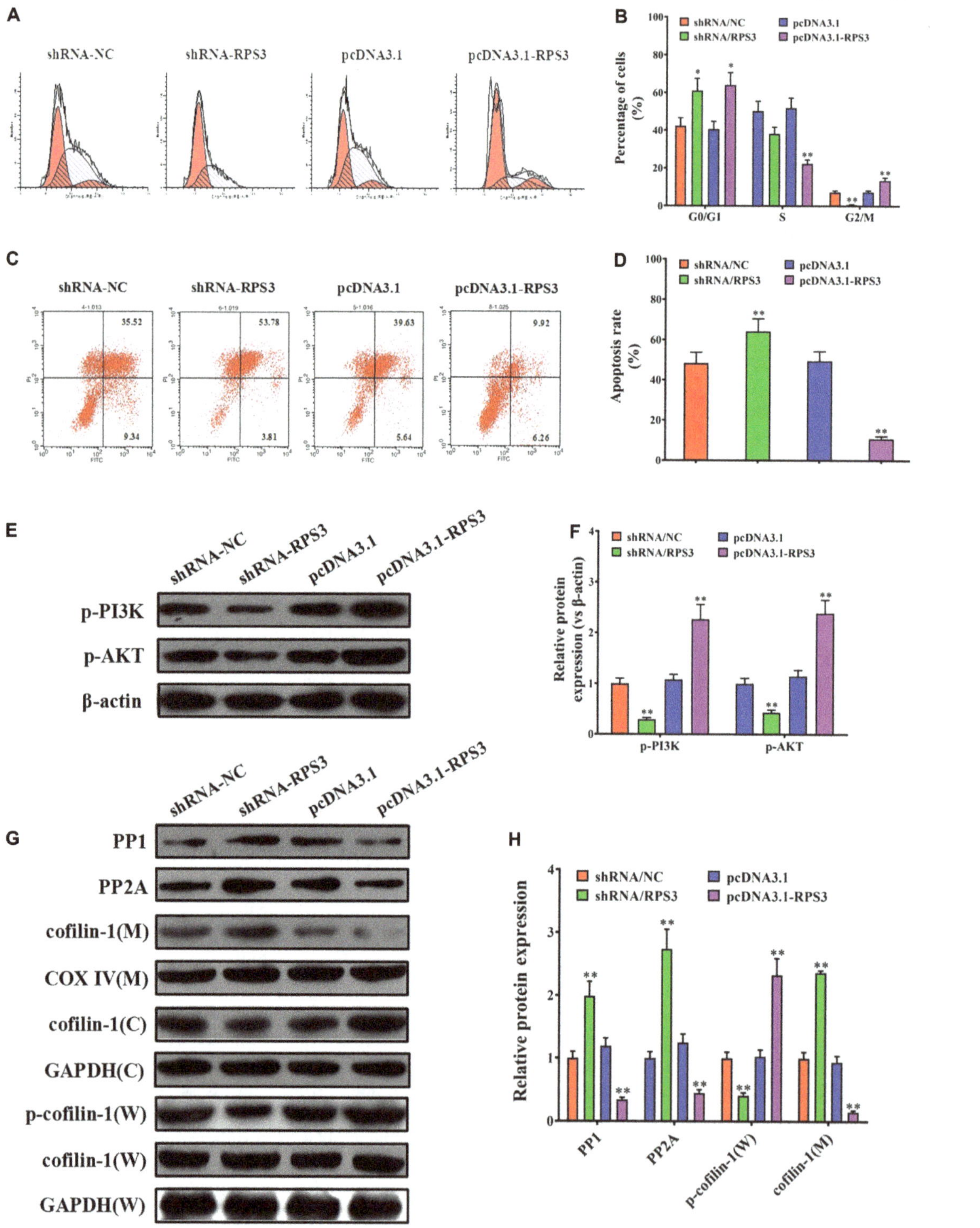

FIGURE 4 | RPS3-rich exosomes from SGC7901R inhibited the apoptosis of SGC7901S via mitochondrial translocation of p-cofilin-1. **(A,B)** Flow cytometry method and quantitative assay were performed to observe the shift of cell cycles in SGC7901S cells treated with exosomes derived from RPS3-overexpressing or -silencing SGC7901R cells, or their respective controls. **(C,D)** Flow cytometry method and quantitative assay were performed to observe the change of cell apoptosis in SGC7901S cells treated with exosomes derived from RPS3-overexpressing or -silencing SGC7901R cells, or their respective controls. **(E–H)** Whole-cell lysates and mitochondrial and cytosolic proteins were prepared for the detection of p-PI3K, p-AKT, PP1, PP2A, p-cofilin-1, and cofilin-1 in the SGC7901S cells treated with exosomes derived from RPS3-overexpressing or -silencing SGC7901R cells, or their respective controls using western blotting. The levels of each protein were normalized against those of GAPDH (total and cytosolic proteins) or COXIV (mitochondrial proteins). Each experiment was performed at least in triplicate and all the data are shown as mean ± SD. Student's *t*-test was used to analyze the data. $^{*}P < 0.05$, $^{**}P < 0.01$.

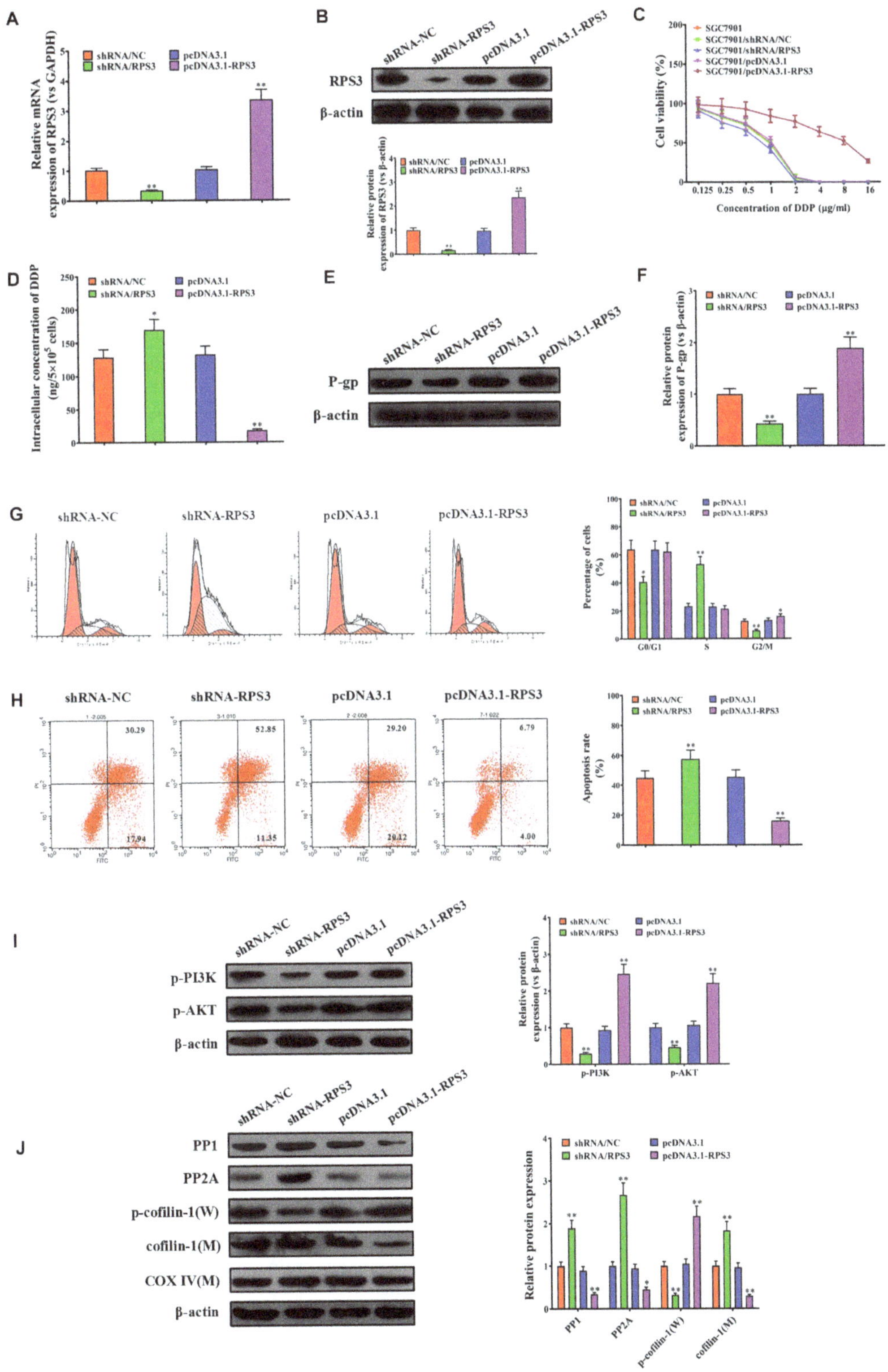

FIGURE 5 | RPS3 overexpression directly in SGC7901S cells increases the DDP resistance of SGC7901S cells. **(A)** RT-qPCR was performed to observe the effect of RPS3 knockdown and overexpression on the mRNA expression of RPS3 in SGC7901S cells. **(B)** Western blotting was performed to observe the effect of RPS3 knockdown and overexpression on the protein expression of RPS3 in SGC7901S cells. **(C)** CCK-8 assay was performed to observe the effect of cisplatin (DDP) on the proliferation of indicated cells: SGC7901S, SGC7901S-shRNA/NC, SGC7901S + SGC7901S-shRNA/RPS3, SGC7901S-pcDNA3.1, and SGC7901S-pcDNA3.1-RPS3. The concentrations of DDP used for the drug dose-response curve analysis of indicated cells were 0, 125, 250, 500, 1,000, 2,000, 4,000, 8,000,

(Continued)

FIGURE 5 | Continued
and 16,000 μg/L. Each experiment was performed in triplicate. **(D)** ICP-MS analysis was applied to investigate the effect of RPS3 knockdown and overexpression on the DDP concentration in the cellular of SGC7901S cells. **(E,F)** Western blotting and quantitative analysis were performed to observe the effect of RPS3 knockdown and overexpression on the P-gp protein expression in SGC7901S cells. β-Actin was used as cellular control. **(G)** Flow cytometry and quantitative assay were performed to observe the shift of cell cycles in SGC7901S cells treated with RPS3-overexpressing or -silencing, or their respective controls. **(H)** Flow cytometry and quantitative assay were performed to observe the change of cell apoptosis in SGC7901S cells treated with RPS3-overexpressing or -silencing, or their respective controls. **(I,J)** Western blotting and quantitative assays of p-PI3K, p-AKT, PP1, PP2A, p-cofilin-1, and cofilin-1 proteins in the SGC7901S cells treated with RPS3-overexpressing or -silencing, or their respective controls. The level of each protein was normalized against those of β-actin (total proteins) or COXIV (mitochondrial proteins). Each experiment was performed at least in triplicate, and all the data are shown as mean ± SD. Student's *t*-test was used to analyze the data. $^{*}P < 0.05$, $^{**}P < 0.01$.

enhances the chemotherapy resistance of cells through the PI3K-AKt signaling pathway.

Impact of RPS3-Rich Exosomes From SGC7901R Cells on the Growth of Subcutaneous Xenograft of SGC-7901S Cells in Nude Mice

To explore whether RPS3-rich exosomes from SGC7901R cells inhibited the pro-apoptotic effect of cisplatin *in vivo*, we employed a subcutaneous xenograft of SGC7901 cells in nude mouse models. As shown in **Figure 6A**, pretreatment of exosomes derived from RPS3-overexpressing SGC7901R cells reduced the inhibitory effect of cisplatin on the tumor growth in compared with cisplatin (0.6 mg/kg) alone, while the pretreatment of exosomes derived from RPS3-silencing SGC7901R cells did the opposite effect (**Figure 6A**). The final tumor resection and weight calculation also showed that pretreatment of exosomes derived from RPS3-overexpressing SGC7901R cells following incubation with cisplatin showed the highest tumor weight compared with cisplatin alone, while the pretreatment of exosomes derived from RPS3-silencing SGC7901R cells following incubation with cisplatin did the opposite effect (**Figures 6B,C**). Next, ICP-MS analysis was applied to investigate the cisplatin concentration in the subcutaneous xenograft of SGC7901S cells with indicated treatments. The results showed that pretreatment of exosomes derived from RPS3-overexpressing SGC7901R cells following incubation with cisplatin showed the highest levels of cisplatin concentration in the xenograft tumor compared with cisplatin alone, while the pretreatment of exosomes derived from RPS3-silencing SGC7901R cells following incubation with cisplatin did the opposite effect (**Figure 6D**).

In **Figure 6E**, pretreatment of exosomes derived from RPS3-overexpressing SGC7901R cells following incubation with DDP showed the least apoptotic tumor cells in the xenograft tumor compared with DDP alone, while the pretreatment of exosomes derived from RPS3-silencing SGC7901R cells following incubation with DDP did the opposite effect. Additionally, we detected the expression of p-PI3K, p-Akt, PP1, and PP2A in the xenograft tumor tissues by immunohistochemistry (IHC). The IHC images demonstrated that pretreatment of exosomes derived from RPS3-overexpressing SGC7901R cells following incubation with DDP showed the highest expression levels of p-PI3K and p-AKT and the lowest expression levels of PP1 and PP2A in the xenograft tumor compared with DDP alone, while the pretreatment of exosomes derived from RPS3-silencing SGC7901R cells following incubation with DDP did the opposite effect (**Figure 6F**). Finally, we detected the p-cofilin-1 expression by immunofluorescence in the subcutaneous xenograft of SGC7901S cells with indicated treatments. The results showed that pretreatment of exosomes derived from RPS3-overexpressing SGC7901R cells following incubation with DDP showed the highest expression levels of p-cofilin-1 in the xenograft tumor compared with DDP alone, while the pretreatment of exosomes derived from RPS3-silencing SGC7901R cells following incubation with DDP did the opposite effect (**Figure 6G**).

All the above data suggested that RPS3-rich exosomes from SGC7901R cells blocked the inhibitory effect of DDP on the growth of subcutaneous xenograft in nude mice by enhancing the cisplatin chemoresistance in SGC7901S cells.

DISCUSSION

Cisplatin has been widely used in tumor therapy, but the development of chemoresistance is often observed in patients with tumors (Guo et al., 2015; Zhang and Fan, 2017). At present, cisplatin resistance in tumors has been reported to be associated with underlying mechanisms, including increased drug efflux, alteration of intercellular signaling, tubulin mutation, and overexpression of β-tubulin isotype composition (Kavallaris, 2010; Vergara et al., 2012). Recently, it has been demonstrated that drug-resistant cancer cells could transmit chemoresistant phenotypes to chemosensitive cancer cells via exosomes (Sharma, 2017). Whether the acquisition of cisplatin resistance by gastric cancer cells occurs in this way remains unknown.

Among the main components in exosomal cargo, some molecules have been discovered acting as the vital regulating effect on chemoresistance (Cui et al., 2013; Soldevilla et al., 2014; Liu et al., 2016; Zeng et al., 2017). Exosomal miRNAs, lncRNAs, mRNA, and proteins could be shuttled from chemoresistant to chemosensitive cancer cells to transmit chemoresistance. For example, exosomal miR-222-3p from the gemcitabine-resistant lung cancer line A549 enhanced gemcitabine resistance in parental sensitive cells (Wei et al., 2017). Qu et al. (2016) identify lncARSR as a mediator of sunitinib resistance in renal cell carcinoma by acting as a competing endogenous RNA for miR-34 and miR-449, thereby increasing the expression of their targets AXL and c-MET. Exosomes from glioblastoma cancer cells harboring a protein tyrosine phosphatase receptor type Z1-MET fusion conferred temozolomide resistance on parental cells

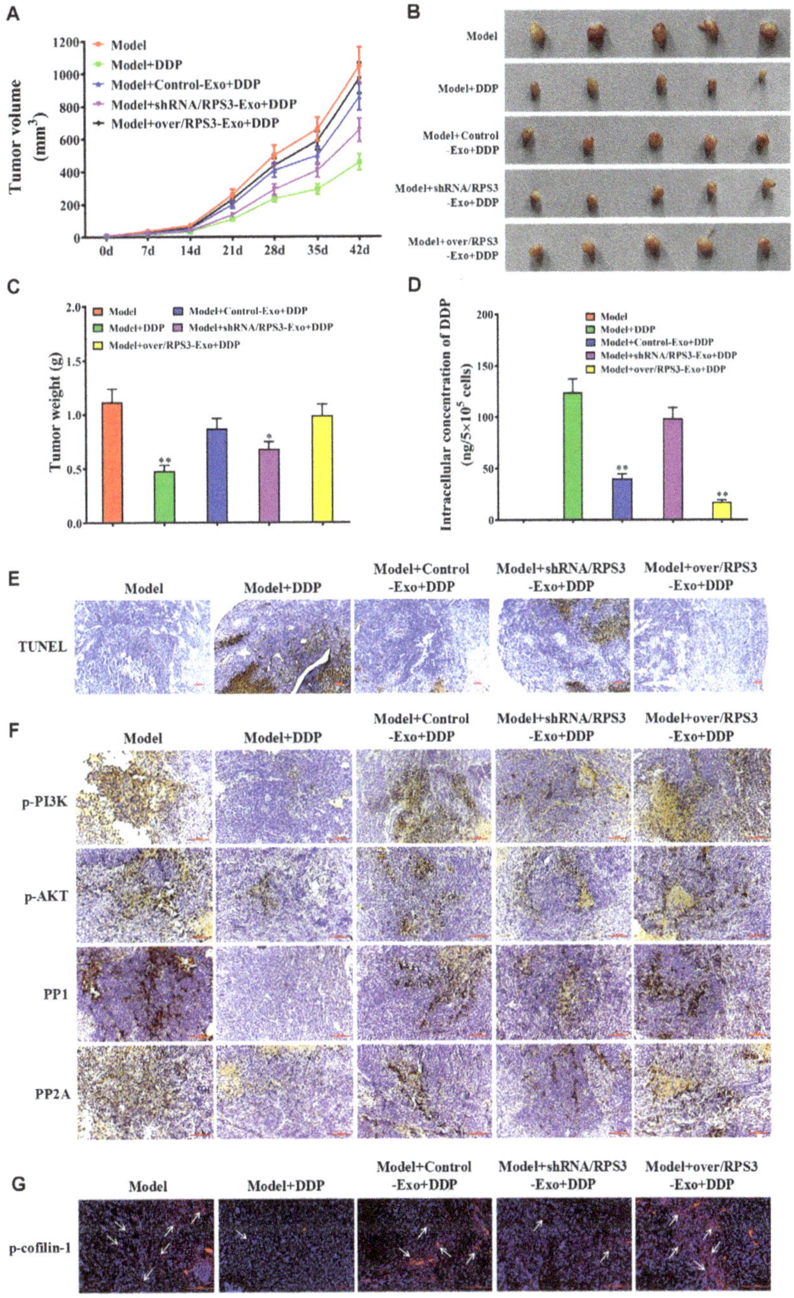

FIGURE 6 | Impact of RPS3-rich exosomes from SGC7901R on the growth of subcutaneous xenograft of SGC-7901S. **(A)** Xenografts of SGC-7901S cells with indicated treatments performed on nude mice. SGC-7901S cells were pretreated with exosomes from RPS3-overexpressing or -silencing SGC-7901R cells, or control SGC-7901R cells. The length and width of the subcutaneous tumors were measured every 7 days. **(B,C)** Tumors were surgically removed from nude mice and weighed after administration for 35 days. $^*P < 0.05$, $^{**}P < 0.01$, in contrast to model groups treated with DDP alone. **(D)** ICP-MS analysis was applied to investigate the DDP concentration in the subcutaneous xenograft of SGC7901S cells with indicated treatments. **(E)** TUNEL assay was performed to observe the apoptosis of tumor cells in the subcutaneous xenograft of SGC7901S cells with indicated treatments. Scale bar, 100 μm. **(F)** The xenograft tumor tissues in mice of all groups were subjected to immunohistochemistry analysis using the antibody of p-PI3K, p-AKT, PP1, and PP2A. Scale bar, 100 μm. **(G)** Immunofluorescence detection of the expression of p-cofilin-1 in the subcutaneous xenograft of SGC7901S cells with indicated treatments. Scale bar, 100 μm. Each experiment was performed at least in triplicate and all the data are shown as mean ± SD. Student's *t*-test was used to analyze the data. $^*P < 0.05$, $^{**}P < 0.01$.

(Zeng et al., 2017). These findings demonstrated that exosomes could transfer intercellular drug resistance from drug-resistant to drug-sensitive cancer cells.

To investigate the mechanism of cisplatin resistance in gastric cancer cells, the cisplatin-resistant gastric cancer cell line SGC7901R was established in the present study. SGC7901R cell-derived exosomes could be effectively taken up by cisplatin-sensitive SGC7901S cells, and the receptor cells exhibited remarkably chemoresistance phenotypes. Consistently, it was demonstrated that SGC7901R-derived exosomes conferred a cisplatin-resistant phenotype in SGC7901S cells. Presently, a large number of differentially expressed molecules in the exosomes are discovered by RNA sequencing or proteomics, many of which are potentially associated with chemoresistance; however, quite a lot of them are little investigated.

In this study, cisplatin-resistant gastric cancer cell line SGC7901R was determined by LC-MS/MS with increased exosomal levels of RPS3 protein. RPS3, a component of the 40S ribosomal small subunit, is mainly involved in ribosomal maturation and initiation of translation (Schafer et al., 2006). RPS3 has various extra-ribosomal functions, including cell signaling (Kim et al., 2011), transcriptional regulation (Wan et al., 2007), and DNA repair (Kim et al., 2013). In addition, both upregulation and intrinsic dysfunctions in ribosomes result in an increased incidence of tumors, and RPS3 is involved in radioresistance or invasion of tumor cells (Kim et al., 2007; Kool et al., 2008). Huang et al. (2019) showed that Vitamin D promotes the cisplatin sensitivity of oral squamous cell carcinoma by inhibiting LCN2-modulated NF-κB pathway activation through RPS3. Zhao et al. (2019) unveiled a novel extra-ribosomal role of RPS3 in facilitating hepatocarcinogenesis via the posttranscriptional regulation of SIRT1 expression and proposes that the RPS3/SIRT1 pathway serves as a potential therapeutic target in HCC. A previous study showed that RPS3 was secreted into the extracellular environment in a dimeric form. All the reported data suggested that RPS3 may be a putative marker for malignant tumors.

Our data demonstrated that RPS3 protein was enriched in SGC7901R exosomes and could be delivered into SGC7901S cells. Overexpression of RPS3 directly in SGC7901S cells can also result in similar phenotypic effects as treatment with SGC7901R exosomes, which are then capable of inducing the malignant phenotype in the sensitive cells. A further mechanism study demonstrated that cisplatin-resistant gastric cancer cell-derived exosomal RPS3 could enhance the chemoresistance through the PI3K/Akt-mediated mitochondrial translocation of cofilin-1. The suppression of PI3K/Akt (LY294002) dramatically attenuated RPS3-induced DDP resistance and cofilin-1 mitochondrial translocation in GC. Cofilin-1, a 19-kDa ubiquitous actin-modulating protein, exists in two states, activated (cofilin-1) and inactivated (p-cofilin-1) (Vartiainen et al., 2002). The de-phosphorylation of p-cofilin-1 can induce degradation of F-actin to G-actin and promote the translocation of cofilin-1 to the mitochondria, triggering mitochondrial apoptosis (Tang et al., 2016). Many studies demonstrated that high-expression levels of cofilin-1 in many cancers correlated with tumor metastasis, chemotherapy resistance, and poor prognosis (Zhang Y. et al., 2015; Wang et al., 2019). In our previous studies, we have demonstrated that activation of PI3K/Akt can reduce the expression of the phosphoric acid lipases, PP1, PP2A, and SSH, then activate the de-phosphorylation of p-cofilin-1 and mitochondrial translocation of cofilin-1 and finally activate mitochondrial damage and induce the mitochondrial apoptosis of cisplatin-resistant gastric cancer cells (Tang et al., 2016). Previous studies demonstrated that changes in cofilin-1 or p-cofilin-1 patterns played an important role in multidrug resistance in tumor cells (Zhang et al., 2012; Li et al., 2013). All the findings demonstrated that cisplatin-resistant gastric cancer cells communicate with sensitive cells through the delivery key exosomal protein RPS3 and the activation of PI3K-Akt-cofilin-1 signaling pathway.

CONCLUSION

In summary, our present study demonstrated that RPS3 protein expression levels were significantly elevated in SGC7901R cells, which was selectively sorted into SGC7901R cell-derived exosomes. Exosomal delivery of RPS3 protein may induce chemoresistance phenotypes from cisplatin-resistant gastric cancer cells to sensitive cancer cells by regulating the PI3K-Akt-cofilin-1 signaling pathway. Therefore, exosomal RPS3 protein in cisplatin-resistant gastric cancer cells may thus be a promising strategy to overcome cisplatin resistance in gastric cancer.

ETHICS STATEMENT

The animal study was reviewed and approved by Animal Experimentation Ethics Committee of Shanghai University of Traditional Chinese Medicine.

AUTHOR CONTRIBUTIONS

Q-FT, HZ, and SC were responsible for designing the experiments and research supervision. M-YS, BX, and Q-XW were responsible for conducting experiments, acquisition of data, and analysis. SC and W-LC carried out the statistical analysis. M-YS and Q-XW wrote the manuscript. All authors reviewed and approved the final version.

ACKNOWLEDGMENTS

We thank Professor Ming Guan from Department of Clinical Laboratory and Central Laboratory, Huashan Hospital, Shanghai Medical School, Fudan University.

REFERENCES

Antunes, A. T., Goos, Y. J., Pereboom, T. C., Hermkens, D., Wlodarski, M. W., Costa, L. D., et al. (2015). Ribosomal protein mutations result in constitutive p53 protein degradation through impairment of the AKT pathway. *PLoS Genet.* 11:e1005326. doi: 10.1371/journal.pgen.1005326

Bandari, S. K., Purushothaman, A., Ramani, V. C., Brinkley, G. J., Chandrashekar, D. S., Varambally, S., et al. (2018). Chemotherapy induces secretion of exosomes loaded with heparanase that degrades extracellular matrix and impacts tumor and host cell behavior. *Matrix Biol.* 65, 104–118. doi: 10.1016/j.matbio.2017.09.001

Bray, F., Ferlay, J., Soerjomataram, I., Siegel, R. L., Torre, L. A., and Jemal, A. (2018). Global cancer statistics 2018: GLOBOCAN estimates of incidence and mortality worldwide for 36 cancers in 185 countries. *CA Cancer J. Clin.* 68, 394–424. doi: 10.3322/caac.21492

Brinton, L. T., Sloane, H. S., Kester, M., and Kelly, K. A. (2015). Formation and role of exosomes in cancer. *Cell Mol. Life Sci.* 72, 659–671. doi: 10.1007/s00018-014-1764-3

Butera, G., Pacchiana, R., and Donadelli, M. (2018). Autocrine mechanisms of cancer chemoresistance. *Semin. Cell Dev. Biol.* 78, 3–12. doi: 10.1016/j.semcdb.2017.07.019

Colombo, M., Raposo, G., and Théry, C. (2014). Biogenesis, secretion, and intercellular interactions of exosomes and other extracellular vesicles. *Annu. Rev. Cell Dev Biol.* 30, 255–289. doi: 10.1146/annurev-cellbio-101512-122326

Cui, S. Y., Wang, R., and Chen, L. B. (2013). MicroRNAs: key players of taxane resistance and their therapeutic potential in human cancers. *J. Cell Mol. Med.* 17, 1207–1217. doi: 10.1111/jcmm.12131

Guo, Z. Q., Wang, X. J., Lin, R. B., Chen, L., Fan, N. F., Chen, Y., et al. (2015). Paclitaxel-based regimens as first-line treatment in advanced gastric cancer. *J. Chemother.* 27, 94–98. doi: 10.1179/1973947814Y.0000000169

Huang, Z. X., Zhang, Y., Li, H. G., Zhou, Y. F., and Huang, Z. Q. (2019). Vitamin D promotes the cisplatin sensitivity of oral squamous cell carcinoma by inhibiting LCN2-modulated NF-κB pathway activation through RPS3. *Cell Death Dis.* 10:936. doi: 10.1038/s41419-020-2389-0

Kavallaris, M. (2010). Microtubules and resistance to tubulin-binding agents. *Nat. Rev. Cancer* 10, 194–204. doi: 10.1038/nrc2803

Kawahata, T., Kawahara, K., Shimokawa, M., Sakiyama, A., Shiraishi, T., Minami, K., et al. (2020). Involvement of ribosomal protein L11 expression in sensitivity of gastric cancer against 5-FU. *Oncol. Lett.* 19, 2258–2264. doi: 10.3892/ol.2020.11352

Kim, H. D., Kim, T. S., and Kim, J. (2011). Aberrant ribosome biogenesis activates c-Myc and ASK1 pathways resulting in p53-dependent G1 arrest. *Oncogene* 30, 3317–3327. doi: 10.1038/onc.2011.47

Kim, Y., Kim, H. D., and Kim, J. (2013). Cytoplasmic ribosomal protein S3 (rpS3) plays a pivotal role in mitochondrial DNA damage surveillance. *Biochim. Biophys. Acta* 1833, 2943–2952. doi: 10.1016/j.bbamcr.2013.07.015

Kim, Y., Yoon, J. W., Xiao, X., Dean, N. M., Monia, B. P., and Marcusson, E. G. (2007). Selective down-regulation of glioma-associated oncogene 2 inhibits the proliferation of hepatocellular carcinoma cells. *Cancer Res.* 67, 3583–3593. doi: 10.1158/0008-5472.CAN-06-3040

Kool, M., Koster, J., Bunt, J., Hasselt, N. E., Lakeman, A., Van, S. P., et al. (2008). Integrated genomics identifies five medulloblastoma subtypes with distinct genetic profiles, pathway signatures and clinicopathological features. *PLoS One* 3:e3088. doi: 10.1371/journal.pone.0003088

Kreger, B. T., Johansen, E. R., Cerione, R. A., and Antonyak, M. A. (2016). The enrichment of survivin in exosomes from breast cancer cells treated with cisplatin promotes cell survival and chemoresistance. *Cancers* 8:111. doi: 10.3390/cancers8120111

Lavilla, I., Costas, M., Miguel, P. S., Millos, J., and Bendicho, C. (2009). Elemental fingerprinting of tumorous and adjacent non-tumorous tissues from patients with colorectal cancer using ICP-MS, ICP-OES and chemometric analysis. *Biometals* 22, 863–875. doi: 10.1007/s10534-009-9231-6

Li, M., Yin, J., Mao, N., and Pan, L. (2013). Upregulation of phosphorylated cofilin 1 correlates with taxol resistance in human ovarian cancer in vitro and in vivo. *Oncol. Rep.* 29, 58–66. doi: 10.3892/or.2012.2078

Liu, C. C., He, X. G., Liu, X. W., Yu, J., Zhang, M., Yu, F. D., et al. (2019). RPS15A promotes gastric cancer progression via activation of the Akt/IKK-β/NF-κB signalling pathway. *J Cell. Mol. Med.* 23, 2207–2218. doi: 10.1111/jcmm.14141

Liu, X., Fu, Q., Du, Y., Yang, Y., and Cho, W. C. (2016). MicroRNA as regulators of cancer stem cells and chemoresistance in colorectal cancer. *Curr. Cancer Drug Targets* 16, 738–754. doi: 10.2174/1568009616666151118114759

Livak, K. J., and Schmittgen, T. D. (2001). Analysis of relative gene expression data using real-time quantitative PCR and the 2(-Delta Delta C(T)) method. *Methods* 25, 402–408. doi: 10.1006/meth.2001.1262

Meehan, K., and Vella, L. J. (2016). The contribution of tumour-derived exosomes to the hallmarks of cancer. *Crit. Rev. Clin. Lab. Sci.* 53, 121–131. doi: 10.3109/10408363.2015.1092496

Ning, K., Wang, T., Sun, X., Zhang, P. F., Chen, Y., Jin, J., et al. (2017). UCH-L1-containing exosomes mediate chemotherapeutic resistance transfer in breast cancer. *J. Surg. Oncol.* 115, 932–940. doi: 10.1002/jso.24614

Qin, Z., Wang, P. Y., Wan, J. J., Zhang, Y., Wei, J., Sun, Y., et al. (2020). MicroRNA124-IL6R mediates the effect of nicotine in inflammatory bowel disease by shifting Th1/Th2 balance toward Th1. *Front. Immunol.* 11:235. doi: 10.3389/fimmu.2020.00235

Qu, L., Ding, J., Chen, C., Wu, Z. J., Liu, B., Gao, Y., et al. (2016). Exosome-transmitted lncARSR promotes sunitinib resistance in renal cancer by acting as a competing endogenous RNA. *Cancer Cell.* 29, 653–668. doi: 10.1016/j.ccell.2016.03.004

Ruivo, C. F., Adem, B., Silva, M., and Melo, S. A. (2017). The biology of cancer exosomes: insights and new perspectives. *Cancer Res.* 77, 6480–6488. doi: 10.1158/0008-5472.CAN-17-0994

Schafer, T., Maco, B., Petfalski, E., Tollervey, D., Battcher, B., Aebi, U., et al. (2006). Hrr25-dependent phosphorylation state regulates organization of the pre-40S subunit. *Nature* 441, 651–655. doi: 10.1038/nature04840

Sharma, A. (2017). Chemoresistance in cancer cells: exosomes as potential regulators of therapeutic tumor heterogeneity. *Nanomedicine* 12, 2137–2148. doi: 10.2217/nnm-2017-0184

Soldevilla, B., Rodriguez, M., San, M. C., Garcia, V., Fernandez, P. R., Gil, C. B., et al. (2014). Tumor-derived exosomes are enriched in ΔNp73, which promotes oncogenic potential in acceptor cells and correlates with patient survival. *Hum. Mol. Genet.* 23, 467–478. doi: 10.1093/hmg/ddt437

Sousa, D., Lima, R. T., and Vasconcelos, M. H. (2015). Intercellular transfer of cancer drug resistance traits by extracellular vesicles. *Trends Mol. Med.* 21, 595–608. doi: 10.1016/j.molmed.2015.08.002

Sun, M. Y., Xu, B., Wu, Q. X., Cai, S., Chen, W. L., Li, D., et al. (2020). Cisplatin-resistant gastric cancer cells promote the chemoresistance of cisplatin-sensitive cells via exosomal RPS3 mediated PI3K-Akt-cofilin-1 signaling axis. *Res. Square* [Epub ahead of print].

Tang, Q. F., Sun, J., Yu, H., Shi, X. J., Lv, R., Wei, H. C., et al. (2016). The zuo jin wan formula induces mitochondrial apoptosis of cisplatin-resistant gastric cancer cells via cofilin-1. *Evid. Based Complement. Alternat. Med.* 2016:8203789. doi: 10.1155/2016/8203789

Vartiainen, M. K., Mustonen, T., Mattila, P. K., Ojala, P. J., Thesleff, I., Partanen, J., et al. (2002). The three mouse actin-depolymerizing factor/cofilins evolved to fulfill cell-type-specific requirements for actin dynamics. *Mol. Biol. Cell.* 13, 183–194.

Vergara, D., Tinelli, A., Iannone, A., and Maffia, M. (2012). The impact of proteomics in the understanding of the molecular basis of Cisplatin-resistance in ovarian tumors. *Curr. Cancer Drug Targets* 12, 987–997. doi: 10.2174/156800912803251171

Wan, F., Anderson, D. E., Barnitz, R. A., Snow, A., Bidere, N., Zheng, L., et al. (2007). Ribosomal protein S3: a KH domain subunit in NF-kappaB complexes that mediates selective gene regulation. *Cell* 131, 927–939. doi: 10.1016/j.cell.2007.10.009

Wang, F., Wu, D. L., Xu, Z. P., Chen, J. X., Zhang, J. Y., Li, X. J., et al. (2019). miR-182-5p affects human bladder cancer cell proliferation, migration and invasion through regulating cofilin 1. *Cancer Cell. Int.* 19:42. doi: 10.1186/s12935-019-0758-5

Wei, F., Ma, C. Y., Zhou, T., Dong, X. C., Luo, Q. H., Geng, L., et al. (2017). Exosomes derived from gemcitabine-resistant cells transfer malignant phenotypic traits via delivery of miRNA-222-3p. *Mol. Cancer* 16:132. doi: 10.1186/s12943-017-0694-8

Wu, Q., Gou, Y. W., Wang, Q. M., Jin, H. F., Cui, L. N., Zhang, Y. G., et al. (2011). Downregulation of RPL6 by siRNA inhibits proliferation and cell cycle progression of human gastric cancer cell lines. *PLoS One* 6:e26401. doi: 10.1371/journal.pone.0026401

Zeng, A. L., Yan, W., Liu, Y. W., Wang, Z., Hu, Q., Nie, E., et al. (2017). Tumour exosomes from cells harbouring PTPRZ1-MET fusion contribute to a malignant phenotype and temozolomide chemoresistance in glioblastoma. *Oncogene* 36, 5369–5381. doi: 10.1038/onc.2017.134

Zhang, D., and Fan, D. (2017). Multidrug resistance in gastric cancer: recent research advances and ongoing therapeutic challenges. *Expert Rev. Anticancer Ther.* 7, 1369–1378. doi: 10.1586/14737140.7.10.1369

Zhang, H., Wang, Y., Xing, F. J., Wang, J. C., and Gao, Z. L. (2012). Overexpression of LIMK1 promotes migration ability ofmultidrug-resistant osteosarcoma cells. *Oncol. Res.* 19, 501–509. doi: 10.3727/096504012X13286534482511

Zhang, J., Li, S., Li, L., Li, M., Guo, C., Yao, J., et al. (2015). Exosome and exosomal microRNA: trafficking, sorting, and function. *Genom. Proteomics Bioinform.* 13, 17–24. doi: 10.1016/j.gpb.2015.02.001

Zhang, Y., Liao, R. Y., Li, H., Liu, L., Chen, X., and Chen, H. M. (2015). Expression of cofilin-1 and transgelin in esophageal squamous cell carcinoma. *Med. Sci. Monit.* 2015, 2659–2665. doi: 10.12659/MSM.895242

Zhao, L. J., Cao, J. Z., Hu, K. X., Wang, P. H., Li, G. D., He, X. D., et al. (2019). RNA-binding protein RPS3 contributes to hepatocarcinogenesis by post-transcriptionally up-regulating SIRT1. *Nucleic Acids Res.* 47, 2011–2028. doi: 10.1093/nar/gky1209

15

SYVN1-MTR4-MAT2A Signaling Axis Regulates Methionine Metabolism in Glioma Cells

Lude Wang[1], Bin Hu[2], Kailing Pan[1], Jie Chang[1], Xiaoya Zhao[1], Lin Chen[1], Haiping Lin[1], Jing Wang[1], Gezhi Zhou[3], Wenxia Xu[1] and Jianlie Yuan[3]**

[1] Central Laboratory, Affiliated Jinhua Hospital, Zhejiang University School of Medicine, Jinhua, China, [2] Department of Pathology, Affiliated Jinhua Hospital, Zhejiang University School of Medicine, Jinhua, China, [3] Department of Neurosurgery, Affiliated Jinhua Hospital, Zhejiang University School of Medicine, Jinhua, China

***Correspondence:**
Wenxia Xu
Xuwenxia@zju.edu.cn
Jianlie Yuan
yuanjianlie@zju.edu.cn

Methionine is one of the essential amino acids. How tumor cells adapt and adjust their signal transduction networks to avoid apoptosis in a methionine-restricted environment is worthy of further exploration. In this study, we investigated the molecular mechanism of glioma response to methionine restriction, providing a theoretical basis for new treatment strategies for glioma.

Methods: We constructed methionine-restriction-tolerant cells in order to study the response of glioma to a methionine-restricted environment. The transcriptome analysis of the tolerant cells showed significant changes in MAT2A. Western blotting, immunohistochemistry, quantitative real-time PCR, colony formation assays, and other experiments were used to verify the role of MAT2A in glioma genesis. In addition, the regulatory mechanism of MAT2A mRNA nuclear export was investigated by transfection, plasma nucleation separation, and co-immunoprecipitation.

Results: Under methionine restriction, glioma cells showed high expression of MAT2A, and an inhibitor of MAT2A reduced the proliferation of tumor cells. The expression of MAT2A was positively correlated with World Health Organization-grade glioma. High expression of MAT2A was related to increased transfer of its mRNA out of the nucleus. The expression of nuclear export regulatory molecule MTR4 could affect the export of MAT2A mRNA. In a methionine-restricted environment, ubiquitination of MTR4 was enhanced, and thus its protein level was reduced. The E3 ubiquitin ligase was verified to be SYVN1.

Conclusion: In summary, methionine restriction leads to increased ubiquitination of MTR4, which promotes the transfer of MAT2A mRNA out of the nucleus and MAT2A protein expression. MAT2A promotes histone methylation, prompting cells to proliferate in a methionine-restricted environment.

Keywords: methionine metabolism, glioma, MAT2A, MTR4, SYVN1

Abbreviations: ATP, adenosine triphosphate; CM, complete medium; CQ, Chloroquine; CT, computed tomography; HCC, hepatocellular carcinoma; IHC, immunohistochemistry; NXF1, nuclear RNA export factor 1; NXT1, nuclear transport factor 2 like export factor 1; MAT2A, methionine adenosyltransferase 2A; MRM, methionine-restricted medium; MRT, methionine-restriction tolerant; MTR4, Mtr4 exosome RNA helicase; qRT-PCR, quantitative real-time PCR; PMSF, Phenylmethanesulfonyl fluoride; SAM, S-adenosylmethionine.

INTRODUCTION

Glioma is the most common type of primary brain tumor, accounting for approximately 81% of primary intracranial tumors (Ostrom et al., 2014). Although relatively rare, glioma causes significant mortality and morbidity. Currently, surgery and chemoradiotherapy are the main treatments for patients with glioma. However, patients have poor survival despite these treatments, and no major breakthrough has been made in glioma treatment recently (Riabovol et al., 2019). Therefore, there is a vital and urgent need to identify the molecular mechanisms underlying glioma occurrence to enable the exploration of novel strategies for glioma treatment.

In recent years, the role of metabolic reprogramming in tumors has captured increasing attention owing to the development of metabolomics technology and the discovery of tumor metabolites through metabolomics (Poljsak et al., 2019). Metabolites, in addition to serving as substrates for energy generation and anabolism, can regulate the expression of oncogenes and tumor suppressor genes and change epigenetic status (KaelinJr., and McKnight, 2013; Pavlova and Thompson, 2016; Ducker and Rabinowitz, 2017). Therefore, the causal relationship between gene expression and metabolism plays an important part in tumor development (Jain et al., 2012; Xia et al., 2017; Nencioni et al., 2018).

Methionine is one of the essential amino acids in the human body and is involved in the synthesis of many important proteins (Sanderson et al., 2019). The rapid proliferation of glioma cells requires abundant protein; therefore, large amounts of methionine must be ingested and utilized. Based on this theory, ^{11}C-MET computed tomography (CT) can serve as a crucial measure for glioma diagnosis and treatment (Glaudemans et al., 2013; Luckerath et al., 2015; He et al., 2019). Methionine reacts with adenosine triphosphate (ATP) to generate S-adenosylmethionine (SAM) under the catalysis of MAT2A (LeGrosJr., Halim et al., 2000). Then SAM, catalyzed by methyltransferase, transfers its methyl group to methyl group receptors such as proteins, DNA, RNA, and other biological macromolecules, thereby methylating them. Moreover, the methionine cycle enables SAM to regenerate methionine through multiple enzymatic reactions (Wang et al., 2019; **Figure 1A**); MAT2A is the first rate-limiting enzyme of this cycle. The role of MAT2A in a variety of cancers has been elucidated, in particular, liver cancer (Anstee and Day, 2012; Pajares et al., 2013); however, its counterpart in glioma remains unclear.

Whether a newly synthesized RNA is exported to the cytoplasm or degraded is of extreme significance to the precise expression of genes. A competition model has been introduced to explain the mechanism that determines these outcomes. In this model, nuclear RNA export factor 1 (NXF1)/nuclear transport factor 2-like export factor 1 (NXT1) and the TREX complex (Chi et al., 2013), the key factor of which is ALYREF (Masuda et al., 2005; Shi et al., 2017), work together to mediate the mRNA nuclear export process (Strasser et al., 2002; Carmody and Wente, 2009). Furthermore, the multi-subunit exosome complex, which has endonuclease and 3′-to-5′ exonuclease activity, is responsible for degrading RNA of aberrant structure or quantity (Andersen et al., 2013). RNA helicase MTR4 is a dispensable cofactor of the exosome complex (Lubas et al., 2011; Meola et al., 2016). When RNA becomes mature, ALYREF competes with MTR4 to bind to ARS2, a component of the 5′-cap-binding complex; the "winner" is recruited to the mature mRNA (Fan et al., 2017). In other words, the competition between ALYREF and MTR4 determines the destiny of the RNA inside the nucleus. However, little is known about the balance between RNA export to the cytoplasm and RNA degradation in the process of tumor metabolism regulation.

Here, in order to explore the metabolic reprogramming of glioma cells in a low-methionine environment, methionine-restriction-tolerant (MRT) cells were constructed. Sequencing showed that their metabolites and mRNA expression profiles were significantly changed, with MAT2A expression significantly increased in the tolerant cells. We demonstrated the important roles of MAT2A in promoting glioma tumorigenesis and cancer metabolic reprogramming. In addition, we found that ubiquitination of MTR4 in a low-methionine environment was the cause of the high levels of export of MAT2A mRNA to the cytoplasm, leading to MAT2A overexpression. Our results provide a new molecular mechanism for understanding the response of glioma cells to methionine restriction.

MATERIALS AND METHODS

Reagents and Inhibitors

RPMI-1640 medium powder (31800-105) and fetal bovine serum (FBS, 11011-8611) were purchased from Gibco (Invitrogen, United States). Streptomycin and penicillin (GNM15140) were purchased from Genome (Hangzhou, China). RPMI-1640 medium w/o amino acids powder (R8999-04A) was obtained from United States Biological (United States).

PF9366 (25 μM final concentration), actinomycin D (5 μg/mL final concentration), cycloheximide (a general inhibitor of protein synthesis; 25 μM final concentration), MG-132 (25 μM final concentration), CQ (25 μM final concentration), and PS-341 (25 μM final concentration) were purchased from MCE (China).

Cell Culture

Human glioma cell lines U251, U87, and HEK293T were obtained from the Type Culture Collection of the Chinese Academy of Sciences (Shanghai, China). U251 and U87 cells were cultured in RPMI-1640 medium containing 10% FBS, 100 μg/mL streptomycin, and 100 U/mL penicillin and used to prepare cells in the complete medium (CM) group. The methionine-restriction cell model was established as follows: RPMI-1640 w/o amino acids medium powder with 19 amino acids was added as standard, the amount of methionine was reduced from 15 mg/L to 3.75 mg/L (Moore et al., 1967) to prepare a methionine-restricted medium (MRM). Cells cultured in MRM for ~20 days were denoted U251-M or U87-M, whereas those cultured with MRM for a short time were used to prepare the MRM group. All cell cultures were maintained in a 5% CO_2 humidified incubator at 37°C.

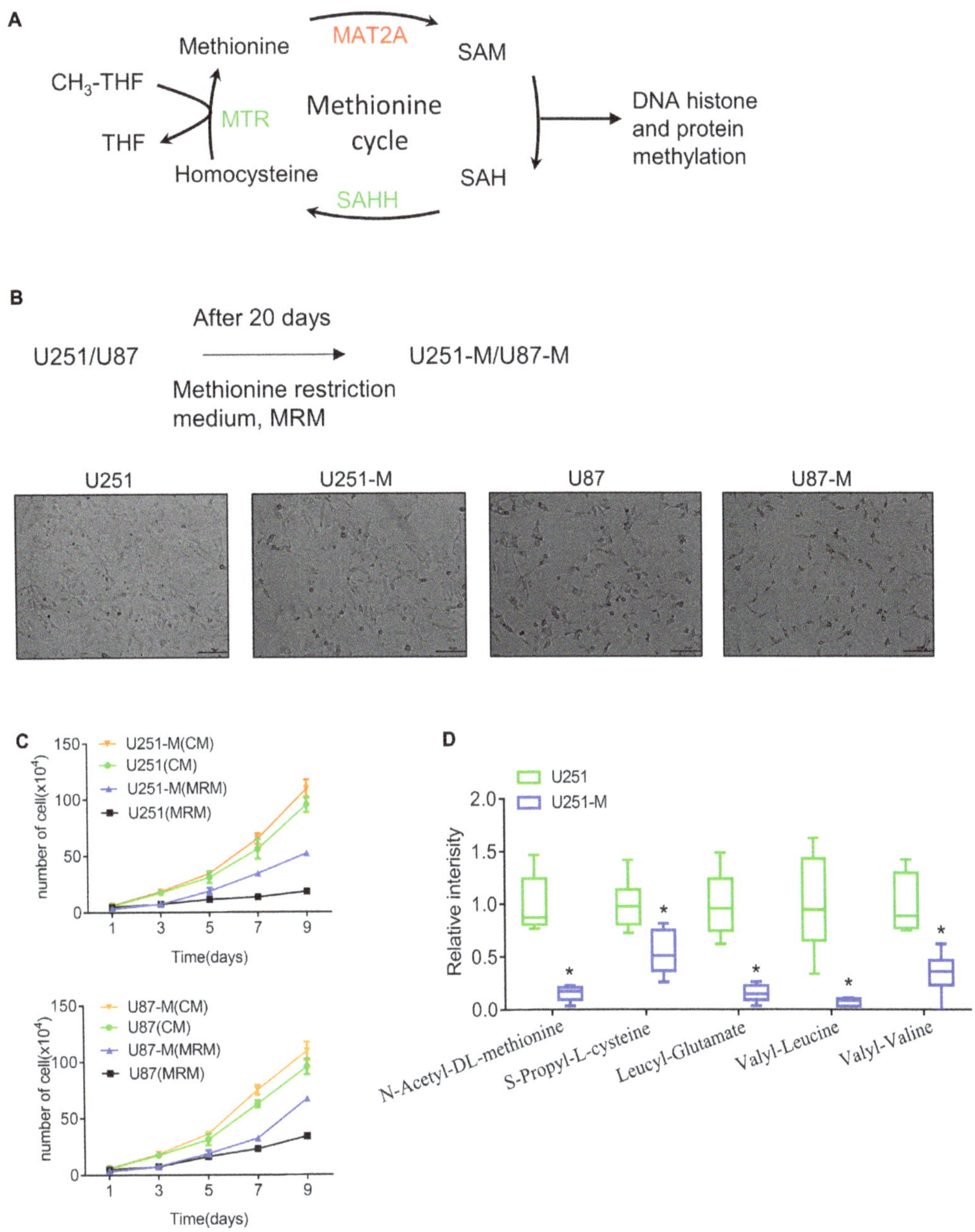

FIGURE 1 | Establishment of MRT glioma cells. **(A)** Schematic of the methionine cycle. Methionine reacts with ATP under the catalysis of MAT2A to produce the universal methyl donor SAM. SAM provides methyl groups for DNA histone and protein methylation, which is then transferred to SAH. SAH is hydrolyzed by the catalyzation of SAHH to generate homocysteine, which is then converted to methionine with methyl donation from tetrahydrofolate (THF). **(B)** Schematic of construction of MRT glioma cells. **(C)** Proliferation of U251-M and U87-M cells cultured with CM and MRM was analyzed by cell counting (n = 3 biologically independent experiments). Differences between the two groups were calculated by two-way ANOVA. Data are presented as mean ± s. d., and P-values are indicated. **(D)** Changes of several amino acids between U251 and U251-M cells. $^*p < 0.05$.

Cell Proliferation, Edu, and Colony Formation Assays

For the cell proliferation assay, glioma cell lines were plated in 24-well plates at a density of 3 × 10^4 cells per well and cultured in 500 μL medium for 24 h. Subsequently, the medium was replaced with fresh CM or MRM. Cell numbers were counted at multiple time points (1, 3, 5, 7, and 9 days).

The Edu assay was performed using a Cell Proliferation Detection Kit (Beyotime, China) following the manufacturer's protocol. Briefly, glioma cells were seeded at a density of 3 × 10^4 cells per well in 24-well plates and treated for 24 h. Then, the medium was replaced with 20 μM Edu solution for 2 h. Cells were fixed with 4% paraformaldehyde, then incubated with phosphate-buffered saline (PBS) containing 0.3% Triton X-100 for 15 min. After the addition of 100 μL/well Click solution for 30 min, cells were rinsed three times with PBS and then observed with a fluorescence microscope.

For colony formation analysis, cells were grown in six-well plates at a density of 500 cells per well. After ~2 weeks of culture, the colonies were fixed with 4% paraformaldehyde and stained with crystal violet. A low-power microscope was used to count the number of colonies, with 50 cells designated as a colony. The size of a colony was analyzed using colony counting software.

Quantitative PCR Analysis

Total RNA was isolated using TRIzol reagent (Life Technologies, CA, United States) according to the manufacturer's instructions. A NanoDrop 2000 (Thermo Fisher Scientific) instrument was used to quantify total RNA. First, 1 μg of total RNA was reverse transcribed to cDNA using a PrimeScript RT Master Mix kit (Takara). Then, the mRNA expression level was determined by quantitative real-time PCR (qRT-PCR) using SYBR Green Master Mix (Takara) on a Light Cycler 480 II system (Roche), followed by calculation with the standard $2^{-\Delta\Delta Ct}$ relative quantification method. The primers for MAT2A, SAHH, MTR, MTR4, METTL16, and β-actin were synthesized by TSINGKE Biological Technology (Beijing, China). β-actin was used as an internal reference for RNA integrity.

For the preparation of cytoplasmic and nuclear extracts, cells were processed according to a slightly modified version of a previously published protocol (Vermeulen et al., 2010). Briefly, cells were harvested, washed once with PBS, resuspended in 100 μL of lysis buffer A (10 mM HEPES-KOH pH 7.9, 1.5 mM $MgCl_2$, 10 mM KCl, 0.2% NP-40, 1X Roche protease inhibitors, 1 U/mL NEB RNase inhibitors) and left for 10 min on ice. After 40 strokes with a Dounce homogenizer, cells were centrifuged for 15 min at 3750 rpm. The supernatant (representing the cytoplasmic extract) was collected, 1 mL TRIzol was added, and mRNA was extracted by the above method.

The PCR primers were as follows:
MAT2A-F 5′-ATGAACGGACAGCTCAACGG-3′,
MAT2A-R 5′-CCAGCAAGAAGGATCATTCCAG-3′,
SAHH-F 5′-GCATGTCTGACAAACTGCCC-3′,
SAHH-R 5′-ACCACTGCACCTCAGCA-3′,
MTR-F 5′-TGCTCTCACTGCTCCCAAAAA-3′,
MTR-R 5′-CATCAAAACGTTTCCCTGCCT-3′,
MTR4-F 5′-AACGGGAGGCGTCAAAAGAC-3′,
MTR4-R 5′-TCTTCAGACCTTCGGGTTGC-3′,
METTL16-F 5′-TCAATTGGAAGCCAAGGGAGT-3′,
METTL16-R 5′-ACCCCTTGTATGCGAAGCTC-3′,
β-actin-F 5′-ACTCTTCCAGCCTTCCTTCC-3′, and
β-actin-R 5′-CGTCATACTCCTGCTTGCTG-3′.

Immunohistochemistry Analysis of Tumor Samples

A tumor tissue microarray was obtained from the Affiliated Hospital of Xuzhou Medical University. Anti-MAT2A (ab189208) from Abcam was used for immunohistochemistry analyses. Immunohistochemistry was performed by the Department of Pathology of the Affiliated Jinhua Hospital, Zhejiang University School of Medicine. Samples were subsequently scored by visual assessment as "+1," "+2," or "+3," according to the staining intensity for MAT2A. Associations between MAT2A staining and clinicopathological factors of patients with glioma, including age, gender, World Health Organization (WHO) grade, and histologic type, were evaluated by χ^2-test.

Gene Transfection and RNA Interference

The flag-MTR4 plasmid was constructed by TSINGKE Biological Technology (Beijing, China). The SYVN1 plasmid was purchased from Sino Biological (China). Glioma cells were plated overnight in six-well plates at a density of 3 × 10[1] cells per well, and then the plasmid was transfected into cells with Lipofectamine® 2000 reagent (Invitrogen, United States). DNA was diluted to a final concentration of 1 μg plasmid DNA per 100 μL medium before supplementation with 2 μL DNA transfection reagent. After incubation for 15 min, the DNA complex was added to the cells in a dropwise manner. After incubation for 1–3 days at 37°C, the transfected cells were harvested for further analysis.

Cells were seeded in six-well plates at 40–60% confluence and transfected with short interfering RNA (siRNA) (50 nM) with Lipofectamine RNAiMAX reagent (Life Technologies, CA, United States) in Opti-MEM medium (Invitrogen) according to the manufacturer's protocol. The transfected cells were incubated at 37°C for 1–3 days before harvesting. The siRNAs for MAT2A were designed by and purchased from RiboBio (Guangzhou, China); their sequences were as follows:

si-MAT2A#1 GAGCAACAGTCACCAGATA

si-MAT2A#2 GTGGCAAAATCCCTTGTTA

si-MTR4#1 GCAAGTGCTTCGAGATGCA

si-MTR4#2 GCAGCATAATTCGTTGTAT

si-SYVN1#1 CCATCTTCATCAAGTATGT

si-SYVN1#2 CCGTATGGATGTCCTTCGT

si-METTL16#1 GCCGGACAGTACCTGTTTA

si-METTL16#2 CCGCCTAGTTCTGTTAATA

Western Blotting and Co-immunoprecipitation

To prepare whole protein samples, cells were lysed and extracted with RIPA lysis buffer containing 1% PMSF (Phenylmethanesulfonyl fluoride). Then, lysates of 20–30 μg were loaded onto 8% or 12% sodium dodecyl sulfate polyacrylamide gels for electrophoresis, and the separated proteins were transferred to polyvinylidene fluoride membranes. After being blocked with 5% skim milk in Tris-buffered

[1]https://www.oncomine.org

saline containing 0.1% Tween-20 (TBST) for 2 h at room temperature, the membranes were incubated with primary antibody overnight at 4°C. On the second day, the membranes were washed with TBST and then incubated with peroxidase-labeled secondary antibodies for 1 h. Immunoreactivity was determined using enhanced chemiluminescence reagents and visualized on a Bio-Rad ChemiDoc XRS system. β-actin served to normalize protein levels.

Protein Antibodies Used for Western Blotting

For the co-immunoprecipitation assay, glioma cells were washed with PBS and lysed with lysis buffer (Thermo Fisher Scientific, United States), and the lysates were pretreated with protein A/G beads (Thermo Fisher Scientific, United States) for 1 h at 4°C. The cell lysates were incubated with anti-MTR4 (10 μg) and anti-SYVN1 (10 μg) antibodies overnight at 4°C. Then, the supernatant was precipitated with protein A/G overnight at 4°C to precipitate the immune complexes. After washing the complexes six times with cell lysis buffer, the samples were analyzed via western blotting.

Antibodies	Source	Catalog no.	Dilution
MAT2A	Abcam	ab189208	1:2000
H3K4me3	CST	9751	1:2000
H3K9me3	CST	13969	1:2000
H3K27me3	CST	9733	1:2000
Histone H3	CST	4499	1:2000
MTR4	Abcam	ab70551	1:2000
Aly/Ref	Abcam	ab202894	1:2000
SYVN1	Proteintech	13473-1-AP	1:1000
Ub	Beyotime	AF1705	1:1000
β-actin	Beyotime	AF003	1:1000

Metabolomic Analyses

Sample Preparation and Extraction of Quality Control (QC) Samples

To guarantee the quality of the non-targeted bioanalytical data, QC samples were used for method validation. QC samples were prepared from a mixture of 20 μL per sample. QC samples were extracted using the sample extraction method described above. The QC specimens were analyzed every six samples throughout the whole analysis procedure.

Data Processing

Raw data files were pretreated with procedures including peak finding, alignment, filtering, and normalization to total area. A three-dimensional data set consisting of sample information, peak intensities, peak retention time, and mass-to-charge ratio (m/z) was obtained. Retention time and m/z data were used as identifiers of each ion. Moreover, peaks with missing values (ion intensity = 0) in more than 80% of samples were removed in order to obtain consistent variables. Then, the resultant data matrices were imported into SIMCA14.1 (Umetrics, Umeå, Sweden) software for multivariate statistical analysis. Analytic methods including principal components analysis and orthogonal partial least-squares discriminant analysis (OPLS-DA) were used for metabolite profile analysis.

Biomarker Identification and Metabolic Pathway Analysis

The OPLS-DA model was used to visualize the metabolic differences between the model group and control group. Variables with VIP > 1 in the OPLS-DA model, as well as those with $p|\text{corr}|$ value > 0.58 in the S-plot and those with confidence interval crossing zero in the jack-knifed loading plot, were considered to be potential biomarkers. The potential biomarkers were identified using Agilent Mass Hunter Qualitative Navigator (Agilent, United States) combined with the HMDB database[2], Kyoto Encyclopedia of Genes and Genomes (KEGG)[3], and lipid maps database[4]. The pathway analysis used MetaboAnalyst 3.0[5].

RNA-Sequencing Analysis

TRIzol reagent (Carlsbad, CA, United States) was used to extract total RNA from three independent samples of cells. RNA sequencing was performed by KaiTai-Bio (Hangzhou, China). RNA-seq libraries were constructed using an Illumina TruSeq RNA sample preparation kit (RS-122-2001) and sequenced using an Illumina HiSeq 2000 system with a read length of 50 base pairs with paired ends. RNA-seq reads were mapped to the human genome (hg19) using TopHat (Trapnell et al., 2009). Only those reads mapped to unique genomic locations and with <5% mismatches were analyzed further. We used FPKM (Trapnell et al., 2010) to measure gene transcripts, and DEGSeq (Wang et al., 2010) to identify differentially expressed genes. The differentially expressed genes were counted and annotated using the NCBI, UniProt, gene ontology, and KEGG databases to obtain detailed descriptions.

Quantification and Statistical Analysis

The data were presented as mean ± SEM of at least three independent experiments. Statistical analyses were performed via GraphPad prism software (San Diego, CA, United States). One-way analysis of variance (ANOVA), which was followed by a *post hoc* test, was used for multiple comparisons. $P < 0.05$ was considered to be statistically significant.

RESULTS

Establishment of MRT Glioma Cells

Methionine is an essential amino acid, and its lack causes cell growth arrest. In order to explore the reaction of glioma cells to a methionine-restricted environment, MRM (with a methionine concentration of 3.75 mg/L in contrast to 15 mg/L in normal medium) was used to culture glioma cells. In this way, MRT glioma cells were established and denoted U251-M and U87-M, respectively (**Figure 1B**). After cultivation in

[2]http://www.hmdb.ca
[3]http://www.genome.jp/kegg
[4]https://www.lipidmaps.org/
[5]http://www.MetaboAnalyst.ca/

MRM for 9 days, there was no apparent increase in the numbers of parental cells (U251 and U87). However, MRT cells (U251-M and U87-M) had a stronger proliferation ability than the corresponding parental cells (**Figure 1C**). To thoroughly investigate the mechanism underlying this phenomenon, we performed metabolomic sequencing on parental U251 cells and MRT U251-M cells. The sequencing results showed statistically significant differences in levels of 45 metabolites between the two cell types (**Supplementary Figure 1A**), including 36 metabolites that were downregulated and nine that were upregulated (**Supplementary Table 1**). Levels of multiple amino acids were changed, including methionine, leucine, and valine (**Figure 1D**). Many metabolites related to lipid metabolism and glucose metabolism, including trihydroxystearic acid, pantothenic acid, folic acid, furfuryl thioacetate, and nicotinamide, also showed changes (**Supplementary Table 1**). These results indicated that the MRT glioma cells had been successfully constructed and that their metabolism had been remodeled.

Transcriptome Comparison Showed Upregulation of MAT2A in MRT Glioma Cells and Parental Glioma Cells

To further reveal the genes whose expression levels changed with metabolic reprogramming, transcriptome sequencing was performed on U251 and U251-M cells. The results showed that 363 genes were upregulated and 655 genes were downregulated (**Supplementary Figures 1B,C**). KEGG pathway analysis of these differentially expressed genes showed that they were markedly enriched in metabolic pathways, as illustrated in the bubble plot in **Figure 2A**. Further gene set enrichment analysis (GSEA) of the sequencing results showed that methionine metabolism pathways were downregulated (**Figure 2B**), whereas pathways related to glucose and lipid metabolism were upregulated (**Supplementary Figure 1D**). Based on analysis of the high-throughput data, the 50 genes with the largest fold change in expression levels were used to plot a heatmap. Among them, the metabolic enzyme of the methionine cycle, MAT2A, attracted our attention (**Figure 2C**). Therefore, we tested the expression levels of MAT2A and two other metabolic enzymes of the methionine cycle, SAHH, and MTR, in U251-M by qRT-PCR and found that the mRNA level of MAT2A was significantly elevated, whereas those of SAHH and MTR increased comparatively less (**Figure 2D**). Furthermore, as the cultivation time in MRM was increased up to 24 h, the mRNA level of MAT2A in U251 gradually increased (**Figure 2E**). Besides, both mRNA and protein levels of MAT2A in U251 and U87 cells showed marked increases after cultivation in MRM for 24 h (**Figures 2F,G**). Based on these findings, we speculated that MAT2A might have a crucial role in the response of U251 and U87 cells to a methionine-restricted environment.

MAT2A Is Required for Glioma Cells

Previous studies have reported that MAT2A was able to promote the proliferation, invasiveness, and metastasis of various tumor cells and was closely related to patients' prognosis (Marjon et al., 2016; Murray et al., 2019), but its role in glioma cells remained unknown. Consequently, preliminary research was carried out to investigate this. PF9366 is known to inhibit MAT2A by embedding into its spatial structure (Quinlan et al., 2017). Treatment with PF9366 at a concentration of 25 μM (**Supplementary Figure 2A**) significantly inhibited the proliferation ability of U251-M and U87-M cells (**Figures 3A,B**). We then transiently transfected siRNA into U251 and U87 glioma cells, which were harvested 48 h after transfection for qRT-PCR and cell proliferation assays. The qRT-PCR results confirmed that there was a significant decrease in MAT2A expression in both U251-M and U87-M cells compared with the control group (**Supplementary Figure 2B**). The transfected U251-M and U87-M cells exhibited decreased cellular growth (**Figures 3C,D**). We also investigated the role of MAT2A in glioma migration. The results of the wound-healing assays showed no significant difference in healing speed between the PF9366-processed and MAT2A-knockdown cells and the corresponding controls (**Supplementary Figure 2C**). These results suggest that MAT2A is an important molecule that enables glioma cells to survive in a methionine-restricted environment. We performed transcriptome sequencing analysis to determine the differences in gene expression between untreated U251-M cells and those treated with PF9366 and found 186 upregulated genes and 125 downregulated genes (**Supplementary Figures 2D,E**). KEGG pathway analysis of these differentially expressed genes showed that they were involved in pathways including Wnt signaling, TNF signaling, MAPK signaling, and glioma (**Figure 3E**). GSEA analysis of the data showed that metabolic pathways including methionine metabolism and glucose metabolism were downregulated, whereas metabolic pathways related to DNA replication were upregulated (**Supplementary Figure 2F**). We further performed metabolomic analysis on U251-M cells with and without PF9366 treatment. Differences were observed between the two groups for more than 100 metabolites, and 12 differentially identifiable metabolites were identified (**Supplementary Table 2** and **Supplementary Figure 2G**). The differential metabolites were mainly enriched in sphingolipid metabolism (**Figure 3F**). Changes in MAT2A will directly affect levels of SAM, thereby influencing the methylation of biomolecules. Therefore, we examined the abundance of methylated histones. In comparison with U251-M cells, the majority of histone methylation marks in both PF9366-processed and MAT2A-knockdown cells were greatly downregulated (**Figure 3G**). The above results show that in a methionine-restricted environment, glioma cells regulate the methylation of biological macromolecules by regulating the expression of MAT2A, enabling the cells to survive in a methionine-restricted environment.

Increased MAT2A Expression Was Significantly Associated With WHO Grade in Glioma

To determine the clinical significance of MAT2A in patients with glioma, we performed data mining and analyzed MAT2A expression data downloaded from the publicly available Oncomine database (an online cancer microarray database)[5]. MAT2A gene expression analysis based on seven databases

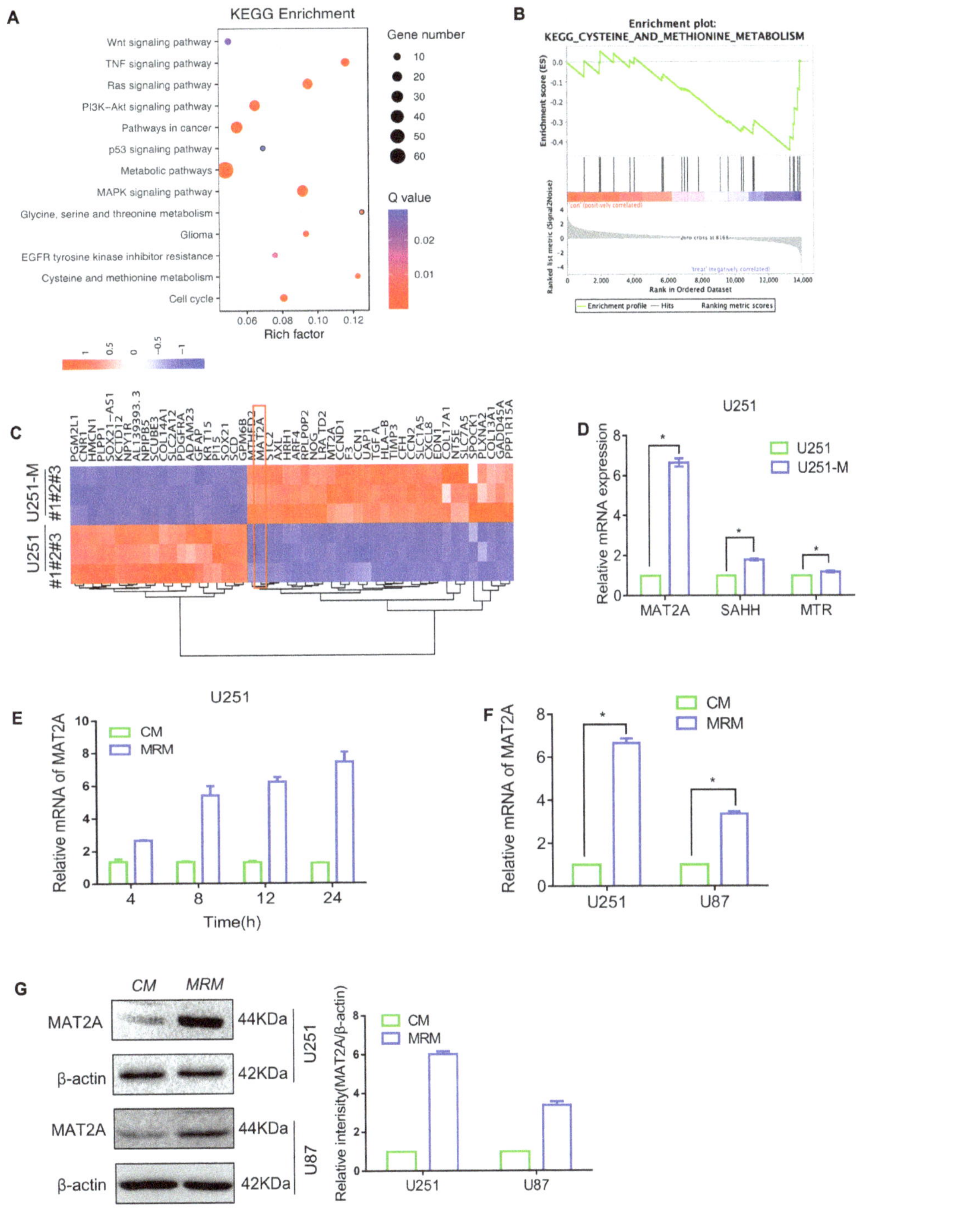

FIGURE 2 | Transcriptome comparison showing upregulation of MAT2A in MRT glioma cells and parental glioma cells. **(A)** KEGG enrichment of different signaling pathways in U251 and U251-M glioma cells. **(B)** GSEA plot depicting enrichment of downregulated genes in cysteine and methionine metabolism. **(C)** Heatmap of the top 50 differentially expressed genes between U251 and U251-M. **(D)** Expression of MAT2A, SAHH, and MTR in U251 and U251-M glioma cells, evaluated via RT-PCR. mRNA was normalized to β-actin and plotted relative to the control. **(E)** U251 cells were cultured in MRM for the indicated times (4, 8, 12, and 24 h), and MAT2A mRNA was detected by RT-PCR. **(F)** Relative mRNA of MAT2A was evaluated by RT-PCR in U251 and U87 glioma cells cultured in CM or MRM. **(G)** Western blotting for MAT2A in U251 and U87 glioma cells following culture in CM or MRM. β-actin was used as an internal control. The left graph is a quantized graph. *$p < 0.05$.

exhibited four databases with a significant *P*-value ($P < 0.01$) and gene ranks in the top 10% among all differentially expressed genes. In these databases, MAT2A was upregulated in tumor tissues of glioma compared with normal tissues (**Figure 4A**). We evaluated MAT2A expression in microarray tissues from 410 glioma cancer patients using immunohistochemistry staining

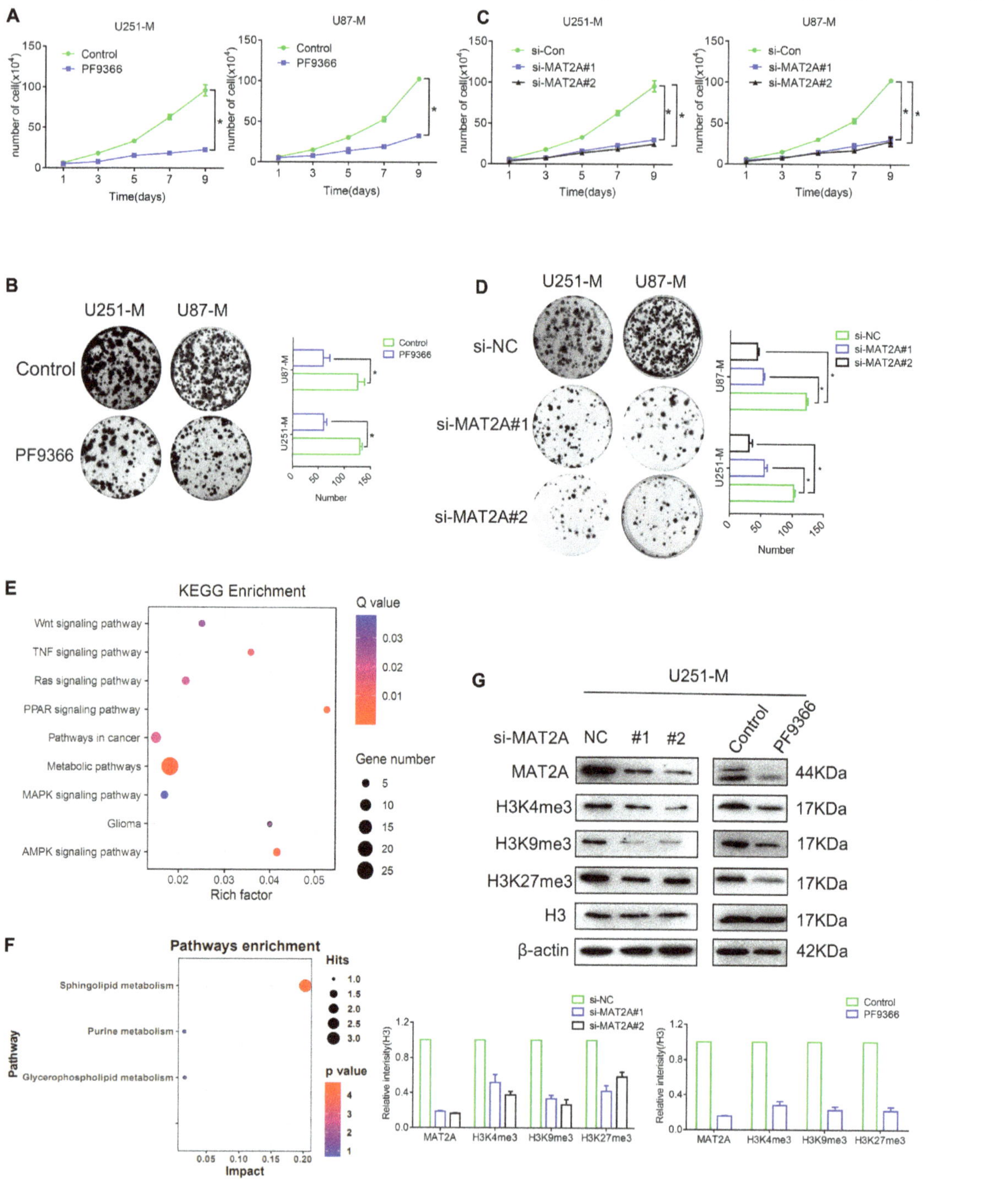

FIGURE 3 | MAT2A is required by glioma cells. **(A)** Proliferation of cells with MAT2A inhibited by PF9366 and control cells was analyzed by cell counting. **(B)** Colony formation assay for control cells and cells with MAT2A inhibited by PF9366. Differences between the two groups were calculated by a two-tailed, unpaired *t*-test. Data are presented as mean ± s. d., and *P*-values are indicated ($n = 3$ biologically independent samples). **(C)** Proliferation of MAT2A-knockdown and control cells was analyzed by cell counting. **(D)** Colony formation assay for control and MAT2A-knockdown cells. **(E)** KEGG enrichment of different signaling pathways in U251 and PF9366-processed U251-M cells. **(F)** Enrichment of differential metabolites in signaling pathways in U251 and PF9366-processed U251-M cells. **(G)** Protein levels of modified histones in MAT2A-knockdown and PF9366-processed U251-M cells. Histone H3 was used as a loading control. Independent blots were repeated at least three times with similar results. A quantized graph is shown below. $^{*}p < 0.05$.

(**Supplementary Figure 3A**). As shown in **Figure 4B**, MAT2A protein was found to be intracellularly localized. The intensity of staining in glioma tissue varies from patient to patient. In addition, histological type and WHO grade are important factors affecting the prognosis of glioma patients. We investigated whether the expression of MAT2A was related to these factors.

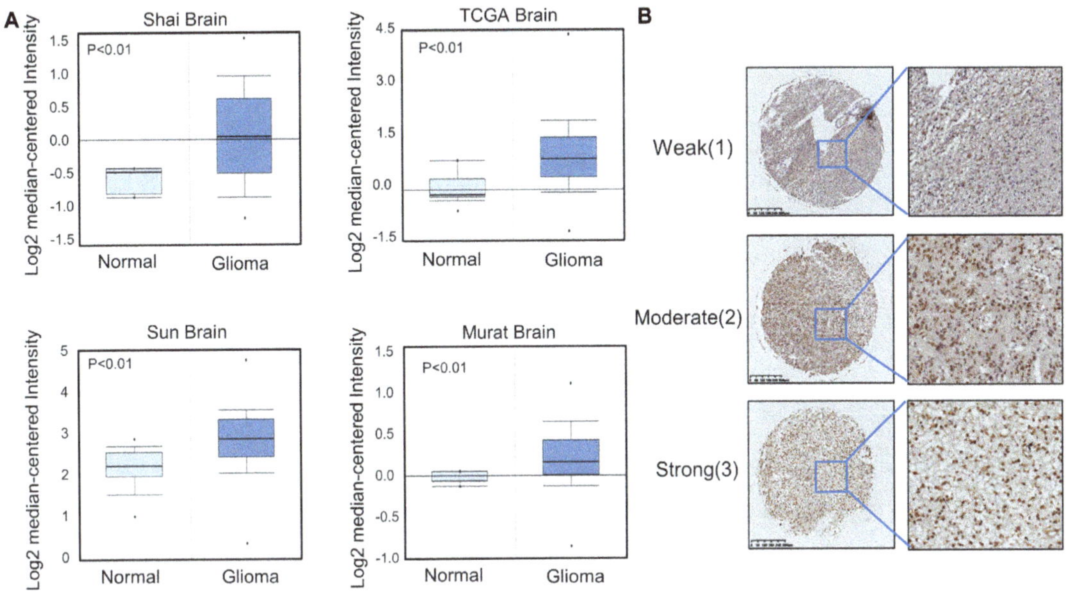

C

Variable	MAT2A staining intensity			
	1	2	3	P. Value
All cases	154	206	50	
Age				
≤42 years	78 (39.59)	95 (48.22)	24 (12.18)	0.696
>42 years	76(35.68)	111 (52.11)	26 (12.21)	
Gender				
Male	73 (30.42)	131(54.58)	36(15.00)	0.001
Female	81 (47.65)	75 (44.12)	14 (8.24)	
WHO grade				
I	22 (64.71)	9 (26.47)	3 (8.82)	<0.001
II	81 (41.54)	101 (51.79)	13 (6.67)	
III	33 (28.21)	61 (52.14)	23 (19.66)	
IV	18 (28.13)	35 (54.69)	11 (17.19)	
Histological type				
Astrocytoma	119 (38.14)	159 (50.96)	34 (10.90)	0.262
Glioblastoma	12 (25.00)	29 (60.42)	7 (14.58)	
Oligodendroglioma	14 (48.28)	11 (37.93)	4 (13.79)	
Medulloblastoma	6 (37.50)	6 (37.50)	4 (25.00)	
Ependymoma	3 (60.00)	1 (20.00)	1 (20.00)	

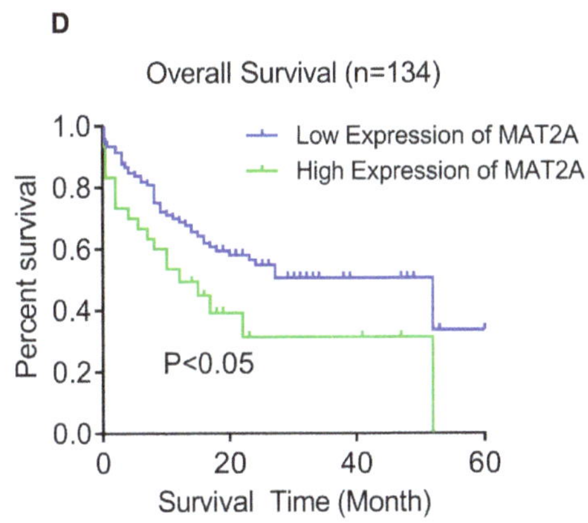

FIGURE 4 | Increased MAT2A expression was significantly associated with WHO grade of glioma. **(A)** Oncomine data mining analysis of MAT2A mRNA levels in four different datasets between normal tissues and glioma. **(B)** Representative images of MAT2A immunohistochemical staining. From top to bottom: weak, moderate, and strong MAT2A staining in glioma tissue. **(C)** MAT2A staining and clinicopathological characteristics of 410 glioma patients. Categorical variables were compared using χ^2-test or Fisher's exact test. **(D)** Kaplan–Meier overall survival curves for glioma patients with low ("+1," "+2") and high ("+3") expression of DKC1 ($P < 0.05$, log-rank test).

As shown in **Figure 4B**, the tissue staining intensity was classified into weak (1), moderate (2), and strong (3) levels; of the 410 histological glioma tissues analyzed, 154 tissues (37.5%) showed weak immunostaining, 206 tissues (50.2%) showed moderate immunostaining, and 50 tissues (12.3%) showed strong immunostaining (**Figure 4C**). Statistical analysis of the staining results and patient information showed that the expression of MAT2A in glioma tissues was significantly positively correlated with WHO grade ($P < 0.001$) but not with age or histological type. To further study the effects of MAT2A on the clinical outcomes of patients with glioma, we constructed Kaplan–Meier survival curves for overall survival (**Figure 4D**). The high MAT2A expression group had a shorter survival time than the low expression group. The difference in the overall survival rate between patients with low and high MAT2A expression was statistically significant ($P < 0.05$).

MTR4 Regulates the Release of MAT2A mRNA From the Nucleus

Fan et al. (2017) discovered that competition between ALYREF and MTR4 determines whether mRNA inside the nucleus is destined for export or degradation (**Figure 5A**). Thus, we detected protein levels of MTR4 and ALYREF in U251 and found an apparent reduction in MTR4 in the MRM group (**Figure 5B**). We also overexpressed the MTR4 through transfection with a

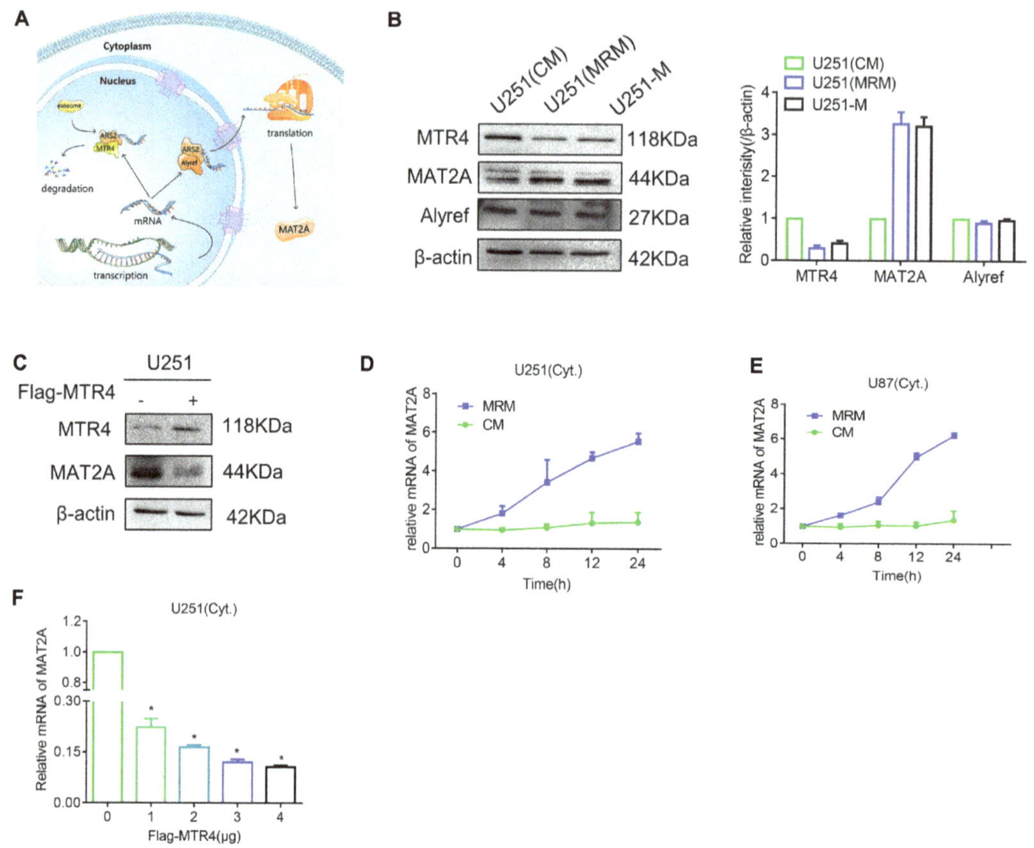

FIGURE 5 | MTR4 regulates the release of MAT2A mRNA from the nucleus. **(A)** Schematic diagram of the fate of RNA in the nucleus. If an mRNA can effectively recruit ALYREF, it will exit the nucleus smoothly and efficiently. Conversely, MTR4 may bind to ARS2, and then recruit exosomes to degrade it. **(B)** Western blotting for MAT2A, MTR4, and ALYREF in U251-M and U251 cells following culture in CM or MRM. β-actin was used as an internal control. **(C)** U251 cells were transfected with MTR4, and immunoblotting analysis was performed with the indicated antibodies. **(D,E)** U251 and U87 cells were cultured with MRM for 0, 4, 8, 12, and 24 h; the cytoplasm and nucleus were separated; and cytoplasm mRNA levels of MAT2A were analyzed by qRT-PCR. **(F)** U251 cells were transfected with MTR4 (0, 1, 2, 3, or 4 μg); again the cytoplasm and nucleus were separated, and cytoplasm mRNA levels of MAT2A were analyzed by qRT-PCR. $^*p < 0.05$.

Flag-MTR4 plasmid and noted that levels of MAT2A protein declined (**Figure 5C**). To further identify the reason for the change in MAT2A expression, we treated U251 cells with MRM for different times and separated the cytoplasm from the nucleus so that the level of MAT2A mRNA in the cytoplasm could be examined. The results showed that the level of MAT2A mRNA in the cytoplasm progressively increased over time (**Figures 5D,E**). In addition, Flag-MTR4 at several concentrations was transfected into the U251 cells to elevate the expression of MTR4 to different extents; as the expression of MTR4 increased, the level of MAT2A mRNA in the cytoplasm decreased (**Figure 5F** and **Supplementary Figures 3C,D**). This indicated that the increased level of MAT2A was due to reduced expression of MTR4 in glioma cells, which boosted the combination of MAT2A mRNA with ALYREF, resulting in the export of MAT2A mRNA.

SYVN1 Interacts With and Ubiquitinates MTR4

Next, we considered the reason for the decreased expression level of MTR4 in glioma cells in response to methionine restriction. Generally, the expression of genes is regulated by transcriptional regulation (Salminen et al., 2016), post-transcriptional regulation, and protein post-translational modification (Lamoliatte et al., 2017). Hence, we first measured levels of MTR4 mRNA in a methionine-restricted environment; no obvious decrease was observed compared with the CM group (**Figure 6A**). Next, glioma cells were treated with cycloheximide, which is a general inhibitor of protein synthesis (Chesnokov and Mertvetsov, 1990). The subsequent half-life analyses showed a more marked decline in MTR4 protein levels in the MRM group (**Figure 6B**). This suggested that protein post-translational modification might play a substantial part in regulating dynamic changes of MTR4.

Ubiquitination is the most universal means of protein degradation in eukaryotic cells. The ubiquitination reaction catalyzed by specific ubiquitin enzymes is capable of efficiently mediating the target protein into the 26S proteasome to complete the degradation reaction. We found that proteasome inhibitors MG-132 and PS341 could completely reverse the decrease in MTR4 protein levels caused by methionine restriction stimulation, whereas the autophagy inhibitor CQ could not

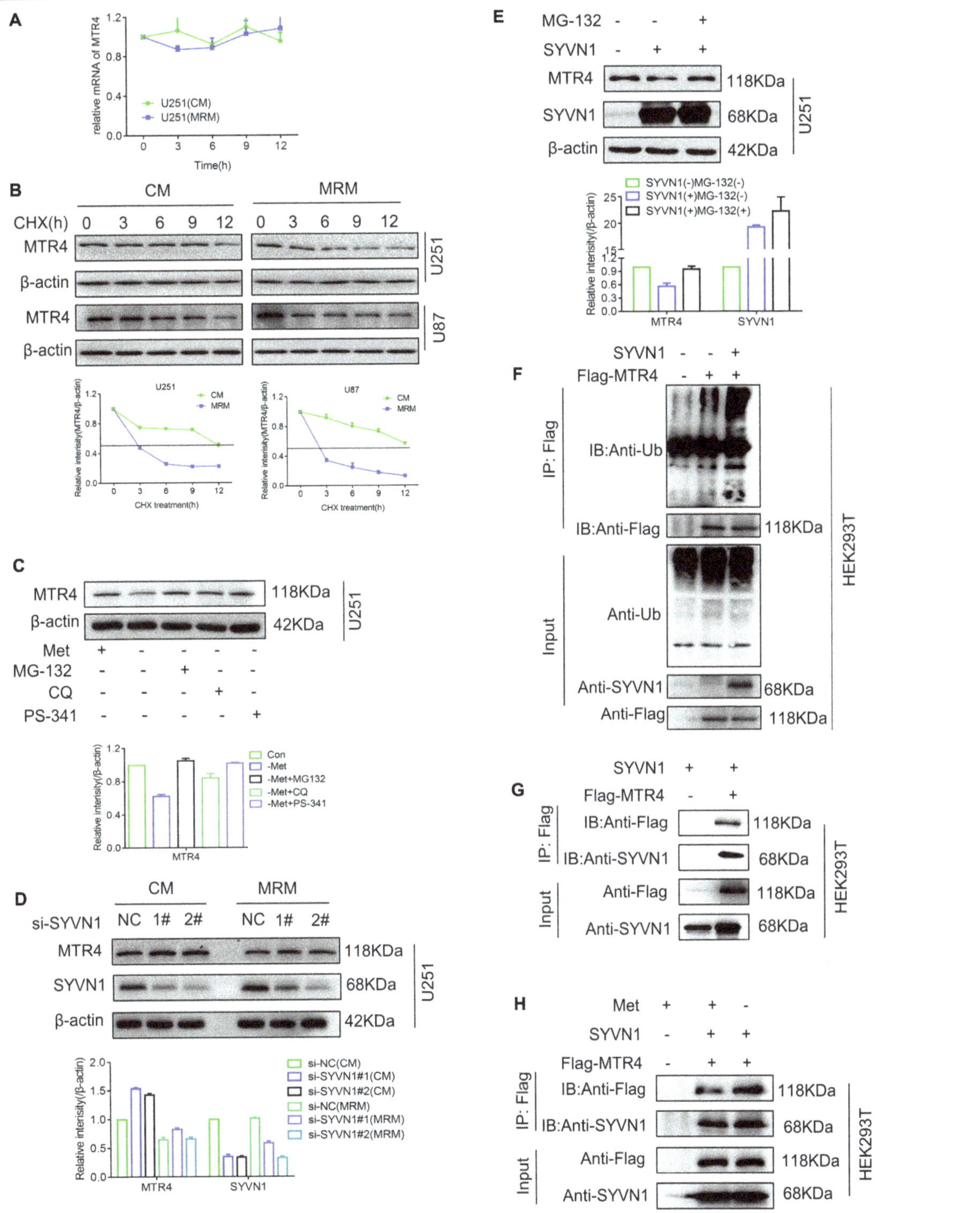

FIGURE 6 | SYVN1 interacts with and ubiquitinates MTR4. **(A)** qRT-PCR analysis of MTR4 mRNA in U251 cultured in MRM. **(B)** U251 and U87 cells stably expressing MTR4 were treated with cycloheximide (25 μg/mL), cultured in CM or MRM, and harvested at the indicated times; protein levels of MTR4 were analyzed by immunoblotting. β-actin was used as an internal control. **(C)** U251 stably expressing MTR4 were treated with MG132, CQ, and PS341 for 6 h following culture in CM or MRM, and cell lysates were immunoblotted as indicated. β-actin was used as an internal control. **(D)** Immunoblotting analysis of MTR4 protein expression in U251 cells depleted of SYVN1 by siRNA. A quantized graph is shown below the immunoblots. **(E)** U251 cells transfected with control and SYVN1 were left untreated or treated with MG132 (25 μmol/L) for 4 h, followed by immunoblotting of cell lysates as indicated. β-actin was used as an internal control. **(F)** HEK293T cells were transfected with Flag-MTR4 and SYVN1. Extracts were immunoprecipitated with anti-Flag treated protein A/G beads and examined by immunoblotting.
(G) HEK293T cells were transfected with Flag-MTR4 and SYVN1. Extracts were immunoprecipitated with anti-Flag-treated protein A/G beads and examined by immunoblotting. SYVN1 was found to interact with MTR4. **(H)** HEK293T cells were transfected with Flag-MTR4 and SYVN1 and cultivated with MRM for 24 h. Extracts were immunoprecipitated with anti-Flag treated protein A/G beads and examined by immunoblotting.

(**Figure 6C**). These results implied that the decrease in MTR4 protein was probably mediated by the ubiquitination pathway. The E3 ubiquitin ligase of MTR4 protein was predicted using the UbiBrowser website[6]; the possibilities included SYVN1, ZEB2, TRIM5, NEDD4L, and MDM2 (**Supplementary Figure 3E**). A series of screening experiments showed that there were no significant changes in levels of MTR4 protein in the cells with knockdown of E3 ubiquitin ligase SYVN1 following treatment with MRM (**Figure 6D**). Meanwhile, overexpression of SYVN1 could enhance ubiquitination of MTR4, thereby reducing MTR4 protein levels of U251, whereas MG-132 restored them (**Figures 6E,F**).

We then asked whether SYVN1 modulated MTR4 by directly interacting. We co-transfected exogenous MTR4 and SYVN1 into HEK293T cells; a co-immunoprecipitation assay showed that MTR4 indeed physically interacted with SYVN1 (**Figure 6G**). At the same time, we tested the expression of SYVN1 in resistant cells and MRM-cultured cell species (**Supplementary Figure 3F**) and found that SYVN1 did not change much, but SYVN1 bound to MTR4 increased in MRM-cultured cells (**Figure 6H**). In conclusion, it is SYVN1 that directly interacts with MTR4 to ubiquitinate it in a methionine-restricted environment.

DISCUSSION

In recent years, our understanding of malignant tumors has undergone a gradual change from "genetic disease" to "metabolic disease" (Wishart, 2015), and metabolic reprogramming has been recognized as one of the ten characteristics of tumors (Sun et al., 2018). Metabolic changes constitute a selective advantage for tumor growth, proliferation, and survival. Metabolic processes produce energy and anabolic substrates to sustain cell survival and proliferation. Tumor cells metabolize to meet the energy, biosynthesis, and oxidation-reduction reaction requirements of rapid and continuous proliferation. Methionine is an essential amino acid involved in protein synthesis, regulation of protein function, and methylation reactions (McIsaac et al., 2016). Dietary restriction of methionine has anti-aging and anti-obesogenic properties and influences cancer outcomes through controlled and reproducible changes to one-carbon metabolism (Hasek et al., 2013; Lees et al., 2014; Ables et al., 2015; Gao et al., 2019). Tumor cells are generally methionine dependent owing to the nature of their continuous proliferation. In our study, MRT cells were constructed to simulate a deficiency of methionine in glioma cells. Detection of the proliferation of MRT cells showed that they could proliferate normally in MRM, whereas their proliferation in CM was faster than that of parental cells. Sequencing of the transcriptome showed that MAT2A was enriched in multiple signaling pathways, including cell growth pathways. The metabolome of the MRT cells was detected, showing that metabolite levels changed significantly, including those involved in amino acid metabolism, sugar metabolism, and lipid metabolism. This confirmed the successful construction of the MRT cells and demonstrated that their metabolism was altered.

Methionine adenosyltransferase genes encode enzymes responsible for the biosynthesis of SAM – the principal biological methyl donor and precursor of polyamines and glutathione (Pajares and Markham, 2011; Maldonado et al., 2018). Mammalian systems express two genes, MAT1A and MAT2A, which encode MATα1 and MATα2, the catalytic subunits of the MAT isoenzymes, respectively. MAT1A is mainly expressed in the liver. Conversely, MAT2A is widely distributed in non-parenchymal cells of the liver and extrahepatic tissues (Maldonado et al., 2018; Murray et al., 2019). Changes in MAT2A directly affect levels of SAM, thereby affecting the methylation of biological macromolecules. Histone methylation plays an important part in regulating gene transcription (Gong and Miller, 2019). In liver cancer, MAT2A is closely related to cell proliferation signals, thereby regulating cell cycle progression (Zhao et al., 2018). Silencing the expression of MAT2A in the HepG2 cell line could reduce intracellular SAM and limit polyamine biosynthesis, preventing leptin's pro-survival signal, which is essential for cell growth. However, MAT2A has not been studied extensively in glioma. We found that MAT2A was significantly increased in a low-methionine environment. After inhibiting MAT2A with PF9366 or knocking out MAT2A with siRNA, cell proliferation was significantly inhibited. Combined with database and tissue microarray analysis, these results showed that MAT2A expression was positively correlated with glioma WTO grade. Survival curves showed that the expression of MAT2A was also related to the prognosis of patients. MAT2A may thus be used as a therapeutic target for glioma and an indicator to predict prognosis.

Subsequently, we explored the mechanism underlying the increase in expression of MAT2A in a methionine-restricted environment. This process starts with transcription. After the pre-mRNA produced by transcription is processed and matured in the nucleus, it is translated into protein in the ribosome following a controlled exit process. RNA that cannot exit the nucleus smoothly is degraded in the nucleus (Carmody and Wente, 2009). Pendleton et al. (2017) confirmed that in a methionine-deficient environment, m6A modification of METTL16-mediated MAT2A pre-mRNA increases, thereby promoting its maturity. Shima et al. (2017) confirmed that in a methionine-deficient environment, cells increase their expression of MAT2A mRNA to maintain SAM levels by enhancing the stability of MAT2A mRNA. We verified the conclusions of these two studies through simple experiments (**Supplementary Figures 3G,H**). We found no report on the controlled nucleation process of MAT2A mRNA. According to the current mainstream theory of RNA-controlled export, competition between MTR4 and ALYREF determines the nuclear export or degradation of mRNA in the nucleus (Fan et al., 2017). Yu et al. (2020) demonstrated the important roles of MTR4 in promoting hepatocellular carcinoma (HCC) tumorigenesis and cancer metabolic reprogramming by regulating HCC-relevant alternative splicing events through recruiting PTBP1 to its target pre-mRNAs. In the current study, we found that MTR4 expression was downregulated in a low-methionine

[6]http://ubibrowser.nb.org/

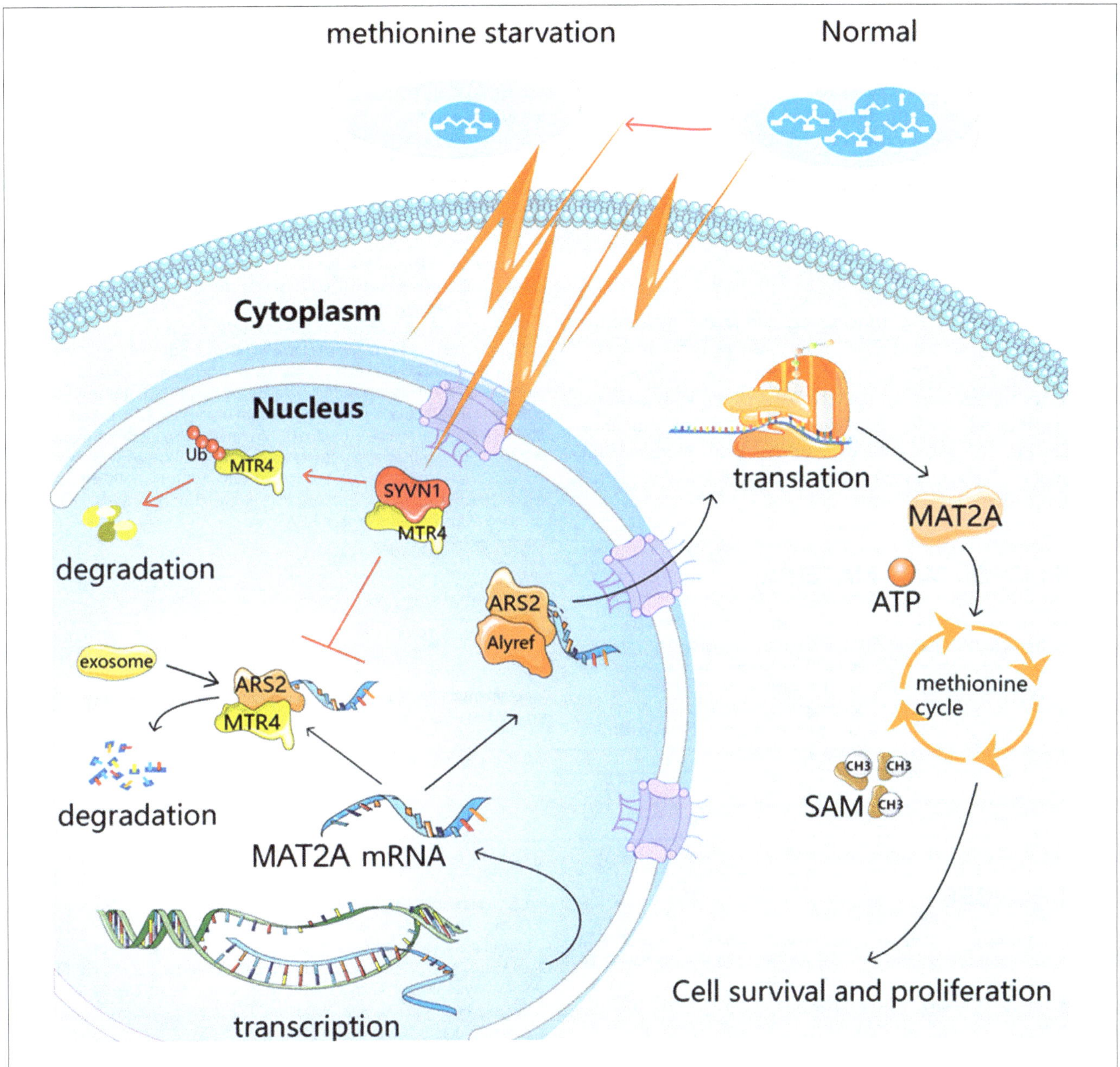

FIGURE 7 | Schematic hypothesis.

environment. Furthermore, levels of MAT2A mRNA in the cytoplasm of cells cultured in MRM and CM were detected at different times; levels of mRNA in the MRM group increased significantly compared with those in the CM group. High expression of MTR4 also affected levels of MAT2A mRNA in the cytoplasm. Therefore, we propose that MTR4 regulates the nuclear export of MAT2A mRNA. We also found that MTR4 regulates not only MAT2A but also other proteins. We believe that MTR4 plays an important part in the adaptation of glioma cells to a low-methionine environment. Owing to the lack of methionine, which is an important raw material for protein synthesis, the RNA nuclear regulation mechanism may preferentially allow genes related to cell survival and growth to be transcribed and translated, while mRNAs of genes that are relatively unimportant to cells will undergo accelerated degradation. This research group will conduct in-depth research on this issue in future studies.

Then, we investigated the mechanism by which MTR4 expression is decreased in the response of glioma cells to methionine restriction. Gene expression is regulated mainly through transcription regulation (Salminen et al., 2016), post-transcription regulation, and regulation of protein post-translational modification (Lamoliatte et al., 2017). We found that MTR4 responded to the methionine-restricted environment through ubiquitination. We also identified its E3 pantothenate ligase as SYVN1.

In summary, methionine restriction leads to enhanced binding of MTR4 and SYVN1, and increased ubiquitination; promotes the transfer of MAT2A mRNA out of the nucleus; increases MAT2A protein expression; accelerates the methionine cycle; and promotes cell proliferation in a methionine-restricted environment. This study provides a scientific basis for revealing the methionine metabolism characteristics of glioma cells and corresponding targeted therapy strategies (**Figure 7**).

AUTHOR CONTRIBUTIONS

LW: carried out the experiments and wrote the manuscript. BH: tissue microarray. KP, JC, and XZ: assisted with the experiments. LC: assisted with metabonomics analysis. HL: assisted with transcriptome analysis. JW: assisted with analyzed the experimental results. GZ: clinical information guidance. WX and JY: designed the experiments and modified the manuscript. All authors contributed to the article and approved the submitted version.

SUPPLEMENTARY MATERIAL

Supplementary Figure 1 | (A) Liquid chromatography-mass spectrometry (LC-MS)-based metabolite profiles of U251 and U251-M glioma cells based on electrospray positive ion mode. **(B)** Heatmap of global mRNA expression profiles of U251 (*n* = 3) and U251-M (*n* = 3) cells. **(C)** Volcano plot of differential mRNA expression (363 upregulated and 655 downregulated mRNAs) in U251 (*n* = 3) and U251-M (*n* = 3) cells. **(D)** GSEA plot depicting the enrichment of genes in fatty acid metabolism, biosynthesis of unsaturated fatty acids, and glycosaminoglycan degradation.

Supplementary Figure 2 | (A) Half-maximal inhibitory concentration (IC_{50}) of PF9366 used to treat U251 and U87 cells. **(B)** QRT-PCR analysis of MAT2A mRNA in U251 and U87 cells transfected with MAT2A siRNA. **(C)** Representative images of wound healing in MAT2A-knockdown and PF9366-processed U251-M cells. **(D)** Heatmap of differential mRNA expression in U251-M (*n* = 3) and U251-M cells treated with PF9366 (*n* = 3). **(E)** Volcano plot of differential mRNA expression (363 upregulated and 655 downregulated mRNAs) in U251-M (*n* = 3) and U251-M cells treated with PF9366 (*n* = 3). **(F)** GSEA plot depicting the enrichment of genes in cysteine and methionine metabolism, starch and sucrose metabolism, and DNA replication. **(G)** LC-MS-based metabolite profiles between U251-M and U251-M treated with PF9366 based on electrospray positive ion mode.

Supplementary Figure 3 | (A) Immunohistochemical staining of MAT2A (*n* = 410). **(B)** The proliferation of U251-M cells after transfection with Flag-MTR4. **(C)** U251 cells were transfected with MTR4 (0, 1, 2, 3, or 4 μg), followed by immunoblotting of cell lysates as indicated. β-actin was used as an internal control. **(D)** U251 cells were transfected with MTR4 (0 μg, 0.25 μg, 0.5 μg, 0.75 μg, or 1 μg), and then the cytoplasm and nucleus were separated, cytoplasm mRNA levels of MAT2A were analyzed by qRT-PCR. **(E)** The predicted results of MTR4 E3 ubiquitin ligase. **(F)** Western blotting for SYVN1 in U251-M and U251 cells following complete medium (CM) or methionine restriction medium (MRM). β-actin was used as an internal control. **(G)** qRT-PCR analysis of METTL16 and MAT2A mRNA in U251 cells transfected with METTL16 siRNA. **(H)** U251 cells were treated with actinomycin D (5 μg/mL), cultivated in CM or MRM, and harvested at the indicated times; mRNA levels of MAT2A were analyzed by qRT-PCR.

Supplementary Table 1 | Identities of differential metabolites between U251 and U251-M.

Supplementary Table 2 | Identities of differential metabolites between U251-M and U251-M+PF9366.

REFERENCES

Ables, G. P., Ouattara, A., Hampton, T. G., Cooke, D., Perodin, F., Augie, I., et al. (2015). Dietary methionine restriction in mice elicits an adaptive cardiovascular response to hyperhomocysteinemia. *Sci. Rep.* 5:8886.

Andersen, P. R., Domanski, M., Kristiansen, M. S., Storvall, H., Ntini, E., Verheggen, C., et al. (2013). The human cap-binding complex is functionally connected to the nuclear RNA exosome. *Nat. Struct. Mol. Biol.* 20, 1367–1376. doi: 10.1038/nsmb.2703

Anstee, Q. M., and Day, C. P. (2012). S-adenosylmethionine (SAMe) therapy in liver disease: a review of current evidence and clinical utility. *J. Hepatol.* 57, 1097–1109. doi: 10.1016/j.jhep.2012.04.041

Carmody, S. R., and Wente, S. R. (2009). mRNA nuclear export at a glance. *J. Cell Sci.* 122, 1933–1937. doi: 10.1242/jcs.041236

Chesnokov, V. N., and Mertvetsov, N. P. (1990). [The effect of translation inhibitor cycloheximide on expression of mammalian genes]. *Biokhimiia* 55, 1276–1278.

Chi, B., Wang, Q., Wu, G., Tan, M., Wang, L., Shi, M., et al. (2013). Aly and THO are required for assembly of the human TREX complex and association of TREX components with the spliced mRNA. *Nucleic Acids Res.* 41, 1294–1306. doi: 10.1093/nar/gks1188

Ducker, G. S., and Rabinowitz, J. D. (2017). One-Carbon metabolism in health and disease. *Cell Metab.* 25, 27–42. doi: 10.1016/j.cmet.2016.08.009

Fan, J., Kuai, B., Wu, G., Wu, X., Chi, B., Wang, L., et al. (2017). Exosome cofactor hMTR4 competes with export adaptor ALYREF to ensure balanced nuclear RNA pools for degradation and export. *EMBO J.* 36, 2870–2886. doi: 10.15252/embj.201696139

Gao, X., Sanderson, S. M., Dai, Z., Reid, M. A., Cooper, D. E., Lu, M., et al. (2019). Dietary methionine influences therapy in mouse cancer models and alters human metabolism. *Nature* 572, 397–401. doi: 10.1038/s41586-019-1437-3

Glaudemans, A. W., Enting, R. H., Heesters, M. A., Dierckx, R. A., van Rheenen, R. W., Walenkamp, A. M., et al. (2013). Value of 11C-methionine PET in imaging brain tumours and metastases. *Eur. J. Nucl. Med. Mol. Imaging* 40, 615–635. doi: 10.1007/s00259-012-2295-5

Gong, F., and Miller, K. M. (2019). Histone methylation and the DNA damage response. *Mutat. Res.* 780, 37–47. doi: 10.1016/j.mrrev.2017.09.003

Hasek, B. E., Boudreau, A., Shin, J., Feng, D., Hulver, M., Van, N. T., et al. (2013). Remodeling the integration of lipid metabolism between liver and adipose tissue by dietary methionine restriction in rats. *Diabetes* 62, 3362–3372. doi: 10.2337/db13-0501

He, Q., Zhang, L., Zhang, B., Shi, X., Yi, C., and Zhang, X. (2019). Diagnostic accuracy of (13)N-ammonia PET, (11)C-methionine PET and (18)F-fluorodeoxyglucose PET: a comparative study in patients with suspected cerebral glioma. *BMC Cancer* 19:332. doi: 10.1186/s12885-019-5560-1

Jain, M., Nilsson, R., Sharma, S., Madhusudhan, N., Kitami, T., Souza, A. L., et al. (2012). Metabolite profiling identifies a key role for glycine in rapid cancer cell proliferation. *Science* 336, 1040–1044. doi: 10.1126/science.1218595

Kaelin, W. G. Jr., and McKnight, S. L. (2013). Influence of metabolism on epigenetics and disease. *Cell* 153, 56–69. doi: 10.1016/j.cell.2013.03.004

Lamoliatte, F., McManus, F. P., Maarifi, G., Chelbi-Alix, M. K., and Thibault, P. (2017). Uncovering the SUMOylation and ubiquitylation crosstalk in human cells using sequential peptide immunopurification. *Nat. Commun.* 8: 14109.

Lees, E. K., Krol, E., Grant, L., Shearer, K., Wyse, C., Moncur, E., et al. (2014). Methionine restriction restores a younger metabolic phenotype in adult mice with alterations in fibroblast growth factor 21. *Aging Cell* 13, 817–827. doi: 10.1111/acel.12238

LeGros, H. L. Jr., Halim, A. B., Geller, A. M., and Kotb, M. (2000). Cloning, expression, and functional characterization of the beta regulatory subunit of human methionine adenosyltransferase (MAT II). *J. Biol. Chem.* 275, 2359–2366. doi: 10.1074/jbc.275.4.2359

Lubas, M., Christensen, M. S., Kristiansen, M. S., Domanski, M., Falkenby, L. G., Lykke-Andersen, S., et al. (2011). Interaction profiling identifies the human nuclear exosome targeting complex. *Mol. Cell* 43, 624–637. doi: 10.1016/j.molcel.2011.06.028

Luckerath, K., Lapa, C., Albert, C., Herrmann, K., Jorg, G., Samnick, S., et al. (2015). 11C-Methionine-PET: a novel and sensitive tool for monitoring of early response to treatment in multiple myeloma. *Oncotarget* 6, 8418–8429. doi: 10.18632/oncotarget.3053

Maldonado, L. Y., Arsene, D., Mato, J. M., and Lu, S. C. (2018). Methionine adenosyltransferases in cancers: mechanisms of dysregulation and implications for therapy. *Exp. Biol. Med. (Maywood)* 243, 107–117. doi: 10.1177/1535370217740860

Marjon, K., Cameron, M. J., Quang, P., Clasquin, M. F., Mandley, E., Kunii, K., et al. (2016). MTAP deletions in cancer create vulnerability to targeting of the MAT2A/PRMT5/RIOK1 axis. *Cell Rep.* 15, 574–587. doi: 10.1016/j.celrep.2016.03.043

Masuda, S., Das, R., Cheng, H., Hurt, E., Dorman, N., and Reed, R. (2005). Recruitment of the human TREX complex to mRNA during splicing. *Genes Dev.* 19, 1512–1517. doi: 10.1101/gad.1302205

McIsaac, R. S., Lewis, K. N., Gibney, P. A., and Buffenstein, R. (2016). From yeast to human: exploring the comparative biology of methionine restriction in extending eukaryotic life span. *Ann. N. Y. Acad. Sci. U.S.A.* 1363, 155–170. doi: 10.1111/nyas.13032

Meola, N., Domanski, M., Karadoulama, E., Chen, Y., Gentil, C., Pultz, D., et al. (2016). Identification of a nuclear exosome decay pathway for processed transcripts. *Mol. Cell* 64, 520–533. doi: 10.1016/j.molcel.2016.09.025

Moore, G. E., Gerner, R. E., and Franklin, H. A. (1967). Culture of normal human leukocytes. *JAMA* 199, 519–524. doi: 10.1001/jama.199.8.519

Murray, B., Barbier-Torres, L., Fan, W., Mato, J. M., and Lu, S. C. (2019). Methionine adenosyltransferases in liver cancer. *World J. Gastroenterol.* 25, 4300–4319. doi: 10.3748/wjg.v25.i31.4300

Nencioni, A., Caffa, I., Cortellino, S., and Longo, V. D. (2018). Fasting and cancer: molecular mechanisms and clinical application. *Nat. Rev. Cancer* 18, 707–719. doi: 10.1038/s41568-018-0061-0

Ostrom, Q. T., Bauchet, L., Davis, F. G., Deltour, I., Fisher, J. L., Langer, C. E., et al. (2014). The epidemiology of glioma in adults: a "state of the science" review. *Neuro Oncol.* 16, 896–913. doi: 10.1093/neuonc/nou087

Pajares, M. A., Alvarez, L., and Perez-Sala, D. (2013). How are mammalian methionine adenosyltransferases regulated in the liver? A focus on redox stress. *FEBS Lett.* 587, 1711–1716. doi: 10.1016/j.febslet.2013.04.034

Pajares, M. A., and Markham, G. D. (2011). Methionine adenosyltransferase (s-adenosylmethionine synthetase). *Adv. Enzymol. Relat. Areas Mol. Biol.* 78, 449–521. doi: 10.1002/9781118105771.ch11

Pavlova, N. N., and Thompson, C. B. (2016). The emerging hallmarks of cancer metabolism. *Cell Metab.* 23, 27–47. doi: 10.1016/j.cmet.2015.12.006

Pendleton, K. E., Chen, B., Liu, K., Hunter, O. V., Xie, Y., Tu, B. P., et al. (2017). The U6 snRNA m(6)A methyltransferase METTL16 regulates SAM synthetase intron retention. *Cell* 169, 824–835.e14.

Poljsak, B., Kovac, V., Dahmane, R., Levec, T., and Starc, A. (2019). Cancer etiology: a metabolic disease originating from life's major evolutionary transition? *Oxid. Med. Cell. Longev.* 2019:7831952.

Quinlan, C. L., Kaiser, S. E., Bolanos, B., Nowlin, D., Grantner, R., Karlicek-Bryant, S., et al. (2017). Targeting S-adenosylmethionine biosynthesis with a novel allosteric inhibitor of Mat2A. *Nat. Chem. Biol.* 13, 785–792. doi: 10.1038/nchembio.2384

Riabovol, O. O., Tsymbal, D. O., Minchenko, D. O., Lebid-Biletska, K. M., Sliusar, M. Y., Rudnytska, O. V., et al. (2019). Effect of glucose deprivation on the expression of genes encoding glucocorticoid receptor and some related factors in ERN1-knockdown U87 glioma cells. *Endocr. Regul.* 53, 237–249. doi: 10.2478/enr-2019-0024

Salminen, A., Kaarniranta, K., and Kauppinen, A. (2016). Hypoxia-Inducible histone lysine demethylases: impact on the aging process and age-related diseases. *Aging Dis.* 7, 180–200. doi: 10.14336/ad.2015.0929

Sanderson, S. M., Gao, X., Dai, Z., and Locasale, J. W. (2019). Methionine metabolism in health and cancer: a nexus of diet and precision medicine. *Nat. Rev. Cancer* 19, 625–637. doi: 10.1038/s41568-019-0187-8

Shi, M., Zhang, H., Wu, X., He, Z., Wang, L., Yin, S., et al. (2017). ALYREF mainly binds to the 5′ and the 3′ regions of the mRNA in vivo. *Nucleic Acids Res.* 45, 9640–9653. doi: 10.1093/nar/gkx597

Shima, H., Matsumoto, M., Ishigami, Y., Ebina, M., Muto, A., Sato, Y., et al. (2017). S-Adenosylmethionine synthesis is regulated by selective N(6)-adenosine methylation and mRNA degradation involving METTL16 and YTHDC1. *Cell Rep.* 21, 3354–3363. doi: 10.1016/j.celrep.2017.11.092

Strasser, K., Masuda, S., Mason, P., Pfannstiel, J., Oppizzi, M., Rodriguez-Navarro, S., et al. (2002). TREX is a conserved complex coupling transcription with messenger RNA export. *Nature* 417, 304–308. doi: 10.1038/nature746

Sun, L., Suo, C., Li, S. T., Zhang, H., and Gao, P. (2018). Metabolic reprogramming for cancer cells and their microenvironment: beyond the Warburg effect. *Biochim. Biophys. Acta Rev. Cancer* 1870, 51–66. doi: 10.1016/j.bbcan.2018.06.005

Trapnell, C., Pachter, L., and Salzberg, S. L. (2009). TopHat: discovering splice junctions with RNA-Seq. *Bioinformatics* 25, 1105–1111. doi: 10.1093/bioinformatics/btp120

Trapnell, C., Williams, B. A., Pertea, G., Mortazavi, A., Kwan, G., van Baren, M. J., et al. (2010). Transcript assembly and quantification by RNA-Seq reveals unannotated transcripts and isoform switching during cell differentiation. *Nat. Biotechnol.* 28, 511–515. doi: 10.1038/nbt.1621

Vermeulen, M., Eberl, H. C., Matarese, F., Marks, H., Denissov, S., Butter, F., et al. (2010). Quantitative interaction proteomics and genome-wide profiling of epigenetic histone marks and their readers. *Cell* 142, 967–980. doi: 10.1016/j.cell.2010.08.020

Wang, L., Feng, Z., Wang, X., Wang, X., and Zhang, X. (2010). DEGseq: an R package for identifying differentially expressed genes from RNA-seq data. *Bioinformatics* 26, 136–138. doi: 10.1093/bioinformatics/btp612

Wang, Z., Yip, L. Y., Lee, J. H. J., Wu, Z., Chew, H. Y., Chong, P. K. W., et al. (2019). Methionine is a metabolic dependency of tumor-initiating cells. *Nat. Med.* 25, 825–837.

Wishart, D. S. (2015). Is cancer a genetic disease or a metabolic disease? *EBioMedicine* 2, 478–479. doi: 10.1016/j.ebiom.2015.05.022

Xia, S., Lin, R., Jin, L., Zhao, L., Kang, H. B., Pan, Y., et al. (2017). Prevention of dietary-fat-fueled ketogenesis attenuates BRAF V600E tumor growth. *Cell Metab.* 25, 358–373. doi: 10.1016/j.cmet.2016.12.010

Yu, L., Kim, J., Jiang, L., Feng, B., Ying, Y., Ji, K. Y., et al. (2020). MTR4 drives liver tumorigenesis by promoting cancer metabolic switch through alternative splicing. *Nat. Commun.* 11:708.

Zhao, C., Wu, H., Qimuge, N., Pang, W., Li, X., Chu, G., et al. (2018). MAT2A promotes porcine adipogenesis by mediating H3K27me3 at Wnt10b locus and repressing Wnt/beta-catenin signaling. *Biochim. Biophys. Acta Mol. Cell Biol. Lipids* 1863, 132–142. doi: 10.1016/j.bbalip.2017.11.001

16

Pan-Cancer Analysis of NOS3 Identifies its Expression and Clinical Relevance in Gastric Cancer

Dan Zou [1], Zhi Li [2], Fei Lv [1], Yi Yang [3], Chunjiao Yang [1], Jincheng Song [1,4], Yang Chen [5], Zi Jin [6], Jinpeng Zhou [7], Yang Jiang [7,8], Yanju Ma [9], Zhitao Jing [7], Yu Tang [9] and Ye Zhang [1]*

[1] The First Laboratory of Cancer Institute, The First Hospital of China Medical University, Shenyang, China, [2] Department of Medical Oncology, The First Hospital of China Medical University, Shenyang, China, [3] Laboratory Animal Center, China Medical University, Shenyang, China, [4] Lymphoma and Myeloma Diagnosis and Treatment Center, The Second Affiliated Hospital of Dalian Medical University, Dalian, China, [5] Department of Respiratory and Infectious Disease of Geriatrics, The First Hospital of China Medical University, Shenyang, China, [6] The First Department of Oncology, Shenyang Fifth People's Hospital, Shenyang, China, [7] Department of Neurosurgery, The First Hospital of China Medical University, Shenyang, China, [8] Department of Neurosurgery, Shanghai General Hospital, Shanghai Jiao Tong University School of Medicine, Shanghai, China, [9] Department of Medical Oncology, Cancer Hospital of China Medical University, Liaoning Cancer Hospital & Insititute, Shenyang, China

***Correspondence:**
Ye Zhang
zhangyecmu@163.com

Background: *NOS3* (endothelial NOS, *eNOS*) is a member of the nitric oxide synthase (NOS) enzyme family, mainly participating in nitric oxide (NO) generation. *NOS3* has been reported to inhibit apoptosis and promote angiogenesis, proliferation, and invasiveness. However, the expression pattern of *NOS3* and its diagnostic and prognostic potential has not been investigated in a pan-cancer perspective.

Methods: Data from the Genotype-Tissue Expression (GTEx), the Cancer Genome Atlas (TCGA), the Cancer Cell Line Encyclopedia (CCLE), and the Cancer Therapeutics Response Portal (CTRP) were employed and *NOS3* expression was comprehensively analyzed in normal tissues, cancer tissues, and cell lines. Immunohistochemical staining of tissue sections were used to validate the prognostic role of *NOS3* in gastric cancer patients. GSVA and GSEA analyses were performed to investigate signaling pathways related to *NOS3* expression.

Results: In normal tissues, *NOS3* was expressed highest in the spleen and lowest in the blood. *NOS3* expression was increased in stomach adenocarcinoma (STAD) and significantly associated with poor prognosis of patients. Immunohistochemical staining validated that *NOS3* was an independent prognostic factor of gastric cancer. Several canonical cancer-related pathways were found to be correlated with *NOS3* expression in STAD. The expression of NOS3 was related to the response to QS-11 and brivinib in STAD.

Conclusions: *NOS3* was an independent prognostic factor for patients with STAD. Increased expression of *NOS3* influenced occurrence and development of STAD through several canonical cancer-related pathways. Drug response analysis reported drugs to suppress NOS3. NOS3 might be a novel target for gastric cancer treatment.

Keywords: NOS3, pan-cancer, gene expression, gastric cancer, eNOS

INTRODUCTION

NOS3 (endothelial NOS, eNOS) is a member of the nitric oxide synthase (NOS) enzyme family, which is a cluster of catalytic enzymes that mainly participate in nitric oxide (NO) generation (1). The *NOS3* protein is encoded by the *NOS3* gene, located on chromosome 7q36.1. Usually, *NOS3* protein is constitutively expressed in cells in an inactive state. Following the increase in calcium (Ca^{2+}) concentration in cells, it can be activated by combining with the CaM protein. In addition, the direct combination of *NOS3* with caveolin-1 (CAV-1) and heat shock protein 90 (HSP90) and the phosphorylation (Ser-1177) of *NOS3* by PI3K/Akt signaling can modulate the activity of *NOS3* protein (2–4).

NOS3 protein was initially found to participate in NO generation, mainly in endothelial cells, and is associated with cardiovascular diseases such as hypertension, atherosclerosis, and diabetes mellitus (5). In recent years, *NOS3* has been found to play various roles in malignant tumors, such as inhibiting apoptosis and promoting angiogenesis, proliferation, invasiveness, and immunosuppression (6–8). Circulating *NOS3* levels were inversely correlated with progression-free survival and overall survival (OS) of metastatic colorectal cancer patients (9). Another research in mesenchymal colorectal cancer patients reported that *NOS3* upregulation occurs after Apc loss, which was associated with poor prognosis (10). In breast cancer, the increasing expression of *NOS3* was reported to be a pro-angiogenic factor (11). It was found to promote angiogenesis via PI3K/Akt/mTOR pathway, and enhance the migration and invasion via NOS3-NO-sGC-cGMP signaling in breast cancer cells (12, 13). In pancreatic cancer, *NOS3* promoted tumor maintenance through the PI3K-Akt-NOS3-RAS (wild type) pathway (14). *NOS3* inhibition by the inhibitor N(G)-nitro-L-arginine methyl ester (L-NAME) could suppress pancreatic ductal adenocarcinoma cancer (PDAC) tumor growth (15). *NOS3* activation was reported to promote the antiandrogen-resistant growth through NO-mediated AR suppression in prostate cancer (PCa) (16). And *NOS3* was found to participate in promoting aggressive phenotype of PCa, resulting in poor prognosis in PCa patients (17). In addition, Trachootham et al. found that non-tumorigenic epithelial cells from oral and ovarian tissue could be induced to become invasive in stroma containing p53-deficient fibroblasts, through NOS3/RNS/ICAM1 signaling (18). NOS3 was also found to participate in oncogenic inflammation and immunosuppression of tumors through NOTCH1-PI3K/AKT-NOS3 axis (19). *NOS3* expression inhibition was involved in cervical cancer cell sensitivity to radiotherapy (20). Additionally, many studies have reported that *NOS3* gene polymorphisms are associated with risk for cancer progression, cancer susceptibility and drug response (21–23). However, research by Smeda et al. reported that *NOS3* activity and phosphorylation reduction was an early event in the lung metastasis of breast cancer, preceding the onset of the mesenchymal phenotype (EndMT) (24). *NOS3* participated in the enhancement of Taxol chemosensitivity with astragaloside IV treatment in breast cancer as a downstream target of caveolin-1 (25). These studies suggest that *NOS3* may perform multiple functions depending on different tumor types, and genetic background. Studies on *NOS3* expression in tumors are still scarce, and the functions of *NOS3* in tumor pathogenesis, especially in gastric cancer, are not comprehensively understood.

By applying data from the Genotype-Tissue Expression (GTEx; https://www.gtexportal.org/home/), the Cancer Genome Atlas (TCGA; https://portal.gdc.cancer.gov/) and the Cancer Cell Line Encyclopedia (CCLE; https://portals.broadinstitute.org/ccle/), the expression level of *NOS3* in 30 different normal human tissues and 33 different tumors types, as well as the corresponding normal tissues and 1,457 cancer cell lines was systematically analyzed. We investigated the relationship between *NOS3* expression and the clinical phenotypes of patients for all cancers and then separately for each cancer type. Subsequently, GSVA and GSEA analyses were performed to investigate signaling pathways related to *NOS3* expression. Subsequently, *NOS3* protein level was individually assessed in gastric cancer tissues. Ultimately, the correlation between *NOS3* expression level in 664 cancer cells and cell response to 544 drugs was analyzed to explore the potential of *NOS3* as a therapeutic target.

MATERIALS AND METHODS

Download of TCGA and GTEx Datasets

TOIL GTEx and TCGA (primary tumor and normal tissues) gene expression RNA-seq data (IlluminaHiSeq: log2-normalized_count+ 1) and TCGA phenotype data, containing 9359 TCGA tumor tissues, 727 TCGA normal tissues and 7792 GTEx normal tissues, were obtained from UCSC Xena (https://xena.ucsc.edu/). TOIL reprocesses raw GTEx and TCGA RNA-seq data to correct for batch effects and to allow for the merging of samples across GTEx and TCGA datasets for pan-analyses (26).

Analyses of *NOS3* Differential Expression in Tumor and Normal Tissues

To analyze the differential expression of *NOS3* between TCGA tumors and normal tissues, *t*-test was applied for tumor types with at least two normal tissues. The median gene expression level was employed to calculate the fold change. Then, the log2-fold change (cancer vs. normal) was employed as the x-axis and -log10 *p*-value was employed as the y-axis to produce a Volcano plot for each tumor type. The expression profiles *NOS3* mRNA within and between tumor types were graphed using GraphPad Prism (version 7) (San Diego, CA, USA).

Analyses of *NOS3* Expression and Clinical Phenotypes

NOS3 expression levels among different tumor stages (TNM stage) were assessed by *t*-test (for two groups) and ANOVA analyses (for three and more groups). To assess the relationship of *NOS3* expression to overall survival (diagnosis to death), the median of *NOS3* expression in each tumor was used as cutoff value to divide patients into two groups, and Cox proportional hazards models were employed. OS time was defined as the time from the day at diagnosis to the date of death (dead patients) or the date of the last follow-up. Cox proportional hazards model was used to generate hazard ratio (HR) and 95% confidence interval (CI) for each cancer types. Kaplan-Meier survival analysis and the log-rank test was applied to calculate *p*-value. A forest plot was constructed to visually display the hazard ratio (HR) and 95% CI for each tumor type. $p < 0.05$ was considered a significant correlation. The survival curve and forest plot were generated by GraphPad Prism.

GSEA and GSVA Analyses

Gene Set Enrichment Analyses (GSEA) was performed by GSEA v4.1.0 (www.broadinstitute.org/gsea) to detect discrepantly enriched signaling pathways between *NOS3* higher and lower group. The gene set "c2.cp.kegg.v7.1.symbols.gmt" from MSigDB gene set was selected as reference gene set. Signaling pathways with normalized $p < 0.05$, normalized enrichment score (NES) >1.5 and false discovery rate (FDR) $q < 0.25$ was considered as statistically significant.

We utilized the R package "GSVA" to perform Gene Set Variation Analysis (GSVA) analyses of *NOS3* expression to find the pathways most associated with *NOS3* expression. $P < 0.05$ was regarded as statistically significant. The gene set "c2.cp.kegg.v7.1.symbols.gmt," was selected as the reference gene set. Signaling pathways commonly enriched by GSEA and GSVA analysis were considered to be potential pathways related to *NOS3* expression.

Cell Lines *NOS3* Expression

NOS3 mRNA expression, promoter DNA methylation, and copy number data were downloaded from the Cancer Cell Line Encyclopedia (CCLE, https://portals.broadinstitute.org/ccle/), which contained RNA-seq data, DNA methylation data from the matching reduced representation bisulfite sequencing (RRBS) and copy number data of 1,457 human cancer cell lines. *NOS3* expression levels among different cell lines of different cancer types were investigated. Box plots and scatter plots were downloaded from the CCLE website. The relation of *NOS3* mRNA to promoter DNA methylation and copy number was evaluated by Spearman correlation analysis.

Drug Responses

The drug response data were obtained from the Cancer Therapeutics Response Portal (CTRP, https://portals.broadinstitute.org/ctrp.v2.1/), which contained the responses of 664 cell lines to 482 drugs. Spearman correlation analyses was also performed to evaluate the association of *NOS3* expression with drug responses (area under the curve, AUC) first for all cell lines together and then individually in STAD. Then, correlation *r*-value was employed as the x-axis and -log10 *p*-value was employed as the y-axis to produce a Volcano plot. NOS3 mRNA was used as x-axis and AUC was used as y-axis to generate a scatter plot. The volcano and scatter plots were plotted using GraphPad Prism.

Immunohistochemical Staining and Result Analysis of Patients

In total, 90 clinical samples from gastric cancer patients were collected from the First Affiliated Hospital of China Medical University (Shenyang, China) from January 2013 to December 2014. Demographic and clinical characteristics such as age at initial diagnosis, gender, initial diagnosis date, and tumor stage were also collected. All the patients provided informed consent. And this study was approved by the ethics committee of the First Affiliated Hospital of China Medical University.

Formalin-fixed tissues were embedded in paraffin and cut into 5-μm thick sections for H&E staining and immunohistochemical staining. The expression level of *NOS3* was detected by streptavidin-peroxidase method. Antigen of de-waxed sections were exposed to 3% H_2O_2 for 10 min at room temperature to quench the endogenous peroxidase activity. Then the tissues were blocked with goat serum for 30 min at room temperature. After incubation with *NOS3* primary antibody (Abcam, 1:100) overnight at 4°C, tissues were incubated with the secondary antibody (10 min) and biotin-labeled horseradish peroxidase (10 min). Next, 3,30-diaminobenzidine tetrahydrochloride (DAB) kit (Maixin, China) was used to visualize the antibody binding. Eventually, immunohistochemical staining was observed under an inverted phase contrast microscope.

Immunoreactivity was dependently evaluated using semi-quantitatively method by two investigators. Five representative regions were randomly selected from the 400-fold field of view of the microscope. The immunoreactive score was determined by the proportion of positive cells and the staining intensity. The proportion of positive cells was scored as follows: <9%, 0; 10–25%, 1; 26–50%, 2; 51–75%, 3; 76–100%, 4. The staining intensity was scored as follows: 0 for no staining, 1 for light yellow, 2 for yellow, and 3 for brown. The final immunoreactive score was the product of the two scores.

Statistical Analyses

For all statistical analyses, a $p < 0.05$ was considered statistically significant. All statistical analyses and visualization were accomplished by using GraphPad Prism 7 and R software (R version 3.6.0).

RESULTS

NOS3 mRNA Expression in Various Normal Tissues and Tumors

To comprehensively analyze *NOS3* expression and distribution in human normal tissues and tumor tissues, we first analyzed *NOS3* mRNA expression level in 30 different normal tissues from GTEx and 33 different tumor tissues from Xena (https://xenabrowser.net/). The expression of *NOS3* was highly variable across different normal tissues and tumor tissues (**Figure 1, Supplementary Figure 1**). In normal tissues, the median *NOS3* expression levels varied from 5.624 (blood) to 12.8 (spleen). Tissues with the highest *NOS3* expression were spleen (12.8 ± 1.391), heart (10.64 ± 1.099), testis (10.59 ± 0.532). Tissues with

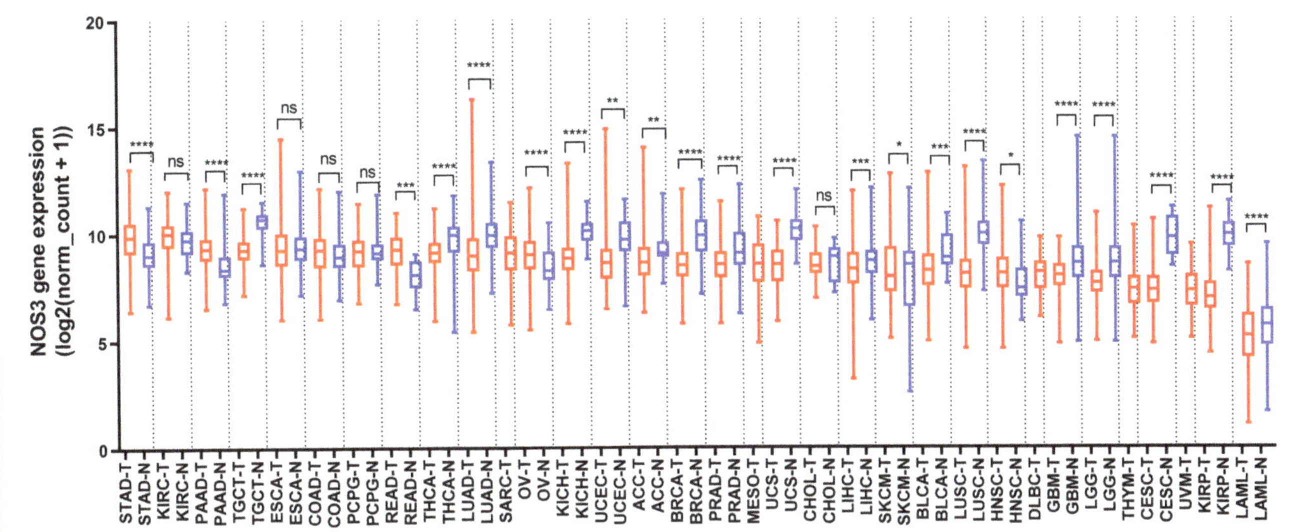

FIGURE 1 | *NOS3* mRNA expression in various normal tissues and tumors. *NOS3* is differentially expressed between tumor and normal tissues in some cancers from TCGA and GTEx databases. Each boxplot represents *NOS3* expression [RNA-seq RSEM, log2(normalized count +1)] across different cancers. Red is for tumors and blue is for normal tissues. The bar represents median expression of tumors or normal tissues and lower and upper box ends represent the 25th and 75th percentile expression. ns, without statistical significance, $^{*}p < 0.05$, $^{**}p < 0.01$, $^{***}p < 0.001$, $^{****}p < 0.0001$, based on Student's *t*-test.

the lowest *NOS3* expression were blood (5.624 ± 1.325), skin (7.904 ± 1.753), pancreas (8.363 ± 1.159).

In tumor tissues, *NOS3* expression levels varied from 9.85 (stomach adenocarcinoma, STAD) to 5.071 (acute myeloid leukemia, LAML). Tumor tissues with the highest *NOS3* expression were STAD (9.85 ± 1.018), kidney renal clear cell carcinoma (KIRC, 9.848 ± 0.9791), pancreatic adenocarcinoma (PAAD, 9.297 ± 0.8167). Tumor tissues with the lowest *NOS3* expression were LAML (5.071 ± 1.591), kidney renal papillary cell carcinoma (KIRP, 7.173 ± 1.14), uveal melanoma (UVM, 7.278 ± 0.9764).

NOS3 mRNA Expression in Tumor Cell Lines

Considering that tissue-based RNA expression detection might be complicated by the non-tumor tissues that are adjacent to tumor cells, we analyzed *NOS3* mRNA expression in 1457 cell lines derived from 26 tumor types in the CCLE database. Initially, *NOS3* expression in different cell lines was checked and the results showed that cell lines from STAD and COAD were the top two cell lines expressing the highest levels of *NOS3* mRNA, and cell lines from nerve system tissues (e.g., GBM and neuroblastoma) and bone tissues (e.g., chondrosarcoma and osteosarcoma) expressed relatively lower *NOS3* mRNA (**Figure 2A**). Interestingly, *NOS3* in STAD was expressed at the highest level both in stomach tissues from TCGA and in stomach cell lines from CCLE. Further analysis of the association between *NOS3* mRNA and promoter DNA methylation level showed a weak correlation (Spearman correlation coefficient = 0.1282, $p = 0.0002$, **Figure 2B**). Spearman correlation analysis between *NOS3* mRNA and copy number did not show statistical significance ($p = 0.1193$, **Figure 2C**). These results indicated that promoter DNA methylation and copy number variants of the *NOS3* gene might not be the main determinant of *NOS3* mRNA levels. *Tumor necrosis factor (TNF)-α* was reported to decrease functional activity of *NOS3* mRNA 3′-untranslated region (3′-UTR), regulating the translation process (27). In this research, we further determined the correlation between TNF-α mRNA and *NOS3* mRNA to verity if *TNF-α* affect transcription process of *NOS3*. However, there was only a weak correlation between them (spearman $r = 0.1119$, $p = 0.003$), suggesting that *TNF-α* might affect expression to a certain extent, but not a decisive factor (**Supplementary Figure 2**).

NOS3 Is Differentially Expressed in Various Tumors and Their Corresponding Normal Tissues

We analyzed *NOS3* mRNA expression levels across tumors and their corresponding normal tissues in 28 tumor types that had three or more normal tissues data based on TCGA and GTEx database (**Figure 1**). *NOS3* mRNA expression in 6 of 28 tumor types, rectum adenocarcinoma (READ), STAD, PAAD, ovarian serous cystadenocarcinoma (OV), skin cutaneous melanoma (SKCM), head and neck squamous cell carcinoma (HNSC), was much higher than that in corresponding normal tissues, with statistical significance. Furthermore, we analyzed fold change (FC) of *NOS3* mRNA between tumor and corresponding normal tissues (**Figures 3A,B**). The FC in READ, STAD, PAAD, OV, SKCM, and HNSC ranged from 1.276 to 2.180. In cancer tissues and cancer cell lines, *NOS3* mRNA expressed highest in STAD. The differential analysis results showed that expression of *NOS3* in cancer tissues is 1.765-fold higher than that of corresponding normal tissues ($p < 0.0001$).

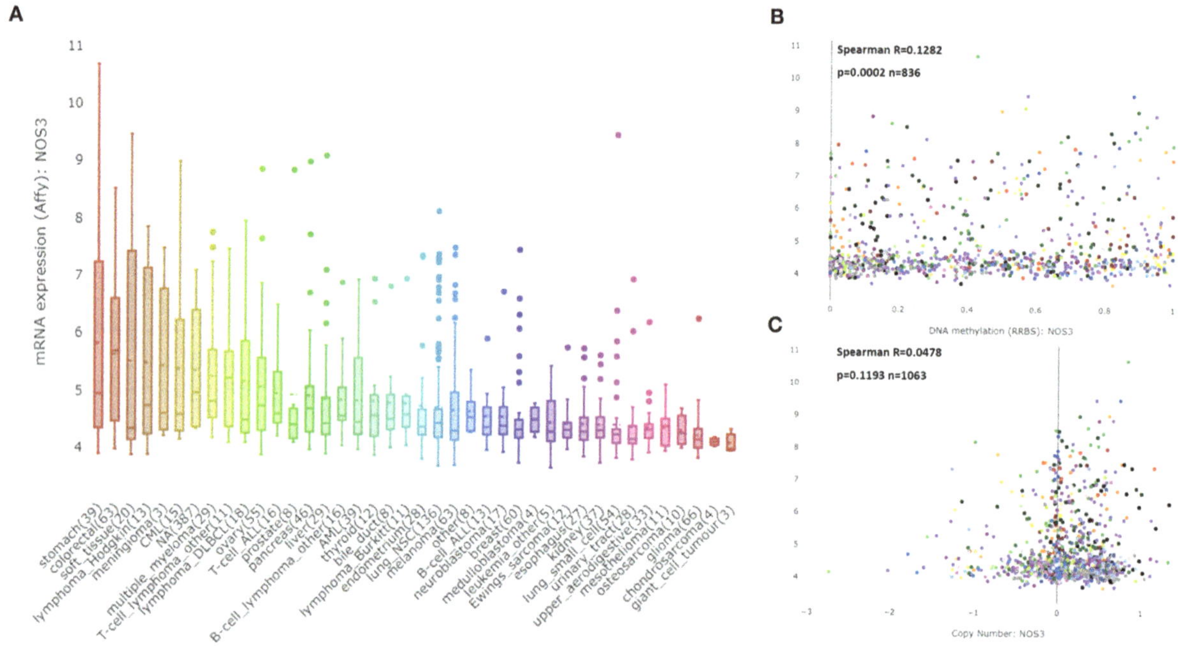

FIGURE 2 | *NOS3* mRNA expression in tumor cell lines. **(A)** *NOS3* mRNA expression across different cell lines from CCLE. **(B)** A scatter plot of promoter DNA methylation and mRNA levels of *NOS3* across different cell lines is shown. **(C)** A scatter plot of copy number variation and mRNA level of *NOS3* across different cell lines. The correlation between two variables is analyzed by Spearman analysis.

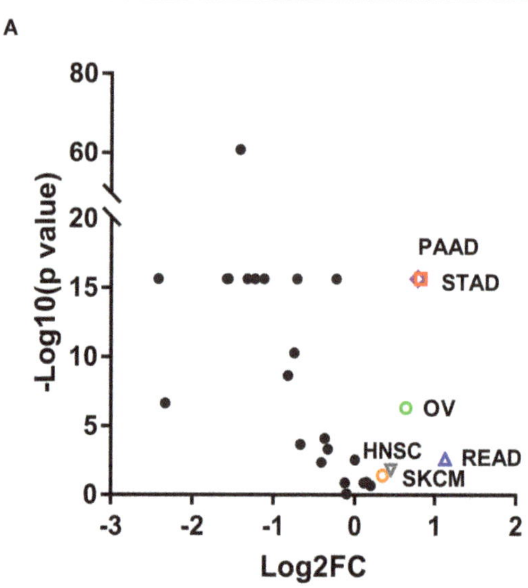

B

Tumor type	Fold change	*p* value
READ	2.180904	0.00231
STAD	1.764566	2.20E-16
PAAD	1.722826	2.20E-16
OV	1.561483	4.81E-07
SKCM	1.368265	0.01406
HNSC	1.276004	0.03885

FIGURE 3 | *NOS3* is differentially expressed in various tumors and their corresponding normal tissues. **(A)** Scatter plot of log2 FC and minus log10(*p*-value) across different cancers. The horizontal line on the Y-axis represents a *p*-value of 0.05. Points above the horizontal line have statistical significance. The vertical line on the X-axis represents log2 FC was−1 or 1, respectively. **(B)** The log2 FC and *p*-value in the six tumor types, which expressed higher NOS3 mRNA level.

Association Between *NOS3* mRNA Expression and Clinical Phenotypes

We analyzed the association between *NOS3* expression and tumor stage in 6 tumor types that had stage information in TCGA. Stages I and II were combined as early stage, and stages III and IV were combined as advanced stage. The result of *t*-test showed that in SKCM, patients with advanced tumor stage expressed higher *NOS3* mRNA levels, indicating that *NOS3* mRNA might positively related to later tumor stage (**Figure 4A**). However, *NOS3* expression in STAD

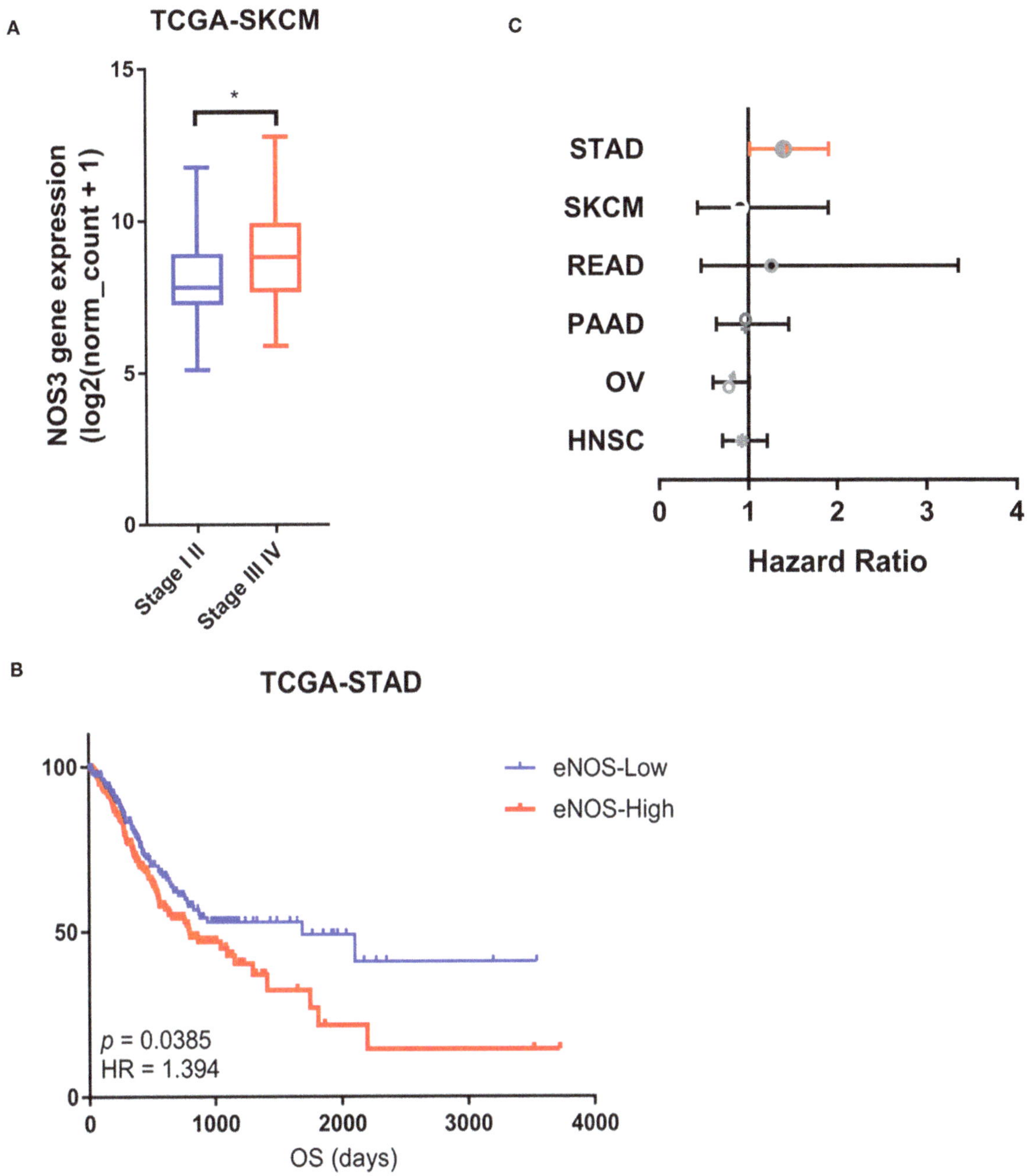

FIGURE 4 | Association between *NOS3* mRNA expression and clinical phenotypes. **(A)** *NOS3* expression between the early and advanced stages in SKCM. *T*-test was applied to analyses in the early stage and advanced stage. $^{*}p < 0.05$. **(B)** The *NOS3* expression level is related to overall survival in STAD. In the survival curves, the red line represents high *NOS3* expression levels and the blue line represents low *NOS3* expression levels. **(C)** A forest plot for survival association of each cancer is shown. The X-axis is the HR, the small points are the estimate of HR for each tumor and the bar represents the 95% confidence interval. Cox proportional hazards models were used to evaluate the association of *NOS3* expression levels on overall survival.

patients did not show difference in early and advanced tumor stage (early stage: mean of *NOS3* expression = 9.888 ± 0.9934; advanced stage: mean = 9.872 ± 1.025, p = 0.6653) (**Supplementary Figure 3**). *NOS3* mRNA in READ, PAAD, OV, and HNSC also showed no correlation with tumor stage.

To analyze the relationship between *NOS3* expression and overall survival of tumor patients, log-rank test was performed in six tumor types. We found that among the six tumor types expressed higher *NOS3* level, *NOS3* mRNA was related to a worse prognosis in patients with STAD (median survival: 1,686 vs. 801, $p = 0.0133385$, HR = 1.394) (**Figure 4B**). However, *NOS3* mRNA did not show correlation with OS in READ, PAAD, OV, SKCM, HNSC (**Figure 4C**).

Increased Expression Level of *NOS3* Was Related to Poor Prognoses of Gastric Cancer Patients

Through the above pan-cancer analysis, we found that *NOS3* has a higher expression level in gastric cancer tissues, and it is significantly related to the poor prognosis of gastric cancer patients. Furthermore, the expression pattern of *NOS3* protein was explored in clinical tissue samples to validate the role of *NOS3* in gastric cancer. Based on *NOS3* protein expression levels, gastric cancer patients ($N = 90$) were divided into *NOS3* positive ($N = 45$) and *NOS3* negative ($N = 45$) group. The relationship of demographic and clinicopathological parameters with *NOS3* expression was analyzed using Chi square analysis. The results showed that *NOS3* expression was related to survival state ($p = 0.049$), but other parameters (gender, age, tumor stage, and grade) showed no correlation with *NOS3* expression (**Table 1**). Kaplan-Meier curves and log-rank test analyses confirmed that patients with positive *NOS3* expression had significantly shorter overall survival (OS) than patients with negative *NOS3* expression ($p = 0.0278$, **Figures 5A,B**). Furthermore, cox proportional-hazards model was used to validate the potential of *NOS3* as a prognostic factor in gastric cancer. Univariate cox regression suggested that *NOS3* expression (HR = 2.166, 95% CI: 1.065–4.405, $p = 0.033$) and tumor stage (HR = 4.775, 95% CI: 2.213–10.302, $p < 0.001$), were related to OS. Multivariate cox regression indicated that *NOS3* expression (HR = 2.416, 95% CI: 1.181–4.941, $p = 0.016$) and tumor stage (HR = 5.101, 95% CI: 2.353–11.058, $p < 0.001$) were independent prognostic factors for OS (**Figure 5C**). In summary, *NOS3* was an independent prognostic factor for patients with gastric cancer.

Mechanism of *NOS3* Influencing the Clinical Outcome in STAD

In order to explore the mechanism underlying *NOS3* affecting clinical outcome of patients with STAD, GSEA and GSVA analyses were performed. Under the conditions of $p < 0.05$, FDR $q < 0.25$ and NES more than 1.5, GSVA and GSEA analyses commonly enriched 27 KEGG signaling pathways (**Figures 6A–H**, **Table 2**). Several canonical signaling pathways generally acknowledged to promote pathological behavior of malignant tumors were involved, such as "KEGG_ABC_TRANSPORTERS," "KEGG_CALCIUM_SIGNALING_PATHWAY," "KEGG_ECM_RECEPTOR_INTERACTION," "KEGG_CYTOKINE_CYTOKINE_RECEPTOR_INTERACTION," "KEGG_CHEMOKINE_SIGNALING_PATHWAY" and "KEGG_MAPK_SIGNALING_PATHWAY." These results indicated that *NOS3* might participate in multiple canonical cancer-related signaling pathways to facilitate STAD.

TABLE 1 | Demographic and clinicopathological parameters of patients with gastric cancer.

		$N = 90$	NOS3 positive	NOS3 negative	p-value
Gender	Male	60	32	28	0.3711
	Female	30	13	17	
Age	<60	40	19	21	0.6714
	≥60	50	26	24	
T stage	T1-2	38	18	20	0.6695
	T3-4	52	27	25	
N stage	N0-1	62	27	35	0.0685
	N2-3	28	18	10	
pStage	I-II	50	23	27	0.3961
	III-IV	40	22	18	
Grade	1	6	3	3	1
	2-3	84	42	42	
Status	Alive	57	24	33	**0.049**
	Dead	33	21	12	

The meaning of bold value is p < 0.05.

Association Between *NOS3* Expression and Drug Sensitivity

To investigate the correlation between *NOS3* mRNA expression and drug sensitivity, *NOS3* expression in 664 cell lines and drug response to 482 drugs were analyzed. Spearman correlation analysis revealed that, "SR8278" was considered to moderately correlate with *NOS3* mRNA expression, with a correlation coefficient >0.3 (**Figure 7A**). A negative correlation indicated that a better response (smaller response AUC value) was correlated with increased expression of *NOS3*. "SR8278" is an antagonist of the transcription factor REV-ERBα, affecting its circadian and metabolic functions. Two other drugs, "GSK.J4" and "CIL55A" had a correlation coefficient >0.2 and were also negatively correlated. Subsequently, Spearman analysis were performed to investigate the correlation of *NOS3* expression with drug response individually in STAD. The results showed that response of cells to QS-11 (correlation coefficient $r = -0.8986$, $p = 0.0278$) and brivanib (correlation coefficient $r = -0.7182$, $p = 0.0162$) was significantly correlated with *NOS3* mRNA level (**Figures 7B,C**).

DISCUSSION

NOS3 has been found to inhibit apoptosis and promote angiogenesis, proliferation, invasiveness, and immunosuppression of malignant tumors. However, because of the limited number of studies on *NOS3* expression in malignant tumors, *NOS3* functions in tumor pathogenesis and development are still not fully understood. And the expression pattern of *NOS3* and its diagnostic and prognostic potential has not been investigated in a pan-cancer perspective. In this study, the expression level of *NOS3* (mainly mRNA) in 30 different normal human tissues, 33 different tumors types as well as their corresponding normal tissues, and 1,457 cancer cell lines was

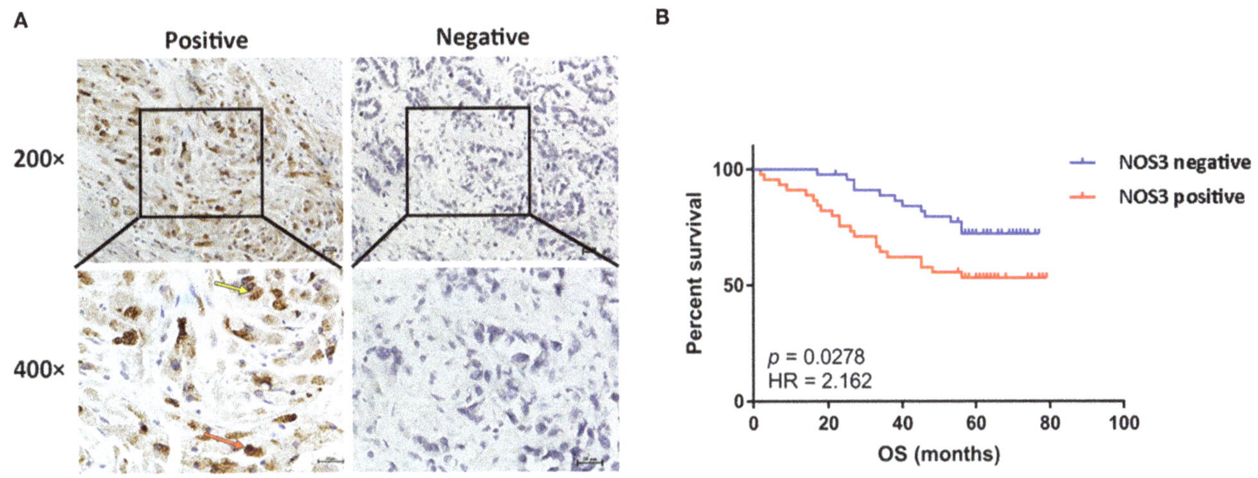

C

	Univariate Cox regression			Multivariate Cox regression		
	HR	95%CI	P Value	HR	95%CI	P Value
NOS3	2.166	1.065-4.405	0.033	2.416	1.181-4.941	0.016
Age	0.981	0.494-1.946	0.956			
Gender	1.078	0.530-2.191	0.836			
Stage (I-II v.s. III-IV)	4.775	2.213-10.302	0.000068	5.101	2.353-11.058	0.000037
Grade	1.433	0.663-3.098	0.360			

FIGURE 5 | *NOS3* was independent prognostic factor of patients with gastric cancer. **(A)** Representative images of positive and negative *NOS3* protein expression in gastric cancer tissues. NOS3 was expressed in cytoplasm (yellow arrow) and nucleus (red arrow) of tumor cells. There were 45 patients stained positive and 45 patients stained negative. The scales bars indicate 20 μm. **(B)** Kaplan-Meier analysis of *NOS3* protein in gastric cancer patients. Patients with higher *NOS3* expression had shorter OS compared with patients with lower *NOS3* expression ($p = 0.0278$, HR = 2.162). **(C)** Univariate and multivariate cox regression showed that higher *NOS3* protein expression and advanced pathological stage were independent prognostic factor in gastric cancer patients.

systematically analyzed, to determine the expression level of *NOS3* in tumor and normal tissues and its role in malignant tumors. We also explored its potential association with clinical characteristics (pathological stage, OS and drug response).

Pan-cancer analysis focused on whole genome can reveal genes that are associated with the occurrence and development of cancer, providing insights into cancer diagnosis, monitoring and treatment (28–30). By analyzing *NOS3* mRNA levels in normal tissues from GTEx, we found that *NOS3* was expressed at the highest level in the spleen and was expressed at the lowest level in the blood. According to the Human Protein Atlas (www.proteinatlas.org) database, the *NOS3* protein level in the spleen was also the highest, which was consisted with our results. And research has reported that *NOS3* is mainly upregulated in endothelial progenitor cells (EPCs) of the spleen, exerting beneficial functions on atherosclerosis, angiogenesis, and vascular repair (31, 32). And in 33 tumor types involved in this study, *NOS3* mRNA was expressed highest in STAD. Analyses in cancer cell lines showed that *NOS3* was expressed at quite high levels in COAD and STAD cell lines. Previous research showed that *NOS3* promoter DNA methylation could reduce *NOS3* mRNA level (33). Copy number variations (CNVs) could also modify gene mRNA expression (34). However, further analyses about promoter DNA methylation and CNVs of *NOS3* gene suggested that neither of the two factors showed a strong statistical correlation with *NOS3* mRNA, indicating that promoter DNA methylation and CNVs of the *NOS3* gene might not be the main determinant of *NOS3* mRNA levels in tumors.

Analyses of TCGA data showed that *NOS3* expression increased in six tumor tissues compared with their corresponding normal tissues. Among the six tumor types, NOS3 related to advanced tumor stage in SKCM. Previous research reported by Panich et al. suggested that NOS3 inhibition could effectively protect against UVA-dependent melanogenesis (35). In addition, patients with higher *NOS3* levels were diagnosed with a later tumor stage in COAD (**Supplementary Figure 4A**). This was consistent with the observation that L-NIO (a *NOS3* inhibitor) inhibited cell growth and angiogenesis in colorectal

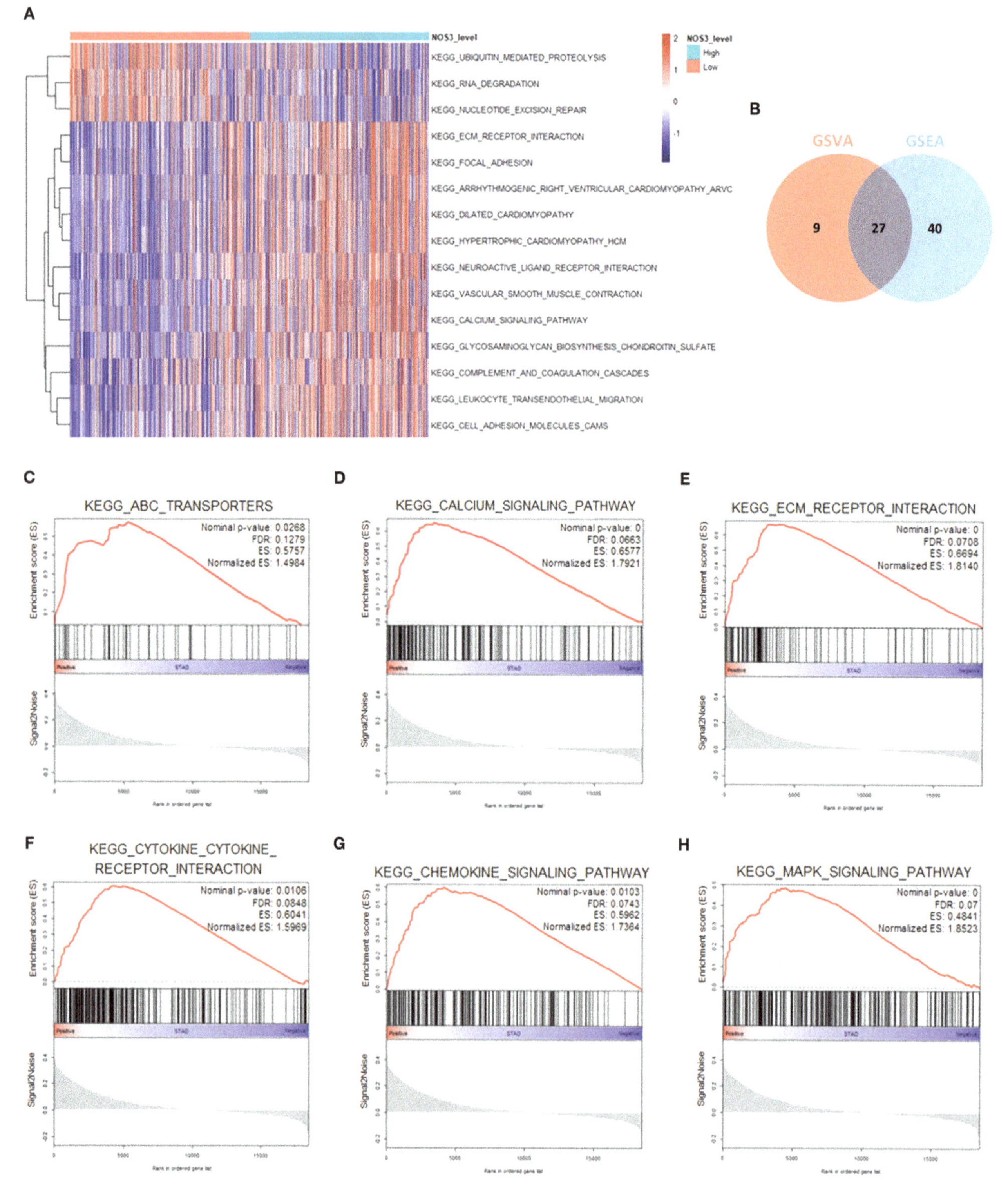

FIGURE 6 | GSEA and GSVA analyses in STAD. **(A)** Top 15 differentially enriched KEGG signaling pathways in higher and lower *NOS3* expression groups analyzed by GSVA in STAD. **(B)** Seven signaling pathways commonly enriched by GSEA and GSVA in STAD. **(C–H)** Signaling pathways enriched by GSEA analyses in STAD.

cancer (36, 37). In BRCA, we also found that the higher expression of *NOS3* mRNA was related to advanced tumor stage (**Supplementary Figure 4B**). These results were consistent with previous researches, which reported that *NOS3* promoted angiogenesis and enhance the migration and invasion in breast cancer cells (11–13).

TABLE 2 | GSVA and GSEA analyses revealed mechanism of *NOS3* participant in occurrence and development of STAD.

Signaling pathways	GSVA	GSEA	
	p-value	NES	*p*-value
KEGG_GLYCOSAMINOGLYCAN_BIOSYNTHESIS_CHONDROITIN_SULFATE	<0.0001	1.48	0.044
KEGG_ECM_RECEPTOR_INTERACTION	<0.0001	1.81	<0.0001
KEGG_DILATED_CARDIOMYOPATHY	<0.0001	1.69	<0.0001
KEGG_VASCULAR_SMOOTH_MUSCLE_CONTRACTION	<0.0001	1.90	<0.0001
KEGG_NEUROACTIVE_LIGAND_RECEPTOR_INTERACTION	<0.0001	1.65	<0.0001
KEGG_CALCIUM_SIGNALING_PATHWAY	<0.0001	1.79	<0.0001
KEGG_FOCAL_ADHESION	<0.0001	2.01	<0.0001
KEGG_HYPERTROPHIC_CARDIOMYOPATHY_HCM	<0.0001	1.73	<0.0001
KEGG_CELL_ADHESION_MOLECULES_CAMS	<0.0001	1.71	0.006
KEGG_ARRHYTHMOGENIC_RIGHT_VENTRICULAR_CARDIOMYOPATHY_ARVC	<0.0001	1.63	0.004
KEGG_LEUKOCYTE_TRANSENDOTHELIAL_MIGRATION	<0.0001	1.99	0.002
KEGG_HEMATOPOIETIC_CELL_LINEAGE	<0.0001	1.60	0.033
KEGG_COMPLEMENT_AND_COAGULATION_CASCADES	<0.0001	1.58	0.012
KEGG_RENIN_ANGIOTENSIN_SYSTEM	<0.0001	1.54	0.025
KEGG_CYTOKINE_CYTOKINE_RECEPTOR_INTERACTION	<0.0001	1.60	0.011
KEGG_AXON_GUIDANCE	<0.0001	1.88	<0.0001
KEGG_CHEMOKINE_SIGNALING_PATHWAY	<0.0001	1.74	0.010
KEGG_PRION_DISEASES	<0.0001	1.51	0.037
KEGG_REGULATION_OF_ACTIN_CYTOSKELETON	<0.0001	1.87	<0.0001
KEGG_VIRAL_MYOCARDITIS	<0.0001	1.55	0.046
KEGG_DORSO_VENTRAL_AXIS_FORMATION	<0.0001	1.77	0.002
KEGG_MAPK_SIGNALING_PATHWAY	<0.0001	1.85	<0.0001
KEGG_ALDOSTERONE_REGULATED_SODIUM_REABSORPTION	<0.0001	1.50	0.035
KEGG_TYPE_II_DIABETES_MELLITUS	<0.0001	1.59	0.012
KEGG_GAP_JUNCTION	<0.0001	1.65	0.004
KEGG_ABC_TRANSPORTERS	<0.0001	1.50	0.027
KEGG_ADIPOCYTOKINE_SIGNALING_PATHWAY	<0.0001	1.62	0.019

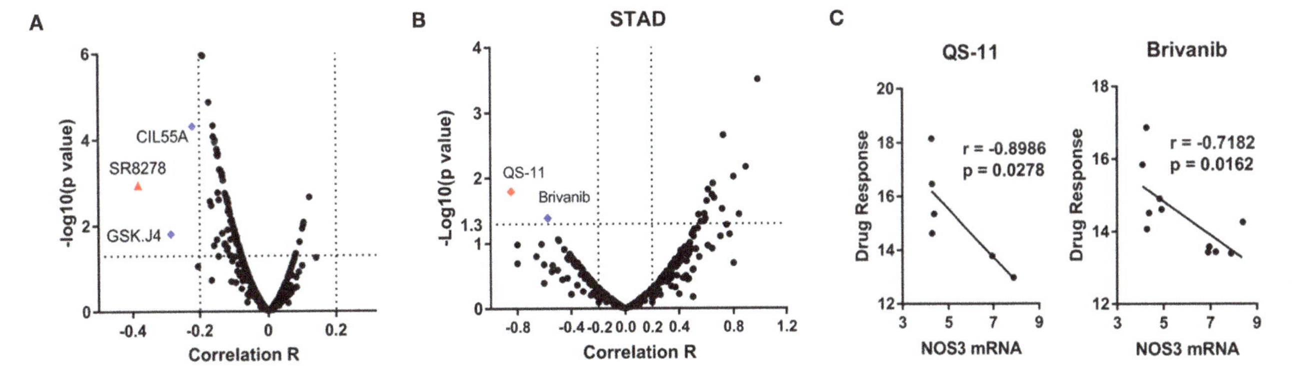

FIGURE 7 | Association between *NOS3* expression and drug sensitivity. **(A)** Volcano plot of the correlation coefficient and minus log10(*p*-value) between *NOS3* expression in all cell lines and 482 drugs. Most of correlations are not significant and in negative direction. The correlation coefficient of "SR8278" is >0.3 (negative, higher expression is correlated with better response represented by smaller AUC). Blue dots are the drugs with correlation coefficients >0.2. **(B,C)** Spearman analysis performed individually in STAD. Volcano plot of the correlation coefficient and minus log10(*p*-value) between *NOS3* expression in STAD cell lines was shown in B (including 23132-87, NCI-N87, MKN-45, MKN-1, HS746T, NUGC-3, MKN-7, IM-95, HGC-27, OCUM-1, FU-97, and AGS cells). The response of cells to QS-11 (correlation coefficient $r = -0.8986$, $p = 0.0278$) and brivanib (correlation coefficient $r = -0.7182$, $p = 0.0162$) was significantly correlated with *NOS3* mRNA level. The scatter plots of QS-11 and brivanib were shown in **(C)**.

There are few researches have reported *NOS3* in STAD. Doi et al. reported in 1999 that the quantity of *NOS3* in gastric cancer tissues was negatively correlated with serosal invasion (38). And *NOS3* has been reported to promote the angiogenic phenotype and predict poor prognosis in STAD (39). In our research, expression level of *NOS3* was significantly increased in STAD tumor tissues, and its expression level was the highest among the tumor types and cancer cell lines involved in this study. Analyses of clinical parameters also showed that *NOS3* predicted poor prognosis, consistent with previous research. These results confirmed the important role of *NOS3* in the development of STAD. Furthermore, experiments and analyses in our gastric cancer tissues also indicated that higher *NOS3* protein level was closely related to shorter OS of gastric cancer patients. *NOS3* was an independent prognostic factor for patients with gastric cancer. However, *NOS3* showed no correlation with tumor stage in mRNA and protein level. It may be due to the limitation of sample size. The sample size needs to be increased for further verification in future research. At present, the mechanism of *NOS3* promoting STAD progression was not clear. Therefore, we further analyzed the potential signaling pathways participating in *NOS3* promoting gastric cancer. The results of GSEA and GSVA analyses suggested that in STAD, several canonical cancer-related pathways were enriched in higher *NOS3* expression group. As key members of "KEGG_ABC_TRANSPORTERS," ATP binding cassette (ABC) transporters were identified to mediate multidrug-resistance (MDR) in acute myeloid leukemia (AML), OV, BRCA, and lung cancer (40, 41). And researches also reported that ATP-binding cassette transporter G1 (ABCG1), a member of ABC transporter family, could modulate the interaction of Cav-1 and *NOS3* protein in endothelial cells (ECs), and increase cell migration through Lyn/Akt/*NOS3* in endothelial progenitor cells (EPCs). "KEGG_CALCIUM_SIGNALING_PATHWAY" contributes to many crucial tumor pathology processes, including proliferation, invasion, cell death, and autophagy in many tumors (42–45). As described above, the increased concentration of Ca^{2+} could induce the combination of CaM protein and *NOS3* protein, and subsequently stimulate the activity of *NOS3* protein (2, 46). We also enriched "KEGG_ECM_RECEPTOR_INTERACTION." Specific interactions between the extracellular matrix (ECM) and cells are mediated by transmembrane molecules, including integrins, proteoglycans, and other cell-surface-associated components. These interactions can lead to malignant biological behavior of tumor cells, such as adhesion, migration, proliferation, and apoptosis (47, 48). A study by Njah et al. found that Agrin interacted with Lrp4-Integrin β1-FAK axis in ECs. This interaction could sustain the VEGFR2 pathway as well as stimulate *NOS3* signaling, and ultimately promote angiogenesis in tumor (49). In addition, "KEGG_CYTOKINE_CYTOKIN E_RECEPTOR_INTERACTION," "KEGG_CHEMOKINE_SI GNALING_PATHWAY,"and"KEGG_MAPK_SIGNALING_ PATHWAY" were also generally recognized as cancer-related signaling pathway. These pathways were widely involved in tumor occurrence and development. The mechanism of these signaling pathways involved in *NOS3* regulation of gastric cancer needs further study.

Currently, research on *NOS3*-targeted medicine is mainly concentrating on cardiovascular and cerebrovascular disease. Many inhibitors and agonists have been found to have satisfactory therapeutic effects. For example, ursolic acid, which has an anti-tumor effect, has been proven to promote *NOS3* phosphorylation and inhibit *NOS3* uncoupling, thereby preventing doxorubicin-induced cardiac toxicity (50). However, the research on and application of *NOS3*-targeted medicine in malignant tumors are still extremely limited. The *NOS3* inhibitor L-NIO was reported to inhibit COAD cell growth and angiogenesis. Another *NOS3* inhibitor, N(G)-nitro-L-arginine methyl ester (L-NAME) was also reported to inhibit PAAD tumor growth (15). In addition, L-NIO could promote the anti-tumor effect of lenvatinib (36, 37). The *NOS3* level was significantly correlated with outcomes of bevacizumab-based chemotherapy in COAD (9, 51). Unfortunately, bevacizumab, L-NIO, and L-NAME were not included in the CTRP database. Our research showed that "SR8278," an antagonist of Rev-ErbAα was negatively correlated with *NOS3* expression, indicating that *NOS3* was the potential target of "SR8278." "SR8278" targeted NR1D1, a nuclear hormone receptor (52), reiterating the potential relationship between *NOS3* and NR1D1. Further analyses in STAD showed that response of STAD cancer cells to QS-11 and brivanib were strongly correlated with *NOS3* expression. QS-11 is an inhibitor of GTPase activating protein of ARF (ARFGAP), increasing ARF1-GTP and ARF6-GTP levels (53). Currently, studies on QS-11 in malignant tumor are very few. Only one research by Zhang et al. reported that the combination of QS-11 and ARFGAP1 protein could stimulate Wnt/β-catenin signaling pathway, resulting in the regulation of cell differentiation, proliferation, and apoptosis (54). Our research suggested that QS-11 may play an important role in STAD by inhibiting NOS3, which requires further research in the future. Brivanib is a dual tyrosine kinase inhibitor used to treat solid tumor in advanced stages. It can selectively target vascular endothelial growth factor receptor (VEGFR) and fibroblast growth factor receptor (FGFR) (55, 56). However, the response of *NOS3* expressed cell to brivanib has not been reported. *NOS3* was a downstream molecular of VEGFR signaling pathway. Thus, we guessed that brivanib might regulate *NOS3* through VEGFR signaling pathway. These results about drug response warrant further investigation.

In conclusion, this research showed that the expression level and clinical significance of *NOS3* was highly cancer-dependent. Analyses in public data sets gastric cancer tissues demonstrated that higher *NOS3* expression was related to poor prognosis of patients with STAD. *NOS3* was an independent prognostic factor for patients with STAD. Increased expression of *NOS3* might influence occurrence and development of STAD through several canonical cancer-related pathways. In addition, *NOS3* expression was related to some therapeutic drugs, such as "SR8278" and "brivanib," which warrant further investigation. These results reported that *NOS3* might participate in occurrence and development of gastric cancer by canonical signaling pathways, suggesting that NOS3 might a novel target for gastric cancer treatment.

DATA AVAILABILITY STATEMENT

Publicly available datasets were analyzed in this study. This data can be found at: UCSC Xena (https://xena.ucsc.edu/), CCLE (CCLE; https://portals.broadinstitute.org/ccle/), and CTRP (https://portals.broadinstitute.org/ctrp.v2.1/).

ETHICS STATEMENT

The studies involving human participants were reviewed and approved by the ethics committee of the First Affiliated Hospital of China Medical University. The patients/participants provided their written informed consent to participate in this study.

AUTHOR CONTRIBUTIONS

YZ, YT, and ZJ: project administration. ZL, FL, and JZ: software. DZ, YC, YM, and ZJ: statistical analysis. JS, CY, and YJ: visualization. DZ and YY: manuscript writing. All authors: contributed to the article and approved the submitted version.

ACKNOWLEDGMENTS

The authors thank the colleges in the First Laboratory of Cancer Institute for data collation and statistical analysis. This manuscript has been released as a pre-print at Research Square (57).

SUPPLEMENTARY MATERIAL

Supplementary Figure 1 | NOS3 mRNA expression level in normal tissues from GTEx database.

Supplementary Figure 2 | A scatter plot of *NOS3* mRNA and *TNF-α* mRNA. The correlation between two variables is analyzed by Spearman analysis.

Supplementary Figure 3 | Association between *NOS3* mRNA expression and tumor stage in STAD. ANOVA analysis showed that tumor stages (stage I-IV) were not related to NOS3 expression, with *p*-value more than 0.05 (mean ± SD: I, 9.63 1.139; II, 10.01 ± 0.8962; III, 9.845 ± 1.014; IV,9.983 ± 1.075) **(A)**. *T*-test also suggested that tumor stages (stage I-II and stage III-IV) showed no connection with NOS3 expression, with *p*-value more than 0.05 (mean ± SD: I-II, 9.888 ± 0.9934; III-IV, 9.872 ± 1.025) **(B)**.

Supplementary Figure 4 | Association between *NOS3* mRNA expression and tumor stage in COAD **(A)** and BRCA **(B)** (*$p < 0.05$, **$p < 0.01$).

Supplementary Table 1 | Case number of all the tumor types.

REFERENCES

Xu W, Liu LZ, Loizidou M, Ahmed M, Charles IG. The role of nitric oxide in cancer. *Cell Res.* (2002) 12:311–20. doi: 10.1038/sj.cr.7290133

Fischmann TO, Hruza A, Niu XD, Fossetta JD, Lunn CA, Dolphin E, et al. Structural characterization of nitric oxide synthase isoforms reveals striking active-site conservation. *Nat Struct Biol.* (1999) 6:233–42. doi: 10.1038/6675

Trane AE, Pavlov D, Sharma A, Saqib U, Lau K, van Petegem F, et al. Deciphering the binding of caveolin-1 to client protein endothelial nitric- oxide synthase (eNOS): scaffolding subdomain identification, interaction modeling, and biological significance. *J Biol Chem.* (2014) 289:13273– 83. doi: 10.1074/jbc.M113.528695

Pritchard KA, Ackerman AW, Ou J, Curtis M, Smalley DM, Fontana JT, et al. Native low-density lipoprotein induces endothelial nitric oxide synthase dysfunction: role of heat shock protein 90 and caveolin-1. *Free Radical Biol Med.* (2002) 33:52–62. doi: 10.1016/S0891-5849(02)00851-1

Xia N, Daiber A, Habermeier A, Closs EI, Thum T, Spanier G, et al. Resveratrol reverses endothelial nitric-oxide synthase uncoupling in apolipoprotein E knockout mice. *J Pharmacol Exp Therap.* (2010) 335:149– 54. doi: 10.1124/jpet.110.168724

Ying L, Hofseth LJ. An emerging role for endothelial nitric oxide synthase in chronic inflammation and cancer. *Cancer Res.* (2007) 67:1407– 10. doi: 10.1158/0008-5472.CAN-06-2149

Song Y, Zhao XP, Song K, Shang ZJ. Ephrin-A1 is up-regulated by hypoxia in cancer cells and promotes angiogenesis of HUVECs through a coordinated cross-talk with eNOS. *PLoS ONE.* (2013) 8:e74464. doi: 10.1371/journal.pone.0074464

Zhang L, Zeng M, Fu BM. Inhibition of endothelial nitric oxide synthase decreases breast cancer cell MDA-MB-231 adhesion to intact microvessels under physiological flows. *Am J Physiol Heart Circul Physiol.* (2016) 310:H1735–47. doi: 10.1152/ajpheart.00109.2016

Marisi G, Scarpi E, Passardi A, Nanni O, Ragazzini A, Valgiusti M, et al. Circulating VEGF and eNOS variations as predictors of outcome in metastatic colorectal cancer patients receiving bevacizumab. *Sci Rep.* (2017) 7:1293. doi: 10.1038/s41598-017-01420-0

Penarando J, Lopez-Sanchez LM, Mena R, Guil-Luna S, Conde F, Hernandez V, et al. A role for endothelial nitric oxide synthase in intestinal stem cell proliferation and mesenchymal colorectal cancer. *BMC Biol.* (2018) 16:3. doi: 10.1186/s12915-017-0472-5

Maniyar R, Chakraborty S, Suriano R. Ethanol enhances estrogen mediated angiogenesis in breast cancer. *J Cancer.* (2018) 9:3874–85. doi: 10.7150/jca.25581

Sharma S, Guru SK, Manda S, Kumar A, Mintoo MJ, Prasad VD, et al. A marine sponge alkaloid derivative 4-chloro fascaplysin inhibits tumor growth and VEGF mediated angiogenesis by disrupting PI3K/Akt/mTOR signaling cascade. *Chem Biol Interact.* (2017) 275:47–60. doi: 10.1016/j.cbi.2017.07.017

Gajalakshmi P, Priya MK, Pradeep T, Behera J, Muthumani K, Madhuwanti S, et al. Breast cancer drugs dampen vascular functions by interfering with nitric oxide signaling in endothelium. *Toxicol Appl Pharmacol.* (2013) 269:121– 31. doi: 10.1016/j.taap.2013.03.011

Lim KH, Ancrile BB, Kashatus DF, Counter CM. Tumour maintenance is mediated by eNOS. *Nature.* (2008) 452:646–9. doi: 10.1038/nature06778

Lampson BL, Kendall SD, Ancrile BB, Morrison MM, Shealy MJ, Barrientos KS, et al. Targeting eNOS in pancreatic cancer. *Cancer Res.* (2012) 72:4472– 82. doi: 10.1158/0008-5472.CAN-12-0057

Yu S, Jia L, Zhang Y, Wu D, Xu Z, Ng CF, et al. Increased expression of activated endothelial nitric oxide synthase contributes to antiandrogen resistance in prostate cancer cells by suppressing androgen receptor transactivation. *Cancer Lett.* (2013) 328:83– 94. doi: 10.1016/j.canlet.2012.09.006

Nanni S, Aiello A, Re A, Guffanti A, Benvenuti V, Colussi C, et al. Estrogen-dependent dynamic profile of eNOS-DNA associations in

Permissions

All chapters in this book were first published by Frontiers; hereby published with permission under the Creative Commons Attribution License or equivalent. Every chapter published in this book has been scrutinized by our experts. Their significance has been extensively debated. The topics covered herein carry significant findings which will fuel the growth of the discipline. They may even be implemented as practical applications or may be referred to as a beginning point for another development.

The contributors of this book come from diverse backgrounds, making this book a truly international effort. This book will bring forth new frontiers with its revolutionizing research information and detailed analysis of the nascent developments around the world.

We would like to thank all the contributing authors for lending their expertise to make the book truly unique. They have played a crucial role in the development of this book. Without their invaluable contributions this book wouldn't have been possible. They have made vital efforts to compile up to date information on the varied aspects of this subject to make this book a valuable addition to the collection of many professionals and students.

This book was conceptualized with the vision of imparting up-to-date information and advanced data in this field. To ensure the same, a matchless editorial board was set up. Every individual on the board went through rigorous rounds of assessment to prove their worth. After which they invested a large part of their time researching and compiling the most relevant data for our readers.

The editorial board has been involved in producing this book since its inception. They have spent rigorous hours researching and exploring the diverse topics which have resulted in the successful publishing of this book. They have passed on their knowledge of decades through this book. To expedite this challenging task, the publisher supported the team at every step. A small team of assistant editors was also appointed to further simplify the editing procedure and attain best results for the readers.

Apart from the editorial board, the designing team has also invested a significant amount of their time in understanding the subject and creating the most relevant covers. They scrutinized every image to scout for the most suitable representation of the subject and create an appropriate cover for the book.

The publishing team has been an ardent support to the editorial, designing and production team. Their endless efforts to recruit the best for this project, has resulted in the accomplishment of this book. They are a veteran in the field of academics and their pool of knowledge is as vast as their experience in printing. Their expertise and guidance has proved useful at every step. Their uncompromising quality standards have made this book an exceptional effort. Their encouragement from time to time has been an inspiration for everyone.

The publisher and the editorial board hope that this book will prove to be a valuable piece of knowledge for researchers, students, practitioners and scholars across the globe.

List of Contributors

Jinqi Lv, Simeng Zhang, Yang Liu, Ce Li, Tianshu Guo, Shuairan Zhang, Zenan Li, Zihan Jiao, Haina Sun and Ling Xu
Department of Medical Oncology, The First Hospital of China Medical University, Shenyang, China
Key Laboratory of Anticancer Drugs and Biotherapy of Liaoning Province, The First Hospital of China Medical University, Shenyang, China
Liaoning Province Clinical Research Center for Cancer, Shenyang, China
Key Laboratory of Precision Diagnosis and Treatment of Gastrointestinal Tumors, Ministry of Education, Shenyang, China

Ye Zhang
The First Laboratory of Cancer Institute, The First Hospital of China Medical University, Shenyang, China

Peng Chen and Zhiwei He
Department of Hepatobiliary Surgery, Renmin Hospital of Wuhan University, Wuhan, China
Department of Hepatic-Biliary-Pancreatic Surgery, The Affiliated Hospital of Guizhou Medical University, Guiyang, China

Jie Wang, Jian Xu and Jianxin Jiang
Department of Hepatobiliary Surgery, Renmin Hospital of Wuhan University, Wuhan, China

Youngmi Kim
Institute of New Frontier Research, College of Medicine, Hallym University, Chuncheon, South Korea

Tao Jiang, Hu Song, Yixin Xu, Renhao Wang and Jun Song
Department of General Surgery, The Affiliated Hospital of Xuzhou Medical University, Xuzhou, China
Institute of Digestive Diseases, Xuzhou Medical University, Xuzhou, China

Li Zheng
State Key Laboratory of Proteomics, Beijing Proteome Research Center, National Center for Protein Sciences, Beijing Institute of Lifeomics, Beijing, China
State Key Laboratory of Food Nutrition and Safety, Tianjin University of Science and Technology, Tianjin, China

Xia Li
The Graduate School, Xuzhou Medical University, Xuzhou, China

Jia Liu
Department of Pathology, The Affiliated Hospital of Xuzhou Medical University, Xuzhou, China

Chenhua Dong, Lianyu Liu and Hongyu Wang
Department of General Surgery, The Affiliated Hospital of Xuzhou Medical University, Xuzhou, China
The Graduate School, Xuzhou Medical University, Xuzhou, China

Shuai Wang
School of Life Sciences, Xuzhou Medical University, Xuzhou, China

Yiming Guan, Yuzhang Du, Guanzheng Wang, Hongquan Gou, Yilun Xue, Jingsong Xu, Enhao Li, Di Wu, Peiqing Xu, Peihua Ni, Dakang Xu and Yiqun Hu
Faculty of Medical Laboratory Science, Ruijin Hospital, School of Medicine, Shanghai Jiao Tong University, Shanghai, China

David W. Chan
Department of Obstetrics and Gynaecology, LKS Faculty of Medicine, The University of Hong Kong, Hong Kong, China

Wangzhi Wei, Wei Zhao and Yu Zhang
Life Science Institute of Jinzhou Medical University, Jinzhou, China

Minjeong Yeon, Hyun Suk Jung and Dooil Jeoung
Department of Biochemistry, College of Natural Sciences, Kangwon National University, Chuncheon, South Korea

Xueyi Jiang, Yankun Chen and Xinyuan Liu
Department of Hepatic-Biliary-Pancreatic Surgery, The Affiliated Hospital of Guizhou Medical University, Guiyang, China

Deepak Pathak, Eunju Kwon and Dong Young Kim
College of Pharmacy, Yeungnam University, Gyeongsan, South Korea

Myeong Seon Jeong
Department of Biochemistry, College of Natural Sciences, Kangwon National University, Chuncheon, South Korea
Chuncheon Center, Korea Basic Science Institute, Chuncheon, South Korea

Yuqiang Li
Department of General Surgery, Xiangya Hospital, Central South University, Changsha, China
National Clinical Research Center for Geriatric Disorders, Xiangya Hospital, Central South University, Changsha, China
Department of General, Visceral and Thoracic Surgery, University Medical Center Hamburg-Eppendorf, Hamburg, Germany

Mengxiang Tian, Dan Wang, Zhongyi Zhou, Qian Pei and Fengbo Tan
Department of General Surgery, Xiangya Hospital, Central South University, Changsha, China
National Clinical Research Center for Geriatric Disorders, Xiangya Hospital, Central South University, Changsha, China

Wenxue Liu
National Clinical Research Center for Geriatric Disorders, Xiangya Hospital, Central South University, Changsha, China
Department of Cardiology, Xiangya Hospital, Central South University, Changsha, China

Yan Huang
Key Laboratory of Protein Chemistry and Developmental Biology of Ministry of Education, College of Life Sciences, Hunan Normal University, Changsha, China
Department of Neurosurgery, Second Affiliated Hospital of Hunan Normal University, Changsha, China
Hunan Provincial Key Laboratory of Neurorestoration, Changsha, China

Cenap Güngör
Department of General, Visceral and Thoracic Surgery, University Medical Center Hamburg-Eppendorf, Hamburg, Germany

Ya Wang and Yuqiao Chen
Institute of Molecular Precision Medicine and Hunan Key Laboratory of Molecular Precision Medicine, Xiangya Hospital, Central South University, Changsha, China
Department of General Surgery, Xiangya Hospital, Central South University, Changsha, China

Shuai Xiao
Department of Gastrointestinal Surgery and Institute of Clinical Medicine, The First Affiliated Hospital, University of South China, Hengyang, China

Kai Fu
Institute of Molecular Precision Medicine and Hunan Key Laboratory of Molecular Precision Medicine, Xiangya Hospital, Central South University, Changsha, China
Department of General Surgery, Xiangya Hospital, Central South University, Changsha, China
Center for Medical Genetics & Hunan Key Laboratory of Medical Genetics, School of Life Sciences, Central South University, Changsha, China
Hunan Key Laboratory of Animal Models for Human Diseases, Central South University, Changsha, China

Lei Wang, Pei Xu, Xiao Xie, Fengqing Hu, Lianyong Jiang, Rui Hu, Fangbao Ding and Haibo Xiao
Department of Cardiothoracic Surgery, Xinhua Hospital Affiliated to Shanghai Jiao Tong University School of Medicine, Shanghai, China

Huijun Zhang
Department of Cardiothoracic Surgery, Huashan Hospital of Fudan University, Shanghai, China

Xing Huang and Gang Zhang
Zhejiang Provincial Key Laboratory of Pancreatic Disease, School of Medicine, Zhejiang University, Hangzhou, China

Xiyang Zhang, Dongbo Jiang, Shuya Yang, Yuanjie Sun and Jingqi Shi
Chenchen Hu, Jingyu Pan, Tianyue Liu, Boquan Jin and Kun Yang Department of Immunology, The Fourth Military Medical University, Xi'an, China

Lin Cui and Xiuqing Wang
Department of Gastroenterology and Hepatology, The Second Affiliated Hospital, Harbin Medical University, Harbin, China

Dekai Zhang
Center for Infectious and Inflammatory Diseases, Texas A&M University, Houston, TX, United States

Yiyi Zhang, Yong Wu, Yong Peng, Jinfu Zhuang, Yuanfeng Yang, Xing Liu and Guoxian Guan
Department of Colorectal Surgery, The First Affiliated Hospital of Fujian Medical University, Fuzhou, China

Qiao Gao
Fujian Maternity and Child Health Hospital, Affiliated Hospital of Fujian Medical University, Fuzhou, China

Weizhong Jiang
Department of Colorectal Surgery, Fujian Medical University Union Hospital, Fuzhou, China

Meng-Yao Sun, Bo Xu, Qiu-Xue Wu and Si Cai
Department of Clinical Laboratory and Central Laboratory, Putuo Hospital, Shanghai University of Traditional Chinese Medicine, Shanghai, China

Wen-Lian Chen
Cancer Institute, Longhua Hospital, Shanghai University of Traditional Chinese Medicine, Shanghai, China

Hui Zhang
Research Center for Traditional Chinese Medicine Complexity System, Institute of Interdisciplinary Integrative Medicine Research, Shanghai University of Traditional Chinese Medicine, Shanghai, China

Qing-Feng Tang
Department of Clinical Laboratory and Central Laboratory, Putuo Hospital, Shanghai University of Traditional Chinese Medicine, Shanghai, China
Department of Clinical Laboratory, Jiading Branch of Shanghai General Hospital, Shanghai, China

Lude Wang, Kailing Pan, Jie Chang, Xiaoya Zhao, Lin Chen, Haiping Lin, Jing Wang and Wenxia Xu
Central Laboratory, Affiliated Jinhua Hospital, Zhejiang University School of Medicine, Jinhua, China

Bin Hu
Department of Pathology, Affiliated Jinhua Hospital, Zhejiang University School of Medicine, Jinhua, China

Yi Yang
Laboratory Animal Center, China Medical University, Shenyang, China

Zhi Li
Department of Medical Oncology, The First Hospital of China Medical University, Shenyang, China

Dan Zou, Fei Lv, Chunjiao Yang and Ye Zhang
The First Laboratory of Cancer Institute, The First Hospital of China Medical University, Shenyang, China

Gezhi Zhou and Jianlie Yuan
Department of Neurosurgery, Affiliated Jinhua Hospital, Zhejiang University School of Medicine, Jinhua, China

Jincheng Song
The First Laboratory of Cancer Institute, The First Hospital of China Medical University, Shenyang, China
Lymphoma and Myeloma Diagnosis and Treatment Center, The Second Affiliated Hospital of Dalian Medical University, Dalian, China

Yang Chen
Department of Respiratory and Infectious Disease of Geriatrics, The First Hospital of China Medical University, Shenyang, China

Zi Jin
The First Department of Oncology, Shenyang Fifth People's Hospital, Shenyang, China

Jinpeng Zhou and Zhitao Jing
Department of Neurosurgery, The First Hospital of China Medical University, Shenyang, China

Yang Jiang
Department of Neurosurgery, The First Hospital of China Medical University, Shenyang, China
Department of Neurosurgery, Shanghai General Hospital, Shanghai Jiao Tong University School of Medicine, Shanghai, China

Yanju Ma and Yu Tang
Department of Medical Oncology, Cancer Hospital of China Medical University, Liaoning Cancer Hospital & Institute, Shenyang, China

Index

www.ingramcontent.com/pod-product-compliance
Lightning Source LLC
LaVergne TN
LVHW082213200926
848484LV00008B/2250